Cognitive Errors and Diagnostic Mistakes

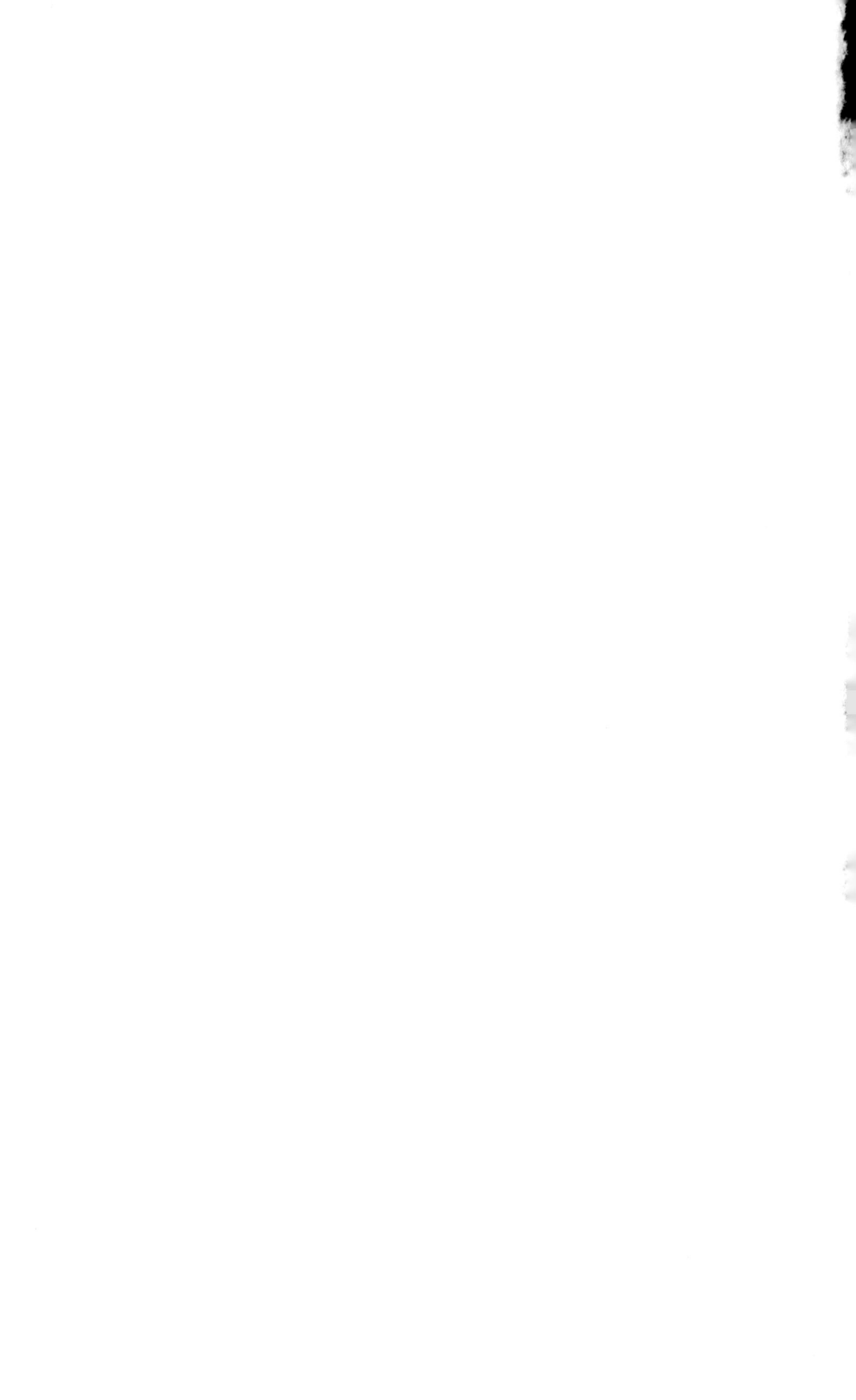

Jonathan Howard

Cognitive Errors and Diagnostic Mistakes

A Case-Based Guide to Critical Thinking in Medicine

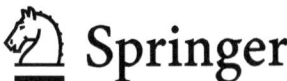 Springer

Jonathan Howard, MD
Neurology and Psychiatry
NYU Langone Medical Center
New York, NY
USA

ISBN 978-3-319-93223-1   ISBN 978-3-319-93224-8   (eBook)
https://doi.org/10.1007/978-3-319-93224-8

Library of Congress Control Number: 2018948736

This Springer imprint is published by the registered company Springer Nature Switzerland AG
The registered company address is: Gewerbestrasse 11, 6330 Cham, Switzerland

Acknowledgment

There are many people without whom this book would not be possible. First of all, I would like to thank Pat Croskerry for being a pioneer in the field of cognitive biases in medicine. His encouragement and thoughts have been invaluable throughout this process. I am grateful that he let me use his definition of many of the cognitive biases. I would like to thank Steven Novella, Harriet Hall, David Gorski, and the entire team at Science Based Medicine. Their work has taught me an enormous amount about skepticism and critical thinking. I would like to thank "Fallacy Man" at "The Logic of Science" and Erik at "Contrive Platitudes" for letting me use their brilliant memes and cartoons. Thanks to GM at, "I Fucking Hate Pseudoscience," for letting me borrow some of his writing. Cindy Harlow deserves angel wings for proofreading and helping to arrange the references along with Allyson Reid. Carol Lynn Curchoe and Dana Bigelow provided invaluable help and suggestions. I would like to thank Gregory Sutorius and the production team at Springer Publishing for recognizing that a book on biases was worth writing in the first place.

Finally, I would like to thank my parents and wife for their support and encouragement.

Disclaimer

None of these cases are real; though many are based loosely on actual cases, names, ages, and genders were changed. In every case, I invented key aspects to make a point. When pictures of people were used, these were obtained from free imaging sites, and there is no relation between the actual person and the medical case.

Contents

About the Author

Jonathan Howard is a neurologist and psychiatrist at NYU and Bellevue. He is the director of neurology and Bellevue Hospital and the neurology clerkship coordinator.

Introduction

We [doctors] do things, because other doctors do so and we don't want to be different, so we do so; or because we were taught so [by teachers, fellows and residents (junior doctors)]; or because we were forced [by teachers, administrators, regulators, guideline developers] to do so, and think that we must do so; or because patient wants so, and we think we should do so; or because of more incentives [unnecessary tests (especially by procedure oriented physicians) and visits], we think we should do so; or because of the fear [by the legal system, audits] we feel that we should do so [so-called 'covering oneself']; or because we need some time [to let nature take its course], so we do so; finally and more commonly, that we have to do something [justification] and we fail to apply common sense, so we do so [1].

Parmar MS.

Summary

"Medical Errors Are No. 3 Cause of US Deaths, Researchers Say," blared the headline [2]. According to an article in the *British Medical Journal*, scientists from Johns Hopkins University claimed that 250,000 Americans die annually from medical errors, a toll exceeded only by cancer and heart disease [3]. A previous report, titled *To Err is Human* issued in 1999 by the US Institute of Medicine, concluded that between 44,000 to 98,000 people die each year as a result of preventable medical errors. Other grim statistics are not hard to find. A study in 2012 of patients in the intensive care unit (ICU) estimated that "40,500 adult patients in an ICU in USA may die with an ICU misdiagnoses annually" [4]. Another study published in 2014 of diagnostic errors in the outpatient setting found that every year, 5% of patients are either misdiagnosed or suffer when clinicians fail to follow up warning signs of serious illness [5]. This amounts to 12 million Americans every year. Another study from the Mayo Clinic found that only 12% of the patients referred there for a second opinion had a complete and correct original diagnosis [6]. The diagnosis was completely changed in 21% of patients.

© Springer International Publishing AG, part of Springer Nature 2019
J. Howard, *Cognitive Errors and Diagnostic Mistakes*,
https://doi.org/10.1007/978-3-319-93224-8_1

While the number of deaths due to medical error are highly debated, mostly because medical errors are difficult to define, there is no question that the consequences of medical errors are enormous. This is especially true given that the majority of errors are likely to result in suffering and injury, but not death, the most dramatic and easily measured outcome. Given this, it is possible that most medical errors go unreported or even unnoticed.

Not only do patients suffer from medical errors, so do the clinicians who make the errors. Most obviously, clinicians can be disciplined, sued, and their careers endangered after an error. Beyond this, most clinicians care intensely about doing their job well and the patients under their care. The pain that clinicians suffer after making an error is known as second victim syndrome. It causes shame, grief, and depression, occasionally intense enough that some devastated clinicians take their own lives [7].

Errors in Medicine

Overall, diagnostic errors are estimated to occur in 10–20% of patients [8]. Errors are most common in fields such as emergency and internal medicine, where large volumes of information must be synthesized in often chaotic environments with time pressures. In contrast, errors are less common (only 2–5%) in specialties such as radiology and pathology, which primarily depend on pattern recognition [9]. Gordon Schiff and colleagues examined 583 diagnostic errors, 162 (28%) of which were rated as major [10]. According to this study, "Errors occurred most frequently in the testing phase (failure to order, report, and follow-up laboratory results) (44%), followed by clinician assessment errors (failure to consider and overweighing competing diagnosis) (32%), history taking (10%), physical examination (10%), and referral or consultation errors and delays (3%)."

Several attempts have been made to further categorize such errors. Lucian Leape and colleagues identified four types of medical errors: diagnostic, treatment, preventive, and other (Fig. 1.1) [11].

Mark Graber and colleagues suggested three categories of diagnostic errors: no-fault errors, system errors, and cognitive errors [12]. No-fault errors occur when a disease is silent, presents in an unusual manner, or imitates another disease. System errors occur due to inefficiencies or gaps in the health care system. A good example of such a systems error occurred with the case of Thomas Eric Duncan. In 2014, he presented to the Texas Health Presbyterian Hospital ER with a fever, headache, abdominal pain, vertigo, and nausea. Although Duncan told a nurse he had recently traveled in Africa and this information was entered in the computer, this was not verbally communicated to the ER doctor in charge of his care. Despite a fever that increased to 103°F, he was sent home with a prescription for antibiotics and Tylenol. Two days later, he returned via ambulance with worsening symptoms. At that time, his travel history raised suspicions that he might be suffering from Ebola, a diagnosis that was later confirmed by the CDC. Two nurses who treated Duncan contracted Ebola, the first people on US soil to contract the infection, and nearly 100 other people were exposed. The nurses had neither the training nor the proper protective treatment to treat someone with such an infection. Duncan himself died several weeks later.

Types of Errors

Diagnostic
    Error or delay in diagnosis
    Failure to employ indicated tests
    Use of outmoded tests or therapy
    Failure to act on results of monitoring or testing

Treatment
    Error in the performance of an operation, procedure, or test
    Error in administering the treatment
    Error in the dose or method of using a drug
    Avoidable delay in treatment or in responding to an abnormal test
    Inappropriate (not indicated) care

Preventive
    Failure to provide prophylactic treatment
    Inadequate monitoring or follow-up of treatment

Other
    Failure of communication
    Equipment failure
    Other system failure

Source: Leape, Lucian; Lawthers, Ann G.; Brennan, Troyen A., et al. Preventing Medical Injury. Qual Rev Bull. 19(5):144–149, 1993.

Fig. 1.1 Medical errors as defined by Leape and colleagues. (Leape LL, Lawthers AG, Brennan TA, Johnson WG. Preventing medical injury. QRB – Qual Rev Bull 1993;19(5):144–149. https://doi.org/10.1016/S0097-5990(16)30608-X.)

According to a nurse's union that reviewed the case, "There was no advance preparedness on what to do with the patient, there was no protocol, there was no system" [13]. Daniel Varga, the chief clinical officer at Texas Health Resources, admitted the multiple errors, saying, "We believe we were very well attuned to the potential risk of Ebola, and that we had communicated that fairly aggressively. What we didn't do is train and simulate for that" [14].

In contrast, cognitive errors occur because of flaws in the thinking of the clinician. In a later study, Graber and colleagues examined 100 instances of diagnostic error in internal medicine. They found that the most common cognitive error was premature closure, which they defined as "the failure to continue considering reasonable alternatives after an initial diagnosis was reached" [15]. Other common errors included faulty context generation, misjudging the salience of findings, faulty perception, and errors arising from the use of heuristics. Errors due to faulty or inadequate knowledge were uncommon.

When a medical error is made, it is unlikely that a single factor in isolation is to blame. Most errors are multifactorial in origin. This model is sometimes called the Swiss cheese model of accident causation, which posits that an error occurs when flaws in safety barriers perfectly align to allow the error to occur (Fig. 1.2).

Graber's study supports this Swiss cheese model. In 93 errors, they found a total of 548 different system-related or cognitive factors, or nearly six errors per

Fig. 1.2 The Swiss cheese model of accident causation posits that, although many layers of defense lie between hazards and losses, there are flaws in each layer that, if aligned, can allow the accident to occur. (Davidmack. Swiss cheese model of accident causation [Image file]. In: Wikipedia. 2014. Retrieved from https://en.wikipedia.org/wiki/Swiss_cheese_model.)

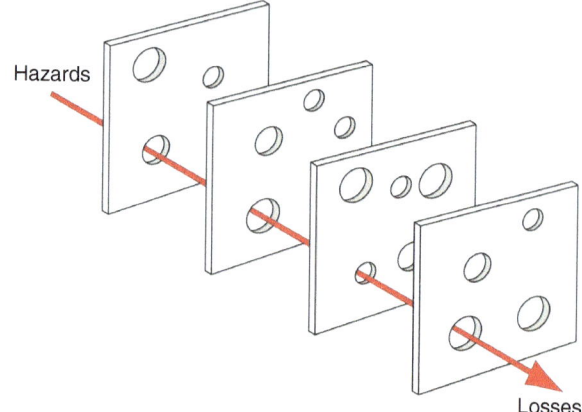

case [15]. System-related factors, such as problems with policies and procedures, inefficient processes, teamwork, and communication, occurred in 65% of the cases. Cognitive errors occurred in 74% of the cases.

Cognitive Biases

Cognitive biases are systematic, unconscious, automatic patterns of thought that sometimes distort thinking and potentially lead to errors. Nearly 200 such biases have been described, though there is no formal list. They can be divided into several different categories: decision-making/behavioral biases, social biases, memory errors, and biases in probability and belief (Fig. 1.3).

We like to think of ourselves as objective, fair, and honest. To be called biased feels like a slight. Yet, taking a broader view, to say we are biased simply means we all see the world from a specific vantage point, based on our beliefs, desires, personality, past experiences, and culture. Having biases does not make us immoral or flawed. Biases make us human.

Many cognitive biases originate from the use of heuristics, which are unconscious mental shortcuts to problem-solving. Heuristics are essentially "rules of thumb." Heuristics and biases are not necessarily bad in and of themselves, especially in situations where there is little time for deliberate thought. In fact, they are absolutely necessary. It would be impossible to live an entirely rational life, coolly weighing the ups and downs of every single decision we must make throughout the day.

Neurologist Antonio Damasio described a man named Elliot whose life was dramatically altered by a brain tumor in his frontal lobe. Prior to the tumor, Elliot had been a successful businessman and devoted husband. Afterwards, his memory and intellect remained perfectly intact, but his ability to feel emotions was obliterated. He could look at emotionally laden pictures and intellectually know he should feel something, but he was utterly unable to do so. As a result of this

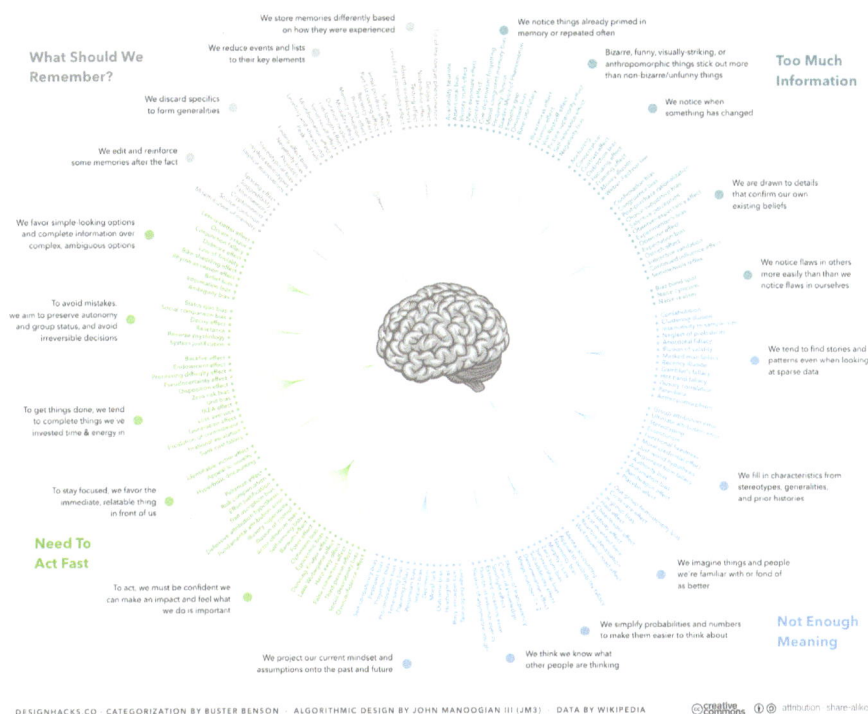

Fig. 1.3 The cognitive bias codex. (Jm3. [John Manoogian III]. Cognitive bias codex – 180+ biases [Image file]. In: Wikimedia commons. 2016. Retrieved from https://commons.wikimedia.org/wiki/File:Cognitive_Bias_Codex_-_180%2B_biases,_designed_by_John_Manoogian_III_(jm3).jpg.)

deficit, he would endlessly deliberate the pros and cons of the most mundane choices. He was frozen, unable to make decisions. As Dr. Damasio wrote, "I began to think that the cold-bloodedness of Elliot's reasoning prevented him from assigning different values to different options and made his decision-making landscape hopelessly flat" [16].

In addition to being necessary, heuristics are often correct. Opposite are two pictures of Barack Obama greeting a championship team. In which picture do you think he was congratulating a basketball team, and in which picture do you think he was congratulating a gymnastics team? (Fig. 1.4).

If you recognize he is congratulating basketball players in the top picture and congratulating gymnasts in the bottom picture, you are correct. You likely assumed that basketball players are taller than gymnasts. Your heuristic served you well.

However, our heuristics can often be wrong. Consider the following scenario created by the pioneering psychologists Amos Tversky and Daniel Kahneman:

"Steve is very shy and withdrawn, invariably helpful, but with little interested in people, or in the world of reality. A meek and tidy soul, he has a need for order and structure, and a passion for detail." Is Steve more likely to be a librarian or a school teacher? [17].

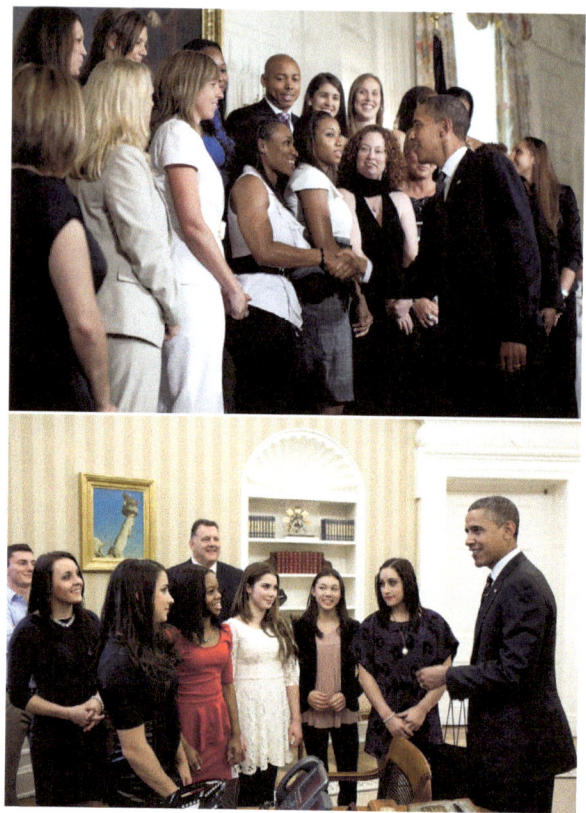

Fig. 1.4 Barack Obama greeting championship teams. (**Top**: Johnson T. Honoring the WNBA champion Phoenix Mercury [Blog post]. 2010. Retrieved from https://obamawhitehouse.archives. gov/blog/2010/07/20/honoring-wnba-champion-phoenix-mercury; **Bottom**: Souza P. President Barack Obama talks with members of the 2012 US Olympic gymnastics teams in the Oval Office [Image file]. In: Wikimedia commons. (n.d.). Retrieved from https://commons.wikimedia.org/ wiki/File:Barack_Obama_with_members_of_the_2012_U.S._Olympic_gymnastics_teams.jpg.)

Many people would answer that Steve is more likely to be a librarian. Certainly, he sounds more like a librarian than a teacher. However, given that there are many more teachers than librarians, and the odds that Steve is an unusual teacher are greater than the odds that he is a stereotypical librarian. Your heuristic served you poorly. (This particular heuristic is termed the representativeness heuristic.) So, while heuristics will often lead to a correct conclusion in a short amount of time, they will occasionally lead you astray. The heuristic that short people are unlikely to be basketball stars will also occasionally be wrong. After all, Muggsy Bogues was only 5 feet 3 inches tall, yet managed to play 14 seasons in the NBA.

Cognitive Biases in Medicine

Heuristics play an important role in medicine. An experienced clinician can often use her knowledge to rapidly assess a patient, render an accurate diagnosis, and start the appropriate treatment. In an emergency, clinicians must use heuristics. When a patient presents with chest pain or the sudden onset of weakness, clinicians don't have the time to deliberate. I, for example, have been treating patients with multiple sclerosis (MS) for the past nine years. Patients with MS often have tremors when they reach for objects, a characteristic speech pattern (called scanning speech), an unsteady gait, and abnormal eye movements. Not infrequently, by observing these signs during the short trip from the waiting room to my office, I am fairly certain that a patient has MS. This is an involuntary process, completely out of my control.

Most of the time, these heuristics serve me well. By the time I am done with a more thorough evaluation, my initial suspicions of MS are usually confirmed. However, the same processes that allow for a rapid, and often correct diagnosis are far from foolproof. I have many patients who have presented with the same constellation of findings as a typical MS patient, who instead have genetic diseases or other inflammatory conditions. As such, whenever I am "sure" that a patient has MS, I do my best to keep an open mind and try to think, "what else might this be?"

This pattern of diagnosis illustrates the dual process theory, which posits that there is a duality to our thinking. It has been most thoroughly described by Kahneman in his book *Thinking Fast and Slow*. In this book, "system I" thinking is rapid, automatic, and emotional, while "system II" is slower, conscious, and logical. While this is a simplification and there are no absolute borders between the two systems, it provides a useful model for human cognition. We spend most of our time using system I thinking, reserving system II thinking for complex problems. While system I thinking is generally perceived to be more responsible for errors than system II thinking, evidence has shown than this is not necessarily the case [18]. Both automatic and analytical thinking can lead to errors at times and both can provide the right answer. While system II may allow us to solve mathematical equations, with system I, we can accurately glean large amounts of information from a scene in milliseconds [19]. You can likely look at someone's face and instantly and involuntarily recognize their emotional state, knowing whether they are friend or foe. There is even some evidence that rapid rendered diagnoses are more accurate than those rendered with greater deliberation [20].

Despite the importance of cognitive biases in our thinking, the idea that medical students and residents should be taught about them is relatively new. Medical training and practice largely subscribe to the rational man (or *homo economicus*) model of human behavior, in which people are felt to rationally pursue optimal outcomes. Although this model used to be widespread, as economists and psychologists started to learn how people actually behave, as opposed to how they should behave if they were perfectly rationally, significant differences emerged between theory and reality. The truth is we often behave quite irrationally, though predictable patterns of irrationality have been discovered. In the words of psychologist Dan Ariely, we are "predictably irrational" [21]. While people often do behave rationally, the idea that humans always do so was long ago abandoned by these disciplines. However, this notion of human rationality largely persists in medicine, perhaps because it was debunked by other professions (the not invented here syndrome).

As a result of adhering to the rational man model in medicine, errors by individual clinicians are generally perceived to be due to a lack of knowledge, skill, or effort. The solution, therefore, is to encourage clinicians to study more and work harder. There is often little consideration given to how intelligent, hard-working people can be systematically misled by their own thought processes. When I went to medical school, there were no courses on biases, rationality, or metacognition (the practice of "thinking about thinking.")

Given this, it is not surprising that systems errors, such as giving a patient the wrong medication or operating on the wrong side of someone's body, have received the most attention from patient-safety advocates. These errors are often glaringly obvious and relatively easy to fix. Perhaps because they are harder to define, measure, and correct, errors due to clinicians' thought processes have received considerably less attention.

This Book

This book is largely based upon cognitive biases as described by Dr. Croskerry. He divided cognitive biases in medicine into several categories as follows [22]:

- **Errors of overattachment to a particular diagnosis.**
  - Anchoring, confirmation bias, premature closure, sunk costs.
- **Errors due to failure to consider alternative diagnoses.**
  - Multiple alternatives bias, representativeness restraint, search satisfying, unpacking principle.
- **Errors due to inheriting someone else's thinking.**
  - Diagnosis momentum, framing effect, bandwagon effect.
- **Errors in prevalence perception or estimation.**
  - Availability bias, ambiguity effect, base-rate neglect, gambler's fallacy, hot-hand fallacy, hindsight bias, playing the odds, posterior probability error, order effects.
- **Errors involving patient characteristics or presentation context.**
  - Fundamental attribution error, affective bias, in-group bias, triage cueing, contrast effect, yin-yang out.
- **Errors associated with physician affect, personality, or decision style.**
  - Commission bias, omission bias, outcome bias, visceral bias, overconfidence, belief bias, ego bias, sunk costs, zebra retreat.

These biases, as well as several others, will be discussed in this book. Many of these biases are inverses of each other, and I have paired them together in the book's organization. Additionally, a number of factors that distort clinicians' practices but are not cognitive biases per se are presented here. These include systems problems in medicine such as perverse financial incentives, fears of medical malpractice, patient satisfaction scores, alarm fatigue, and the impact of the electronic medical record. These are ubiquitous in the lives of every clinician, changing their behavior in both conscious and unconscious ways. The penultimate chapter of the book discusses what, if anything, can be done to minimize the impact of cognitive biases and improve our thinking. Lastly, I will discuss some of the challenges facing researchers as well as clinicians who use the medical literature to make recommendations for their patients. Though many of the cases reflect the fact that I am a neurologist and a psychiatrist who specializes in the treatment of MS, I hope that this book will be useful and interest to clinicians regardless of their specialty.

Many chapters in this book use examples of complementary and alternative medicine (CAM), as a launching point for how human cognition can lead clinicians astray. This is because CAM, when not outright fraudulent, is nothing more than the triumph of cognitive biases over rationality and science. Consider what CAM really means. As actor Tim Minchin said, "By definition, alternative medicine has either not been proved to work or been proved not to work." He also posed the following rhetorical question, "Do you know what they call alternative medicine that's been proved to work? Medicine" (Fig. 1.5).

Pediatrician Paul Offit, perhaps the most vocal defendant of vaccines in the US, expressed a similar sentiment in his book *Do You Believe in Magic?* by writing, "There's no such thing as alternative medicine. There's only medicine that works and medicine that doesn't" [23]. The TV show *Please Like Me* also put it well, with one character saying, "Putting the word 'alterative' before medicine is like point at a dog and saying, 'that's my alternative cat.' It's still not a cat." Not surprisingly, despite billions of dollars spent in the search, almost no alternative treatments have been shown to do any good (Fig. 1.6) [24].

To the modern eye, quackery of the past is very easy to spot (Fig. 1.7).

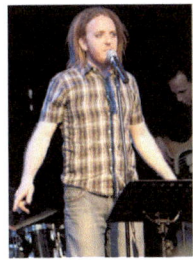

By definition alternative medicine has either not been proved to work or been proved not to work. Do you know what they call alternative medicine that's been proved to work?
Tim Minchin

Fig. 1.5 Tim Minchin gets it right. (Nekonoir. Tim Minchin [Image file]. In: Wikimedia commons. 2007. Retrieved from https://commons.wikimedia.org/wiki/Category:Tim_Minchin.)

Fig. 1.6 (Asdfghjkl. Alternative cat [Image file]. In: Know your meme. (ca. 2016). Retrieved from https://knowyourmeme. com/photos/1046097.)

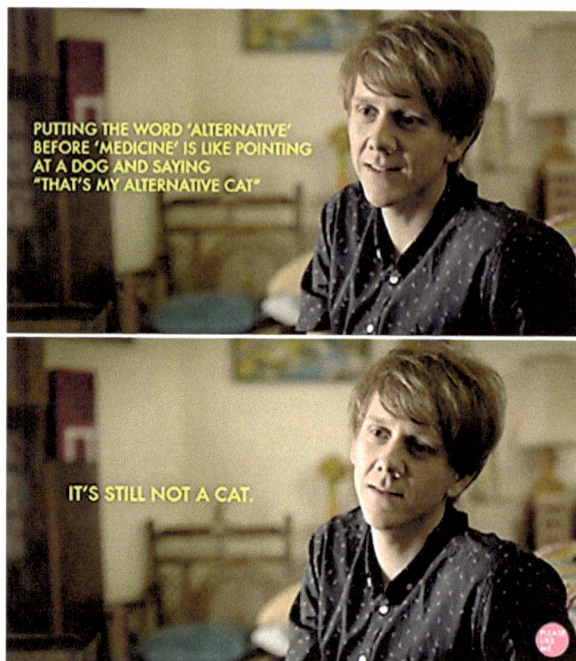

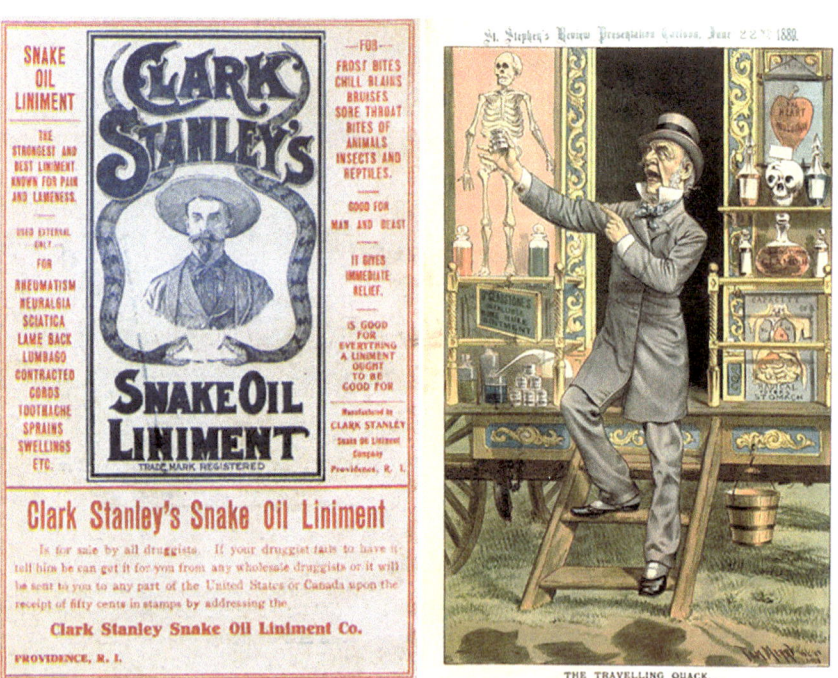

Fig. 1.7 To the modern eye, quackery of the past is very easy to spot. (Clark Stanley' Snake Oil Liniment. [Image file] (original image ca. 1905). In: Here today, here tomorrow varieties of medical Ephemera. 2011. Retrieved from https://www.nlm.nih.gov/exhibition/ephemera/medshow. html; Merry T. The traveling quack [Image file]. In: Deceptology. 1889. Retrieved from http:// www.deceptology.com/2011/01/dr-gladstones-infallible-home-rule.html.)

Fig. 1.8 Dr. Mehmet Oz. (Shankbone D. [David]. Dr. Mehmet Oz [Image file]. In: Wikimedia commons. 2016. Retrieved from https://commons.wikimedia.org/w/index.php?search=dr.+oz&title=Special:Search&go=Go#/media/File:Dr_Oz_(cropped).png.)

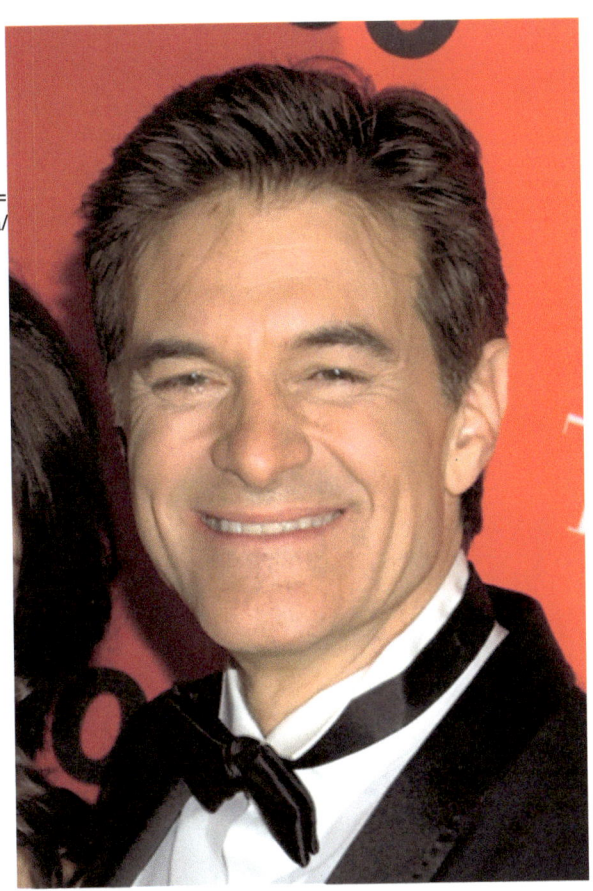

However, with a few well-produced YouTube videos and a well-designed website, an attractive, charismatic CAM practitioner, especially one with legitimate credentials, can fool millions of people (Fig. 1.8). The website sci-ence.org has a great graphic describing the "red flags of quackery." Hopefully readers of this book will gain insight into some of these red flags and the techniques of CAM practitioners (Fig. 1.9).

While some CAM practitioners may be well-intended, this is not always the case. For example, many CAM practitioners celebrated news reports that declared medicine the third leading cause of death in the US, gleefully writing articles with dramatic titles such as "Pharmageddon: Proof Conventional Medicine is a Killing Machine" [25]. CAM practitioner Gary Null even calculated in his book, *Death by Medicine*, that conventional medicine kills 783,936 Americans annually. This would make medicine the single largest cause of death in the US, killing one in every three Americans. This schadenfreude exists because the livelihoods of many CAM practitioners depend on fostering mistrust between patients and mainstream

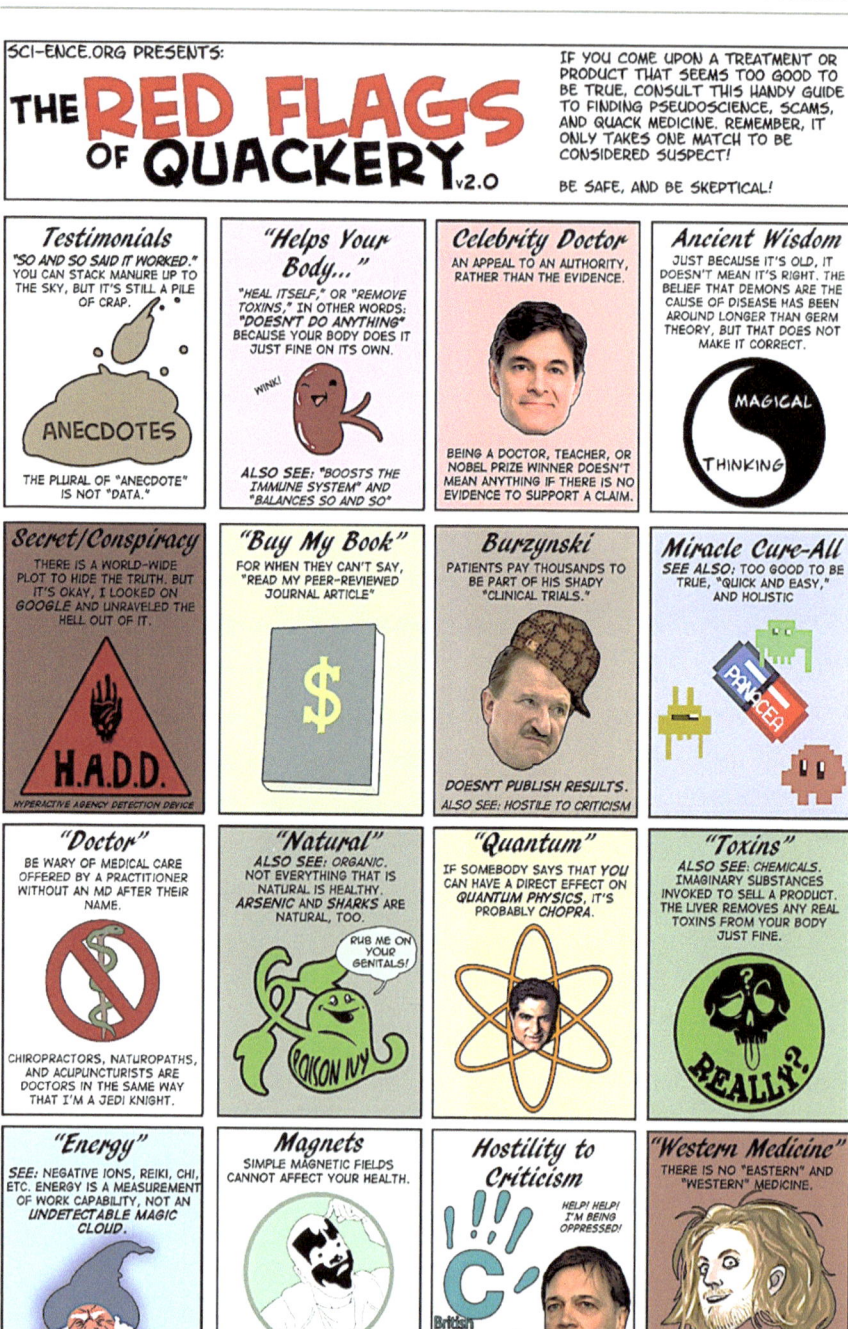

Fig. 1.9 The red flags of quackery. (Maki. The red flags of quackery v 2.0 [Image file]. Sci-Ence. org. 2012. Retrieved from http://sci-ence.org/red-flags2/.)

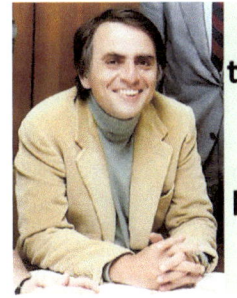

Fig. 1.10 Carl Sagan gets it right. (NASA/JPL. Carl Sagan [Image file]. In: Wikimedia commons. 1979. Retrieved from https://commons.wikimedia.org/wiki/Carl_Sagan#/media/File:Carl_Sagan_Planetary_Society.JPG.)

For me, it is far better to grasp the universe as it really is than to persist in delusion, however satisfying and reassuring.

Carl Sagan

clinicians. At times, the conspiratorial thinking of CAM advocates can venture into delusional thinking. Consider this description of the book *Defy Your Doctor and Be Healed*:

> *Your doctor is not your healer. He is your dealer. This is why diabetes drugs cause full-onset diabetes, cholesterol medications cause sudden-onset heart attacks, and why radiation from cancer screenings causes cancer. The system is primarily designed to be self-perpetuating, and to prevent us from ever being free. There is no money to be made from healthy patients, nor is there profit in having dead patients. The money is made somewhere in the middle, in patients who are alive, but barely* [26].

Overall, I intend this book to be a passionate defense of science and critical thinking. Modern medicine has eliminated or virtually eliminated diseases that have plagued humanity for centuries. We are living longer than ever before, and in most countries of the world, parents do not have to wonder if their children will live to adulthood. An infected wound or broken bone is no longer a death sentence. Almost everyone who reads this book can expect to live into their 80s and beyond. Yet despite the successes, many challenges remain and opportunities for improvement abound (Fig. 1.10).

I hope that these cases and subsequent discussions will illustrate how easy it is for anyone, including smart and well-intended clinicians with years of training and decades of experience, to fall into cognitive traps. I hope that this will spur further discussion of how to minimize cognitive biases and ultimately achieve what we all set out to do: save lives and prevent suffering.

References

1. Parmar MS. We do things because [Rapid response]. BMJ. 2004;328:474. https://doi.org/10.1136/bmj.328.7438.474.
2. Allen M, Pierce O. (2016, May 3). Medical errors are no. 3 cause of U.S. deaths, researchers say. Morning Edition. Retrieved from https://www.npr.org/sections/health-shots/2016/05/03/476636183/death-certificates-undercount-toll-of-medical-errors.
3. Malary MA, Daniel M. Medical error-the third leading cause of death in the US. BMJ. 2016;353:i2139. https://doi.org/10.1136/bmj.i2139.
4. Winters B, Custer J, Galvagno SM, Colantuoni E, Kapoor SG, Lee H, Goode V, Robinson K, Nakhasi A, Pronovost P, Newman-Toker B. Diagnostic error in the intensive care unit: a systematic review of autopsy studies. BMJ Qual Saf. 2012;21(11):894–902. https://doi.org/10.1136/bmjqs-2012-000803.

5. Singh H, Meyer AND, Thomas EJ. The frequency of diagnostic errors in outpatient care: esti-mations from three large observational studies involving US adult populations. BMJ Qual Saf. 2014;23(9):727–31. https://doi.org/10.1136/bmjqs-2013-002627.

6. Zimmerman E. (2017, April 4). Mayo Clinic researchers demonstrate value of sec-ond opinions. Mayo Clinic. https://newsnetwork.mayoclinic.org/discussion/mayo-clinic-researchers-demonstrate-value-of-second-opinions/.

7. Saavedra SM. (2015, Nov 25). Remembering Kimberly Hiatt: a casualty of second victim syn-drome. NursesLab.com. https://nurseslabs.com/remembering-kimberly-hiatt-casualty-second-victim-syndrome/.

8. Graber ML, Wachter RM, Cassel CK. Bringing diagnosis into the quality and safety equations. JAMA. 2012;308(12):1211–2. https://doi.org/10.1001/2012.jama.11913.

9. Berner ES, Graber ML. Overconfidence as a cause of diagnostic error in medicine. Am J Med. 2008;121(5):S2–S23. https://doi.org/10.1016/j.amjmed.2008.01.001.

10. Schiff GG, Hasan O, Kim S, Abrams R, Cosby K, Lambert BL, Elstein AS, Hasler S, Kabongo ML, Krosnjar N, Odwazny R, Wisniewski MF, McNutt RA. Diagnostic error in medicine: analysis of 583 physician-reported errors. Arch Intern Med. 2009;169(20):1881–7. https://doi.org/10.1001/archinternmed.2009.333.

11. Leape LL, Lawthers AG, Brennan TA, Johnson WG. Preventing medical injury. QRB Qua Rev Bull. 1993;19(5):144–9. https://doi.org/10.1016/S0097-5990(16)30608-X.

12. Graber M, Gordon R, Franklin N. Reducing diagnostic errors in medicine: what's the goal? Acad Med. 2002;77(10):981–92. https://doi.org/10.1097/00001888-200210000-00009.

13. Voorhees J. (2014, Oct 14). Everything that went wrong in Dallas. Slate. Retrieved from http://www.slate.com/articles/health_and_science/medical_examiner/2014/10/dallas_ebola_time-line_the_many_medical_missteps_at_texas_health_presbyterian.html.

14. Silverman L, Chavez SM. (Reporters). (n.d.). Learning from Ebola mistakes, North Texas hos-pitals make changes [Audio recording]. In: Becker S. (Producer), KERA News. Retrieved from http://stories.kera.org/surviving-ebola/2015/09/08/learning-from-mistakes-north-texas-hospitals-make-changes/.

15. Graber ML, Franklin N, Gordon R. Diagnostic error in internal medicine. Arch Intern Med. 2005;165(13):1493–9. https://doi.org/10.1001/archinte.165.13.1493.

16. Baer D. (2016, June 14). How only being able to use logic to make decisions destroyed a man's life. The Cut. https://www.thecut.com/2016/06/how-only-using-logic-destroyed-a-man.html.

17. Tversky A, Kahneman D. Judgment under uncertainty: heuristics and biases. Science. 1974;185(4157):1124–31. https://doi.org/10.1126/science.185.4157.1124.

18. Norman GR, Eva KW. Diagnostic error and clinical reasoning. Med Educ. 2010;44(1):94–100. https://doi.org/10.1111/j.1365-2923.2009.03507.x.

19. Alt NP, Goodale B, Lick DJ, Johnson KL. Threat in the company of men: ensemble perception and threat evaluations of groups varying in sex ratio. Soc Psychol Personal Sci. 2017; https://doi.org/10.1177/1948550617731498.

20. Sherbino J, Dore KL, Wood TJ, Young ME, Gaissmaier W, Kreuger S, Norman GR. The rela-tionship between response time and diagnostic accuracy. Acad Med. 2012;87(6):785–891. https://doi.org/10.1097/ACM.0b013e318253acbd.

21. Ariely D. Predictably irrational. Revised & expanded edition. New York: HarperCollins Publishers; 2009

22. Croskerry P. 50 cognitive and affective biases in medicine [PDF file]. 2013. Retrieved from http://sjrhem.ca/wp-content/uploads/2015/11/CriticaThinking-Listof50-biases.pdf.

23. Offit PA. Do you believe in magic? The sense and nonsense of alternative medicine. New York: HarperCollins Publishers; 2013.

24. Associated Press. (2009, June 10). $2.5 billion spent, no alternative cures found. Retrieved from http://www.nbcnews.com/id/31190909.

25. Fassa P. (n.d.). Pharmageddon: proof conventional medicine is a killing machine. Retrieved September15,2018fromhttps://realfarmacy.com/pharmageddon-proof-conventional-medicine-killing-machine/.

26. Corriher CT, Corriher SC. Defy your doctor and be healed. Mocksville: HealthWyze.org; 2013.

Ambiguity Effect

Case

George was a 24-year-old man who presented with confusion and lethargy for three days. An MRI revealed multiple demyelinating lesions consistent with multiple sclerosis (MS). Many of the lesions enhanced with the administration of contrast, indicating active inflammation (Fig. 2.1).

George was started on methylprednisolone, a steroid used to decrease inflammation. He received this medication for three days with no improvement. His case was presented in academic rounds where several other neurologists suggested treating him with high doses of cyclophosphamide, a chemotherapeutic agent. The neurologist in charge of his care was only vaguely familiar with this medication and instead opted to treat him with a more prolonged course of methylprednisolone. He was then discharged him to a rehabilitation facility. While there, he deteriorated to the point where he developed difficulty expressing himself and trouble swallowing. He was readmitted to the hospital where a repeat MRI showed several new demyelinating lesions. A different neurologist treated him with cyclophosphamide. Although he lost his hair and had to be isolation for a week due to low white blood cells, he gradually improved over the course of two weeks, and a third MRI showed complete resolution of the active inflammation.

What Dr. Cohen Was Thinking

This was an unusual and extreme case. I've read about cases of fulminant neuro-inflammatory diseases like this, but had never seen one myself. I have treated run-of-the-mill cases of MS with steroids many times. So that was my first instinct when I met George, and I still think it was the right one. However, my mistake was not moving on to a more aggressive treatment when he failed to improve. I knew some of the senior doctors had used chemotherapy to treat such cases in the past. Though they suggested this to me, I was unable to find more than a few cases in the scientific literature to support the use of such a powerful medication. Cyclophosphamide is chemotherapy, and I'm not an oncologist. I don't use chemotherapy, and I still have the same visceral, negative reaction to that word as the

© Springer International Publishing AG, part of Springer Nature 2019

J. Howard, *Cognitive Errors and Diagnostic Mistakes*,

https://doi.org/10.1007/978-3-319-93224-8_2

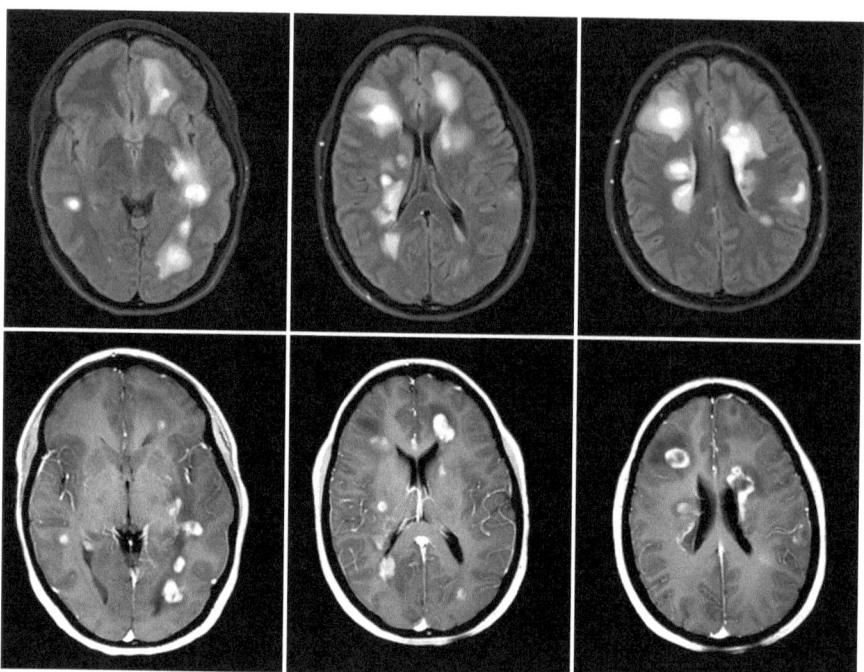

Fig. 2.1 Axial FLAIR and post-contrast T1-weighted images showing multiple inflammatory lesions throughout the brain

general public. Cyclophosphamide is a medication with potentially serious side effects, so it should not be used casually. However, this is the type of case for which there simply aren't large scientific studies to guide treatment. With George, I let my fear of a potential problem prevent me from treating a real problem that was staring me in the face. I stuck with what I knew rather than take a chance on an unfamiliar treatment.

Discussion

The ambiguity effect is due to decision makers' avoiding options when a probability is unknown. In the same way that familiarity generates comfort (the mere exposure effect), novelty can generate discomfort. Many people prefer to return to the same restaurants or vacation spots rather than take a chance on something new.

In medicine, there is often an irreducible uncertainty and ambiguity, which can be associated with uncertainty and avoidance. In considering options on a differential diagnosis, for example, this would be illustrated by a tendency to select options for which the probability of a particular outcome is known over an option for which the probability is unknown. The probability may be unknown because of lack of knowledge or because the means to obtain the probability (a specific test) is unavailable. Similarly, when initiating a treatment, clinicians naturally prefer those with known, familiar risks to those with unknown risks.

Fig. 2.2 Which urn would you chose?

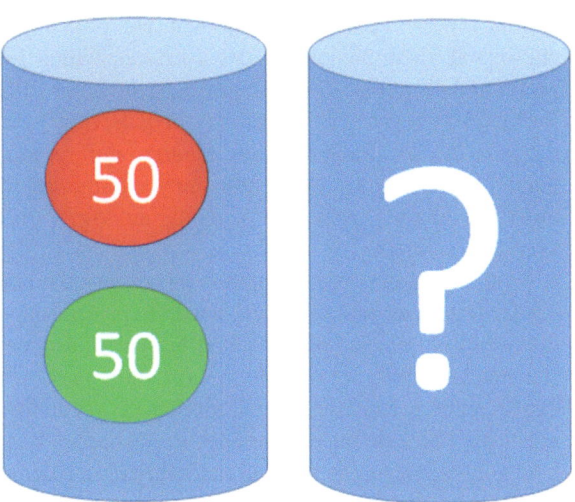

The ambiguity effect was coined by the economist Daniel Ellsberg and is also known as the "Ellsberg paradox." His insight was that people often prefer to take a known risk, even if that risk is not a particularly good option, over a relatively unknown risk. Uncertainty can be extremely disconcerting and making a decision to change can be difficult. For example, most people choose a secure job with a regular paycheck over the unknowns of a business venture, even one with a potentially large payoff.

Consider the following thought experiment, proposed by Chip Heath and Amos Tversky. There are two urns, each with 100 balls [1]. One urn has 50 red balls and 50 green balls, while the other urn has an unknown mixture of balls of each color. If you correctly guess the color of the ball you win $20. Which urn would you chose? (Fig. 2.2).

Objectively, with the information provided, the two urns are the same, and the odds of winning the $20 is 50%. Yet, most people chose the urn with the known mixture of 50 red and green balls over an urn with an unknown mixture.

The ambiguity effect is often encountered in sports, where coaches may make decisions hoping not to win a game, but rather not to lose it. For example, they may opt for a safe play with a small reward, such as kicking a field goal on fourth down, rather than a riskier play with the potential for greater benefit. Statisticians have studied this particular scenario in detail and indeed found that professional football coaches are often too timid when it comes to going for it on fourth down. When told about this analysis, former Steeler's coach Bill Cowher responded:

> It's easy to sit there and apply a formula, but it's not always the easiest thing to do on a Sunday. There's so much more involved with the game than just sitting there, looking at the numbers and saying, 'OK, these are my percentages, then I'm going to do it this way,' because that one time it doesn't work could cost your team a football game, and that's the thing a head coach has to live with, not the professor [2].

He's right. It is easy to make the safe choice of kicking a field goal, when the alternative is unknown probability, even when the alternative is a potentially greater reward, namely a touchdown. His philosophy also demonstrates the psychological phenomenon of loss aversion, which refers to people's tendency to prefer avoiding losses over acquiring equivalent gains. In other words, the pain of losing $100 is greater than the joy of receiving $100. In the case in this chapter, the pain of potentially harming George with an unknown treatment (cyclophosphamide) would have outweighed any satisfaction in benefitting him. Indeed, the most fundamental principle of medicine, "first, do no harm," is essentially loss aversion codified.

In sports, almost every situation has occurred countless of times before and thus can be translated into relatively accurate probabilities. However, in medicine, rare diseases, complicated patients, conflicting studies, and new discoveries make such statistical certainly impossible in most situations. For this reason, the loss aversion displayed by football coaches is similar to, but subtly different from the ambiguity effect as clinicians may experience it. If coaches had to choose between kicking a field goal or having the football randomly placed somewhere on the field, this might better approximate the ambiguous decisions clinicians often have to make.

Closely related to the ambiguity effect, is the status quo bias, a natural preference for the current state of affairs, which serves as a reference point from which deviations are perceived as risky and unnecessary. Barack Obama was vilified by many people for passing healthcare reform, for example, but once it became ingrained as normal for many Americans, there was a similar resistance to anyone who proposed significant alterations to this plan. As the expression goes, "better the devil you know than the devil you don't."

Steven Levitt, an economist, showed how "forcing" people to make a decision with an unknown outcome rather than stick with the status quo may be beneficial in some situations [3]. He identified people who had trouble making decisions about significant life events, such as whether they should change their job or breakup with their significant other. He then asked them to make these decisions based on a virtual coin toss ("heads" meant change, "tails" meant stay.) Over the course of his year-long study, 20,000 virtual coins were flipped. Following the dictates of the experiment, people who flipped a coin to "heads" were 25% more likely to make a change than those who got "tails." Those who made a change, regardless of whether the coin toss prompted them to do so, reported they were significantly happier than those who made no change. Dr. Levitt said his results demonstrate a "substantial bias against making changes when it comes to important life decisions, as evidenced by the fact that those who do make a change report being no worse off after two months and much better off six months later."

Conclusion

The amount of uncertainty differs greatly from one patient to another and one medical specialty to another. A clinician who performs the same few procedures every day might not encounter a wide variety of patients, whereas an ER clinician, dealing with an international population of patients, will likely see dozens of different conditions each shift. However, every clinician will treat patients where there are not clear algorithms to aid with diagnosis nor large clinical trials to guide treatment.

In such instances, it is natural for clinicians to default to conditions and treatments that carry the least uncertainty. While I don't think any patient would be happy to hear that their treatment was decided by a coin toss, clinicians should do their best not to avoid a diagnosis or a potentially beneficial treatment simply because it is unfamiliar to them.

The ambiguity effect may affect patients as well. As the converse of ambiguity is clarity, clinicians who wish to convince skeptical patients of the wisdom of a proposed course of action are advised to explain it to them as clearly and concisely as possible.

References

1. Tversky A. In: Shafir E, editor. Preference, belief, and similarity: selected writings. Cambridge: The MIT Press; 2003.
2. NYT 4th Down Bot. (2014, Sept 4). 4th down: when to go for it and why. The New York Times. Retrieved from https://www.nytimes.com/2014/09/05/upshot/4th-down-when-to-go-for-it-and-why.html.
3. Levitt SD. Heads or tails: the impact of a coin toss on major life decisions and subsequent happiness. The National Bureau of Economic Research. 2016 Aug; NBER Working Paper No. 22487. https://doi.org/10.3386/w22487.

Case

James was a 56-year-old man who arrived to the ER after being thrown from his motorcycle. He was taken to a trauma center and was unable to move his legs. A CT scan showed a significant spinal cord injury. The neurosurgeon started him on high-dose, intravenous methylprednisolone, a steroid commonly used in neurological diseases to decrease inflammation, as this had been the hospital protocol for the past 15 years. James developed a urinary tract infection several days later and never regained movement in his legs.

What Dr. Liang Was Thinking

The use of steroids in patients with acute spinal cord injuries has a complicated history. Several trials done in the 1990s showed steroids might benefit patients, and treating them with this medication became the standard of care. Our hospital developed a protocol, and we all routinely gave steroids to patients with acute spinal cord injuries without a second thought.

However, over the years, the quality of these studies began to be questioned, and the benefits of steroid treatment began to be doubted. The Congress of Neurological Surgeons put out a statement in 2002 that steroid therapy "should only be undertaken with the knowledge that the evidence suggesting harmful side effects is more consistent than any suggestion of clinical benefit" [1].

I certainly was not alone in my continued use of steroids, however. A survey by the Canadian Association of Emergency Physicians in 2001 revealed that 75% of respondents were using methylprednisolone either "because everyone else does" or out of fear of litigation for failing to do so. Another survey in 2006 found 90.5% of doctors used steroids in acute spinal cord injuries, though only 24.1% felt this improved clinical outcomes. The main justifications for this were fear of a lawsuit and "institutional protocol" [2].

© Springer International Publishing AG, part of Springer Nature 2019   21
J. Howard, *Cognitive Errors and Diagnostic Mistakes*,
https://doi.org/10.1007/978-3-319-93224-8_3

Finally, in 2013, the American Association of Neurological Surgeons and Congress of Neurological Surgeons put out an unambiguous policy stating that the use of steroids in acute spinal cord injury is not recommended [3]. Another survey of surgeons, in 2014, showed a significant decrease in the use of steroids in acute spinal cord injuries. However, in some clinical scenarios, over 50% of surgeons said they would still use them. When asked why, "26% thought that steroids improved neurological recovery, 19.2% used steroids to adhere to institutional protocol, and 25.6% stated they did not think steroids were beneficial but used them because of medicolegal concerns" [4].

After reviewing all the evidence, I have now come to agree with the following statement by the Canadian Association of Emergency Physicians: "Physicians should not feel intimidated into prescribing high-dose methylprednisolone for acute spinal cord injuries" [5]. I took a lot of flak when I finally decided not to give steroids to these patients. We had been doing it for so long, and it violated the hospital's policy. But I had to do what was right. Medicine is a changing field. Studies are conducted, evidence changes, and hopefully, practices change as well. So who knows? Maybe in a few years a study will be done showing that steroids are beneficial after all in certain patients. Until then, however, I should treat my patients according to the best evidence, not according to an outdated "institutional protocol" and certainly not because I don't want to be the odd man out.

Case

Luisa was a 45-year-old woman who presented with the acute onset of right-sided weakness. An MRI revealed a stroke in her left frontal lobe. Investigation into the etiology of the stroke revealed 60% narrowing of her left internal carotid artery. Though guidelines suggest operating only when there is at least 70% narrowing, the chief of vascular surgery felt that because of her young age, she would benefit from an operation to open up her artery. During a discussion of her case in a weekly conference, none of the junior team members objected to his plan. Though they were aware of the guidelines, team members who were privately initially skeptical of the surgery came to embrace it after hearing their chief propose it and another senior faculty member defend it. Unfortunately, Luisa suffered a second stroke during the surgery and her case was reviewed in a morbidity conference. It turned out that many junior clinicians harbored doubts about the wisdom of the surgery, but were afraid to speak up, believing they were alone in this regard.

What Dr. Abiola Was Thinking

I was a junior resident when Luisa came into the hospital. When I first heard the chief of vascular surgery propose surgery for Luisa, I thought she was either making a big mistake or some new study had been published that I had not read. It turns out she was acting well outside established guidelines for when to operate, but I was afraid to say anything. No one else spoke up, and I didn't want to violate protocol or risk making a fool of myself in public. It turns out that almost everyone in the room disagreed with her decision to operate, but we were all afraid to contradict the boss. Several people who were initially opposed to the operation, at least privately, said that they had become convinced by the silence of others into supporting her decision. In our defense, the chief was not someone who tolerated dissent, having publically berated several people who had previously questioned her judgment. I can't promise that I'll start shouting every time I feel a senior surgeon is making an error. But I also know there are consequences to keeping quiet too.

Discussion

The authority bias occurs when the opinions and instructions of authority figures are unquestionably accepted and followed. The bandwagon effect, or the tyranny of the majority, is the tendency for people to adopt ideas and customs because of the behavior of others around them. It explains why beliefs, fads, and trends spread, as individuals change their behavior in response to the crowd. As a belief becomes more widespread, others also jump on "bandwagon," often regardless of the objective truth. These biases can negatively impact patient care when clinicians unthinkingly and inappropriately follow the instructions of authority figures or behavior of their peers.

We all imagine ourselves as independent thinkers, immune to influence of crowds and authority figures. We want to believe that us are unique and that our beliefs are the result of careful thought and deliberation. Similarly, we readily believe that others are conformists, easily influenced by the masses and powerful people. However, the evidence suggests for almost of us, our independence is largely an illusion. After all, we usually dress like our peers, watch the same movies, read the same books, buy the same products, and live in similar houses. I can speculate that almost everyone reading this owns a smart phone, spends time on social media, and sometimes watches videos on YouTube, probably of cats.

Similarly, you hold many of your most cherished opinions largely because other people around you hold them and you've grown up with them. If you're a liberal Democrat, the odds are likely that your parents and their friends were too. If you're highly religious, it's almost certain your parents were as well. Like most people in Western countries, you probably strongly believe in free speech, democracy, equal rights for women, and the right to a fair trial. So do I, and I am not suggesting that these are mere cultural artifacts, the way horseshoes are considered good luck. However, these beliefs were shaped largely by our common culture and upbringing. Many people around the world don't believe in these principles, reflecting how their beliefs were shaped by their environment. Do you honestly think that if you had grown up in North Korea you would have the same values you do today?

Moreover, you almost certainly believe many myths and urban legends because they have been repeated in the culture and you never thought to question them. Did you know that no accused witches were burned in Salem, Massachusetts? Did you know that fortune cookies were brought to the US from Japan, and they are actually rare in China? Did you know that sugar does not cause hyperactive behavior in children? Did you know hair and fingernails stop growing after a person's death? Did you know Thomas Edison did not invent the lightbulb? Wikipedia has a fascinating page of such "common misconceptions," many of them related to health and medicine [6]. It's worth looking at this list to see how many things you "know" to be true are based on passively accepting what you've been told. None of this makes you a thoughtless sheep. It means that conformity is a powerful regulator of human thought and that you are normal, without the time or inclination to thoroughly investigate every piece of information you've ever been told.

On a societal level, the bandwagon effect and information cascades can lead individuals to behave in extraordinary ways, with both positive and disastrous results. Scottish journalist Charles Mackay reported such behavior in his book *Extraordinary Popular Delusions and the Madness of Crowds*, published in 1841. He described economic bubbles, pseudoscientific fads, religious fanaticism, and literal witch hunts that plagued our ancestors. As the housing market crash of 2008 showed, people still rush to invest in the latest money-making scheme, creating massive economic bubbles that have the potential to devastate entire economies when they pop. Before the internet, otherwise well-adjusted people literally fought over the latest holiday toy as happened in 1983, when parents battled in store aisles to buy Cabbage Patch Kids for their children. Revolutions, such as those that began in the Arab world in 2010, can arise rapidly and spread widely, seemingly out of nowhere. More dramatically, people commit atrocities during wartime that would be unimaginable to them during peace.

Several of the most seminal studies in the history of psychology have demonstrated the power of the bandwagon effect and authority bias, with dramatic and sometimes horrifying results. The most famous and disturbing study of the authority bias was conducted by psychologist Stanley Milgram in 1961. His experiment consisted of a study subject, a confederate who appeared to be another study volunteer, and the person running the experience. The study subject was given the role of "teacher" while the study confederate, who was said to have a "heart condition," was given the role of "learner." The two were then separated by a thin wall. The job of the teacher was to give a series of increasingly stronger electric shocks to the learner every time he made an error on a word memorization task (Fig. 3.1).

Of course, the shocks were fake, but the actor who played the role of the learner would bang on the wall, complain about his heart condition, and ask that the experiment stop. Eventually, the learner stopped responding at all. If the teacher said he no longer wished to administer the electric shocks, the experimenter would give the following instructions:

1. Please continue.
2. The experiment requires that you continue.
3. It is absolutely essential that you continue.
4. You have no other choice, you must go on.

If the teacher inquired about the safety of the learner, the experimenter replied, "Although the shocks may be painful, there is no permanent tissue damage, so please go on." If the teacher reported the learner wanted to stop, the experimenter replied, "Whether the learner likes it or not, you must go on until he has learned all the word pairs correctly, so please go on." The experiment stopped only if the teacher refused to continue after the fourth command.

So what would you do if you were the teacher? Of course, you would stop once it became clear the learner was being hurt and didn't want to continue. Everyone feels that way about themselves when they read about this experiment. Prior to the experiment, Milgram asked 14 Yale psychology students to predict the results. He also reportedly informally asked psychiatrists and other professionals their opinion about how subjects would behave. They estimated that only about 4% of the teachers would inflict the maximum voltage, with one psychiatrist predicting that everyone would ask to cease the experiment once the learner requested it [7]. In reality, 65% (26 of 40) of people in Milgram's original study proceeded to give the learner a maximum shock. Videos of his experiment are available on YouTube and they are chilling to watch. The teachers are clearly uncomfortable and many express concern about the learner. Nonetheless, most, but not all people, continue to inflict shocks on the learner even after he screams in pain and begs for the experiment to stop [8]. Milgram's experiments have been repeated by many others, and his findings have been largely been replicated [9]. Most recently, a study of 80 people from Poland, conducted in 2015, found that 90% of subjects were willing to give the maximum shock to the learner [10]. Interestingly the physical proximity of the experimenter to the teacher plays the largest role in ensuring obedience.

Dr. Milgram explained his results by saying that the teachers are willing to shock the learners because they have transferred the blame to the experimenter and no

Fig. 3.1 Illustration of the setup of a Milgram experiment. The experimenter (E) convinces the subject ("Teacher" T) to give what he believes are painful electric shocks to another subject, who is actually an actor ("Learner" L). (Fred the Oyster. Milgram experiment [Image file]. In: Wikimedia commons. 2014. Retrieved from https://commons.wikimedia.org/wiki/File:Milgram_experiment_v2.svg.)

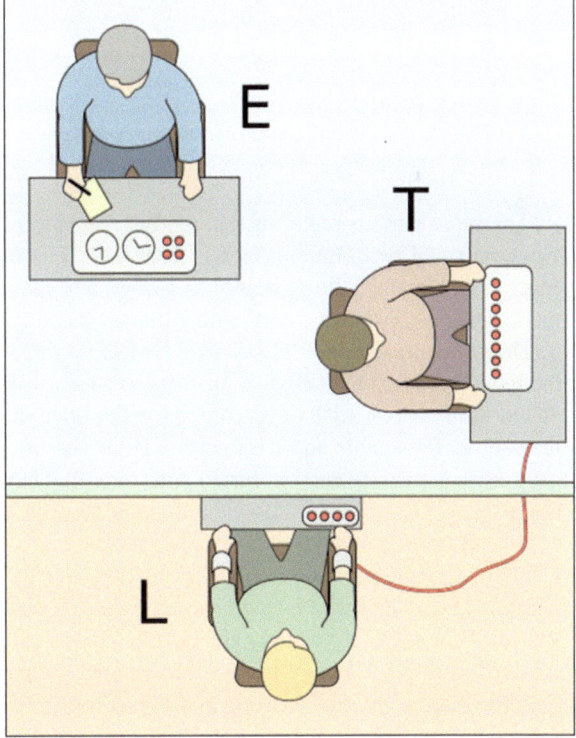

Fig. 3.2 The lines used in Dr. Asch's conformity study. (Fred the Oyster. One of the pair of cards used in the experiment [Image file]. In: Wikipedia. 2014. Retrieved from https://en.wikipedia.org/wiki/Asch_conformity_experiments#/media/File:Asch_experiment.svg.)

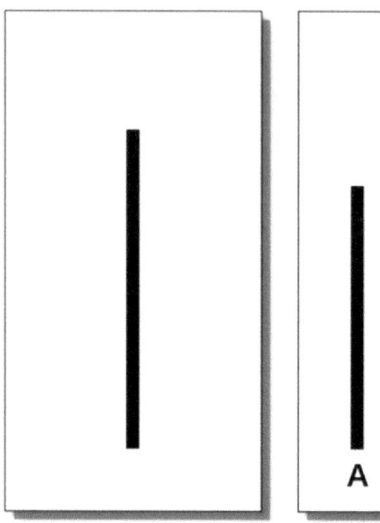
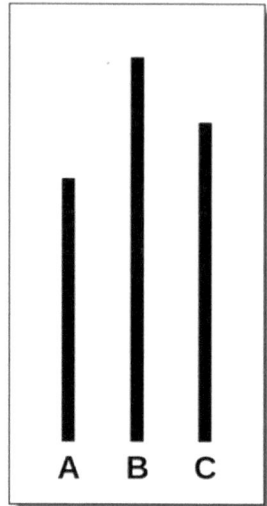

longer see themselves as individual agents who are responsible for their own actions. He wrote:

> *The essence of obedience consists in the fact that a person comes to view themselves as the instrument for carrying out another person's wishes, and they therefore no longer see themselves as responsible for their actions. Once this critical shift of viewpoint has occurred in the person, all of the essential features of obedience follow. [Thus] the major problem for the subject is to recapture control of his own regnant processes once he has committed them to the purposes of the experimenter* [11].

The most famous study of the bandwagon effect and the power of conformity was conducted by Solomon Asch in 1951 [12]. His study involved one subject and seven confederates who appeared as study participants, but were in on the experiment. They were shown a card with a line on it and another card with three lines on it. Their task was simple; to say which of these three lines was the same length as the line on the first card (Fig. 3.2).

On the first two trials, everyone gave the obvious, correct answer, establishing themselves as reliable and trustworthy. However, after that, all of the confederates gave the same wrong answer. Faced with a conflict between what they saw and what the group reported, only 25% of the study subjects consistently defied the group consensus on the length of the line. Even the presence of one person, a "true partner" who was willing to break with the group and give the correct answer, dramatically increased the rate at which study subjects were willing to give the obviously correct answer, with only 5% of study subjects then answering with the incorrect majority. Another example is the "elevator experiment," which appeared on the TV show Candid Camera in 1962 [13]. In the episode titled *Face the Rear*, (which can be viewed on YouTube) unknowing individuals entered an elevator where everyone else was facing backwards. Despite this being a completely unnatural thing to do, many individuals "went with the crowd" and rode the elevator facing away from the doors.

In behavioral economics, such behavior is called an information cascade. It occurs when a person makes a decision based on the behavior of others, ignoring their own private information. A person who makes a decision as part of an information cascade has observed how others have chosen before him. The behavior of others is easy to observe, though their reasons for having made their choice remain opaque. We may assume that others know what they are doing and may follow their behavior. This behavior helps explain the rapid rise and fall of trends and fads. Marketers try to take advantage of information cascades by persuading so-called "thought-leaders" to use their products. In medicine, pharmaceutical companies are eager to have prominent clinicians and celebrities associated with their products, hoping to create a positive cascade.

The bandwagon effect may also affect people not just with a specific decision, but with regard to the overall culture and work environment. Group attitudes and norms are "contagious." We are unconsciously influenced by the attitudes and behaviors of those around us. We have all found ourselves in an unpleasant group before, perhaps one of many angry airline passengers waiting for a delayed flight. The tension can be palpable, and we may find our own anxiety rising in response to that of the strangers next to us. Similarly, experiences such as sporting events and performances are enjoyable largely because the excitement of the crowd spreads to us all. Could you imagine being the only audience member for a rock concert, for example? Even if your favorite band was playing, the experience would be odd and utterly incomplete without the roar of the crowd and shared enthusiasm of strangers.

Psychologists have demonstrated that people unwittingly adopt social norms and practices related to their surroundings. In one study, researchers placed paper fliers on 139 cars in a hospital parking lot [14]. When the parking lot was scattered with litter, which had placed there by the researchers, nearly half of people threw the flier on the ground. However, when the parking garage was cleaned ahead of time, only about 10% of people dropped the flier on the ground. It's not hard to see how this behavior manifests itself in your life. Are you the same person at a solemn religious service as you are at a rock concert or child's birthday party? Probably not. When you are with your boss, do you act differently than you do on a first date or seeing old college friends? Probably so. You automatically adjust to the environment in which you find yourself and unconsciously adopt the norms and behaviors of those around you. As such, there are multiple versions of "you" depending on your surroundings.

Perhaps the most famous demonstration of the power of group attitudes and behaviors was the Stanford prison experiment, conducted by Philip Zimbardo in 1973 (although some questions have recently been raised about its methodology) [15]. He recruited 24 male, college students who were then randomly assigned to either the role of prisoner or guard in a simulated prison he had set up in a basement of the psychology department. The "prisoners" were "arrested" at home and taken to the police station where they fingerprinted and photographed. They were then blindfolded and taken to Zimbardo's "prison" where they were stripped, deloused, and changed in prison garb. The "guards" were similarly dressed to suit their roles and instructed to take steps to command the prisoners' respect and maintain law and order. Within hours, each group started to behave according to its perceived role. The guards started to abuse the prisoners, and the prisoners started to behave in a submissive manner. Over the next few days the guards proceeded to humiliate, berate, and at times outright torture the prisoners. The prisoners began to act according to their role as well, staging a revolt. Several prisoners had nervous breakdowns. Zimbardo himself lost sight of the experiment and began to perceive himself as the prison's warden. The experiment lasted six days before an outside observer recognized the horror it had become and demanded that it stop. Experiments like these show that there are many versions of ourselves depending on the environment in which we find ourselves. Most people will readily conform to the roles society expects them to play and will alter their behavior to fit in with those around them.

Several horrific, real-world examples of the Stanford prisoner experiment and Milgram's authority experiment have occurred since 9/11. The first of these was the Abu Ghraib prison incident where American soldiers tortured and murdered several prisoners during the Iraq war. Prison guards Lynndie England, Sabrina Harman, Charles Graner, and several others were sentenced to prison terms ranging from three months to 10 years for their role in these events. In a letter home describing the abuse Harman wrote:

> They've been stripping "the fucked up" prisoners and handcuffing them to the bars. Its pretty sad. I get to laugh at them and throw corn at them. I kind of feel bad for these guys even if they are accused of killing US soldiers. We degrade them but we don't hit and thats a plus even though Im sure they wish we'd kill them. They sleep one hour then we yell and wake them—make them stay up for one hour, then sleep one hour—then up etc. This goes on for 72 hours while we fuck with them. Most have been so scared they piss on themselves. Its sad. It's a little worst than Basic training ie: being naked and hand-cuffed... [16].

Graner, the ringleader of the abuse, had worked as a prison guard previously and had several previous allegations of severe abuse. England and Harman, however, had no such histories and seem to have led average, mundane lives prior to coming under the influence of Graner. Another guard revealed the power of bandwagon effect with regard to taking pictures, saying, "Everyone in theatre had a digital camera. Everyone was taking pictures of everything, from detainees to death" (Fig. 3.3) [16].

Another example of these biases occurred with psychologists Bruce Jessen and James Mitchell, who created and implemented the "enhanced interrogation" techniques used on prisoners in CIA custody after 9/11. These techniques included waterboarding, sleep deprivation, and stress positions, such as being locked in a coffin or being handcuffed to a wall so prisoners could not sit down for several days in a row. It is not clear that any valuable intelligence was obtained from their punishments. Dr. Jessen defended his actions as countless others have done before him, saying "We were soldiers doing what we were instructed to do" [17]. With eerie echoes of the explanations offered by the participants in the Milgram experiment, he said "Jim and I didn't want to continue doing what we were doing. They kept telling me every day a nuclear bomb was going to be exploded in the US and that because I had told them to stop, I had lost my nerve and it was going to be my fault if I didn't continue."

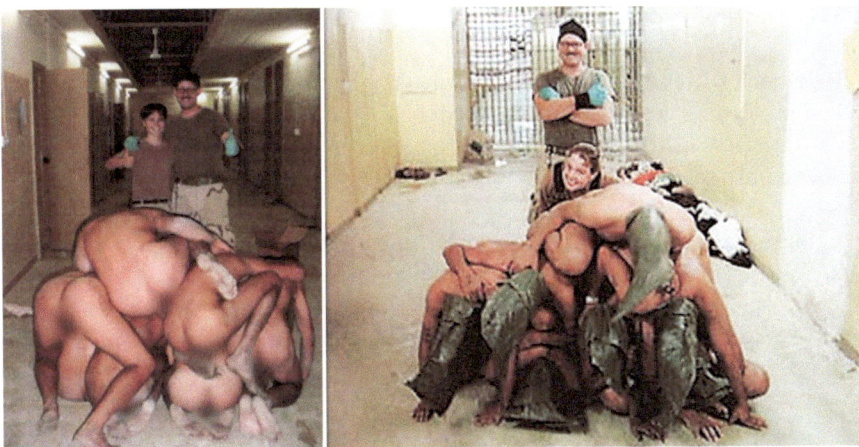

Fig. 3.3 Scenes of torture from the Abu Ghraib prison. (Graner and England. [Image file]. In: Wikipedia. 2003. Retrieved from https://en.wikipedia.org/wiki/Charles_Graner#/media/File:Abu_Ghraib_53.jpg; Graner and Sabrina Harman. [Image file]. In: Wikipedia. (ca. 2003–2004). Retrieved from https://en.wikipedia.org/wiki/Charles_Graner#/media/File:Abu_Ghraib_48.jpg.)

Milgram did not feel that the subjects in his experiment were evil or aberrant. Rather, he felt that they were:

Ordinary people, simply doing their jobs, and without any particular hostility on their part, can become agents in a terrible destructive process. Moreover, even when the destructive effects of their work become patently clear, and they are asked to carry out actions incompatible with fundamental standards of morality, relatively few people have the resources needed to resist authority [7].

I'll concede that if Drs. Jessen and Mitchell truly believed their efforts were necessary to prevent a nuclear apocalypse that might kill millions of people, they were not operating under ordinary circumstances. However, their behavior illustrates Milgram's observation that ordinary people can be manipulated into doing extraordinary things under the proper conditions.

The bandwagon effect and authority bias also occur with the process of group decision-making, which often leads to suboptimal outcomes. Groupthink is a phenomenon that occurs when individuals in a group silence themselves due to a reluctance to challenge authority or break group cohesion. This creates an echo-chamber, which can be exacerbated if group members isolate themselves from outside influences. Psychologist Irving Janis pioneered the study of groupthink [18]. He specifically studied seminal events in American history, such as the Japanese attack on Pearl Harbor in 1941 and the attempted invasion of Cuba in 1961(Bay of Pigs) to show how groupthink can lead to disastrous outcomes. He identified eight symptoms indicative of groupthink:

Overestimating the strength and righteousness of the group

1. Unquestioned belief in the morality of the group.
2. Excessive optimism and a belief of invulnerability encouraging risk taking.

Closed-mindedness

3. Rationalizing or ignoring warnings that might challenge the group's beliefs.
4. Stereotyping those who are opposed to the group as amoral or incompetent.

Pressure to conform

5. Illusions of unanimity among group members as silence is viewed as agreement.
6. Self-censorship of ideas that vary from the group consensus.
7. Pressure to conform placed on any member who deviates from the group.
8. Self-appointed members ("mindguards") who shield others from dissenting information.

While it is intuitive to think that a group's decision may reflect the average view of its constituent members, this is often not the case. In group settings, a phenomenon known as group polarization often occurs. It refers to the tendency for a group to make decisions that are more extreme than the initial inclination of its members. This helps to explain why groups often end up with more extreme views than the individual members. At its most extreme, groups of people commit acts of violence that would likely be unimaginable to each group member individually. David Schkade and colleagues demonstrated the effects of group polarization [19]. They collected a group of conservative and liberal citizens and both individually and anonymously asked them their opinions on contentious political issues, such as gay rights and affirmative action. After each group deliberated the issues, the subjects were again individually and anonymously asked their opinions, and the group was asked for a consensus opinion. They found:

1. The individual group member's initial opinions were less extreme than the group's opinion after discussion occurred. Similarly, after discussion, the liberals became more liberal and the conservatives became more conservative as individuals.
2. Discussion increased agreement within groups. Prior to discussion, individuals within each group showed a broader range of opinion than afterwards.
3. The opinions of the two groups ended up further apart after deliberation. Whereas initially there was some overlap between group members, this largely vanished after discussion.

Another way in which groups can make poor decisions is known as pluralistic ignorance. It occurs when most people in a group privately reject a belief or norm, but publically accept it, incorrectly believing that they are in the minority. If most people in a group have incorrect views about a group belief, then this view fails to accurately represent the true belief of the group. As a result of pluralistic ignorance, many people see themselves as fundamentally different from their peers, when in fact this may not be the case. It most commonly occurs with longstanding, ingrained social norms or when there is a vocal, enthusiastic minority espousing a viewpoint.

Deborah Prentice and Dale Miller provided an example of pluralistic ignorance through their study of attitudes towards excessive alcohol consumption at Princeton University [20]. They queried students, many of whom did not want to participate in such debauchery. These students wrongly assumed that their reluctance to drink excessively placed them in the minority. However, they often did so rather than face possible rejection. Pluralistic ignorance can surface with more consequential matters as well. Hubert O'Gorman examined surveys from 1968 and found that most whites at the time did not believe in segregation [21]. However, they incorrectly thought they were in a minority in this belief, helping segregation to continue longer than it would have otherwise. On certain issues today, such as gun control, a quiet majority of people favor policies that are highly unlikely to become laws. This is because gun control opponents are more vocal and passionate than gun control advocates.

To see how pluralistic ignorance may affect clinicians, imagine a senior clinician asking during rounds if anyone disagrees with her thoughts about a case. If she is greeted by silence this may indeed mean the junior clinicians all agree with her. Alternatively, it may mean several people disagree, but they are afraid to voice their opinion, not wanting to be the odd man out.

A related phenomenon to pluralistic ignorance is known as the Abilene paradox, which was coined by Jerry Harvey in 1974 [22]. It similarly refers to how a group can collectively make a choice that is counter to the desires of most or all of the people in the group. Harvey used the following parable to demonstrate the paradox:

> On a hot afternoon visiting in Coleman, Texas the family is comfortably playing dominoes on a porch, until the father-in-law suggests that they take a trip to Abilene [53 miles north] for dinner. The wife says, "Sounds like a great idea." The husband, despite having reservations because the drive is long and hot, thinks that his preferences must be out-of-step with the group and says, "Sounds good to me. I just hope your mother wants to go." The mother-in-law then says, "Of course I want to go. I haven't been to Abilene in a long time."

> The drive is hot, dusty, and long. When they arrive at the cafeteria, the food is as bad as the drive. They arrive back home four hours later, exhausted.

> One of them dishonestly says, "It was a great trip, wasn't it?" The mother-in-law says that, actually, she would rather have stayed home, but went along since the other three were so enthusiastic. The husband says, "I wasn't delighted to be doing what we were doing. I only went to satisfy the rest of you." The wife says, "I just went along to keep you happy. I would have had to be crazy to want to go out in the heat like that." The father-in-law then says that he only suggested it because he thought the others might be bored.

> The group sits back, perplexed that they together decided to take a trip which none of them wanted. They each would have preferred to sit comfortably, but did not admit to it when they still had time to enjoy the afternoon.

Harvey felt that the Abilene paradox resulted from an inability to manage agreement, not conflict. In contrast to groupthink, where group members are pleased with the outcome, in the Abilene paradox, group members are dissatisfied with the outcome. Additionally, they are not plagued by poor thinking per se, but rather a desire to maintain group cohesion and not "rock the boat."

On a large scale, pluralistic ignorance can best be overcome through public education. For example, letting students know that they are in the majority if they don't want to drink excessively will make them feel more comfortable in their decision not to do so. Additionally, leaders can encourage open dissent, creating an environment where those who disagree are not punished or shunned. On an individual level, people should speak up when they feel a mistake is being made. Though they may feel alone in their dissent, this may not actually be the case.

Medicine is as prone as any other field to both fashion and tradition, neither of which has a place in what should be a science-driven enterprise. Because of the bandwagon effect, clinicians may too rapidly adopt trendy new treatments or fail to abandon longstanding practices that are no longer supported by the evidence. Once a treatment or test becomes widespread, it can often become entrenched and difficult to question, especially if it is endorsed by prominent clinicians.

The harm of the bandwagon effect can be seen in one of medicine's great cautionary tales, the frontal lobotomy. In 1935 Egas Moniz (1874–1955), a Portuguese doctor, learned about two aggressive chimpanzees who had become quite docile after lesions were made to their frontal lobes. He had seen this for himself in soldiers who sustained frontal lobe injuries in battle. This led to him consider that a similar procedure might benefit mentally ill patients. Later that year, along with neurosurgeon Almeida Lima, he devised a surgical procedure to sever white matter connections in the frontal lobes of people with depression and schizophrenia. In his first 20 cases, he reported seven cures, seven improvements, and six non-responders [23]. After performing 40 procedures, Moniz concluded that "prefrontal leukotomy is a simple operation, always safe, which may prove to be an effective surgical treatment in certain cases of mental disorder" [24].

In a time when effective treatments for psychiatric disorders did not exist beyond electroconvulsive therapy, his findings were a potentially revolutionary development. Most hospitals for the mentally ill at this time resembled medieval dungeons, and patients suffered greatly. Some were heavily sedated with opiates or barbiturates. At other times, they were physically restrained or immersed in baths for prolonged periods. Moniz rushed to spread news of his work, presenting his findings at a meeting several weeks later and publishing them the next year. In 1949, he was awarded the Nobel Prize for this work.

The procedure was soon taken up with great gusto around the world, particularly in the US by a neurosurgeon, James Watts (1904–1994), and a neuropsychiatrist Walter Freeman (1895–1972), though he lost his surgical license after a patient died on the operating table (Fig. 3.4).

In 1946, Dr. Freeman developed a procedure known as a transorbital lobotomy, in which a metal pick, called a leucotome, was inserted into the corner of each eye-socket. A hammer was then used to drive it into the brain where he would sever white matter fibers connecting the frontal lobe to the thalamus. He travelled around the country in a van he called the "lobotomobile," sometimes performing dozens of lobotomies daily, without a mask or gloves. Of course, informed consent was nothing like it is today. In 1949,

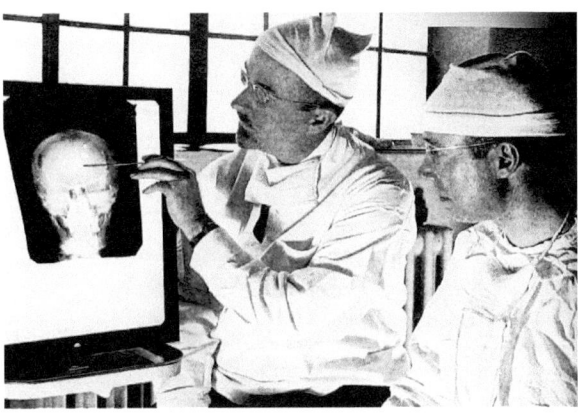

Fig. 3.4 Walter Freeman and James Watts. (Ewing HA. (Harris). Dr. Walter Freeman, left, and Dr. James W. Watts study an X ray before a psychosurgical operation [Image file]. In: Wikimedia commons. 2013. Retrieved from https:// commons.wikimedia.org/ wiki/Category:Lobotomy#/ media/File:Turning_the_ Mind_Inside_Out_ Saturday_Evening_Post_24_ May_1941_a_detail_1.jpg.)

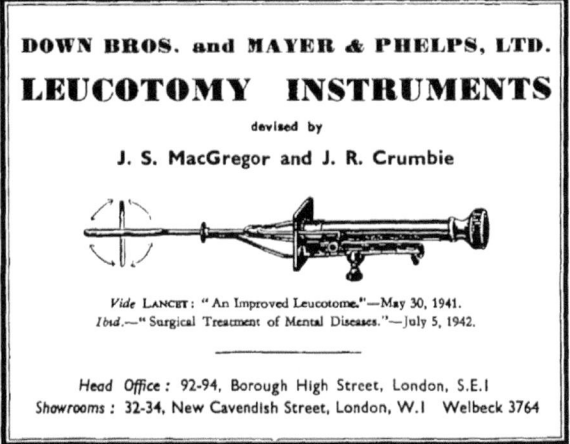

Fig. 3.5 An advertisement for a leucotome. (Bonkersinstitute. Leuco-tome, a tool for performing leucotomies [Image file]. In: Wikimedia commons. 2007. Retrieved from https:// commons.wikimedia.org/ wiki/Category:Lobotomy#/ media/File:Leucotome.gif.)

5,074 procedures were performed in the US, and by 1951 more than 18,600 people had been lobotomized [25]. Tens of thousands of people were lobotomized in other countries as well. Dr. Freeman performed the procedure nearly 3,500 times himself, including on several children. His career ended in 1967 after a patient, Helen Mortensen, died of a brain hemorrhage after receiving her third lobotomy (Fig. 3.5).

Although the procedure did benefit some patients, it came at a terrible price for many others. As Jay Hoffman said in 1949:

These patients are not only no longer distressed by their mental conflicts but also seem to have little capacity for any emotional experiences - pleasurable or otherwise. They are described by the nurses and the doctors, over and over, as dull, apathetic, listless, without drive or initiative, flat, lethargic, placid and unconcerned, childlike, docile, needing pushing, passive, lacking in spontaneity, without aim or purpose, preoccupied and dependent [26].

Other patients developed epilepsy after the procedure. Rarely, they died. President John F. Kennedy's sister Rosemary was famously damaged by the procedure,

Fig. 3.6 A T1-weighted MRI in a patient who had frontal leucotomies. (Gaillard F. (Frank). 65-year old man with history of OCD treatment in 1970s [Image file]. In: Wikimedia commons. 2016. Retrieved from https://commons. wikimedia.org/wiki/ Category:Lobotomy#/media/ File:Frontal-leukotomy.jpg.)

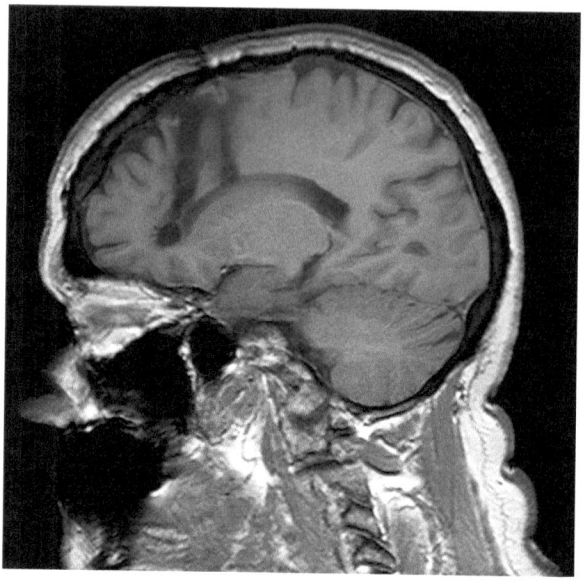

needing full-time care for the rest of her life. As its harms became more apparent and the development of antipsychotic medications offered an effective alternative, the procedure stopped being performed. Today, "lobotomy" is a word associated with cartoonish, evil doctors turning patients into zombies. Victor Swayze, a psychiatrist, cautioned appropriately, "If we learn nothing else from that era, it should be recognized that more rigorous, prospective long-term studies of psychiatric outcome are essential to assess the long-term outcomes of our treatment methods" (Fig. 3.6) [27].

While it is easy to disparage lobotomists in retrospect, the bandwagon effect still impacts clinicians today. All too often, trendy, high-tech treatments and procedures proliferate precisely because they are novel, fancy, and make intuitive sense. For many clinicians, an unbiased evaluation of such treatments is often complicated by the fact that they are highly remunerative (the financial bias). At times, the safety and efficacy of many such treatments are ultimately not borne out by formal studies. In the late 1990s, a device called a laparoscopic power morcellator became widely used to remove uterine fibroids. Unfortunately, it had the potential to spread hidden cancer cells, leading to avoidable deaths. In the past few years, infusions of platelet-rich therapies (PRT) have become popular treatment for a number of orthopedic ailments, in part due to endorsements by celebrity athletes. One clinic boasts of its success with the treatment, describing it as a "revolutionary new treatment that relieves pain by promoting long lasting healing of musculoskeletal conditions using the healing power of your own body" [28]. Multiple patient testimonials are used as evidence of the "success" of this clinic and others like it. Despite the enthusiasm, formal evidence that PRTs actually help patients is lacking. A Cochrane review in 2014 concluded "there is currently insufficient evidence to support the use of PRT for treating musculoskeletal soft tissue injuries" [29]. PRT features what John

Fig. 3.7 Just because bloodletting was popular doesn't mean it was effective. (Wellcome Collection Gallery. An ill man who is being bled by his doctor [Image file]. In: Wikimedia commons. (n.d.). Retrieved from https://commons.wikimedia.org/wiki/Category:Caricatures_of_physicians#/media/File:An_ill_man_who_is_being_bled_by_his_doctor._Coloured_etching_Wellcome_V0011195.jpg.)

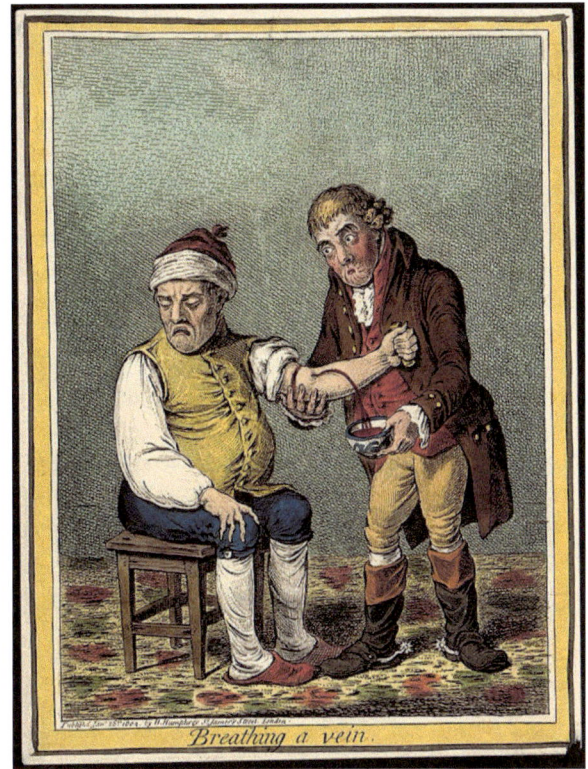

Bergfeld called the Orthopedic Triad of "famous athlete, famous doctor, untested treatment" [30].

Perhaps no greater example of the bandwagon effect in recent times is the use of coronary artery stents. In 2004, over one million stent procedures were performed in the US. Though the procedure can be life-saving in patients with acute heart attacks, no benefit had been demonstrated in patients with stable coronary artery disease, though such patients constituted approximately 85% of stent recipients. In 2007, a large, randomized study demonstrated that the procedure offered no advantage compared to medical management alone in patients with stable coronary artery disease [31]. Later studies showed that not only did the stents fail to prevent heart attacks and save lives, they also failed to relieve chest pain in patients with stable angina (Fig. 3.7) [32].

As an example of how the bandwagon effect can drive medical practice, consider the following story related by David Brown, a cardiologist. He presented data to a group of cardiologists from large, randomized controlled trials showing that coronary artery stents were not superior to noninvasive treatments in patients with stable coronary artery disease. Despite this, when presented with a case where a stent would be inappropriate, many cardiologists nonetheless said they would consider this intervention. When asked why, one replied, "Well, we know what we do" [33].

Additionally, the power of the bandwagon effect and authority bias to influence behaviors applies not just with specific treatments and procedures, but also the overall culture of hospitals and clinics. Whether or not team members relate to each other in a respectful way and whether patients are treated with kindness is similarly "contagious." Any clinician with enough experience will have worked in an environment where shortcomings were dealt with by ridicule and shame. Questions were discouraged, and obedience to authority was the norm. Such environments create an incentive to hide or minimize errors, to the detriment of patients. At its most extreme, humiliation and belittlement can cause depression and burnout, leading clinicians to leave medicine, abuse substances, and in exceptional circumstances, commit suicide.

I have worked in environments where the attending doctors yelled at the senior residents, who then yelled at the interns, who then yelled at the medical students. Everyone was on edge and miserable, and this filtered down to the patients. While the patients weren't yelled at, they were disparaged behind their backs and not treated with empathy. Almost every clinician will eventually witness a patient being mocked, and may feel pressure to "join in the fun." An anonymous medical student wrote an essay in the Annals of Internal Medicine, describing a time when a surgeon saved the life of a Latina patient, but then began to "celebrate" in an inappropriate way:

> Dr. Canby raises his right hand into the air. He starts to sing 'La Cucaracha.' He sings, 'La cucaracha, la cucaracha, dada, dada, dada-daaa.' It looks like he is dancing with her. He stomps his feet, twists his body, and waves his right arm above his head. All the while, he holds her, his whole hand still inside her vagina. He starts laughing. He keeps dancing. And then he looks at me. I begin to sway to his beat. My feet shuffle. I hum and laugh along with him. Moments later, the anesthesiologist yells, 'Knock it off, assholes!' And we stop [34].

In a similar incident, anesthesiologist Tiffany Ingham was accidently recorded telling a sedated patient, "After five minutes of talking to you in pre-op, I wanted to punch you in the face and man you up a little bit" [35]. After continuing to insult the sleeping man, calling him a "retard," she later joked, "I'm going to mark 'hemorrhoids' even though we don't see them and probably won't." Indeed, she did mark down this false diagnosis in his chart. Another doctor in the case joined in the "fun," saying about a rash on his genitals "As long as it's not Ebola, you're okay." Though I suspect some team members were uncomfortable with this behavior, like the subjects in Zimbardo's study, no one was willing to speak up and put a stop to clearly inappropriate behavior.

Fortunately, these types of cases are unusual. Much more commonly, I've worked in environments where clinicians relate to each other respectfully. Mistakes are not ignored, but they are handled with an eye towards fixing the problem, not punishing the clinician who erred. Junior clinicians can challenge their elders without fear of retribution. These behavioral norms filter to down to even the most difficult patients, who are then treated with professionalism.

Although complementary and alternative medicine (CAM) practitioners thrive on an illusion of independence, within its own confines, the bandwagon bias is incredibly powerful there as well. In the world of CAM, various vitamins, herbs,

Fig. 3.8 The bogeymen of alternative medicine are nothing new. (Unholy Three [Image file]. In: Wikimedia commons. (n.d.). Retrieved Sept 15, 2018 from https://commons.wikimedia.org/wiki/File:Unholy_three.png.)

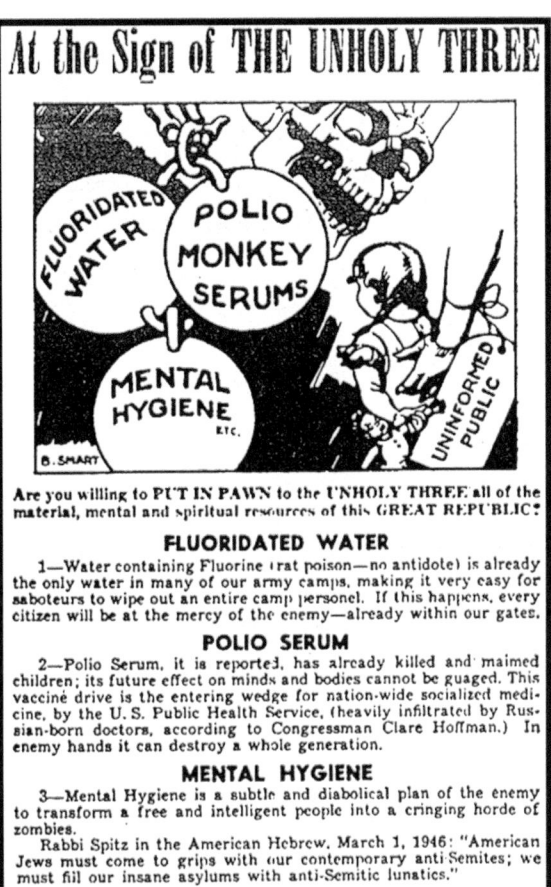

oils, and detox regimens routinely jostle with each other as miracle cures for all that ails humanity. Yesterday kale cured everything, today it is turmeric, and tomorrow it will be something else. Conversely, fluoride, gluten, psychiatric medications, and vaccines rotate as the underlying cause for most diseases. CAM practitioners routinely embrace these same myths in lockstep. As this poster from 1955 shows, these bogeymen have been scapegoated for decades (Fig. 3.8) [36].

A key difference between mainstream medicine and CAM however, is that clinicians who practice science-based medicine eventually bow to the evidence and abandon outdated practices. As evidence of this, we don't perform lobotomies anymore. Additionally, from 2009 to 2014, the number of coronary stents in the US decreased from 21,781 to 7,921 and the percentage deemed "inappropriate" decreased from 26.2% to 13.3% in response to a guideline titled *Appropriate Use Criteria for Coronary Revascularization* [37]. In contrast, CAM practitioners will

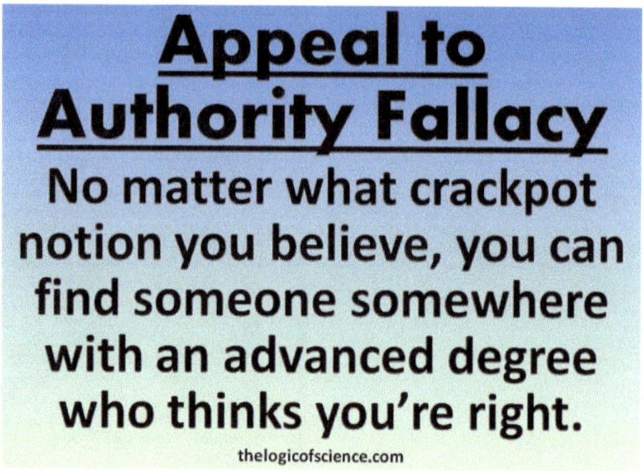

Fig. 3.9 I agree. (The Logic
of Science. Appeal to
authority [Image file]. 2017.
Retrieved from https://
thelogicofscience.files.
wordpress.com/2015/10/
appeal-to-authority-fallacy.
jpg.)

never produce a document on the appropriate use criteria for "turmeric detoxes."
They alter their behaviors primarily in response to what their customers are willing
to pay; and this is based on fads, fears, and the bandwagon effect (Fig. 3.9).

Despite the powerful experiments and real-world cautionary tales reported thus far,
the group is often an appropriate place to be. When traveling in a foreign country, if
the locals exiting a train all walk in one direction, it makes sense to assume that they
know something you don't and follow along. We've all agreed that red means stop and
green means go. We don't get to individually decide what day of the week we want it
to be. Doing what other people are doing around you is common in medicine, and this
is usually for a good reason. Every clinician starts out as the most junior person on the
totem pole in an environment that contains a host of ingrained ideas, customs, and
practices. Many of these are based on decades of clinical experience or formal, science-based policies. No clinician can thoroughly review every hospital policy and
practice guideline, deciding for themselves which to follow and which to ignore.
Clinicians may make thousands of decisions about a single patient over the course of
a hospitalization. No one has the time or expertise to evaluate the entirely of the evidence supporting or refuting each and every one of these practices.

Similarly, more often than not, there is reason to trust authorities. When I fly, I do
not challenge either the pilot or the personnel in charge of security, even though my
life is literally in their hands. If I were to suddenly find myself working in a different
profession, perhaps a mechanic's shop or construction site, I would do my best to do
exactly what everyone else was doing. I would assume that the people there knew a
lot more than I did, and before I suggested any changes, I'd want to gain plenty
experience and expertise myself. I hope young clinicians do the same. Would any
patient want to be cared for by a newly minted intern who decided she was going to
ignore hospital protocol and the wisdom of senior clinicians to "think for myself?"
Of course not.

Additionally, with a little thought, we can understand the conformity of people
in Asch's study on the length of lines. They were faced with a choice between two
highly improbable scenarios; either their own perception or the perception of seven

other seemingly healthy, honest people was completely skewed. I suspect that if seven other presumably competent and honest clinicians saw a finding on an MRI that I could not, I too would go along with the group. My most reasonable response would be to get my eyes examined, rather than to assume the other clinicians were incompetent or hallucinating. Similarly, if while walking to work tomorrow, masses of people started running in the opposite direction with a fearful look in their eyes, I'd probably join in the herd. I'd assume they knew something important I didn't and that being an "independent" thinker could carry grave risks.

Moreover, group decision-making does not always lead to suboptimal decisions, and for many situations, a group may be preferable to an individual. While the archetype of the lone genius captures our imagination, for many of humanity's most monumental achievements, collaboration has allowed for successes that no individual could have achieved on his own. Not only does working in a group allow for increased knowledge and skills, occasionally it can save us from our own cognitive biases. According to a model of human cognition known as argumentative theory, proposed by Hugo Mercier and Dan Sperber, reason evolved primarily to help us win arguments, not to solve problems [38]. We reason primarily to convince other people we are right and to evaluate and defend ourselves against the arguments of others. This model explains several of our cognitive flaws, namely confirmation bias, the tendency we all have to search for information that will confirm our preexisting beliefs. A natural consequence of this is that at times, an individual will not solve problems as well as a group, as long as that group contains members with diverse viewpoints. As Dr. Mercier explained [39]:

People mostly have a problem with the confirmation bias when they reason on their own, when no one is there to argue against their point of view. What has been observed is that often times, when people reason on their own, they're unable to arrive at a good solution, at a good belief, or to make a good decision because they will only confirm their initial intuition.

On the other hand, when people are able to discuss their ideas with other people who disagree with them, then the confirmation biases of the different participants will balance each other out, and the group will be able to focus on the best solution. Thus, reasoning works much better in groups. When people reason on their own, it's very likely that they are going to go down a wrong path. But when they're actually able to reason together, they are much more likely to reach a correct solution.

A practical demonstration of this has been shown with the cognitive reflection test, developed by Shane Frederick [40]. It asks the following brain teasers:

1. A bat and a ball cost $1.10 in total. The bat costs $1.00 more than the ball. How much does the ball cost?
2. If it takes five machines five minutes to make five widgets, how long would it take 100 machines to make 100 widgets?
3. In a lake, there is a patch of lily pads. Every day, the patch doubles in size. If it takes forty eight days for the patch to cover the entire lake, how long would it take for the patch to cover half of the lake?

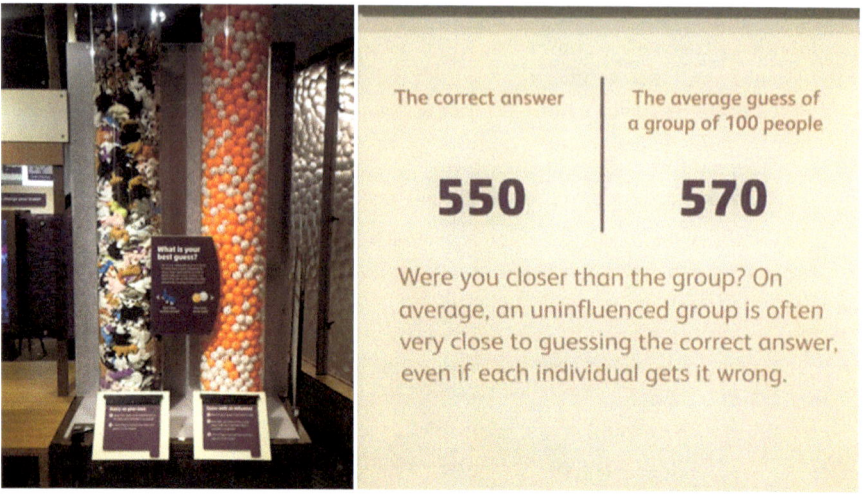

The correct answer | The average guess of a group of 100 people

550 | 570

Were you closer than the group? On average, an uninfluenced group is often very close to guessing the correct answer, even if each individual gets it wrong.

Fig. 3.10 A group of 100 people did quite well, on average, at estimating the number of stuffed animals in a container

The answers are: five cents, five minutes, and forty seven days. Many people do quite poorly on these tests, and about one-third of people get no correct answers. However, when people are allowed to work together in groups of three or more, no one gets any answer wrong. At least one person in the group figures out the correct answer and can explain it to his teammates.

Moreover, large groups of people are often better at coming to a correct answer to a problem when their individual answers are averaged. A display at the Boston Museum of Science shows that a group of people trying to guess the number of toys in a container came very close to the correct answer (Fig. 3.10). Raphael Silberzahn and Eric Uhlmann have similarly demonstrated that the combined results from groups of researchers given access to the same data set, may do better than any single group in minimizing bias and reporting accurate results [41].

Finally, the bandwagon effect can be harnessed to improve medical care as well. Largely because of the bandwagon effect, clinicians are much more reluctant now than in the past to inappropriately prescribe opioids and antibiotics, but more likely to perform routine safety measures such as washing their hands. A study by Daniella Meeker found that sending e-mails to doctors comparing them to their peers with the lowest rate of inappropriate antibiotic use, was successful in reducing the inappropriate use of antibiotics [42]. In contrast, other techniques, including "physician and patient education, computerized clinical decision support, and financial incentives" had only a modest impact. Similarly, the *Clean Your Hands* campaign, which sought to publicize and normalize routine hand washing in the UK, led to dramatic declines in acquired hospital infections [43]. A similar campaign at Vanderbilt University increased hand washing rates from 52% to 89% [44]. It was based largely by creating a cultural shift promoting hand washing. Hospital leaders adopted the program as a quality improvement measure, and their compensation depended in part on its success. A financial incentive was also offered to hospital departments, but only if every person in their division performed well. Tom Talbot, the chief epidemiologist, said, "The concept was we're in this together" [45].

Conclusion

Clinicians should be on guard for practices that continue simply because "everyone else does them." When faced with an outdated policy that continues due to inertia, especially one that negatively impacts patients, clinicians should try to change the policy. Similarly, unless they feel that there is sufficient evidence of its safety and efficacy, clinicians should avoid joining a stampede to adopt a new practice simply because others are doing so. While no one wants to be the last to adopt an effective new test or treatment, early scientific findings can be easily over-hyped, leading clinicians to prematurely put them into widespread use.

In a group setting, clinicians need to be aware of the deleterious effects of groupthink. Janis devised several strategies to minimize groupthink:

- Leaders should not express their opinion at the outset to avoid biasing the team.
- Discussion with outside experts should be encouraged, and outsiders should be invited into the group.
- Organizations should have more than one team trying to solve the same problem.
- Group leaders should not attend all group meetings.
- All effective alternatives should be examined.
- A rotating team member should be designated as the devil's advocate whose job is to disagree with the plan of care. This would free this person from the need to conform to the majority opinion.

Senior clinicians and those in leadership positions should strive to create an environment where dissenting opinions can be easily voiced. Leaders should also be aware of how their attitudes and behavior towards other members of the team and patients can spread to those around them. Rather than go with the crowd, clinicians should strive to be aware of the general environment in which they practice and identify any areas that conflict with their ideals or standards of professionalism. Finally, while independent thought should be encouraged, as long as diverse viewpoints are represented, group problem solving has many potential advantages to individual actors.

Social Loafing and Diffusion of Responsibility

Case

Lana was a 65-year-old woman with schizophrenia who presented to the ER with disturbing auditory hallucinations. She had not taken her anti-psychotic medication for several months and wanted to admit herself to the hospital in order to restart them. A standard battery of admission labs were drawn at that time. The next morning, having spent the night in the ER, Lana said that she felt a bit better and requested to sign herself out of the hospital. As she was not deemed a danger to anyone, she was allowed to do so. Her labs revealed severe anemia. Although not necessarily an acute emergency, this result should trigger further evaluation in a woman her age. This lab result was either never noticed or followed-up, and three months later, Lana was diagnosed with colon cancer, a condition that commonly presents with anemia.

What Dr. Sethi Was Thinking

I was the third and last psychiatrist to see Lana. She had arrived at 10 AM and was evaluated by the morning psychiatrist who ordered the initial labs. Shortly after this, she was seen by the medical doctor who performed a physical exam and wrote that Lana was "cleared for admission pending labs." At 9 PM, the overnight psychiatrist arrived. I arrived at 9 AM the next day, and Lana requested to leave shortly after this. Three other doctors had seen Lana before me, and I was certain that one of them must have reviewed her labs. The ER was busy, and I didn't have the time to review the labs of patients who had already been there for 24 hours. In a review of this case, each one of us thought another doctor either had reviewed her labs or would do so later on.

Discussion

A relatively recent development in medicine is the expansion of the medical team. A single clinician is almost never in charge of a patient's care. During hospital rounds, it is not uncommon to see groups of ten or more people at the patient's bedside. Various disciplines may be represented, including doctors, nurses, social workers, pharmacists, and medical students. While these diverse specialties allow for unique perspectives on a patient's care, several problems may arise as a result. Though ultimate responsibility always lies with the attending doctor of the admitting service, in large groups, people may experience deindividuation where they have a decreased sense of individual responsibility. This is compounded by the fact that team members may change frequently from one shift to the next, especially in ERs. An excess number of clinicians involved in a patient's care may lead to two problematic phenomena: social loafing and diffusion of responsibility.

Social loafing occurs when individuals put forth less effort to achieve a task when working in a group than when working individually. It is one of the prime reasons why the collective efforts of groups can be less than the combined effort of individual team members. The first demonstration of social loafing was performed by Max Ringelmann in 1913. He found that when a group of men pulled on a rope, they pulled with less effort than when they pulled individually (Fig. 3.11).

Bibb Latané performed similar experiments measuring the volume at which people shouted or clapped. He showed that people wearing headphones and blindfolds put forth less effort when they thought they were part of a group than when they thought they were making noise alone. Similar findings have been observed in a

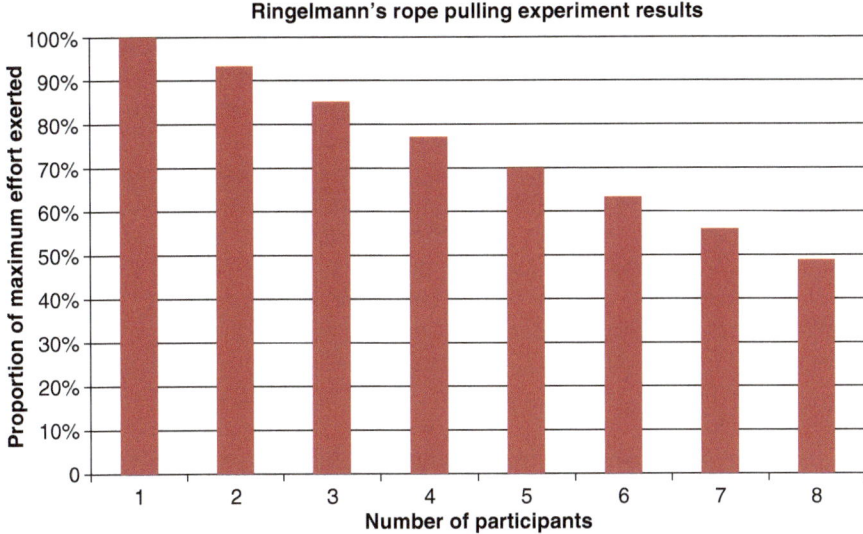

Fig. 3.11 Individuals pulled with less force when part of a large team then when alone or part of a small team. (Teslawlo. Ringelmann's rope pulling experiment results graph. In: Wikimedia commons. 2011. Retrieved from https://upload.wikimedia.org/wikipedia/commons/3/3b/RingelmannExperimentResults.png.)

variety of different tasks and across different cultures. Social loafing is more likely to occur in large, anonymous groups where people can "fly under the radar." As Latané wrote, "If the individual inputs are not identifiable the person may work less hard. Thus, if the person is dividing up the work to be performed or the amount of reward he expects to receive, he will work less hard in groups" [46].

A similar phenomenon is known diffusion of responsibility. This is the psychological phenomenon in which people are less likely to take responsibility for a problem when others are nearby. People may erroneously assume that someone else is responsible for taking action or has already done so. A more specific example is the bystander effect, which occurs as people are less likely to offer help to someone in need or react to a dangerous situation when others are present [47]. John Darley and Bibb Latané demonstrated the power of the bystander effect in a classic experiment in 1968 [48]. In their study, eight groups of three students each were placed in a room that began to fill with smoke. Five out of the eight groups didn't report the smoke, and often did not react at all, even when it became so thick they started to cough. Subsequent experiments showed that a single person responded to the smoke 75% of the time. However, when accompanied by two apathetic actors, subjects responded only 10% of the time, staying in the room rubbing their eyes as it filled with smoke. (Compelling videos of this experiment are available on YouTube) [49]. In real disasters, the bystander effect has had devastating consequences. In one study of 271 survivors of the 9/11 terrorist attacks, only 8.6% of people fled as soon as the alarm was raised [50]. The average person delayed their escape by nearly 8 minutes while others waited up to 30 minutes. Undoubtedly many people who died could have survived had they fled the buildings immediately. The common phenomenon of a group of people collectively not reacting to an emergency has been called a negative panic. It has been documented in disasters in which hundreds of people have died [51].

Like many other psychological phenomena, the bystander effect seems something likely to affect other people. However, we are all vulnerable to it. Imagine, for example, finding someone lying face down while hiking in the woods. Is there any doubt that you would stop to check on them and offer assistance? Now, imagine seeing someone lying down on a busy city sidewalk with dozens of other people walking by as if nothing were amiss. Almost certainly, you would walk past this person as well, rendering no aid. The blasé attitude of your fellow pedestrians may lull you into thinking that there is no emergency or that someone else has already called for help.

Indeed, research shows that in an emergency, people are more likely to act if they are alone than with other people. This is especially the case if the person in need of help is a stranger and there is some ambiguity about whether the person is suffering a true emergency. In one experiment, subjects were paired with an actor who feigned a seizure via an intercom [52]. When the subjects thought they alone knew about the seizure, 85% reported it to the lead experimenter. In contrast, when the subjects thought that four other people were present on the discussion, only 31% did so. Real world examples have shown that people are less likely to call for help when witnessing a drug overdose if four or more bystanders were also present [53]. Diffusion of responsibility also helps explain why individuals in hierarchical organizations may commit atrocities as part of a large group that they would never commit individually. Such people experience deindividuation and do not feel responsible for their actions.

A tragic demonstration of diffusion of responsibility occurred with the case of Esmin Green. She was a 49-year-old woman who presented with "agitation and psychosis." She waited for nearly 24 hours in a Brooklyn psychiatric ER, where she collapsed due to a blood clot in her lungs. A security camera showed the patient on the floor while several hospital workers appeared indifferent to her fate (Fig. 3.12).

Unfortunately, it can be unclear in medicine exactly who is responsible for a patient's care. Imagine a patient who comes to the ER with abdominal pain. An intern orders an abdominal CT "just to make sure." The patient is given medications for indigestion, receives the CT scan, soon feels much better, and requests to leave. As she arrived shortly before a shift change, she is discharged by a different ER team and told to follow-up with her primary care doctor. By the time the official CT report is available, the patient has left the ER. If the CT shows a significant abnormality, whose job is it to ensure this result is not neglected- the radiologists, the intern who ordered the CT, the initial attending ER doctor, the attending ER doctor who discharged the patient, or patient's primary care doctor? It's not always clear.

A tragic example of such a communication failure occurred at New York University (NYU) Langone Medical Center in 2012 when 12-year-old Rory

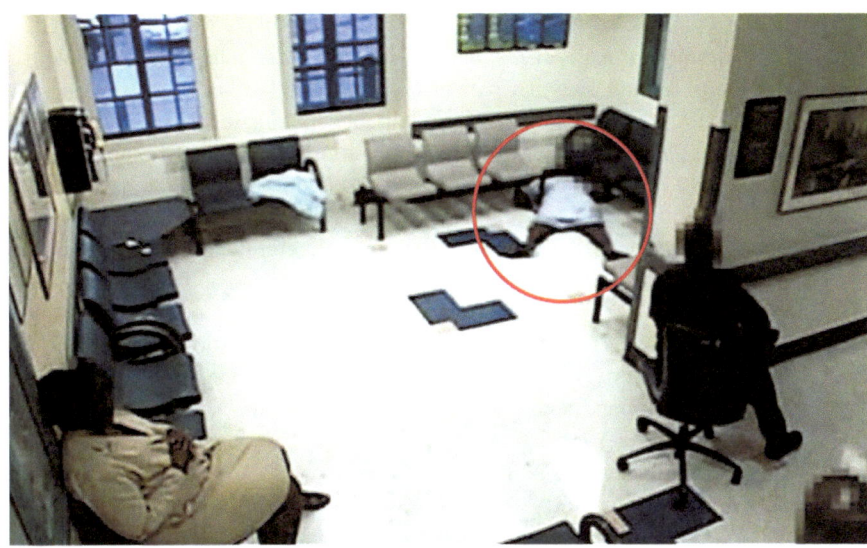

Fig. 3.12 People watch and stare while Esmin Green lies dead on the floor. (Hill RG. DOI's investigation into the circumstances surrounding the death of Esmin Green [PDF file]. Department of Investigation: City of New York. 2009. Retrieved from https://www1.nyc.gov/assets/doi/downloads/pdf/pr_esmingreen_finalrpt.pdf.)

Staunton presented with fever and a high heart rate after cutting his arm while playing basketball [54]. His white blood cells were extremely high, indicating a potentially life-threatening bacterial infection. However, this result did not come back until after Rory had been discharged home, his symptoms attributed to a stomach virus. The significant lab result was not communicated to either Rory's parents or his pediatrician. At home, Rory continued to deteriorate and despite being brought back to the hospital, died three days later of septic shock. As a result of Rory's death, NYU developed procedures to make sure all lab results were reviewed prior to a patient discharge, and New York State passed "Rory's Regulations," which established protocols for the early identification and treatment of sepsis. A study by Christopher Seymour and colleagues published in 2017 found that these regulations were successful in reducing the number of deaths due to sepsis [55].

Diffusion of responsibility can be combatted in several ways, mostly by assigning people clearly defined tasks. If someone finds themselves needing help in a crowd, they are more likely to receive if it they ask a specific person for help ("You! Call 911!") than if they ask for help in general ("Someone! Call 911!"). In medicine, it is important that team members have clearly defined roles and responsibilities. During a trauma code, for example, the roles of each team member are predefined on a daily basis. Each clinician is ideally standing in a specific place, ready to perform their assigned task without confusion about who is responsible for what.

Conclusion

Social loafing and diffusion of responsibility occur when individuals do not work as hard or conscientiously when part of a group. The lack of effort may be conscious, as people do not want to do more than their fair share of work, or it may be unconscious, as they may erroneously assume someone else is responsible for or has responded to a problem. Several factors may reduce social loafing and diffusion of responsibility. When people believe in the importance of the task and the value of the group, they are less likely to engage in social loafing [56]. Similarly, it is less likely to occur when group members feel everyone is pulling their weight. This minimizes the "sucker effect," which occurs when a team member feels duped for working hard while others are shirking their duty. Additionally, having team members work in relatively small groups with clearly delineated responsibilities helps ensure that important tasks do not slip through the cracks. In small subgroups, people will feel less anonymous. Knowing that their hard work will be recognized and their laziness will be noticed helps ensure team members will give maximal effort. Setting clear work standards and measuring individual performance within a group also minimizes social loafing, as does allowing team members to choose their role.

Reactance Bias

Case

Mario was a 23-year-old man who presented to the ER with the acute onset of low back pain that started after he helped move furniture for a friend. He said that the pain shot down his right leg and he was unable to walk as a result. He reported having tried over-the-counter pain medications without any effect. An MRI showed a mild disc herniation in the lumbar spine, and he was given acetaminophen and oxycodone (Percocet™) in the ER with significant relief. In violation of a new ER policy, which limited prescriptions of such medications to a three-day supply, Mario was given a prescription for 30 pills. He returned the next day via ambulance after he was found unconscious at home, having overdosed on his medications.

What Dr. Ivanov Was Thinking

I have been practicing medicine for 30 years. Administrators who either have never cared for patients, or have not done so for many years, are always coming out with new "policies and procedures" with no thought for how it impacts patients or those of us who actually have to carry them out. Their main concerns are money and efficiency. My main concern is the patient in front of me. So when I read about the new policy severely limiting our use of pain medications, I threw it in the trash, like I do most policies. Unfortunately, the policy added multiple steps to ordering such medicines on the electronic health record, so I was reminded of it every shift no matter how hard I tried to ignore it.

This particular policy was established by our hospital's "risk management" department, which consists mainly of lawyers who are out to protect the hospital, not care for patients. I considered myself to be a pretty good judge about who needed pain medications and who was looking to get high. I thought that this policy would unfairly limit the amount of medications patients would receive and would deluge our ER with patients needing refills once they ran out of their medications. In the past, I might have given someone like Mario a less powerful medication or a smaller supply of Percocet. But I was pissed at the restrictions that were being placed on us, and I gave him, and several other patients, enough medication to last several weeks. I didn't want them coming back.

However in retrospect, this policy turned out to be a reasonable and well-thought out response to a significant problem. The administrators who made this policy had access to data showing that prescriptions, such as the one I wrote, were a significant factor in a number of recent overdoses. I was more concerned with protecting my autonomy than I was with caring for my patients.

Case

Susan was a 23-year-old woman who presented with a severe headache over her entire head. She had several miscarriages in the past, but was otherwise healthy. She had gone to bed with a mild headache but got up several times in the middle of the night to vomit. She went to the ER the next morning when the headache became intolerable. She was tearful on examination, both because of the pain and because she had read on the internet that her headache was concerning for a brain tumor. She was uncomfortable and tearful, but otherwise her examination was normal. She had no risk factors for infectious diseases and did not have a fever. The ER doctor ordered a CT scan to "reassure the patient," which was normal. Susan requested an MRI "to be sure," but was told that if she had a brain tumor it would have been seen on the CT scan. The doctor felt that Susan was anxious and possibly suffering from a migraine. She was given a treatment for migraines and discharged home. She went to a different ER later that evening where a doctor was concerned enough to get a brain MRI. This revealed a clot in the venous system of her brain, a serious condition that explained her headaches.

What Dr. Levine Was Thinking

Had Susan not mentioned that she had done an internet search and was fearful she had a brain tumor, there is a good chance I would have taken her more seriously. Susan's self-diagnosis and her demand that a brain tumor be ruled out set the entire stage for our clinical encounter. I always bristle a bit when patients tell me which tests I should order. I didn't even feel a CT scan was needed, but I did it because Susan was so worried. Once that came back as normal, I was able to tell Susan that she didn't have a brain tumor. Yet this was not my job. My job was to figure out what was wrong with her. CT scans are not sensitive enough to detect certain other conditions. Sinus venous thrombosis is an unusual condition, and I don't fault myself for not thinking of that specifically. Yet, had Susan not done internet research and "diagnosed" herself with a brain tumor, and had she not requested an MRI, there is every expectation I would have pursued further diagnostic tests. Had I given in to her demands, I felt I would be "caving in." Certainly, I am not obligated to order tests that I feel are inappropriate just because a patient demands them. Yet, I shouldn't refuse to do them for this reason either.

Discussion

The reactance bias is the tendency towards doing something different from the group and authority figures because they are seen as threatening autonomy and constraining freedom of choice. As a result of the reactance bias, norms, regulations, and protocols are flouted to provide the rule-breaker with a sense of superiority and independence. Some people have a contrarian personality, with a self-identity based largely on doing the opposite of what they feel is mainstream or conventionally accepted behavior. They chafe at rules, conventions, and instructions, opposing them regardless of whether or not this is rational. The reactance bias is well illustrated by the folktale of *Br'er Rabbit and the Tar Baby* [57]. In this story, Br'er Rabbit is captured by a fox. The clever rabbit pleads, "Drown me! Roast me! Hang me! Do whatever you please. Only please, Br'er Fox, please don't throw me into the briar patch." This witless Fox, thinking he is inflicting a great punishment on his nemesis, tosses Br'er Rabbit into the briar patch, his home, and the rabbit escapes.

Though independent thought should obviously be encouraged, at times, the reactance bias can motivate people to behave in incredibly foolish and dangerous ways. For example, some people object to seat belts and motorcycle helmets simply because they are required by law. One such rebel, Derek Kieper, wrote in his college newspaper that "No law, or set of laws, has made the government more intrusive and ridiculous than seat belt legislation" [58]. "It is my choice what type of safety precautions I take," he wrote. "There seems to be a die-hard group of non-wearers out there who simply do not wish to buckle up no matter what the government does. I belong to this group." Though reasonable people may question the legitimacy of the government's forcing adults to wear seat belts, the fact that seat belts save lives is beyond dispute. Sadly, Mr. Kieper paid for his contrarian thinking when he died at age 21 in a car accident while not wearing a seat belt [59]. Two other occupants of the car who were wearing seat belts survived. Similarly, motorcyclist Philip Contos died while participating in a ride to protest mandatory helmet laws. According to new accounts, "State police say evidence at the scene plus information from the attending medical expert indicated Contos would have survived had he been wearing a helmet as required by state law" [60].

Like those who oppose motor vehicle safety measures because the government requires them, some clinicians rebel against rules and authority figures, violating protocols because they view them as a threat to their independence. Surgical oncologist and science blogger David Gorski refers to such clinicians as "Brave Maverick Doctors" [61]. Brave Maverick Doctors are a staple of medical dramas, where they are portrayed as heroically standing up for their patients against incompetent or indifferent bureaucrats. Wikipedia says about Gregory House, the tortured genius of the TV show *House*, that his "flouting of hospital rules and procedures frequently leads him into conflict with his boss, hospital administrator and Dean of Medicine" [62]. Similarly, Wikipedia describes the leading doctor in *M*A*S*H*- Hawkeye Pierce, by saying he has "little tolerance for military red tape and customs, feeling they get in the way of his doing his job." On the TV show *ER*, Doug Ross "doesn't handle authority well," and in one episode, gives a baby a medication "in violation of hospital policy and the law." These doctors risk their careers to do what they feel is right for their patients, and in the fantasyland of TV, their rebellion always turns out to be correct.

The business aspects of medicine often trigger the reactance bias in clinicians, many of whom like to imagine that financial concerns have no place in the care of their patients. Suneel Dhand wrote an essay titled *The Time a 28-Year-Old MBA Told a Physician Where to Round First* that provides an excellent example of the reactance bias. Dr. Dhand relates the story of a colleague by writing:

> He told me that his group, which is essentially run by non-clinicians, is completely (and unsurprisingly) focused on the bottom line only. Administrators aggressively monitor their physicians' whereabouts and try to review all of their patient interactions (mostly how it pertains to billing). To cut a long story short, he told me that the administration for some reason or another wanted him to round first on a particular floor. He didn't think it was the right thing to do for patient care (apparently another floor frequently had patients who required closer and more immediate attention), and it culminated in him basically being scolded by a 28-year-old MBA who informed him that he had to round on that particular floor first, like it or not" [63].

On the face of it, this MBA sure sounds like a jerk, and not someone I would want bossing me around. But perhaps this young MBA had done a detailed analysis of hospital workflow and there was a perfectly valid reason for asking the doctor to make rounds in a certain order. Perhaps if the doctor took the advice of the MBA, he could quickly round on the stable patients and actually spend more time with the patients who require "closer and more immediate attention." Or perhaps the doctor incorrectly felt that patients on a particular floor were stable, when in fact they were rather ill on occasion. Perhaps there had been several bad outcomes because the doctor neglected these patients.

Even if the MBA was only concerned about money, this is far from an irrelevant consideration. Perhaps this hospital's poor finances meant it couldn't hire desperately needed nurses or fix broken machines. Perhaps it was even in danger of closing, like several hospitals near me have done recently. I sure hope my hospital has MBAs worrying about its finances. Because of the reactance bias of the author, the possibility that the MBA might have a valid suggestion wasn't even considered. Note also how this article commits the fallacy of "poisoning the well." In this fallacy, irrelevant and negative information is given about an individual so that nothing the target person says is taken seriously. In this instance, the mere fact of introducing the antagonist as a "28-year-old MBA" biases the reader against his proposals and in favor of the doctor. Yet, rounding in a particular order is a good idea, or not, regardless of who proposes it.

At its most extreme, the reactance bias can lead some clinicians to completely reject science-based medicine and instead embrace the pseudoscience underlying complementary and alternative medicine (CAM). Their desire to feel "independent" and in rebellion against the mainstream medical establishment leads them to extol quack treatments such as coffee enemas and turmeric infusions, while rejecting well-established treatments such as vaccines, the vitamin K shot in newborns, antibiotics, and even insulin for diabetics. The only unifying philosophy of such clinicians is a rejection of medicine and science for the sake of rejecting what is derisively called "conventional" medicine. Such CAM practitioners do not think for themselves, but rather reflexively oppose mainstream medicine for the sole purpose of being oppositional. One could easily imagine that if vaccines were suddenly declared unsafe and banned, many CAM practitioners would reverse course and extol them as a suppressed, miracle cure. Similarly, if coffee enema detoxes became widely embraced by the mainstream medical community, I have little doubt that CAM practitioners would then reject the entire concept of "detoxing" as pseudoscience. A satirical article titled *Mother Requests Vitamin K Shot, Until She Learns it is Universally Recommended* perfectly captures the mindset of CAM devotees who support or oppose medical treatments based on their opposition to authority [64]. In this article, a fictional mother demands the vitamin K shot for her baby until she learned that it is recommended by the "CDC, FDA, WHO, UNICEF, and the American Academy of Pediatrics" (Fig. 3.13).

Indeed, the anti-vaccine movement has tried to grow its ranks largely by trying to take advantage of the reactance bias in the general public. "Personal freedom" and "parental choice" have become a prime rallying cry for those who spread pseudoscience. Anti-vaccine doctor Toni Bark, for example, argued against a California law requiring vaccines for schoolchildren by saying, "Only the parent knows how their child reacts to things. We don't understand who is going to have a negative reaction to vaccines, therefore we must have parental choice. There must be a barrier between big pharma and your children. And that barrier has to be the parent" [65]. She even compared vaccines to unethical medical experiments by writing,

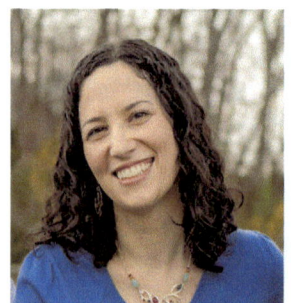

The "alternative" in alternative medicine is not any particular treatment. The "alternative" is a perceived reality with no burden of proof, no accountability, no grounding, no grounding in what we know to be real, and an insistence of being in opposition to the scientific consensus.

Alison Bernstein

Fig. 3.13 Alison Bernstein gets it right. (Bernstein A. Alison Bernstein [Image file]. Michigan State University: Neuroscience Program. (n.d.). Retrieved from https://neuroscience.natsci.msu.edu/about-us/directory/faculty/alison-i-bernstein-phd/.)

Kelly Brogan MD - Holistic Psychiatrist
15 February 2015 · 🌐

"I came to the conclusion that this is medical fascism"

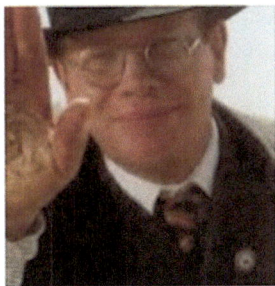

**Unvaccinated today....Jews 1940 Budapest

From the movie: "Indiana Jones" I was quite concerned about the article from TIME Magazine on Feb 11, 2015. The writer, Joe Matthew, called for the outing of parents who don't vaccinate in the pie...

ANNEDACHEL.COM

Fig. 3.14 Anti-vaccine doctor Kelly Brogan comparing laws promoting vaccines to the fate of Jews in Nazi Germany. (Brogan K. [Kelly Brogan MD]. "I came to the conclusion that this is medical "fascism." [Facebook status update]. 2015. Retrieved from https://www.facebook.com/KellyBroganMD/posts/363124607227727.)

"After Nazi Germany, the Nuremberg laws were changed to forbid forced medical procedures. The Helsinki accord is very clear; all patients have the right to informed consent prior to medical procedures. There is no informed consent for vaccination as it is, we really should not be moving backwards" [66]. Though no children are forcibly vaccinated against the will of their parents in the US, Dr. Bark feels that vaccines are akin to "forced medical procedures" and should be rejected, in part, for this reason. Unfortunately, Dr. Bark is not an outlier, and comparisons between vaccines and the Holocaust are not uncommon in the anti-vaccine movement (Fig. 3.14).

This contrarian thinking has worked its way into state governments where important policies are decided based on the reactance bias. In 2017, Rep. Bill Zedler, a member of the Texas Freedom Caucus, introduced legislation that would prevent foster children from being vaccinated during initial medical exams. Though he endorsed multiple anti-vaccine tropes during debate on his bills, his fundamental argument was framed when he asked the question, "Is it the parents' decision to decide, or is it the state's?" [67].

Like those who reject seat belts and motor cycle helmets, clinicians and politicians afflicted by the reactance bias reject vaccines because they are both universally recommended by medical organizations and often required by governments to attend public schools (though most states have easily obtainable exemptions). As with seat belts, the power of the government to enforce vaccines is a matter of legitimate debate about which reasonable people can disagree. However, this legal question has nothing to do with whether vaccines are safe and effective. Knowing they can't win on scientific merits, anti-vaccine crusaders take advantage of the reactance bias to reframe the issue as one of personal freedom.

Patients can also elicit the reactance bias in clinicians. The trope of patients who diagnose themselves with a serious disease after consulting "Dr. Google" is quite real. There is even a term, cyberchondria, to describe people who use the internet to become convinced that mundane symptoms, such as a cough, reflect a dire diagnosis, such as lung cancer. Certain clinicians may react to this by dismissing patient's concerns, feeling they are being undermined or that their clinical expertise is being challenged. Gary Bevill, a family physician, expressed a common sentiment by saying, "I like to think I'm semi-wired. But as a general rule, the early symptom checkers, I basically hated with a passion" [68].

Yet, just because a patient's internet search convinced them they have a brain tumor, doesn't mean they don't, in fact, have a brain tumor or another serious condition. Importantly, there is evidence that doctors who have a participatory decision-making style have a better relationship with their patients. Sherrie Kaplan and colleagues surveyed 7,730 patients from the practices of 300 doctors [69]. They found that one-third of patients who rated their doctor poorly in terms of participatory style changed doctors over the course of a year, while only 15% who rated their doctor highly changed doctors.

Conclusion

Clinicians who violate the rules and defy authority figures for the sake of preserving their own autonomy are no better than clinicians who mindlessly obey. A clinician who prioritizes her own sense of independence is putting herself first, not her patients. Protocols and rules should be obeyed (or occasionally ignored) based on what is in the patient's best interest, not on what satisfies a clinician's need to feel subversive and independent.

References

1. Hadley MN, Walters BC, Grabb PA, Oyesiku NM, Przybylski GJ, Resnick DK, Ryken TC. Pharmacological therapy after acute cervical spinal cord injury. Neurosurgery. 2002;50(Supplement 3):S63–72. https://doi.org/10.1097/00006123-200203001-00013.
2. Eck JC, Nachtigall D, Humphreys CS, Hodges SD. Questionnaire survey of spine surgeons on the use of methylprednisolone for acute spinal cord injury. Spine. 2006;31(9):E250–3. https://doi.org/10.1097/01.brs.0000214886.21265.8c.
3. Hurlbert RJ, Hadley MN, Walters BC, Aarabi B, Dhall SS, Gelb DE, Rozzelle CJ, Ryken TC, Theodore N. Pharmacological therapy for acute spinal cord injury. Neurosurgery. 2013;72(Supplement 3):93–105. https://doi.org/10.1227/NEU.0b013e31827765c6.
4. Schroeder GD, Kwon BK, Eck JC, Savage JW, Hsu WK, Patel AA. Survey of cervical spine research society members on the use of high-dose steroids for acute spinal cord injuries. Spine. 2014;39(12):971–7. https://doi.org/10.1097/BRS.0000000000000297.
5. Cass D. (n.d.). Methylprednisolone for acute spinal cord injury is not a standard of care; it is only a treatment option [Position statement]. Retrieved 15 Sept 2018 from https://web.archive.org/web/20180309201904/http://caep.ca/resources/position-statements-and-guidelines/steroids-acute-spinal-cord-injury.

6. List of common misconceptions (2018, July 22). In: Wikipedia. Retrieved 15 Sept 2018 from https://en.wikipedia.org/w/index.php?title=List_of_common_misconceptions&oldid=851428920.

7. Milgram S. (1974). The perils of obedience. Retrieved 15 Sept 2018 from https://web.archive.org/web/20101216075927/http://home.swbell.net/revscat/perilsOfObedience.html.

8. Matt. (2016, Dec 12). The Milgram experiment [Video file]. Retrieved from https://www.youtube.com/watch?v=wdUu3u9Web4&.

9. Blass T. The Milgram paradigm after 35 years: some things we now know about obedience to authority. J Appl Soc Psychol. 1999;29(5):955–78. https://doi.org/10.1111/j.1559-1816.1999.tb00134.x.

10. Society for Personality and Social Psychology. (2017, Mar 14). Conducting the Milgram experiment in Poland, psychologists show people still obey. ScienceDaily. Retrieved from https://www.sciencedaily.com/releases/2017/03/170314081558.htm.

11. Nissani M. A cognitive reinterpretation of Stanley Milgram's observations on obedience to authority. Am Psychol. 1990;45(12):1384–5. https://doi.org/10.1037/0003-066X.45.12.1384.

12. Asch SE. Effects of group pressure upon the modification and distortion of judgments. In: Guetzhow H, editor. Groups, leadership and men; research in human relations. Oxford, UK: Carnegie Press; 1951. p. 177–90.

13. Kent T. (n.d.). Bethany's elevator experiment a case of backward research [Reprint]. Bethany Lutheran College. Retrieved from https://www.blc.edu/news/bethanys-elevator-experiment-case-backward-research#.WFc7MNIrIdU.

14. Cialdini RB, Reno RR, Kallgren CA. A focus theory of normative conduct: recycling the concept of norms to reduce littering in public places. J Pers Soc Psychol. 1990;58(6):1015–26.

15. McLeod SA. (2017). Stanford prison experiment. Simply Psychology. Retrieved 15 Sept 2018 from https://www.simplypsychology.org/zimbardo.html.

16. Gourevitch P, Morris E. (2008, Mar 24). Exposure: the woman behind the camera at Abu Ghraib. The New Yorker. Retrieved from https://www.newyorker.com/magazine/2008/03/24/exposure-5.

17. The Editorial Board. (2017, June 23). The torturers speak. The New York Times. Retrieved from https://www.nytimes.com/2017/06/23/opinion/cia-torture-enhanced-interrogation.html.

18. Schmidt A. (2013, May 21). Groupthink. In: Encyclopædia Britannica. Retrieved 15 Sept 2018 from https://www.britannica.com/science/groupthink#ref1181070.

19. Schkade D, Sunstein CR, Hastie R. What happened on deliberation day? Calif Law Rev. 2006;95(3):915–40. https://doi.org/10.15779/Z38740Z.

20. Prentice DA, Miller DT. Pluralistic ignorance and alcohol use on campus: some consequences of misperceiving the social norm. J Pers Soc Psychol. 1994;64(2):243–56. https://doi.org/10.1037/0022-3514.64.2.243.

21. O'Gorman HJ. Pluralistic ignorance and white estimates of white support for racial segregation. Public Opin Q. 1975;39(3):313–30. https://doi.org/10.1086/268231.

22. Harvey JB. The Abilene paradox: the management of agreement. Organ Dyn. 1974;3(1):63–80. https://doi.org/10.1016/0090-2616(74)90005-9.

23. Tierney AJ. Egas Moniz and the origins of psychosurgery: a review commemorating the 50th anniversary of Moniz's Nobel Prize. J Hist Neurosci. 2000;9(1):22–36. https://doi.org/10.1076/0964-704X(200004)9:1;1-2;FT022.

24. Jansson B. (1998, Oct 29). Antonio Caetano de Abrue Freire Egas Moniz. The Nobel Prize. Retrieved from https://www.nobelprize.org/prizes/medicine/1949/moniz/article/.

25. Shorter E. A history of psychiatry: from the era of the asylum to the age of prozac. New York: John Wiley & Sons; 1997.

26. Hoffman JL. Clinical observations concerning schizophrenic patients treated by prefrontal leukotomy. N Engl J Med. 1949;241(6):233–6. https://doi.org/10.1056/NEJM194908112410604.

27. Swayze VW. Frontal leukotomy and related psychosurgical procedures in the era before anti-

psychotics (1935-1954): a historical overview. Am J Psychiatr. 1995;152(4):505–15. https://doi.org/10.1176/ajp.152.4.505.

28. Platelet Therapy (PRP). (n.d.). New platelet rich plasma treatment provides lasting musculoskeletal pain relief. StemCell Arts. Retrieved 15 Sept 2018 from https://stemcellarts.com/regenerative-procedures-2/regenexx-scp/.

29. Moraes VY, Lenza M, Tamaoki MJ, Faloppa F, Belloti JC. Platelet-rich therapies for musculoskeletal soft tissue injuries. Cochrane Database Syst Rev. 2014;2014(4). https://doi.org/10.1002/14651858.CD010071.pub3.

30. Kolata G. (2011, Sept 4). As sports medicine surges, hope and hype outpace proven treatments. The New York Times. Retrieved from https://www.nytimes.com/2011/09/05/health/05treatment.html.

31. Boden WE, O'Rourke RA, Teo KK, Hartigan PM, Maron DJ, Kostuk WJ, Knudtson M, Dada M, Casperson P, Harris CL, Chaitman BR, Shaw L, Gosselin G, Nawaz S, Title LM, Gau G, Blaustein AS, Booth DC, Bates ER, Spertus JA, Berman DS, Mancini GB, Weintraub WS. Optimal medical therapy with or without PCI for stable coronary disease. N Engl J Med. 2007;356(15):1503–16. https://doi.org/10.1056/NEJMoa070829.

32. Al-Lamee R, Thompson D, Dehbi H, Sen S, Tang K, Davies J, Keeble T, Mielewczik M, Kaprielian R, Malik IS, Nijjer SS, Petraco R, Cook C, Ahmad Y, Howard J, Baker C, Sharp A, Gerber R, Talwar S, Assomull R, Mayet J, Wensel R, Collier D, Shun-Shin M, Thom SA, Davies JE, Francis DP. Percutaneous coronary intervention in stable angina (ORBITA): a double-blind, randomised controlled trial. Lancet. 2018;391(10115):31–40. https://doi.org/10.1016/S0140-6736(17)32714-9.

33. Epstein D. (2017, Feb 22). When evidence says no, but doctors say yes. ProPublica. Retrieved https://www.propublica.org/article/when-evidence-says-no-but-doctors-say-yes.

34. Anonymous. Our family secrets. Ann Intern Med. 2015;163(4):321. https://doi.org/10.7326/M14-2168.

35. Jackman T. (2015, June 23). Anesthesiologist trashes sedated patient – and it ends up costing her. The Washington Post. Retrieved from https://www.washingtonpost.com/local/anesthesiologist-trashes-sedated-patient-jury-orders-her-to-pay-500000/2015/06/23/cae05c00-18f3-11e5-ab92-c75ae6ab94b5_story.html.

36. Unholy Three [Image file]. (n.d.). In: Wikimedia Commons. Retrieved 15 Sept 2018 from https://commons.wikimedia.org/wiki/File:Unholy_three.png.

37. Desai NR, Bradley SM, Parzynski CS, Nallamothu BK, Chan PS, Spertus JA, Patel MR, Ader J, Soufer A, Krumholz HM, Curtis JP. Appropriate use criteria for coronary revascularization and trends in utilization, patient selection, and appropriateness of percutaneous coronary intervention. J Am Med Assoc. 2015;314(19):2045–53. https://doi.org/10.1001/jama.2015.13764.

38. Mercier H, Sperber D. Why do humans reason? Arguments for an argumentative theory. Behav Brain Sci. 2011;34(2):57–74. https://doi.org/10.1017/S0140525X10000968.

39. Brockman J. (2011). The argumentative theory: a conversation with Hugo Mercier. Edge. Retrieved from https://www.edge.org/conversation/hugo_mercier-the-argumentative-theory.

40. Frederick S. Cognitive reflection and decision making. J Econ Perspect. 2005;19(4):25–42.

41. Silberzahn R, Uhlmann EL. Crowdsourced research: many hands make tight work. Nature. 2015;526:189–91. https://doi.org/10.1038/526189a.

42. Meeker D, Linder JA, Fox CR, Friedberg MW, Persell SD, Goldstein NJ, Knight TK, Hay JW, Doctor JN. Effect of behavioral interventions on inappropriate antibiotic prescribing among primary care practices: a randomized clinical trial. JAMA. 2016;315(6):562–70. https://doi.org/10.1001/jama.2016.0275.

43. Stone SP, Fuller C, Savage J, Cookson B, Hayward A, Cooper B, Duckworth G, Michie S, Murray M, Jeanes A, Roberts J, Teare L, Charlett A. Evaluation of the national Cleanyourhands campaign to reduce *Staphylococcus aureus* bacteraemia and *Clostridium difficile* infection in hospitals in England and Wales by improved hand hygiene: four year, prospective, ecological, interrupted time series study. BMJ. 2012;344:e3005. https://doi.org/10.1136/bmj.e3005.

44. 8 Ways Vanderbilt University Medical Center Raised Hand Hygiene Compliance. (2013, Sept 25). Becker's clinical leadership & infection control. Retrieved from https://www.beckershospitalreview.com/quality/8-ways-vanderbilt-university-medical-center-raised-hand-hygiene-compliance.html.

45. Kalb C. (2014, July 21). How a team of doctors at one hospital boosted hand washing, cut infections and created a culture of safety. Yahoo.com News. Retrieved from https://www.yahoo.com/news/clean-hands%2D%2Dvanderbilt-s-hand-washing-initiative-172312795.html.

46. Latane B, Williams K, Harkins S. Many hands make light the work: the causes and consequences of social loafing. J Pers Soc Psychol. 1979;37(6):822–32. https://doi.org/10.1037/0022-3514.37.6.822.

47. Fischer P, Krueger JI, Greitemeyer T, Vogrincic C, Kastenmüller A, Frey D, Heene M, Wicher M, Kainbacher M. The bystander-effect: a meta-analytic review on bystander intervention in dangerous and non-dangerous emergencies. Psychol Bull. 2011;137(4):517–37. https://doi.org/10.1037/a0023304.

48. Latané B, Darley JM. Group inhibition of bystander intervention in emergencies. J Pers Soc Psychol. 1968;10(3):215–21. https://doi.org/10.1037/h0026570.

49. McDermott M. (2007, Sept 15). The smoke filled room study [Video file]. Retrieved from https://www.youtube.com/watch?v=KE5YwN4NW5o.

50. Glendinning L. (2008, Sept 9). 9/11 survivors put off evacuation to shut down computers, study finds. The Guardian. Retrieved from https://www.theguardian.com/world/2008/sep/09/september11.usa.

51. Barthelmess S. (1988). Coming to grips with panic [PDF file]. Flight Safety Foundation: Cabin Crew Safety, 23(2). Retrieved from https://flightsafety.org/ccs/ccs_mar-apr88.pdf.

52. Darley JM, Latané B. Bystander intervention in emergencies: diffusion of responsibility. J Pers Soc Psychol. 1968;8(4, Pt. 1):377–83. https://doi.org/10.1037/h0025589.

53. Tobin KE, Davey MA, Latkin CA. Calling emergency medical services during drug overdose: an examination of individual, social and setting correlates. Addiction. 2005;100(3):397–404. https://doi.org/10.1111/j.1360-0443.2005.00975.x.

54. Dwyer J. (2012, July 18). After boy's death, hospital alters discharging procedures. The New York Times. Retrieved from http://www.nytimes.com/2012/07/19/nyregion/after-rory-stauntons-death-hospital-alters-discharge-procedures.html.

55. Seymour CW, Gesten F, Prescott HC, Friedrich ME, Iwashyna TJ, Phillips GS, Lemeshow S, Osborn T, Terry KM, Levy MM. Time to treatment and mortality during mandated emergency care for sepsis. N Engl J Med. 2017;376(23):2235–44. https://doi.org/10.1056/NEJMoa1703058.

56. Zaccaro SJ. Social loafing: the role of task attractiveness. Personal Soc Psychol Bull. 1984;10(1):99–106. https://doi.org/10.1177/0146167284101011.

57. Schlosser SE. (n.d.). Brer Rabbit and the Tar Baby. Americanfolklore.net. Retrieved 15 Sept 2018 from http://americanfolklore.net/folklore/2010/07/brer_rabbit_meets_a_tar_baby.html.

58. Kieper D. (2004, Sept 17). Individual rights buckle under seat belt laws. The Daily Nebraskan. Retrieved from http://www.dailynebraskan.com/derek-kieper-individual-rights-buckle-under-seat-belt-laws/article_76ccbd44-86bc-5380-bb25-f10cdebb5698.html.

59. Mabin B. (2005, Jan 3). I-80 crash claims UNL student's life. Lincoln Star Journal. Retrieved from http://journalstar.com/news/local/i%2D%2Dcrash-claims-unl-student-s-life/article_d61cc109-3492-54ef-849d-0a5d7f48027a.html.

60. Raja N. (2011, July 4). Bareheaded motorcyclist dies in helmet protest. CNN. Retrieved from http://www.cnn.com/2011/US/07/04/new.york.motorcyclist.death/.

61. Gorski D. (2015, Dec 14). Worshiping at the altar of the Cult of the Brave Maverick Doctor. Science-Based Medicine. Retrieved from https://sciencebasedmedicine.org/worshiping-at-the-altar-of-the-cult-of-the-brave-maverickdoctor/.

62. House [Television series]. (n.d.). In: Wikipedia. Retrieved 15 Sept 2018 from https://en.wikipedia.org/wiki/House.

63. Dhand S. (2016, May 11). The time a 28-year-old MBA told a physician where to round first [Blog post]. KevinMD.com. Retrieved from https://www.kevinmd.com/blog/2016/05/the-time-a-28-year-old-mba-told-a-physician-where-to-round-first.html.
64. McSheep S. (2016, Feb 17). Mother requests Vitamin K shot, until she learns it is universally recommended. The Science Post. Retrieved from http://thesciencepost.com/mother-requests-vitamin-k-shot-until-she-learns-it-is-universally-recommended/67/.
65. Dachel A. (2015, Aug 19). Dr. Toni Bark endorses referendum to repeal CA SB277. Age of Autism. Retrieved from http://www.ageofautism.com/2015/08/dr-toni-bark-endorses-referendum-to-repeal-ca-sb277.html.
66. Bark T. (2015, Feb 21). Do not remove vaccine exemptions – Some children die from vaccines. Vaccine Impact. Retrieved from http://vaccineimpact.com/2015/dr-toni-bark-m-d-do-not-remove-vaccine-exemptions-some-children-die-from-vaccines/.
67. Drash W. (2017, May 12). Texas lawmakers spar over 'anti-vaccine measure'. CNN. Retrieved from http://www.cnn.com/2017/05/11/health/texas-house-vaccinations/index.html.
68. Butterfield S. (2013). Patients increasingly checking 'Dr. Google'. ACP Internist. Retrieved 15 Sept 2018 from https://acpinternist.org/archives/2013/11/dr-google.htm.
69. Kaplan SH, Greenfield S, Gandek B, Rogers WH, Ware JE Jr. Characteristics of physicians with participatory decision-making styles. Ann Intern Med. 1996;124(5):497–504. https://doi.org/10.7326/0003-4819-124-5-199603010-00007.

Confirmation Bias, Motivated Cognition, the Backfire Effect

4

Case

Patricia was a 49-year-old woman who presented with confusion while drinking at a bar. Her friend said that she had been behaving normally, but was later found on the bathroom floor "not making sense." On examination, she was lethargic and confused. She gave short answers to questions and did not know the location or date. She was able to name some common objects, but could not sustain attention to participate in a meaningful conversation. She fell asleep when she was not examined and could only be briefly aroused with noxious stimuli. A head CT was normal as was basic blood chemistry.

The ER doctor felt that the patient's presentation was due to intoxication of some sort. A blood alcohol level was 123 mg/dL, though her friend said that Patricia normally drank this much on Friday nights and had never had this problem before. Patricia was treated with thiamine on the premise that that she had Wernicke's encephalopathy, a vitamin-deficiency syndrome characterized by altered mental status that is common in chronic alcoholics. She was also given flumazenil, which reverses overdose on a type of sedatives known as benzodiazepines, and naltrexone, which reverses the soporific effects of opiates. Neither of these treatments had any effect. A toxicology was positive for tetrahydrocannabinol (THC), the active ingredient of marijuana.

Patricia was admitted to the hospital for presumed alcohol intoxication. She had not improved by the next day. A neurologist ordered an MRI, which showed strokes in both thalami. This is an uncommon stroke syndrome that causes disorientation, confusion, hypersomnolence, deep coma, mutism, amnesia, speech, and language dysfunction (Fig. 4.1).

What Dr. Balint Was Thinking

I strongly suspected that Patricia has used some drug, which accounted for her altered mental status. Though I did order a head CT, my investigations and treatments were otherwise dedicated to proving this hypothesis right. I checked an alcohol level and gave her thiamine. I checked a urine toxicology screen and gave her

© Springer International Publishing AG, part of Springer Nature 2019   57
J. Howard, *Cognitive Errors and Diagnostic Mistakes*,
https://doi.org/10.1007/978-3-319-93224-8_4

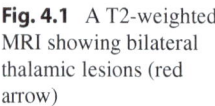
Fig. 4.1 A T2-weighted
MRI showing bilateral
thalamic lesions (red
arrow)

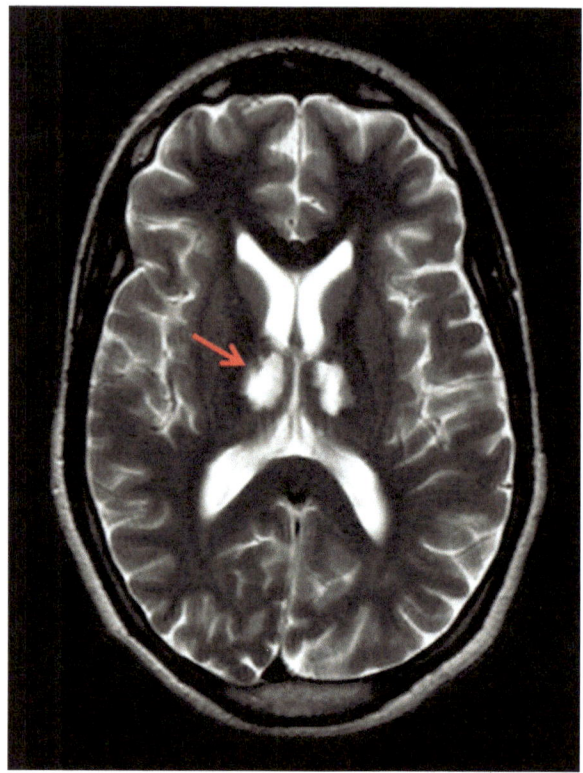

treatments to reverse several drug overdoses. These were dangerous and potentially treatable causes of her symptoms- and of course few things are more common for an ER doctor than an intoxicated patient with altered mental status. These were certainly the right steps initially. If a patient presented like Patricia again, I would probably do the same thing again.

Yet, I stopped too soon. I never stopped to think: assuming this is *not* a drug overdose of some kind, what tests would I need to run to prove that. The fact that she was intoxicated and had THC in her urine also caused me to only consider a drug overdose, though the fact that she was mildly intoxicated and had smoked marijuana at some point in the past few days did not protect her against other diseases. When an intern pointed out to me that there was no intoxicant in her lab work that could have explained her presentation, this only made me more convinced that she had ingested something, albeit something that our lab was not equipped to detect. Not every drug appears on a toxicology screen. Even if she did not intentionally take a drug, we occasionally treat women who have been given "date-rape" drugs at bars.

Certainly, the ultimate cause of her symptoms was a very uncommon stroke syndrome, and I don't think I could have been faulted for not thinking specifically of a bilateral thalamic stroke! Yet, had I seriously considered a diagnosis other than a drug ingestion, I might have ordered an MRI in the ER and she could have received treatment for an acute ischemic stroke.

Discussion

In a study titled *Motivated Skepticism in the Evaluation of Political Beliefs* Charles Taber and Milton Lodge's described the confirmation of six predictions [1]:

1. **Prior attitude effect.** Subjects who feel strongly about an issue, even when encouraged to be objective, will evaluate supportive arguments more favorably than contrary arguments.
2. **Disconfirmation bias**. Subjects will spend more time and cognitive resources denigrating contrary arguments than supportive arguments.
3. **Confirmation bias**. Subjects free to choose their information sources will seek out supportive rather than contrary sources.
4. **Attitude polarization**. Exposing subjects to an apparently balanced set of pro and con arguments will exaggerate their initial polarization.
5. **Attitude strength effect**. Subjects voicing stronger attitudes will be more prone to the above biases.
6. **Sophistication effect**. Knowledgeable subjects, because they possess greater ammunition with which to counter-argue incongruent facts and arguments, will be more prone to the above biases.

This chapter discusses those biases that allow us to see what we want to see, believe what we want to believe, and deny what we want to reject.

Confirmation Bias and Motivated Reasoning

Confirmation bias is the tendency to actively seek out evidence to support a pre-existing belief rather than look for disconfirming evidence to refute it. According to sociologist Steven Hoffman, "rather than search rationally for information that either confirms or disconfirms a particular belief, people actually seek out information that confirms what they already believe" [2]. When President Donald Trump withdrew from the Paris climate accord, his spokeswoman Kellyanne Conway said, "He started with a conclusion, and the evidence brought him to the same conclusion" [3]. This is confirmation bias, and we are all vulnerable to it. Confirmation bias has important implications for scientific and political discourse, especially in our fragmented media landscape where people chose their information sources, isolating themselves from challenging viewpoints.

Imagine you get into a debate with your friend at dinner. You strongly believe more restrictive gun control laws will do nothing to lower crime. Your friend argues the opposite. You're not an expert in this area and can't cite studies to support your claim although you know you've seen many of them. The argument ends in a stalemate, and you leave dinner believing more passionately than before that you are right. As soon as you're alone, you pull out your phone and Google "gun control laws don't work." Bingo! Up pop 10 articles supporting your position. You read them with great satisfaction, knowing you were right all along. Maybe you read the first few paragraphs of an article that supports gun control, but conclude that its core tenets have been refuted by what you've already read and that it's not worth finishing. Meanwhile, your friend does the same thing, finding many articles showing that gun control laws decrease violence. This is confirmation bias (Fig. 4.2).

One clear example of such confirmation bias is the section on Amazon.com titled "customers who bought this item also bought." Not surprisingly, people who buy one book with a specific vantage point tend to purchase similar books. If a person buys one anti-vaccine book, for example, they're likely to buy other anti-vaccine books. The same is of course true for people who purchase pro-science books (Fig. 4.3).

Psychologist Peter Wason developed several simple tests to show the power of confirmation bias. The "2-4-6" task was the first such experiment. In this study, people are told that the numbers "2, 4, and 6" follow a rule. They are allowed to propose their own three number sequences and are told whether or not those numbers follow the rule. Their job is to guess that rule, with as many sequences as they wish. What numbers would you chose to test your hypothesis? You can test yourself here:

http://www.nytimes.com/interactive/2015/07/03/upshot/a-quick-puzzle-to-test-your-problem-solving.html

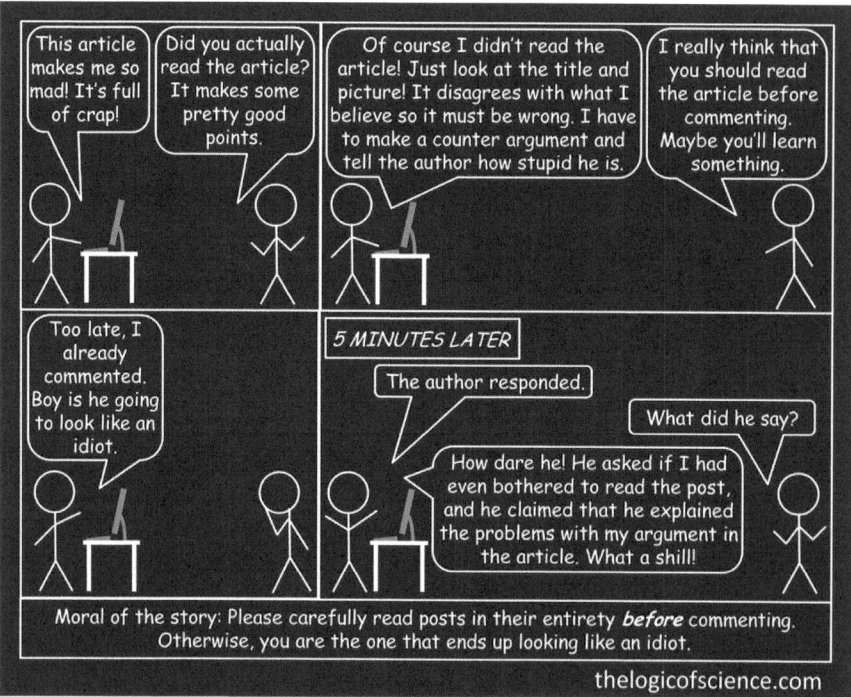

Fig. 4.2 Confirmation bias in action. (The Logic of Science. Few things annoy me more than writing a post only to have people comment with the same arguments that I spent the post debunking. [Facebook status update]. 2017. Retrieved from https://www.facebook.com/thelogicofscience/posts/1924945027736891:0.)

Customers who bought this item also bought

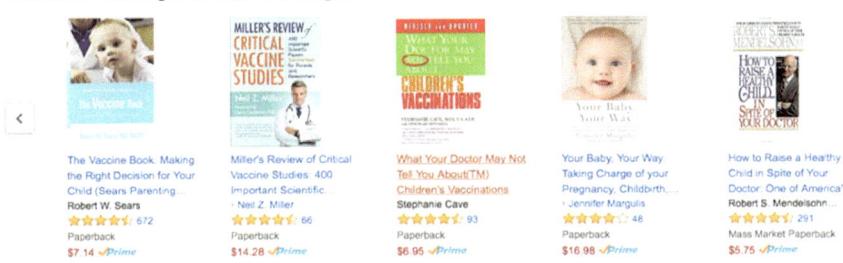

The Vaccine Book: Making the Right Decision for Your Child (Sears Parenting... Robert W. Sears ★★★★☆ 672 Paperback $7.14 ✓Prime

Miller's Review of Critical Vaccine Studies: 400 Important Scientific... Neil Z. Miller ★★★★★ 66 Paperback $14.28 ✓Prime

What Your Doctor May Not Tell You About(TM) Children's Vaccinations Stephanie Cave ★★★★☆ 93 Paperback $6.95 ✓Prime

Your Baby, Your Way: Taking Charge of your Pregnancy, Childbirth,... Jennifer Margulis ★★★★☆ 48 Paperback $16.98 ✓Prime

How to Raise a Healthy Child in Spite of Your Doctor: One of America's... Robert S. Mendelsohn... ★★★★☆ 291 Mass Market Paperback $5.75 ✓Prime

Fig. 4.3 Customers who bought one anti-vaccine book were likely to buy other anti-vaccine book. (Retrieved from Amazon.com.)

Most people naturally assume that the rule is to add two to the previous numbers and guess "8, 10, and 12." While those numbers follow the rule, it is not the rule. Typically, people then continue to guess number sequences such as "10, 14, and 20," which also follow the rule. Most people are content to try to guess the rule, having only proposed number sequences that follow the rule. Few people seek to form a sequence that does *not* satisfy the rule. In other words, few people form a hypothesis and then actively seek to *disprove* it. The tendency to evaluate a hypothesis exclusively through direct testing, while neglecting tests of possible alternative hypotheses is known as the congruence bias. In the "2-4-6" task, finding a sequence of numbers that violates the rule provides essential information to figuring out the rule. The rule, by the way, is extremely simple; each number is larger than the one before it.

Another example of confirmation bias is the four-card selection task, also developed by Wason. In this task, subjects are shown four cards and told each card has a number on one side and a letter on the other. Your task is to figure out which of these cards are worth turning over to determine if the following statement is false: "If a card has a vowel on one side, then it has an even number on the other side" (Fig. 4.4).

Most people feel that "A" and "4" cards are worth turning over. While it is true that the "A" card will help you falsify the statement, turning over the "4" card is not helpful. In contrast, turning over the "7" card could provide essential information. If the "7" card has a vowel on the other side, then the statement would be proven false. Interestingly, this test is trivially easy if social criteria are substituted for numbers and letters. Imagine you are a bartender and want to make sure no one under the age of 21 is drinking alcohol in your bar. Which of the following four people should you investigate, the person drinking beer, the 18-year-old, the person drinking milk, or the 45-year-old? Easy, right?

The desire to gain information that confirms our beliefs extends to more than just games and riddles. In the case presented in this chapter, Dr. Balint used the information that Patricia was mildly intoxicated on alcohol as a reason to search for a toxic ingestion and, other than the head CT, only a toxic ingestion. Furthermore, that she had THC in her urine was used as further evidence that she must have been exposed to some sort of drug. Even when the toxicology screen failed to find evidence of any substance that

Fig. 4.4 The Wason
four-card selection task

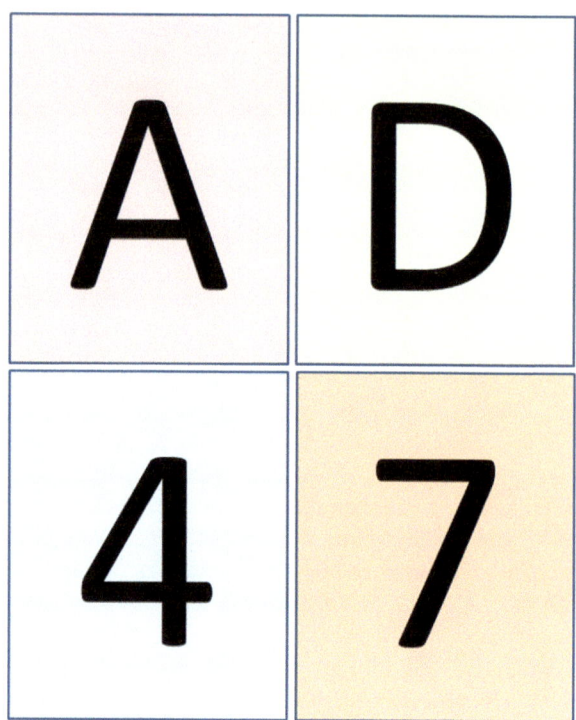

could have caused her presentation, the idea of a toxic ingestion was not discarded. Dr. Balint never considered what test might disprove his theory of a toxic ingestion.

Jonathan Baron and colleagues provided an example of confirmation bias in medical diagnoses [4]. Study subjects were given the following case:

> *A patient has a .8 probability of having Chamber-of-Commerce disease and a .2 probability of Elk's disease. (He surely has one or the other.) A tetherscopic examination yields a posi- tive result in 90% of patients with Chamber-of-Commerce disease and in 20% of patients without it (including those with some other disease). An intraocular smear yields a positive result in 90% of patients with Elk's disease and in 10% of patients without it. If you could do only one of these tests, which would it be? Why?*

The best test to order is the intraocular smear. It would do the best job of both ruling-in and ruling-out the least likely condition. However, 12 of 22 subjects in their study chose the tetherscopic examination, preferring a test with a high probability of a positive result.

Confirmation bias is most likely to occur with topics that are emotionally impor- tant to us. Drs. Taber and Lodge conducted studies that demonstrated the role con- firmation bias has on emotional topics such as gun control and affirmative action. Study subjects were allowed to choose information from groups that either sup- ported or refuted their position. Even when told to be fair-minded, subjects were more likely to read essays that supported their pre-existing opinions. This was

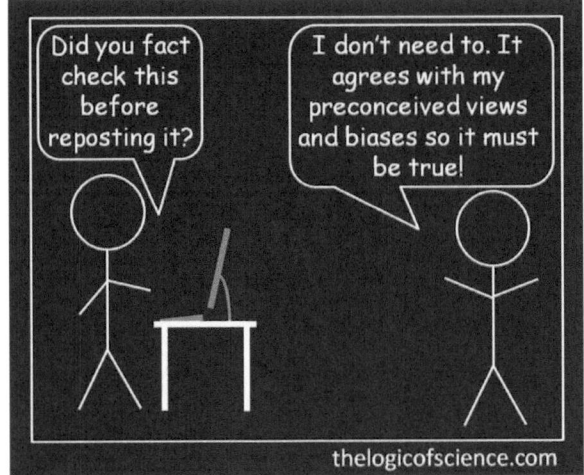

Fig. 4.5 Confirmation bias is common on the internet. (The Logic of Science. This is how myths and conspiracy theories spread [Facebook status update]. 2015. Retrieved from https://www.facebook.com/thelogicofscience/posts/1698242277073835.)

particularly true for subjects with strong baseline opinions and politically knowledgeable subjects. In other words, people sought out information they thought would confirm what they already believed [1].

It is not surprising that confirmation bias is also a significant problem for society at large. The days when everyone got their information from the same trusted anchormen and newspapers are long over. The internet and social media only serve to reinforce echo-chambers of belief. As science communicator David Zaruk said:

> We are living in the Age of Stupid. Social media has built walls around communities of shared ideals (tribes) that confirm people's thinking; and attack, ban or systematically repudiate people with differing ideas. Surrounded in our echo-chambers, our tribal gurus disconnect us from dialogue, raise emotional arguments to the point where anecdote serves as evidence and build trust by elevating fears and vulnerabilities their herd is designed to defend against [5].

Studies support this observation. In an article titled *Debunking in a World of Tribes*, Fabiana Zollo and colleagues examined the online behavior of 54 million Facebook users over a five-year period on both pseudoscience, conspiracy sites and pro-science, debunking sites [6]. They found that there tended to be well-formed and segregated online communities, with little interaction between them (Fig. 4.5). They concluded:

> Our findings show that debunking posts remain mainly confined within the scientific echo chamber and only few users usually exposed to unsubstantiated claims actively interact with the corrections. Dissenting information is mainly ignored and, if we look at the sentiment expressed by users in their comments, we find a rather negative environment.

Furthermore we show that the few users from the conspiracy echo chamber who interact with the debunking posts manifest a higher tendency to comment, in general. However, if we look at their commenting and liking rate—i.e., the daily number of comments and likes—we find that their activity in the conspiracy echo chamber increases after the interaction.

Lastly, the source of information matters. We tend to value information more when we credit ourselves for its discovery. Donald Redelmeier and colleagues investigated how clinicians reacted in two different scenarios involving a personal choice about kidney donation. In the first scenario, the information was provided to the clinician, while in the second scenario, the clinician obtained the information themselves [7]. They discovered that "the pursuit of information can increase its salience and cause clinicians to assign more importance to the information than if the same information was immediately available."

Motivated Reasoning

Confirmation bias leads people not only to seek out information that confirms a pre-existing belief, but also to interpret information in a way that is favorable to their preconceived viewpoints. Information that supports a belief will be readily accepted, a form of confirmation bias called motivated reasoning. Motivated reasoning is well illustrated by the following parable:

A conspiracy theorist dies and goes to heaven. When he arrives at the pearly gates, God is there to receive him. "Welcome. You are permitted to ask me one question, which I will answer truthfully." Without hesitating, the conspiracy theorist asks, "Was the moon landing fake?" God replies, "No, the moon landing was real. NASA astronauts walked on the moon in 1969." The man thinks to himself, "This conspiracy goes even deeper than I thought."

Motivated reasoning is an emotional mechanism that allows people to avoid uncomfortable cognitive dissonance and permits them to hold implausible ideas, such as that Bigfoot exists, or scientifically refuted ones, such as that vaccines cause autism. Motivated reasoning is most likely to occur with longstanding beliefs that have a strong emotional component and with beliefs that have been declared publicly. With such core beliefs, little effort is spared to discredit contradictory information and avoid unpleasant cognitive dissonance. We might like to think that we base our beliefs on the facts. However, just as often, our willingness to accept facts is based on our beliefs.

I witnessed a fascinating example of such motivated reasoning during my residency. One weekend when I was working in the hospital, I received a message that there was a support group for patients suffering from chronic Lyme disease, a medically dubious diagnosis. I had no particular interest in going, but there were sandwiches, so I ran there as fast as I could. It was fascinating to hear multiple patients describe how they had taken ten negative tests for Lyme disease before one finally came back positive. In their minds, the ten negative tests were wrong, while the one positive test was correct. In other words, they *knew* they had Lyme disease and were going to keep testing themselves for it until they got the diagnosis they were already certain they had. I similarly encountered patients who have gone to multiple doctors, a practice called doctor-shopping, searching for one who will give them diagnosis they already "know" they have [8]. These patients are certain they have multiple sclerosis (MS) and will search until they find a doctor who confirms this.

A demonstration of motivated reasoning was performed in 1979 at Stanford. Researchers examined 48 subjects who either supported or opposed the death penalty [9]. They provided them with two fictional studies on the ability of capital punishment to deter crime. One study supported this position, while the other refuted it. The subjects were then asked how convincing the studies were and whether they had swayed their opinions. Almost all subjects said their beliefs did not change, and they expressed a clear preference for the study that supported their original opinion. They lauded evidence from the studies that bolstered their opinion and discarded evidence that contradicted it. Numerous studies since that time have confirmed these findings.

Motivated reasoning is most likely to occur with people who are highly knowledgeable on a particular topic. Such people will be aware of arguments for or against their position. They will be able to marshal strong arguments for what they believe and defend themselves against attacks. Psychologist Dan Kahan demonstrated this phenomenon in a study by asking over 1,500 subjects whether they agreed or disagreed with this statement: "There is solid evidence of recent global warming due mostly to human activity such as burning fossil fuels" [10]. He found that subjects with the lowest scientific knowledge had the least partisan stance. In contrast, liberals with high levels of scientific knowledge were able to find evidence for climate change, while conservatives used their knowledge to argue against it.

In a related experiment, Dr. Kahan and colleagues surveyed over 1,800 subjects on the subject of nanotechnology [11]. They found that subjects with the most scientific intelligence had strong opinions that aligned with their political values, even when their knowledge about nanotechnology was quite low. They specifically found that:

> Peoples' attitudes toward nanotechnology derive from their affective or emotional responses to it. Those who know little or nothing about the concept of "nanotechnology" experience a quick, visceral reaction to it that strongly influences their judgment about the relative size of nanotechnology's potential risks and benefits. That visceral reaction is strongly influenced by their perceptions of more familiar environmental risks, such as those associated with global warming and nuclear power.

Additionally, correcting erroneous beliefs about nanotechnology did little to change their overall opinion of it.

At a basic perceptual level, information and events that we don't want or expect to be true may in some sense be invisible to us. People perceive events depending on their initial viewpoint and frame of reference, a phenomenon known as selective perception. Anyone who has ever watched a sports game with fans of two opposing teams knows the exact same event can be viewed in an entirely different manner depending on which team one is rooting for. A case study of this occurred in 1951 when Princeton played Dartmouth in football [12]. It was a rough, violent game, with multiple broken bones and penalties. After the game, screeds in each college's newspaper blamed the other for the carnage. Albert Hastorf and Hadley Cantril realized that this represented an interesting opportunity. Students from each college were asked to view a film of the game and decide whether it was "rough and dirty" or "clean and fair," and who was to blame if it was dirty. Even after viewing the same exact same footage, students from Princeton overwhelming faulted Dartmouth for the game's violence and vice versa. Hastorf and Cantril concluded:

> In brief, the data here indicate that there is no such "thing" as a "game" existing "out there" in its own right which people merely "observe." The "game" "exists" for a person and is experienced by him only in so far as certain happenings have significances in terms of his purpose. Out of all the occurrences going on in the environment, a person selects those that have some significance for him from his own egocentric position in the total matrix.

That different people watching the same event can come to starkly different conclusions has occurred with much weightier matters than a football game. On July 17, 2014, Eric Garner was approached by the police in Staten Island, New York City, after he was spotted possibly selling cigarettes. Garner did not comply with police instructions and was placed in a chokehold for about 20 seconds, during which he said, "I can't breathe" several times. He soon lost consciousness and was pronounced dead an hour later. The incident was captured on video, prompting outrage and protests. After viewing the footage, Yul-san Liem, co-director of the Justice Committee, an organization that combats police brutality and racism said [13]:

> The video evidence and the medical examiner's report are clear, and together those two things constitute pretty obvious evidence. This man was clearly, brutally taken to the ground by these officers, the video makes pretty clear that there's a chokehold, and the medical examiner report finds the same thing.

However, multiple police officers disagreed with this viewpoint, often in anonymous internet discussions. Someone named Officer Loney wrote, "He was not choked to death. He was taken down by the neck after refusing to comply with the lawful arrest of officers of the NYPD" [14]. Ed Mullins, president of the Sergeants Benevolent Association, agreed with this, saying:

> When you look at the tape that's all over the media, no one talks about the time delay where the officers waited for assistance. There was a greater time delay of assistance, and time for Eric Garner to surrender, than there was any actual scuffle itself. He chose not to. As Pat said, this is not a chokehold. A chokehold is a completely opposite tactic than what you are watching [13].

Like the football game between Princeton and Dartmouth, two different groups of people saw the exact same video and reached markedly different conclusions about what it showed. Each group watched the video with their biases and preconceived notions, primed to reach a conclusion that meshed with what they already knew.

Not surprisingly, the world of complementary and alternative medicine (CAM) offers insight into confirmation bias and motivated reasoning. Consider the writings of anti-vaccine doctor Dr. Joseph Mercola, author of the report *The FDA Exposed* [15]. In this monograph, he claims to tell "The truth about the FDA and why it is no longer fit to safeguard your health." However, when researchers from the FDA found that vaccinated baboons could spread pertussis despite showing no symptoms of the disease, Dr. Mercola trusted and promoted this study. In an essay titled *Whooping Cough Vaccine Not as Effective as Thought and Spreads Through Those Vaccinated,* he used the FDA study to create fear and doubt about the vaccine's efficacy [16]. In contrast to his usual distrust of the FDA, he saw no reason to question its integrity when it produced a finding that confirmed his pre-existing beliefs.

A pattern emerges when studying anti-vaccine doctors, and CAM practitioners when a scientific entity or pharmaceutical company produces evidence that supports vaccines, it is portrayed as corrupt and untrustworthy. In contrast, when these same institutions produce data showing vaccine-limitations, then that evidence is deemed true and irrefutable. Similarly, many anti-vaccine advocates who regularly excoriate pharmaceutical companies and regulatory agencies, simultaneously trust adverse-reactions as reported on the vaccine package insert (Fig. 4.6).

At its most extreme, motivated reasoning can cause people to simply deny any reality that contradicts their desired beliefs. President Trump has an unfortunate habit of labeling any unpleasant information and those who report it as "fake news" (Fig. 4.7).

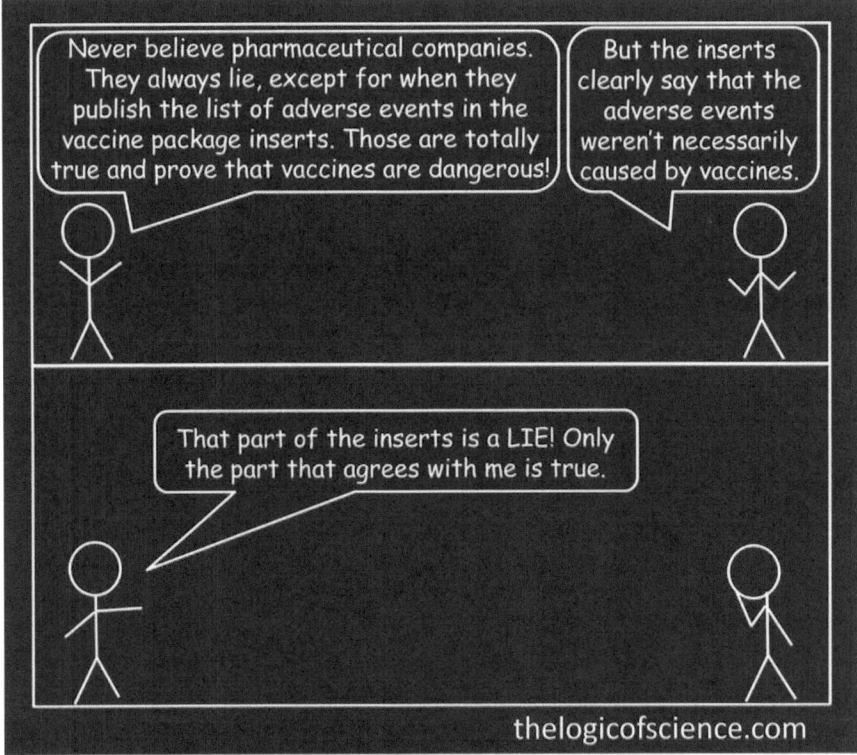

Fig. 4.6 For CAM practitioners pharmaceutical companies are reliable when they want them to be. (The Logic of Science. [Image file, Facebook status update]. 2015. Retrieved from https://www.facebook.com/thelogicofscience/posts/1959614184269975:0.)

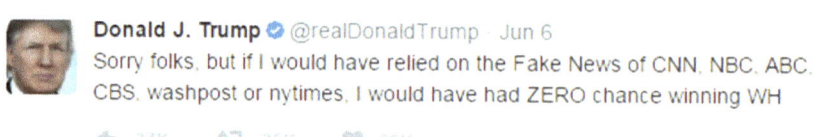

Fig. 4.7   President Donald Trump calling unwanted news, "fake." (RealDonaldTrump. [Donald J. Trump]. (June 6). Sorry folks, but if I would have relied on the Fake news of CNN, NBC, ABC, CBS, washpost or nytimes, I would have had ZERO chance of winning WH [Twitter moment]. Retrieved from https://twitter.com/realdonaldtrump/status/872064426568036353?lang=en.)

As a candidate, President Trump routinely claimed positive job reports put forth by the Bureau of Labor Statistics were fabricated, only to extol positive numbers when he became president. When asked about this, his former spokesman Sean Spicer said, "I talked to the President prior to this and he said to quote him very clearly: 'They may have been phony in the past, but it's very real now'" [17].

Motivated Ignorance and Motivated Skepticism

The corollaries to confirmation bias and motivated reason are known as motivated skepticism and motivated ignorance. Motivated ignorance is the tendency to avoid information that refutes a cherished belief, while motivated skepticism refers to the fact that contradictory information will often be actively rejected when encountered.

Motivated Ignorance

Motivated ignorance, also called information avoidance, occurs when people actively seek to avoid information that may be difficult or unpleasant. People may avoid checking their retirement account when the stock market is in a slump and patients may avoid going to the doctor if they notice an abnormal lump. In one study, subjects were offered a chance to earn $10 as long as they read eight arguments that opposed their view on same-sex marriage [18]. If they read arguments that supported their view, they would only earn $7. As the authors stated, "Greed and curiosity were teamed up against motivated ignorance." In over 60% of the cases, motivated ignorance won. Study subjects said that reading arguments that contradicted their view was "about as unpleasant as taking out the trash or standing in line for 20 minutes." In the interests of full disclosure, I certainly would accept $7 to read a writer whose work I enjoyed rather than receive $10 to read maddening nonsense from a medical conspiracy-theorist.

The most powerful form of motivated ignorance is known as the ostrich effect. This term, used primary by behavioral economists, originates from the myth that ostriches bury their heads in the sand in times of danger. When applied to people, it similarly refers to the tendency to simply ignore information that is potentially dangerous or upsetting. Are there some things that you actively avoid knowing? Do you ever leave bills unopened or neglect to check your bank account if you think the balance is low? Would you really want to know the exact story behind the hamburger that ended up on your plate? Would you really want to know if a product you purchased was made in a sweatshop? Would you want to know if you carried a gene for a fatal, untreatable condition? For most of us, there are certain things we work hard not to know.

Motivated Skepticism

Motivated skepticism occurs when people are more skeptical of claims that they don't believe or don't want to be true than they are of claims they like. I often have patients with MS come to me for a second or third opinion – they want to make sure the bad news is right. In contrast, I have seen many fewer people who were told they're fine and want another opinion to make sure that is the case.

Consider some belief that you hold strongly. Perhaps you are strongly in favor of gun control and have donated money to support it. Now consider you read a study that contradicted a strong component of that belief. Perhaps another country enacted a law very similar to one that you would like to see passed, and found that limiting legal access to guns merely drove their sales underground without actually lowering their numbers. Most likely, your immediate reaction would be to seek to discredit this information rather than modify your belief about the effectiveness of gun control. Indeed, researchers have found that motivated skepticism is a powerful factor in the denial of unpleasant scientific truths such as climate change [19].

A demonstration of motivated skepticism comes from the anti-vaccine, autism advocacy organization SafeMinds. Based on smaller studies showing that vaccines can affect primate neurodevelopment, they spent nearly $250,000 to investigate behavioral and brain changes of rhesus macaques given the standard childhood vaccine-schedule. When, much to their surprise, the vaccines had no effect on the monkeys, they largely refused to accept the results of their own study. As Sallie Bernard, president of SafeMinds, said:

> We feel that embedded within these data sets there are animals that have potentially an adverse reaction to this vaccine schedule that would mirror what happens in human infants. The majority who get vaccines are fine, but we believe there is a subset that have an adverse reaction to their vaccines. By looking at the raw data, not data in aggregate, we may be able to identify the subgroup that had that reaction [20].

In 2012, two articles came to vastly different conclusions about the efficacy of treatments for MS in preventing disability. One concluded that these treatments "significantly reduce the risk of multiple sclerosis progression both in patients with initial high-risk and patients with initial low-risk." The other concluded that "administration of interferon beta was not associated with a reduction in progression of disability." While I have no financial stake in this issue, as an MS specialist I certainly want to feel the treatments I offer help my patients. Which of these two papers do you think I read more closely? What do you think my attitude was in reading the papers? Which do you think I ended up believing?

Importantly, motivated skepticism plays an important role in protecting our beliefs from scam artists and pseudoscience. As such, it should not be viewed as an unequivocal flaw in our cognition. I have read multiple articles on pseudoscience sites on topics I know well. They completely misinterpret scientific studies or are downright dishonest. When I encounter an article on these sites on an unfamiliar topic, I am highly skeptical from the start, hopefully protecting myself from misinformation, even if I cannot readily identify it. Gullible people who believe every conspiracy they read on the internet may suffer from a deficit of motivated skepticism.

Backfire Effect

An outdated model of human cognition, known as the information deficit model, posits that science denial and incorrect beliefs are simply due to a lack of knowledge or understanding. As such, they can be rectified by telling people the facts. While it seems intuitively obvious that facts alone should be powerful enough to correct misinformed beliefs, unfortunately, this is often not the case. This is especially true for beliefs that are longstanding in duration or are integral to a person's self-identity. When people are not emotionally invested in an issue, correcting misinformation with a simple fact almost always suffices. A person who believes that Rio de Janeiro is the capital of Brazil will readily change their mind when given evidence that the capital is actually Brasilia. However, we all know that it is not so easy to correct a misinformed belief with highly polarized issues. Someone who insists that Barack Obama was born in Kenya or that the government is hiding the cure for cancer, is unlikely to have this belief corrected with factual information alone.

The situation is even worse than it appears. Not only do we accept or reject information depending on whether we want it to be true, encountering contradictory information can have the paradoxical effect of strengthening our initial belief rather than causing us to question it. The "backfire effect" is a term coined by Brendan Nyhan and Jason Reifler to describe how many individuals come to hold their original position even more strongly when confronted with evidence that conflicts with their beliefs. They demonstrated this by exposing vaccine-hesitant parents to information explaining the absence of evidence that vaccines cause autism as well as the dangers of measles [21]. While they found that this intervention successfully helped diminish the false belief that vaccines cause autism, it actually "decreased intent to vaccinate among parents who had the least favorable vaccine attitudes." They also showed a similar effect when politically conservative students were given information that contradicted their beliefs about the Iraq War [22]. Their work showed that people tend to dig in their heels and insist even more fervently that their position is true if they sense that their core beliefs are being attacked. They use motivated cognition to preserve their beliefs and defend against the attack.

A related study by Sara Pluviano and colleagues produced similar findings [23]. They examined three common pro-vaccination strategies: contrasting vaccine myths versus facts, employing fact and icon boxes, and showing images of ill, unvaccinated children. They found that:

> *Existing strategies to correct vaccine misinformation are ineffective and often backfire, resulting in the unintended opposite effect, reinforcing ill-founded beliefs about vaccination and reducing intentions to vaccinate...Specifically, we found that the myths vs. facts format, at odds with its aims, induced stronger beliefs in the vaccine/autism link and in vaccines side effects over time, lending credit to the literature showing that countering false informa-*

tion in ways that repeat it may further contribute to its dissemination. Also the exposure to fear appeals through images of sick children led to more increased misperceptions about vaccines causing autism. Moreover, this corrective strategy induced the strongest beliefs in vaccines side effects, highlighting the negative consequences of using loss-framed messages and fear appeals to promote preventive health behaviours. Our findings also suggest that no corrective strategy was useful in enhancing vaccination intention.

The backfire exists in anti-vaccine advocates because their beliefs are rarely derived from facts about vaccines, but rather from feelings about them. The writer Ben Shapiro memorably tweeted that "facts don't care about your feelings" [24]. However, as often as not, our feelings don't care about the facts. In the case of anti-vaccine advocates, these beliefs are an amorphous sense that vaccines are "toxic" or impure, that technology and capitalism are evil, and that nature is inherently benign. As such, arguing against the beliefs of anti-vaccine advocates challenges not just specific beliefs they have about vaccines, but rather core parts of their social identity. Additionally, for most people, even the most overwhelming scientific data is less compelling than a single, close, emotional anecdote in influencing such beliefs. A YouTube video of a young girl who believes she was injured by the Gardasil™ vaccine may do more to influence someone's belief than a study on thousands of people showing the vaccine is safe.

Other researchers have found that public-health messages can backfire as well, a phenomenon termed the boomerang effect. As Sahara Byrne and Philip Hart wrote, "Messages with a specific intent can backfire and cause an increase in the unhealthy or anti-social attitude or behavior targeted for change" [25]. Certain messages can induce a reaction formation, whereby people do the opposite of the intended message in order to preserve a sense of freedom and independence [26].

Researchers have found that the situation may not be so dire and that people are often able to adjust their beliefs when presented with disconfirming factual information [27]. Dr. Nyhan, who discovered the backfire effect, has published work casting doubt on its power [28]. As he correctly observed, "it would be ironic if I dug in my heels" [29]. Certainly, the idea that facts can change people's beliefs is positive news for science-promoters. However, the contradictory findings indicate that more research needs to be done to better delineate the size and scope of the backfire effect.

Mainstream clinicians are not immune to the backfire effect, of course. A clinician who has devoted their career to an operation that is later found to be of no benefit in clinical trials is unlikely to accept this reality overnight. Indeed, after a trial showing that coronary artery stenting was ineffective at relieving chest pain in patients with stable angina, some cardiologists interpreted the data in a manner that supported the procedure. One cardiologist said:

To me actually this study shows angioplasty is quite effective in reducing ischemia, improving [fractional flow reserve] FFR, and in fact I'm actually very pleased with this. It's exactly what I want to do for my patients—improve their blood supply...I promise you, had she studied 400 patients this would be positive because everything was in the right direction [30].

In other words, a study showing that the procedure didn't work was actually evidence the procedure did work!

Cognitive Dissonance

Motivated cognition and the backfire effect serve the valuable purpose of minimizing cognitive dissonance, which is the psychological stress someone experiences when there is a conflict between two or more of their beliefs. Psychologist Leon Festinger proposed cognitive dissonance theory in his book *A Theory of Cognitive Dissonance* published in 1962. He stated that a desire to maintain cognitive consistency can lead to irrational beliefs and maladaptive behaviors.

He demonstrated the backfire effect in a classic psychological investigation called *When Prophecy Fails*, which was based on a cult called The Seekers, headed by a housewife named Dorothy Martin. She predicted that the world would end in a great flood on December 21, 1954. Her followers felt they would be rescued by a spaceship. These true believers had abandoned schools, careers, and family members in preparation for their journey. Dr. Festinger and his colleagues infiltrated the group to study it. When the world didn't end, group members were told that they had "spread so much light that God had saved the world from destruction." Instead of abandoning the group, many members not only remained, but had increased faith in their leader. Since this classic study, similar behavior has been observed in other doomsday cults.

Dr. Festinger noted five conditions are present when someone's belief becomes more intense once it has become disproven:

1. A belief must be held with deep conviction and this must be reflected in their behavior and actions.
2. The believer must have committed themselves to the belief by taking actions that are difficult to undo. The more difficult they are to undo, the greater the believer's dedication.
3. The belief must be sufficiently concerned with the real world so that events may unequivocally refute the belief.
4. Undeniable contradictory evidence must be available and recognized as such by the believer.
5. The believer must have community support to maintain belief when confronted with disconfirming evidence.

Like many biases, confirmation bias and motivated reasoning are easy to spot in others, but nearly impossible to spot in oneself. You probably think of yourself as open-minded and someone who actively seeks out information on all sides of a controversial issue. You likely scoff at the anti-vaccine crusader who clings to their position despite powerful evidence to the contrary. You may cringe in disgust when a politician says unfavorable news is "fake." Surely, you are open-minded and willing to change your mind when presented with compelling evidence that contradicts even your most cherished beliefs. Almost everyone feels this way about themselves.

But, are you really so different? Honestly ask yourself, when was the last time you significantly altered a longstanding belief? When was the last time you actively sought out information that expressed a belief or ideology strongly different from your own? If you are a liberal, when was the last time you read something from a conservative writer? Did you truly approach it with an open mind, or did you only read the headline before you "knew" the article was garbage? I practice confirmation bias every day, though I am only partially aware of it. I routinely read blogs and articles that expose pseudoscience in medicine. While I learn new things all the time from such reading, I do this primarily because it feels good and they tell me what I want to hear.

Despite the power of motivated reasoning and the backfire effect, there are some techniques to minimize these biases, at least when conversing with others. Robb Willer and Matthew Feinberg demonstrated that how we think about many issues, including politicized scientific issues such as climate change, is affected by the frame in which we view them. This school of thought is called moral foundations theory. They found that people can change their minds about an issue as long as it is reframed in a manner that is consistent with their core values. Liberals can support traditional conservative policies if they are reframed to appeal to their values and vice versa. For example, liberals were more likely to support increased military spending if they were told that "through the military, the disadvantaged can achieve equal standing." They were more likely to support making English the official language if they were told that this would decrease the chance immigrants would experience discrimination. Similarly, conservatives were more likely to support liberal positions such as same-sex marriage and universal health care if they were reframed to appeal to their values of authority, group loyalty, purity, traditionalism, religious sanctity, and patriotism [31]. Having said this, it can be very difficult for people to understand the frame by which others view the world. When asked to write a persuasive article to convince conservatives to support same-sex marriage, for example, only 8% of the liberals were able to produce an argument that appealed to conservative values.

John Cook and Stephan Lewandowsky also wrote the following advice when trying to change someone's mind:

> To avoid these "backfire effect," an effective debunking requires three major elements. First, the refutation must focus on core facts rather than the myth to avoid the misinformation becoming more familiar. Second, any mention of a myth should be preceded by explicit warnings to notify the reader that the upcoming information is false. Finally, the refutation should include an alternative explanation that accounts for important qualities in the original misinformation [32].

Conclusion

We are all familiar with the expression, "I'll believe it when I see it." However, because of confirmation bias, "I'll see it when I believe it" is closer to how our minds often function.

Not only do people search out information that confirms their beliefs, but once discovered, there is a strong tendency to accept or reject information based on how well it conforms to our pre-existing beliefs and values. While it is often easy to recognize when others are making these cognitive errors, we are blind to our biases.

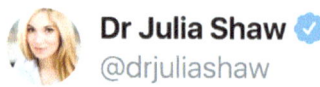

Dr Julia Shaw ✔
@drjuliashaw

Dear science critics:
We are constantly making new
discoveries. If evidence changes we
change our advice.

Don't you wish everyone did this?

Fig. 4.8 Julia Shaw gets it right. (Drjuliashaw. [Dr Julia Shaw]. Dear science critics: we are constantly making new discovers. If evidence changes we change our advice. Don't you wish everyone did this? [Twitter moment]. 2017. Retrieved from https://twitter.com/drjuliashaw/status/922483679997386752.)

We have an internal model of how the world works. We have our notions of right and wrong. We search for information to shore up our beliefs, and we interpret neutral information as being in our favor. When we simply can't mesh uncomfortable facts with a deeply held belief, we may reject those facts and return to our original belief more strongly than before.

Clinicians order tests both to rule-in and rule-out suspected diseases. Confirmation bias can lead people to seek out information that would prove their suspected diagnosis right. It is comforting to get reassuring information that confirms what we already believe. Before making a diagnosis, clinicians should pause and ask themselves not which tests might further confirm their suspected diagnosis, but which tests might refute it. Motivated cognition can also lead clinicians to seek out information that confirms their preconceived beliefs about a diagnosis or treatment. Although it is easier said than done, clinicians should employ conscious strategies to avoid these biases. David Casarett, a palliative care doctor, made two such suggestions: "Before you conclude that a treatment was effective, look for other explanations" and "If you see evidence of success, look for evidence of failure" [33].

While no one is immune to confirmation bias and motivated cognition, people who embrace science and rationality are the most open to having their minds changed by evidence (Fig. 4.8). As Carl Sagan said:

> In science, it often happens that scientists say, 'You know that's a really good argument; my position is mistaken,' and then they would actually change their minds and you never hear that old view from them again. They really do it. It doesn't happen as often as it should, because scientists are human and change is sometimes painful. But it happens every day. I cannot recall the last time something like that happened in politics or religion [34].

Belief Bias

Case

Kristina was a 34-year-old woman who presented to a naturopath for help managing a pregnancy. The naturopath convinced her not to get several recommended vaccines, saying that the effects on her fetus were unknown and that "natural immunity" from vaccine-preventable diseases was beneficial. Unfortunately, a whooping cough outbreak occurred in her community shortly after she delivered, and her son contracted the disease. Though he eventually made a full recovery, he spent several weeks in the neonatal ICU.

What Dr. Ji Was Thinking

I've done a lot of research on vaccines. I read the package insert and am convinced the ingredients were toxic. I also don't trust pharmaceutical companies and the "science" they publish. Many of my patients have children who have been injured by vaccines. Scientists have been wrong before- they even used to say that smoking was safe! Furthermore, diseases such as whooping cough were once a normal part of growing up. Our grandparents weren't afraid of them. And trust me, there is a lot of data showing that vaccines are not safe. A recent survey of mothers discovered:

> Vaccinated children were significantly less likely than the unvaccinated to have been diagnosed with chickenpox and pertussis, but significantly more likely to have been diagnosed with pneumonia, otitis media, allergies and NDDs (defined as Autism Spectrum Disorder, Attention Deficit Hyperactivity Disorder, and/or a learning disability) [35].

When this paper was retracted, it only served to further my belief that it was a threat to the pharmaceutical industry. So, I am sorry that Kristina's baby had a hard time, but now he will have natural immunity to last a lifetime.

Case

Anna was a 44-year-old woman who presented with "brain fog" and indigestion for the past six months. She said that she was unable to focus at work and had little interest in formerly pleasure activities. Basic laboratory work was normal and the patient was treated with an antidepressant with little benefit. She sought treatment with a naturopath who suggested daily coffee enemas. After six weeks, Anna reported feeling more energetic and less depressed.

What Dr. Bonnam Was Thinking

I know that there is little "scientific evidence" to support detoxification with coffee enemas. However, this shows the limitations of science when dealing with a complex, biochemical individual. My goal is not to treat my patients as subjects in a randomized controlled trial. My patients are not trials. They are individuals. In my practice, I have seen coffee enemas increase energy and alertness, stimulate detoxification of congested bile ducts to support the liver, as well as hasten parasite elimination. The scientific method was established to evaluate pharmaceutical products. It was not established to judge non-Western treatments and their effects on the whole person. Treatments such as this threaten powerful interests in the pharmaceutical industry that want every person to take a pill for the rest of their lives. Depression is not an SSRI deficiency, however. I realize that this treatment will never be studied by the pharmaceutical industry since they can't make money from it, and would lose a lot of money if it ever became mainstream.

Discussion

The belief bias is the tendency to evaluate an argument's validity on the basis of whether or not one agrees with the conclusion, instead of whether it is supported by the evidence. It is a form of confirmation bias that occurs when a person's values, ethics, religion, or overall worldview leads to the acceptance of invalid arguments or the rejection of valid ones. It distorts reasoning and prevents the objective evaluation of evidence. It occurs when scientific information is interpreted in light of a deeply held belief, often one with a strong emotional component. Because of the belief bias, many people cling to demonstrably false beliefs and embrace patently absurd ideas.

In medicine, the belief bias causes clinicians to judge scientific studies based on the conclusions they reach, rather than the data itself or the scientific rigor of the study. Because of the belief bias, studies that support a desired position will be unquestionably accepted while those that refute it will be summarily rejected. Additionally, because of the belief bias, clinicians and patients alike may be more predisposed to have success with treatments they fervently believe in (the placebo effect). Richard Asher, an endocrinologist, recognized the power of the belief bias by writing:

> If you can believe fervently in your treatment, even though controlled tests show that it is quite useless, then your results are much better, your patients are much better, and your income is much better, too. I believe this accounts for the remarkable success of some of the less gifted, but more credulous members of our profession, and also for the violent dislike of statistics and controlled tests which fashionable and successful doctors are accustomed to display [36].

A powerful example of the belief bias is seen with a group known as The Association of American Physicians and Surgeons. Despite its rather bland name, this is a right-wing political organization that has espoused multiple beliefs for which there is no scientific evidence. Examples include:

- There is a link between abortions and breast cancer [37].
- Homosexuality is a choice that decreases life expectancy by 20 years [38].
- HIV does not cause AIDS [39].
- Barack Obama may have won the presidency by hypnotizing voters, especially young people and highly educated people [40].
- Vaccines cause autism and are made "using material from aborted babies" [41].

Several prominent politicians are members of this organization, which espouses clearly erroneous medical opinions depending on whether or not they conform to its political persuasions. Its president, Melinda Woofter, made no secret about her disregard for evidence-based medicine, writing in her mission statement in 2016:

> We have witnessed an accelerated transformation of our profession away from individualized patient care toward politicized and collectivized 'evidence-based medicine.' Without a doubt, this one-size-fits-all approach does not work and never can [42].

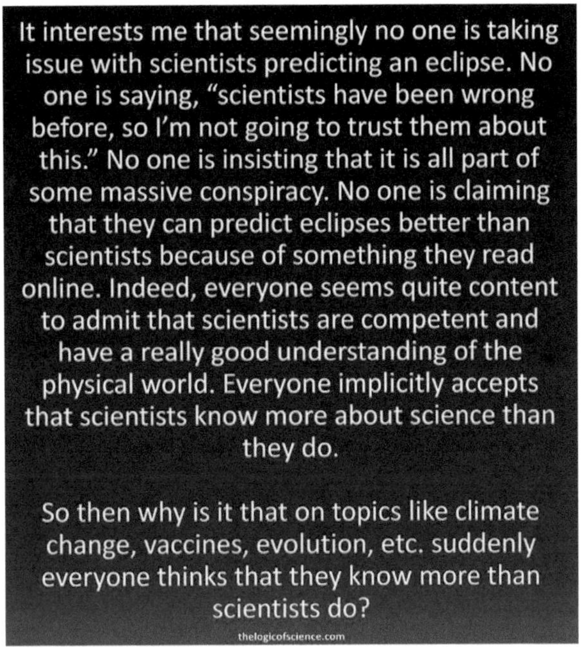

Fig. 4. 9 I agree. (The Logic of Science. [Image file, Facebook status update]. 2017. Retrieved from https://www.facebook.com/thelogicofscience/posts/2027932000771526:0.)

It interests me that seemingly no one is taking issue with scientists predicting an eclipse. No one is saying, "scientists have been wrong before, so I'm not going to trust them about this." No one is insisting that it is all part of some massive conspiracy. No one is claiming that they can predict eclipses better than scientists because of something they read online. Indeed, everyone seems quite content to admit that scientists are competent and have a really good understanding of the physical world. Everyone implicitly accepts that scientists know more about science than they do.

So then why is it that on topics like climate change, vaccines, evolution, etc. suddenly everyone thinks that they know more than scientists do?

thelogicofscience.com

The belief bias is also common in practitioners of CAM, where there is an almost universal tendency to first establish a belief and then judge scientific evidence based on whether or not it supports or refutes this belief. Evidence that support the beliefs of CAM practitioners gets lauded regardless of the quality and rigor of the underlying science. In contrast, evidence that contradicts their beliefs get demonized. Often these beliefs are quasi-religious, extolling the virtues of whatever is perceived as "natural," while simultaneous demonizing pharmaceutical companies and "Western" medical practices (Fig. 4.9).

An example of this can be seen with the CAM website Greenmedinfo. It published an article by Sayer Ji proclaiming *Science Confirms Turmeric as Effective as 14 Drugs* [43] This article proclaims that:

> *Its medicinal properties and components (primarily curcumin) have been the subject of over 5,600 peer-reviewed and published biomedical studies. In fact, our five-year long research project on this sacred plant has revealed over 600 potential preventive and therapeutic applications, as well as 175 distinct beneficial physiological effects.*

While many people felt that Mr. Ji was greatly overstating the strength of the scientific data, at least he was writing in terms that could evaluated and discussed: What does the evidence about turmeric really show? (Fig. 4.10) [44].

In contrast, when a large meta-analysis found no medicinal benefit to turmeric, Mr. Ji then proclaimed the scientific method is like a "religion," and should not apply to turmeric, writing:

> *The RCT (randomized, double-blind, placebo-controlled, human clinical trial) has become the epistemiological holy grail of Scientism and the Medical Monotheism it informs. In this belief system, it doesn't matter if something has had cross-cultural validation as a healing*

agent, even after thousands of years of safe human use; nor does it matter if you personally have experienced (N-of-1) direct and measurable health benefits from consuming it…This Scientism-based belief system is so powerful and all-consuming that sometimes I describe it as the 'Religion that devours all others' [45].

In other words, that turmeric is a powerful medication is a given. When science supports that conclusion, science is wonderful. When science doesn't support that conclusion, it is because science is either corrupt or somehow fundamentally unable to measure turmeric's benefits. First comes the belief, then comes the science (Fig. 4.11).

Fig. 4.10 Claims that a single, miracle substance chance cure multiple diseases are quite old. (Wellcome Collection Gallery. Advertisement for the 'Toxo-Absorbent' cure [Image file]. In: Wikimedia commons. 2014. Retrieved from https://commons. wikimedia.org/wiki/ Category:Quackery#/ media/ File:Quackery;_20th_ century_Wellcome_ L0003567.jpg.)

TOXO-ABSORBENT
THE GREAT DRUGLESS TREATMENT
The most important medical discovery in the world's history.

Diseases can be cured more promptly and with greater certainty without taking medicine in any form.

By the new treatment lingering sickness and premature death can be avoided and mankind can live to a good old age.

THE TOXO-ABSORBENT CURE can be relied on for the cure of any of the following diseases. If suffering from any one of them, write us at once. *See directions for treatment in this book*

Asthma	Typhoid Fever
Bronchitis	Gastritis
Diphtheria	Ulceration of Stomach
Swelled Glands	Chronic Diarrhoea
Hay Fever	Catarrh of Stomach
Catarrh of Throat	Neuralgia of Stomach
Consumption	Kidney Diseases
Inflammation of Lungs	Bright's Disease
Congestions	Abscesses
Pleurisy	Fever Sores
Pneumonia	Varicose Ulcers
Malaria	Blood Poison
Congestion of Liver	Rheumatism
Biliousness	Cancers
Jauridice	Fibroid Tumors
Gall-Stones	Scrofula
Appendicitis	Erysipelas
Peritonitis	Chilblains
Ivy Poison	Syphilis

A list of the diseases which Toxo-Absorbent could be relied (?) on to cure! From a page (reduced more than one-half) of a booklet put out by the Toxo-Absorbent Company.

Fig. 4.11 Isaac Asimov gets it right. (Leonian P. Isaac Asimov [Image file]. In: Wikimedia commons. (n.d.). Retrieved from https://commons. wikimedia.org/wiki/ Isaac_Asimov#/media/ File:Isaac.Asimov01.jpg.)

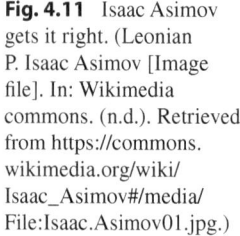

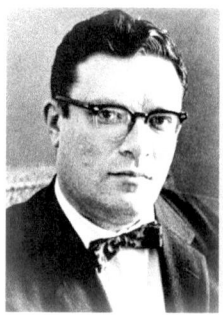

So the universe is not quite as you thought it was. You'd better rearrange your beliefs, then. Because you certainly can't rearrange the universe.

Isaac Asimov

The belief bias is a core part of the anti-vaccine movement. Consider, for example, Suzanne Humphries, a virulently anti-vaccine doctor. She does not believe smallpox was eradicated by vaccines and does not believe the polio virus causes paralysis. She has said "Vaccines are dangerous and should never be injected into anyone for any reason. They are not the answer to infectious diseases" [46]. She also said, "Never has there been a safe vaccine. Never will there be a safe vaccine, and it is not possible to have a safe vaccine" [47].

People like Dr. Humphries are not simply ignorant of the facts of vaccines. Therefore, presenting them with safety and efficacy data about vaccines won't have any impact on their beliefs. There is literally no amount of such information that would convince them that any vaccine is beneficial. It would be like trying to convince someone who keeps a kosher diet that it's fine to eat bacon because it tastes really good. This is because their objections to vaccines are not based on data and science, but rather on belief and philosophy. As vaccine-advocate, Craig Egan, stated:

> *Here's a fun experiment. Ask an anti-vaxxer how they would feel if a vaccine was developed for AIDs or cancer. As long as you ask it simply and straightforward like that, they will almost always say they would be against it. They will be against a hypothetical vaccine that doesn't even exist yet, with no knowledge of its safety or efficacy. That's why arguing about the evidence never gets anywhere; because they don't actually care. They already know it's dangerous and ineffective. Any data claiming otherwise will be viewed as totally corrupt and paid for Big Pharma.*

He also said, "I'll go out of a limb here, and predict that if HIV were ever eradicated through vaccination efforts, twenty years later, the anti-vaccine movement will claim it was never that bad, it was invented to sell vaccines, and it was eradicated through sanitation efforts." I have no doubt he's right.

The belief bias does not just apply to doctors with a right-wing political agenda or CAM practitioners with an anti-science agenda. It can also apply to those who take on powerful interests in a crusade for public health. This subset of the belief bias is known as the white hat bias, a term coined by public health researchers David Allison and Mark Cope. In their words, it is a "bias leading to the distortion of information in the service of what may be perceived to be righteous ends." They examined the purported role of nutritively-sweetened beverages in causing obesity and the purported benefits of breastfeeding. They found a high degree of both cherry-picking the evidence and publication bias in this research. They contend those affected by the white hat bias may "be fueled by feelings of righteous zeal, indignation toward certain aspects of industry, or other factors" (Fig. 4.12) [48].

For example, at my hospital, located in downtown Manhattan, a breastfeeding initiative recently referenced an article in *The Lancet* which stated that "823,000 annual deaths in children under age five could be prevented with universal breastfeeding of infants" [49]. This is true because there are many areas of the world that lack access to clean drinking water. There is no evidence that babies in New York City, where access to clean water is generally not a problem, are dying preventable deaths due to the lack of breastfeeding. In wealthier countries, the benefits of

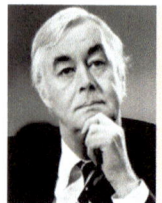 **Everyone is entitled to his own opinion, but not his own facts.**
Daniel Patrick Moynihan

Fig. 4.12 Patrick Monahan gets it right. (US Congress. Pat Moynihan [Image file]. 1998. Retrieved from https://commons.wikimedia.org/wiki/Category:Daniel_Patrick_Moynihan#/media/File:DanielPatrickMoynihan.jpg.)

breastfeeding seem to be extremely mild. Studies of siblings in the same family, where one child was breastfed and the other was not, found no difference in their outcome [50]. This suggests that previous studies showing a benefit to breastfeeding in wealthier counties were marred in part by uncontrolled confounding variables such as race and socioeconomic status. This did not stop a nurse at my hospital from falling prey to the white hat bias, saying about the breastfeeding initiative, "Breastfeeding is the single most preventive modality of care we have available for mothers and infants, affecting babies' lifelong health trajectories." As obstetrician Amy Tuteur wrote, "There's nothing wrong with promoting breastfeeding. But there is something wrong with making spectacular statements about breastfeeding saving hundreds of thousands of lives in the absence of population data to support it" (Fig. 4.13) [51].

On exceptional occasions, some CAM practitioners have adopted a post-modern view of reality, where their beliefs become truth and the scientific method is disparaged in favor of wishes, whims, and desires. Psychiatrist Kelly Brogan, for example, has explicitly discouraged the use of science in medicine saying, "It's time to decide what you believe. Because it's about belief, not about facts, not about science as the final objective" (Fig. 4.14) [52]. She has used this belief to support an anti-vaccine agenda in particular, writing:

> Use logic and reason sparingly – I now understand that science and data only ever reflect our beliefs. They don't create beliefs. I won't convince anyone who is clinging to the Story of Separation that tens of thousands of scientific references undermine the safety and efficacy of pharmaceuticals and vaccines as they are sold to the populace. You have to sit quietly with yourself and feel for your truth. Choose what Story will be yours [53].

Dr. Brogan is not making a factual observation about human nature, recognizing that people interpret information based on how it conforms to their worldview (confirmation bias). She does not recognize this as a flaw in human cognition that impairs our ability to determine the truth and make optimal decisions. Rather, it celebrates the triumph of belief over reason as something to be embraced. It is a wholesale rejection of science, evidence, and rationality as a basis for making medical decisions. This philosophy leads to an inversion of the scientific process, where the belief comes first and evidence comes second. When she published a 23-page

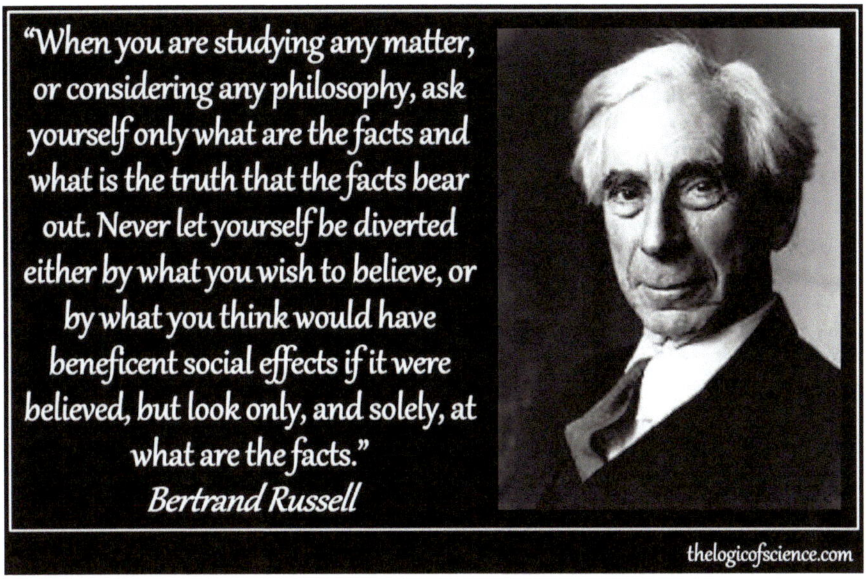

Fig. 4.13 Bertrand Russel gets it right. (The Logic of Science. [Image file, Facebook status update]. 2017. Retrieved from https://www.facebook.com/thelogicofscience/posts/1937246716506722:0.)

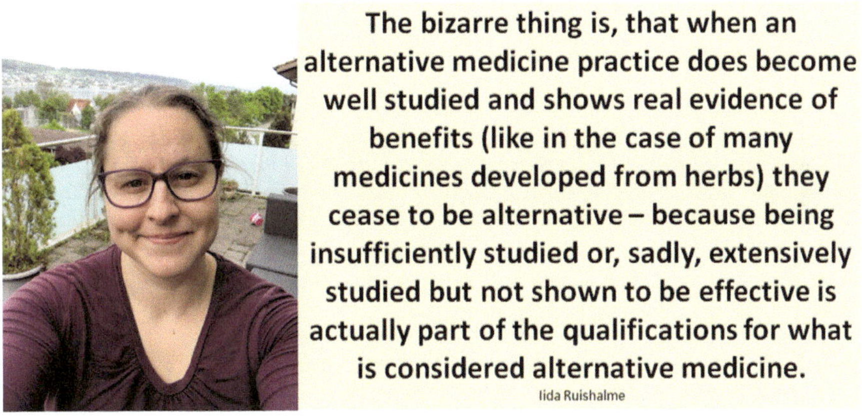

Fig. 4.14 Iida Ruishalme gets it right. (Ruishalme I. (n.d.) Personal photograph.)

booklet on the dangers of vaccines, a pro-vaccine naturopath, Matthew Brignall recognized this, writing:

> I would consider this work to be a canonical example of pseudoscience, or the use of the trappings of science to make a non-science argument. In seventh grade, we all learned that science was a way to ask questions about the world in a way to help to eliminate our biases and beliefs from the assessment. In pseudoscience, however, we start with an answer, and selectively access the work of others to build an argument. She offers us a textbook example of pseudoscience in action [54].

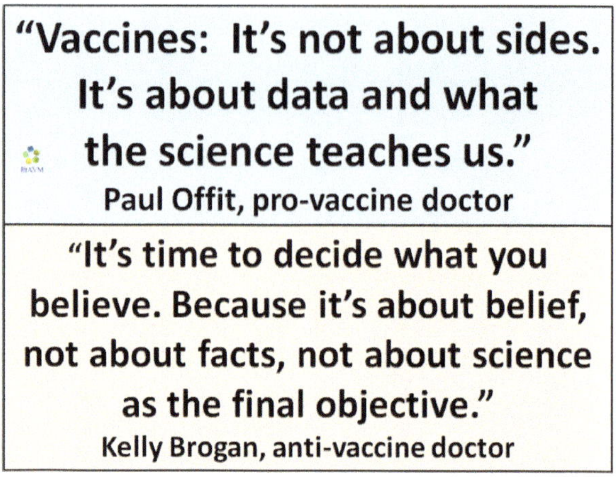

Fig. 4.15 Compare and contrast. (Refutations to Anti-Vaccine Memes. Really, it could not be any clearer than this [Facebook status update]. 2017. Retrieved from https://www.facebook.com/RtAVM/photos/a.414675905269091/1768316569905011/?type=3.)

> "Vaccines: It's not about sides. It's about data and what the science teaches us."
> Paul Offit, pro-vaccine doctor
>
> "It's time to decide what you believe. Because it's about belief, not about facts, not about science as the final objective."
> Kelly Brogan, anti-vaccine doctor

He also noted that financial considerations might be influencing her views, writing:

For my money, the most egregious anti-vaccine propaganda tacks a sales pitch on to the end of the alarmist pseudoscience. Why, it just so happens that Dr. Brogan has a program to help undo the (fake) damage that she claims is done by vaccines. This should tell you all you need to know about her motivations and credibility.

For CAM practitioners like Dr. Brogan, the truth is whatever she wants the truth to be. If science can't confirm her beliefs, then the fault lies with science, not her (Fig. 4.15). True to this philosophy, she wrote:

When Ayurvedic and Chinese medicine interventions attempt to conform to the conventional model of safety and efficacy validation, it is almost surprising to see positive results. Surprising not because I am skeptical about the efficacy of these ancient treatments, but because these modalities employ an individualized assessment of the patient that a trial does not easily 'accommodate.'" [55]

Comedian Stephen Colbert brilliantly mocked this mindset when he coined the word "truthiness." He said about this word:

Now, I'm sure some of the 'word police,' the 'wordinistas' over at Webster's, are gonna say, 'Hey, that's not a word!' Well, anybody who knows me knows that I'm no fan of dictionaries or reference books. They're elitist. Constantly telling us what is or isn't true. Or what did or didn't happen. Who's Britannica to tell me the Panama Canal was finished in 1914? If I wanna say it happened in 1941, that's my right. I don't trust books—they're all fact, no heart … Face it, folks, we are a divided nation … divided between those who think with their head and those who know with their heart … Because that's where the truth comes from, ladies and gentlemen—the gut [56].

Dr. Brogan also has even written that belief itself is the key to good health, suggesting that people become ill because of their beliefs and that patients who don't get better fail to do so because they are too fearful. She wrote:

Believing in your body is the key to resiliency. In my practice, the most important criteria for clinical success is a shared belief system... In many ways, fears that arise around health can be seen as tests of belief. It's easy to see a given circumstance as an exception, an extreme, or a one-time concession...but each and every health experience we are delivered is a dance with our own belief system and a reflection of the trust we have cultivated in our own bodies [57].

The belief bias, especially the wholesale rejection of truth as a meaningful concept, partly explains why facts alone are so ineffective in changing peoples' minds. In all instances where the belief bias is strong, the belief is part of a person's core identity. If you were presented with evidence that Henry Ford did not invent either the car or the assembly line, you would likely readily change your mind about this belief. This is unlikely to be a core, emotional belief of yours that you have publicly defended for years. In contrast, a father who believes vaccines caused autism in his son and then becomes a vocal anti-vaccine crusader, is highly unlikely to be persuaded by even the strongest evidence that vaccines do not cause autism (Fig. 4.16).

When beliefs are based in emotion, facts alone stand little chance. A belief that has been voiced publically and has been held for a long period of time is especially resistant to change. This is because it is rarely the belief alone that is threatened, but rather a person's sense of who they are. Many people cling to irrational beliefs for which there is no evidence because to accept otherwise would mean altering their self-identity. Changing a core beliefs risks alienating people from their family and community.

The neural underpinnings of this reaction have even been elucidated by Jonas Kaplan and colleagues. They presented "liberals with arguments that contradicted their strongly held political and non-political views" [58]. By using functional MRI to measure their brain activity, they found that challenging political beliefs activated brain areas that give rise to personal identity and emotional reaction to threats. This may explain why there are so few examples of prominent political figures or ideologues changing their mind on any issue of great significance. The belief bias may also help explain why seemingly unrelated beliefs track together. People are likely to pick a political party and adopt its positions, rather than consider the merits of the individual issues (Fig. 4.17).

Although Donald Trump's spokeswoman, Kellyanne Conway popularized the phrase "alternative facts," CAM practitioners and those blinded by a political agenda have been long promoted the philosophy that when evidence and science conflict with what they believe to be true, then that is just too bad for evidence and science. Though science is not immune to politics, the entirety of evidence-based medicine is not "politicized and collectivized" as claimed by Dr. Woofter, simply because it doesn't always support what she wants to be true. Using "logic and reason sparingly" to "choose what Story will be yours" as suggested by Dr. Brogan, leads to such absurdities as her belief that "that drug toxicity associated with AIDS treatment may very well be what accounts for the majority of deaths," and recommending daily coffee enemas to treat depression and cancer [59].

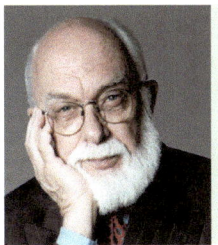

No amount of belief makes something a fact.

James Randi

Fig. 4.16 James Randi gets it right. (Terabyte. James Randi [Image file]. In: Wikimedia commons. 2004. Retrieved from https://commons.wikimedia.org/w/index.php?search=james+randi&title=Special:Search&profile=default&fulltext=1#/media/File:RANDI.jpg.)

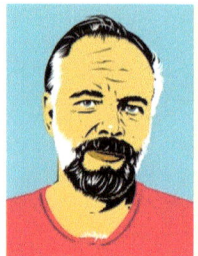

Reality is that which, when you stop believing in it, doesn't go away.
Philip K. Dick

Fig. 4.17 Philip Dick gets it right. (Welsch P. (Pete). Drawn portrait of Philip K Dick [Image file]. In: Wikimedia commons. 2007. Retrieved from https://commons.wikimedia.org/w/index.php?title=Special:Search&search=philip+k+dick&fulltext=1&profile=default#/media/File:Philip_k_dick_drawing.jpg.)

A rational discussion with anyone who rejects the ideal of rationality and literally equates her beliefs with the truth is not possible (Fig. 4.18). As neuroscientist Sam Harris said:

> Water is two parts hydrogen and one part oxygen. What if someone says, "Well, that's not how I choose to think about water"? All we can do is appeal to scientific values. And if he doesn't share those values, the conversation is over. If someone doesn't value evidence, what evidence are you going to provide to prove that they should value it? If someone doesn't value logic, what logical argument could you provide to show the importance of logic? [60]

Perhaps the most extreme consequence of the belief bias is not mere science-denial, but a ban on scientific research. For example, with the backing of the National Rifle Association, the CDC has long been prevented from studying the effects of guns on health. Congressman John Boehner explained this ban by saying, "I'm sorry, but a gun is not a disease. Guns don't kill people — people do. And when people use weapons in a horrible way, we should condemn the actions of the individual and not blame the action on some weapon" [61]. In 2001, president George W. Bush limited federal funding to a small number of embryonic stem cells that were already in existence at the time [62]. Many politicians at the time called for a complete ban on research involving such stem cells. In 2017, the CDC censored seven words ("diversity," "fetus," "transgender," "vulnerable," "entitlement," "science-based" and "evidence-based") in order to maximize the likelihood its proposals would be funded [63].

Importantly, the practice of medicine does not necessitate that clinicians dispense with their beliefs and ethics. Clinicians are not obligated to perform medical procedures that contradict their religion or morals. The American Medical Association recognizes that clinicians are "not defined solely by their profession. They are moral agents in their own right and, like their patients, are informed by and committed to diverse cultural, religious, and philosophical traditions and beliefs." As such, it does not obligate that clinicians treat patients who desire care that is "incompatible with the physician's deeply held personal, religious, or moral beliefs" [64]. However, clinicians must be careful not to let their beliefs affect their interpretation of the scientific facts. A clinician may refuse to perform an abortion on ethical grounds, however they must not mislead patients about the safety of the procedure.

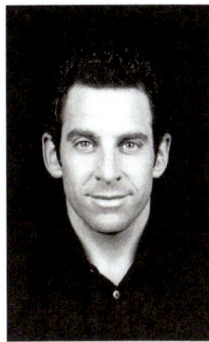

Water is two parts hydrogen and one part oxygen. What if someone says, "Well, that's not how I choose to think about water."? All we can do is appeal to scientific values. And if he doesn't share those values, the conversation is over. If someone doesn't value evidence, what evidence are you going to provide to prove that they should value it? If someone doesn't value logic, what logical argument could you provide to show the importance of logic?

Sam Harris

Fig. 4.18 Sam Harris gets it right. (Harris S. (Sam). Sam Harris [Image file]. (n.d.). Retrieved from https://commons.wikimedia.org/wiki/Sam_Harris#/media/File:Sam_Harris_01.jpg.)

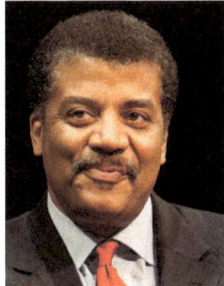

The good thing about science is that it's true whether or not you believe in it.

Neil deGrasse Tyson

Fig. 4.19 Neil gets it right (Press BF. (Bruce F.). Neil deGrasse Tyson on stage with Richard Dawkins at Howard University in Washington D.C. [Image file]. In: Wikimedia commons. 2010. Retrieved from https://commons.wikimedia.org/wiki/Category:Neil_deGrasse_Tyson_facing_front#/media/File:Neil_deGrasse_Tyson_at_Howard_University_September_28,_2010_(cropped_to_collar).jpg.)

Conclusion

The belief bias is the tendency to evaluate information and science based on its conclusion rather than the validity of the evidence or the quality of the research. Due to the belief bias, some clinicians embrace pseudoscientific positions because they mesh with their wishes. Other clinicians take this a step further, deriding the entire concept of science and logic in medicine. No meaningful discussion can be had with such people. As Jonathan Swift said, "It is useless to attempt to reason a man out of a thing he never was reasoned into."

Having said this, clinicians are no different than anyone else when it comes to political, religious, and moral beliefs. The practice of medicine does not necessitate that one dispense with these values. Clinicians are not obligated to perform medical procedures that contradict their religion or morals. However, they must be careful not to let their beliefs affect their interpretation of the facts of medical science. And if science refutes a clinician's cherished belief, then the problem is with that belief, not science. As Neil deGrasse Tyson memorably said, "The good thing about science is that it's true whether or not you believe in it" (Fig. 4.19).

References

1. Taber CS, Lodge M. Motivated skepticism in the evaluation of political beliefs. Am J Polit Sci. 2006;50(3):755–69. https://doi.org/10.1111/j.1540-5907.2006.00214.x.
2. Begley S. (2009, Aug 25). Lies of mass destruction [PDF file]. Newsweek. Retrieved from   http://www.buffalo.edu/content/dam/www/news/imported/pdf/August09/ NewsweekHoffmanMotivatedReasoning.pdf.
3. Parker A, Rucker P, Birnbaum M. (2017, June 1). Inside Trump's climate decision: after fiery debate, he 'stayed where he's always been'. The Washington Post. Retrieved from https://www.washington-post.com/politics/inside-trumps-climate-decision-after-fiery-debate-he-stayed-where-hes-always-been/2017/06/01/e4acb27e-46db-11e7-bcde-624ad94170ab_story.html?utm_term=.bfecd9294b28.
4. Baron J, Beattie J, Hershey JC. Heuristics and biases in diagnostic reasoning: II. Congruence, information, and certainty. Organ Behav Hum Decis Process. 1988;42(1):88–110. Retrieved from https://doi.org/10.1016/0749-5978(88)90021-0.
5. Riskmonger (2017, Oct 24). Glyphosate in the age of stupid [Blog post]. The Risk-Monger. Retrieved from https://risk-monger.com/2017/10/24/glyphosate-in-the-age-of-stupid/.
6. Zollo F, Bessi A, Del Vicario M, Scala A, Caldarelli G, Shekhtman L, Havlin S, Quattrociocchi W. Debunking in a world of tribes. PLoS One. 2017;12(7):e0181821. https://doi.org/10.1371/ journal.pone.0181821.
7. Redelmeier DA, Shafir E, Aujila PS. The beguiling pursuit of more information. Med Decis Mak. 2001;21(5):376–81. https://doi.org/10.1177/0272989X0102100504.
8. Sansone RA, Sansone LA. Doctor shopping: a phenomenon of many themes. Innov Clin Neurosci. 2012;9(11–12):42–6.
9. Lord CG, Ross L, Lepper MR. Biased assimilation and attitude polarization: the effects of prior theories on subsequently considered evidence. J Pers Soc Psychol. 1979;37(11):2098–109. Retrieved from https://doi.org/10.1037/0022-3514.37.11.2098.
10. Kahan DM. Climate-science communication and the measurement problem. Adv Polit Psychol. 2015;34(S1):1–43. https://doi.org/10.1111/pops.12244.
11. Kahan D, Slovic P, Braman D, Gastil J, Cohen G. (2007). Nanotechnology risk perceptions: the influence of affect and values [PDF file]. Woodrow Wilson International Center for Scholars. Retrieved from http://www.nanotechproject.org/file_download/files/ NanotechRiskPerceptions-DanKahan.pdf.
12. Hastorf AH, Cantril H. They saw a game: a case study. J Abnorm Soc Psychol. n.d.;49(1):129. Retrieved from https://doi.org/10.1037/h0057880.
13. Speri A. (2014, Aug 6). A chokehold didn't kill Eric Garner, your disrespect for the NYPD did. Vice News. Retrieved from https://news.vice.com/ article/a-chokehold-didnt-kill-eric-garner-your-disrespect-for-the-nypd-did.
14. Zurcher A. (2014, Dec 4). Eric Garner death: police take to internet in defence of Daniel Pantaleo [Blog post]. BBC News: Echo Chambers. Retrieved from https://www.bbc.com/ news/blogs-echochambers-30323811.
15. The FDA exposed. (n.d.). Mercola. Retrieved 15 Sept 2018 from http://www.mercola.com/ Downloads/bonus/the-FDA-exposed/default.aspx.
16. Whooping cough vaccine not as effective as thought and spreads through those vaccinated. (n.d.). Mercola. Retrieved 15 Sept 2018 from https://articles.mercola.com/sites/articles/ archive/2016/01/26/whooping-cough-vaccine-ineffective.aspx.
17. Diamond J. (2017, Mar 10). Unemployment numbers not 'phony' to Trump anymore. CNN. Retrieved from https://www.cnn.com/2017/03/10/politics/donald-trump-jobs-report-unemployment-numbers-phony/.
18. Frimer J, Skitka L, Motyl M. (2017, Jan 4). Liberals and conservatives have one thing in common: zero interest in opposing views. Los Angeles Times. Retrieved from http://www.latimes. com/opinion/op-ed/la-oe-frimer-skitka-motyle-motivated-ignorance-20170104-story.html.
19. Lewandowsky S, Oberauer K. Motivated rejection of science. Curr Dir Psychol Sci. 2016;25(4):217–22. https://doi.org/10.1177/0963721416654436.
20. Firger J. (2015, Oct 2). Anti-vaxxers accidently fund a study showing no link between autism and vaccines. Newsweek. Retrieved from www.newsweek.com/ anti-vaxxers-accidentally-fund-study-showing-theres-no-link-between-autism-and-379245.

21. Nyhan B, Reifler J, Richey S, Freed GL. Effective messages in vaccine promotion: a random-ized trial. Pediatrics. 2014;133(4):2013–365. https://doi.org/10.1542/peds.2013-2365.
22. Nyhan B, Reifler J. When corrections fail: the persistence of political misperceptions. Polit Behav. 2010;32(2):303–30. https://doi.org/10.1007/s11109-010-9112-2.
23. Pluviano S, Watt C, Della Salla S. Misinformation lingers in memory: failure of three pro-vaccina-tion strategies. PLoS One. 2017;12(7):e0181640. https://doi.org/10.1371/journal.pone.0181640.
24. Shapiro B. [Ben Shapiro]. (2016, Feb 5). Facts don't care about your feelings. [Twitter moment]. Retrieved from https://twitter.com/benshapiro/status/695638866993115136.
25. Byrne S, Hart PS. The boomerang effect a synthesis of findings and a preliminary theoretical frame-work. Ann Int Commun Assoc. 2009;33(1):3–37. https://doi.org/10.1080/23808985.2009.11679083.
26. Ringold DJ. Boomerang effects in response to public health interventions: some unintended consequences in the alcoholic beverage market. J Consum Policy. 2002;25(1):27–63. Retrieved from https://doi.org/10.1023/A:1014588126336.
27. Lewandowsky S, Swire B, Ecker U. The role of familiarity in correcting inaccurate information. J Exp Psychol Learn Mem Cogn. 2017;43(12):1948–61. https://doi.org/10.1037/xlm0000422.
28. Nyhan B, Porter E, Reifler J, Wood T. (2017). Taking corrections literally but not seriously? The effects of information on factual beliefs and candidate favorability. https://doi.org/10.2139/ssrn.2995128.
29. Engber D. (2018, Jan 3). LOL Something matters. Slate. Retrieved from https://slate.com/health-and-science/2018/01/weve-been-told-were-living-in-a-post-truth-age-dont-believe-it.html.
30. Wendling P. (2017, Nov 3). ORBITA: Sham comparison casts doubt on PCI for stable angina. Medscape News. Retrieved from https://www.medscape.com/viewarticle/888011.
31. Feinberg M. From gulf to bridge: when do moral arguments facilitate political influence? Personal Soc Psychol Bull. 2015;41(12):1665–81. https://doi.org/10.1177/0146167215607842.
32. Cook J. (2011, Dec 26). The debunking handbook part 1: the first myth about debunking. ThinkProgress. Retrieved from https://thinkprogress.org/the-debunking-handbook-part-1-the-first-myth-about-debunking-7f2eac1cb33f/.
33. Casarett D. The science of choosing wisely — overcoming the therapeutic illusion. N Engl J Med. 2016;374(13):1203–5. https://doi.org/10.1056/NEJMp1516803.
34. Sagan C. (n.d.). [Personal Quote]. Retrieved 15 Sept 2018 from https://www.goodreads.com/quotes/8385-in-science-it-often-happens-that-scientists-say-you-know.
35. Chawla DS. (2016, Nov 28). Study linking vaccines to autism pulled following heavy criti-cism [Blog post]. Retraction Watch. Retrieved 15 Sept 2018 from https://retractionwatch.com/2016/11/28/study-linking-vaccines-autism-pulled-frontiers-following-heavy-criticism/.
36. Asher R. Talking sense (Lettsomian lecture, 16 Feb, 1959). Transactions of the Medical Society of London, LXXV, 1958-1959. In: Jones FA, editor. Richard Asher talking sense. London: Pitman Medical; 1972.
37. Carroll PS. The breast cancer epidemic: modeling and forecasts based on abortion and other risk factors [PDF file]. J Am Physicians Surg. 2007;12(3):72–8. Retrieved from http://www.jpands.org/vol12no3/carroll.pdf.
38. Lehrman NS. Homosexuality: some neglected considerations [PDF file]. J Am Physicians Surg. 2005;10(3):80–2. Retrieved from http://www.jpands.org/vol10no3/lehrman.pdf.
39. Bauer HH. Questioning HIV/AIDS: morally reprehensible or scientifically warranted? [PDF file]. J Am Physicians Surg. 2007;12(4):116–20. Retrieved from http://www.jpands.org/vol12no4/bauer.pdf.
40. Wonkette. (2010, Sept 27). Rand Paul doctor club. Obama elected by liter-ally hypnotizing voters. Wonkette. Retrieved from https://www.wonkette.com/rand-paul-doctor-club-obama-elected-by-literally-hypnotizing-voters.
41. American Children Need Access to Better Vaccines. (2016, Aug 22). Association of American Physicians and Surgeons. Retrieved from http://aapsonline.org/american-children-need-access-to-better-vaccines/.
42. Woofter M. (2016, Oct 12). What is our mission? [Mission statement]. Association of American Physicians and Surgeons. Retrieved from http://aapsonline.org/presidents-page-what-is-our-mission/.
43. Ji S. (2013, May 13). Science confirms turmeric as effective as 14 drugs. GreenMedInfo. Retrieved from http://www.greenmedinfo.com/blog/science-confirms-turmeric-effective-14-drugs.
44. Hall H. (2014, June 17). Turmeric: tasty in curry, questionable as medicine. Science-Based Medicine. Retrieved from https://sciencebasedmedicine.org/turmeric-tasty-in-curry-questionable-as-medicine/.

45. Ji S. (2017, Feb 2). Forbes leads media attack against turmeric's health benefits [Blog post]. GreenMedInfo. Retrieved from http://www.greenmedinfo.com/blog/forbes-leads-media-attack-against-turmerics-health-benefits.
46. Humphries S. (2011, Feb 5). Vaccines did not save humanity and never will. Vaccination Information Network. https://www.vaccinationinformationnetwork.com/vaccines-did-not-save-humanity-and-never-will-dr-suzanne-humphreys-md/.
47. Null G. (2011, Dec 13). Suzanne Humphries on vaccines [Video file]. Retrieved from https://www.youtube.com/watch?v=efto1LpWkKw.
48. Cope MB, Allison DB. White hat bias: examples of its presence in obesity research and a call for renewed commitment to faithfulness in research reporting. Int J Obes. 2010;34(1):84–8. https://doi.org/10.1038/ijo.2009.239.
49. World Health Organization. (n.d.). Increasing breastfeeding could save 800 000 children and US$ 300 billion every year. Retrieved 15 Sept 2018 from http://www.who.int/maternal_child_adolescent/news_events/news/2016/exclusive-breastfeeding/en/.
50. Colen CG, Ramey DM. Is breast truly best? Estimating the effect of breastfeeding on long-term child wellbeing in the United States using sibling comparisons. Soc Sci Med. 2014;109:55–65. https://doi.org/10.1016/j.socscimed.2014.01.027.
51. Tuteur A. (2016, Jan 29). If breastfeeding saves lives why do countries with the highest infant mortality rates have the highest breastfeeding rates? [Blog post]. The Skeptical OB. Retrieved from http://www.skepticalob.com/2016/01/if-breastfeeding-saves-lives-why-do-countries-with-the-highest-infant-mortality-rates-have-the-highest-breastfeeding-rates.html.
52. Brogan K. (2016). Choose your path: Symptom suppression or health transformation? Kelly Brogan MD. Retrieved 15 Sept 2018 from https://kellybroganmd.com/choose-your-path-suppression-or-transformation/.
53. Brogan K. (2016). Sacred activism: Moving beyond the ego. Kelly Brogan MD. Retrieved 15 Sept 2018 from https://kellybroganmd.com/sacred-activism-moving-beyond-ego/.
54. Brignall M. (2017, Dec 18). Anatomy of an anti-vax screed. NDs for Vaccines. Retrieved from http://ndsforvaccines.com/anatomy-anti-vax-screed/.
55. Brogan K. (n.d.). Weighing treatment options—what informs choices? Kelly Brogan MD. Retrieved 15 Sept 2018 from https://kellybroganmd.com/weighing-treatment-options-what-informs-choices/.
56. Andersen K. (2017, Dec 28). How America lost its mind. The Atlantic. Retrieved 15 Sept 2018 from https://www.theatlantic.com/magazine/archive/2017/09/how-america-lost-its-mind/534231/.
57. Brogan K. (n.d.). How to live a medication free life. Kelly Brogan MD. Retrieved 15 Sept 2018 from https://kellybroganmd.com/how-to-live-a-medication-free-life/.
58. Kaplan JT, Gimbel SI, Harris S. Neural correlates of maintaining one's political beliefs in the face of counterevidence. Sci Rep. 2016;6:39589. https://doi.org/10.1038/srep39589.
59. Brogan K. (n.d.). HIV and pregnancy: pharma abusing women? Kelly Brogan MD. Retrieved 15 Sept 2018 from https://kellybroganmd.com/hiv-pregnancy-pharma-abusing-women/.
60. Harris S. (n.d.). [Personal Quote]. Retrieved 15 Sept 2018 from https://www.goodreads.com/quotes/818485-water-is-two-parts-hydrogen-and-one-part-oxygen-what.
61. Bertrand N. (2015, July 7). Congress quietly renewed a ban on gun-violence research. Business Insider. Retrieved from https://www.businessinsider.com/congressional-ban-on-gun-violence-research-rewnewed-2015-7.
62. Ydstie J, Palca J. (2007, Nov 7). Embryonic stem cells made without embryos [Transcript]. Morning Edition, National Public Radio. Retrieved from https://www.npr.org/templates/story/story.php?storyId=16493814.
63. Branswell H. (2017, Dec 17). CDC director tells staff 'there are no banned words,' while not refuting report. STAT. Retrieved from https://www.statnews.com/2017/12/17/cdc-chief-science-forbidden-words/.
64. American Medical Association. (2016). Chapter 1: opinions on patient-physician relationships [PDF file]. AMA Journal of Ethics. Retrieved 15 Sept 2018 from https://www.ama-assn.org/sites/default/files/media-browser/code-of-medical-ethics-chapter-1.pdf.

Curse of Knowledge

5

Case

Mike was a 67-year-old man who presented with abrupt visual loss in his right eye. He said that he felt like a curtain was being drawn down over this eye. The visual loss was severe, but transient, lasting about a minute.

He was found to have severe stenosis (narrowing) of his right internal carotid artery. The cause of his visual loss was most likely a small plaque that broke off and temporarily occluded the ophthalmic artery, a condition known as amaurosis fugax. Mike was told he needed surgery on his artery, a procedure known as a carotid endarterectomy. His surgery was scheduled for the next day, and when he refused, the vascular surgeon told the patient he was "crazy."

He was discharged the next day and returned three weeks later, having had a large stroke. When asked why he had refused the initial surgery, he said, "the problem was in my eye, why would I let them touch the artery in my neck?"

What Dr. Snow Was Thinking

From a clinical point of view, this was an easy case. Mike had a vascular complication from severe disease of his internal carotid artery, and there is robust literature supporting the need for surgery. However, Mike didn't get this. He was convinced that his problem was in his eye, and he had no idea why we would want to operate on his carotid artery.

I understand that patients aren't experts, but I just couldn't put myself in his shoes to better grasp why he refused the operation. I did try to explain it to him, but I could have done a better job. I had no idea, until it was too late, that he didn't understand the connection between his visual loss and the operation I was proposing. Now, when trying to explain my rationale for operating on patients now, one of my first priorities is to find out what they might or might not understand. Ironically, I have also found interns seem to have more success communicating with patients than I do. I suppose their lack of expertise allows them to better understand the patient's perspective.

© Springer International Publishing AG, part of Springer Nature 2019
J. Howard, *Cognitive Errors and Diagnostic Mistakes*,
https://doi.org/10.1007/978-3-319-93224-8_5

Discussion

The curse of knowledge occurs when a highly informed person is unable see things from the vantage point of a less knowledgeable person. Information may seem so obvious to the high-knowledge person that they are unable to predict how someone lacking that information will behave. The game *Pictionary* involves someone's trying to draw pictures that represent a word or concept printed on a card. If you have ever played this game, it may seem like the people who are trying to guess your drawing are clueless. This is because you are suffering from the curse of knowledge. Experts in a given field are the most likely to be affected by the curse of knowledge. For example, someone who knows the worth of a valuable object is likely to overstate the amount of money someone who is ignorant of its value will pay for it. The curse of knowledge also makes it difficult to fairly evaluate historical events (the hindsight bias). Was the coach who called an onside kick to open up the second half of the Super Bowl a brave genius or a reckless fool? Knowing whether or not the play worked (it did!) will bias our judgment of his decision.

An experiment by psychologist Elizabeth Newton illustrated the curse of knowledge. Study subjects were divided into two groups: tappers and listeners [1]. The tappers chose one of 25 well-known songs (such as "Happy Birthday"), and were asked to tap the song on a table. The listeners had to try to figure out the song. The tappers were also asked to predict how often the listeners would correctly guess the tune. In this experiment, the tappers predicted the listeners would identify the tune 50% of the time. In reality, they were able to do so only 2.5% of the time. The tappers were unable to escape their knowledge of the song they were tapping and so vastly under-estimated the difficulty of the task.

The curse of knowledge also factors into the many issues of cultural competence that clinicians face. The book *The Spirit Catches You and You Fall Down: A Hmong Child, Her American Doctors, and the Collision of Two Cultures* by Anne Fadiman tragically demonstrates the consequences of the curse of knowledge [2]. In the book, a Hmong child named Lia Lee suffers from epilepsy, a condition her parents view as a spiritual gift. They treat her with traditional remedies rather than conventional anti-epileptic medications. Despite dedicated care from a group of pediatricians, Lia suffered a catastrophic seizure, leaving her in a persistent vegetative state. Lia's doctors never knew that her family viewed her seizures as a gift. They did not even consider this a possibility. They, like all of us, were unable to step out of their own cultural boundaries to learn how an illness like epilepsy might be perceived in a different culture.

Overcoming the curse of knowledge is largely impossible; one cannot unlearn what one knows and see things from the vantage point of a novice. The first step in dealing with the curse is to acknowledge that it exists. As psychologist Steven Pinker wrote:

> Anyone who wants to lift the curse of knowledge must first appreciate what a devilish curse it is. Like a drunk who is too impaired to realize that he is too impaired to drive, we do not notice the curse because the curse prevents us from noticing it [3].

Conclusion

Because of the curse of knowledge, the world's experts in a field might have difficulty explaining that field to another person. Their high level of expertise will leave them ignorant of what a non-expert does not know. Clinicians with advanced training often are unable to appreciate a complicated medical diagnosis or treatment decision from the perspective of a non-expert patient. One possible strategy to mitigate the curse of knowledge is for the clinician to ask patients to repeat back their understanding of a diagnosis or proposed treatment, rather than just to assume it was understood. It may also be wise for a senior clinician to include a less-knowledgeable person (an intern or medical student) when talking to patients. The junior person should be encouraged to speak up if they sense that the senior clinician is using inappropriate medical jargon or complex medical concepts that hinder clinician-patient communication. In writing these cases, for example, I have shown them to non-medical people, who have hopefully informed me of medical terms that are familiar to me, but might read like a foreign language to those unfamiliar with them. Finally, when treating patients of a different culture, all attempts should be made to have a member of the treatment team who is familiar with that culture.

References

1. Heath C, Heath D. The curse of knowledge. Harv Bus Rev. 2006;84(12):20–3. Retrieved from https://hbr.org/2006/12/the-curse-of-knowledge.
2. Fadiman A. The spirit catches you and you fall down: a Hmong child, her American doctors, and the collision of two cultures. New York: Farrar, Straus and Giroux; 1997.
3. Pinker S. The sense of style: the thinking person's guide to writing in the 21st century. New York: Penguin Books; 2014.

Decision Fatigue

Case

Ellen was a 45-year-old woman with a history of migraines who presented with "trouble getting out the right words." On exam, she had trouble naming certain objects and saying complicated sentences. She had some mild weakness of her right hand. She was rushed for a CT to rule-out intracranial pathology. The CT was read as normal, and she was diagnosed with a migraine. When a new team of clinicians took over her care after a change of shift, they noticed that the CT had been misread and that there was a clot in her left middle cerebral artery, demonstrating a stroke as the cause of her symptoms. By the time this finding was noticed, too much time had elapsed to give her thrombolytic medications (Fig. 6.1).

What Dr. Ishir Was Thinking

Ellen arrived at the ER at about 7:30 AM, just as I was about the leave. Hers was the last case I read that morning after a 15-hours shift. The abnormality on her CT wasn't exactly subtle, at least in retrospect, but it wasn't glaringly obvious either. I had been looking at scans all night and had only eaten a candy bar. There were several trauma cases that night, so I never got a proper break. When I reviewed Ellen's case with the ER doctor who cared for her, he said that he usually looks at the CT scans himself, but didn't do this her case. She too was at the end of her shift having cared for those trauma cases. I was certainly looking forward to getting something to eat and some much-needed sleep, but I didn't feel impaired in any way. It turns out I was wrong about that.

Discussion

Decision fatigue occurs when someone makes a suboptimal decision due to weariness from having made multiple prior decisions. It is worsened by basic needs such as hunger and sleep deprivation. A famous study of decision fatigue examined 1,112 rulings of Israeli parole judges over a 10-month period. It found that they

Fig. 6.1 A CT scan showing a dense middle cerebral artery on the left (red arrow)

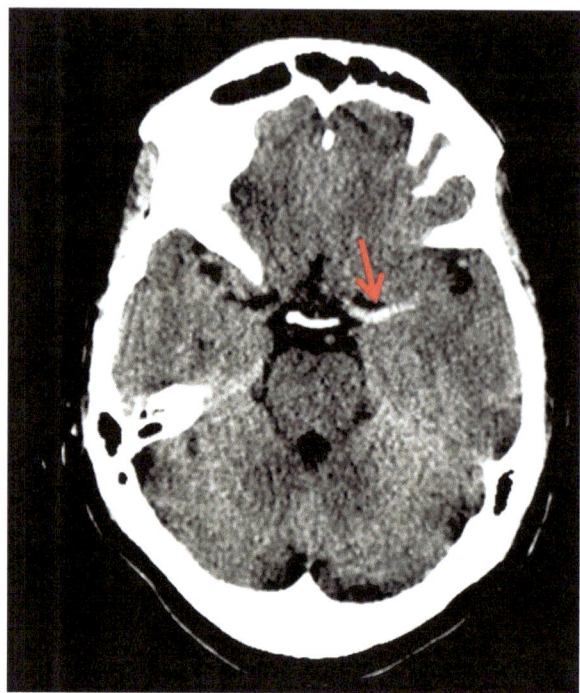

Fig. 6.2 Whether a prisoner was destined for parole depended less on their crime than on whether the judges were well-rested and full. (Danziger S, Levav J, Avnaim-Pesso L. Extraneous factors in judicial decisions [Figure 1]. Proc Natl Acad Sci 2011;108(17):6889–6892. https://doi.org/10.1073/pnas.1018033108.)

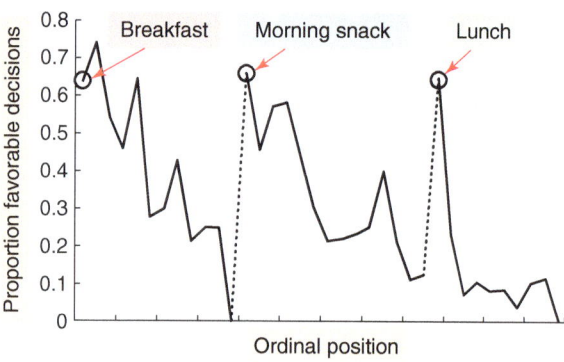

granted a favorable decision to nearly 65% of the prisoners who appeared first [1]. The odds of a favorable decision decreased steadily throughout the morning, such that before lunch, almost no prisoners received a favorable decision. Immediately after a morning snack and lunch, any given prisoner again had about a 65% chance of being granted a favorable decision. After this, the odds gradually decreased to nearly 0% by the end of the day. Rather than consider the merits of each case, the tired judges simply did what was easiest, though they were almost certainly unaware of this (Fig. 6. 2).

Most people choose to solve problems with as little mental effort as possible and are termed cognitive misers. We use mental shortcuts and heuristics as much as possible, a strategy which is often rational given the number of decisions we all make daily. As with physical exertion, people have a limited reserve of mental energy. After engaging in difficult mental tasks, we may become tired and sloppy in our thinking. Recognizing this, some high achievers, such as Barack Obama and Mark Zuckerberg, made a conscious decision to wear similar clothes daily. By limiting the number of decisions they have to make, they hope to reserve their mental energy for more consequential matters [2].

The effects of decision fatigue have been documented in medicine. Jeffrey Linder and colleagues examined 21,867 cases of acute respiratory infections over 18 months in primary care practices [3]. They found that antibiotics were prescribed in 44% of these visits, and the likelihood antibiotics would be prescribed increased throughout the day. Compared to the first hour, the probability of a patient receiving antibiotics increased by 1% in the second hour, 14% in the third hour, and 26% in the fourth hour. As many of the antibiotic prescriptions were inappropriate, the authors concluded that these findings support "the hypothesis that decision fatigue progressively impairs clinicians' ability to resist ordering inappropriate treatments." Dr. Linder wrote about these findings, "The radical notion here is that doctors are people too, and we may be fatigued and make worse decisions toward the end of our clinic sessions" [4]. A similar performance degradation has been found with gastroenterologists performing colonoscopies. One study found that cases performed early in the morning yielded 20% more polyps per patient than later cases [5]. Another study found that their ability to detect polyps deteriorated after only three hours of work [6].

All clinicians will be familiar with the experience of being exhausted beyond belief, driven to the limits of human endurance. Pamela Wible, a doctor and advocate for clinician wellness, has collected multiple sobering anecdotes from sleep-deprived clinicians, detailing both harms to patients and themselves. One told her:

I have made numerous medication errors from being over tired. I also more recently misread an EKG because I was so tired I literally couldn't see straight. She actually had a subarachnoid hemorrhage, and by misreading the EKG, I spent too much time on her heart and didn't whisk her back to CT when she came in code blue. She died [7].

Another said:

I ran a red light driving home in residency after a 36-hour shift. Got pulled over. It was sobering: I was not fit to use my driver's license, but I had just been using my MEDICAL license for over a day non-stop!

Several studies support these anecdotes of exhausted clinicians giving suboptimal care to their patients. A study conducted in 1971 by Richard Friedman and colleagues found that interns who had worked a 24-hour shift made almost twice as many errors interpreting electrocardiograms as did well-rested interns [8]. In a study of 1,412 junior doctors in New Zealand by Phillipa Gander and colleagues,

30% scored "excessively sleepy" on a sleep-rating scale, 42% reported an error in the prior six months due to fatigue, and 24% reported falling asleep while driving home [9]. A survey of 2,737 interns by Laura Barger and colleagues found that:

Fatigue-related preventable adverse events associated with the death of the patient increased by about 300% in interns working more than five extended-duration shifts per month; they were also more likely to fall asleep during lectures, rounds, and clinical activities, including surgery [10].

Two randomized trials from 2004 show how fatigue can impair an intern's performance. A study by Christopher Landrigan and colleagues examined a total of 2,203 patient-days involving 634 admissions. They found that interns made 35.9% more serious medical errors working a traditional schedule (a 24-hour shift every third night), compared to a schedule where the work hours were reduced [11]. A study by Steven Lockley and colleagues of 20 interns working in intensive care units found that reducing their work hours improved their sleep and that well-rested interns had half the rate of attentional failures compared to their sleep-deprived peers [12].

Importantly, there is a universal tendency for people to underestimate how basic physiological states such as fatigue, hunger, depression, addiction, and sexual arousal influence their own attitudes and behaviors, a phenomenon known as the hot-cold empathy gap [13]. The hot-cold empathy is bidirectional.

1. **Hot-to-cold:** People in a hot state, under the influence of powerful bodily drives, fail to grasp how much of their behavior is influenced by their condition. They may act as if their short-term desires reflect their overall preferences. This is why people do things "in the heat of the moment" that are difficult to fathom in a calmer state of mind.
2. **Cold-to-hot:** People in a cold state lack insight into how they might behave in a hot state, minimizing the power of visceral impulses. When we are calm, well-rested, and well-fed, the behavior of people who are angry, tired, and hungry may seem incomprehensible.

Daniel Read and George Loewenstein provided a demonstration of the hot-cold empathy gap by asking three groups of subjects how much money it would take to convince them to experience the pain of immersing their hand in ice water [14]. Subjects who had just immersed their hand (hot state) demanded the most money for doing it again. Subjects who had never done it at all (cold state) demanded the least amount of money, while subjects who had done it a week prior demanded an intermediate payment.

The effects of the hot-cold empathy gap are twofold. First of all, worn-out clinicians are unlikely to appreciate how impaired they are. Secondly, these clinicians are likely to receive little sympathy from well-rested critics. For many clinicians, especially those in the surgical specialties, saying "I'm tired" is essentially equivalent to saying, "I'm incompetent and I don't care." William Halsted, a giant of American medicine and the first surgical chief at Johns Hopkins, gave his residents three days off per year. His work ethic (which was partially fueled by cocaine) persists today. I remember the senior resident during my surgical rotation telling me, "We are surgeons. We don't get tired." This not uncommon attitude is a form of the overconfidence bias, as clinicians behave as if they are superhuman, immune from basic human needs.

Additionally, the general public is unlikely to be sympathetic to tired clinicians. In 2015, someone snapped some pictures of a young doctor sleeping at a desk a 3 AM and wrote, "We are aware that this is a tiring job but doctors are obliged to do their work. There are dozens of patients in need of attention" [15]. Fortunately, hundreds of other doctors responded by defending this exhausted doctor, posting pictures of themselves sleeping at the hospital [16]. Despite this, no patient would want to be cared for by an exhausted clinician. Most people recognize that even clinicians are affected by sleep deprivation.

The movement to legally limit clinicians' working hours began with the death of 18-year-old Libby Zion in Manhattan in 1984. Libby arrived at the ER with a fever, confusion, and abnormal movements. She was given sedatives, one of which interacted with an antidepressant she was taking. This resulted in a condition known as serotonin syndrome. Libby developed a high fever, went into cardiac arrest, and died later that night. The two young doctors in charge of her care were overworked, under-rested, and poorly supervised.

Her father, Sidney Zion, a journalist and lawyer, was able to bring considerable attention to his daughter's case. At the time, residents worked up to 120 hours per week and endured shifts up to 36 hours long. "You don't need kindergarten," he wrote after her death, "to know that a resident working a 36-hour shift is in no condition to make any kind of judgment call – forget about life-and-death" [17]. As a result of Libby's death, New York State passed a law limiting resident doctors' work hours to 80 per week. This law became a model for residents throughout the country when the Accreditation Council for Graduate Medical Education (ACGME) adopted similar regulations in 2003. These rules stated that residents cannot spend more than 80 hours a week on duty (averaged over four weeks), they cannot work over 30 hours at one time, overnight calls cannot be more than every third night, there must be at least 10 hours off-duty between shifts, and one day in seven must be free from all work. Of course, these "limits" still permit residents to work an extreme number of hours. After all, an 80-hours work week averages to over 11 hours every day. Additionally, these regulations do not account for individual variability. Some people simply need more sleep than others.

Despite the undeniable impact fatigue has on clinician performance, formal evidence that reducing resident work hours improves patient outcomes is mixed. Kanaka Shetty and Jayanta Bhattacharya examined 1,268,738 medical patients both before and after the ACGME work hour regulations were implemented. They found work hour reductions were associated with a 0.25% reduction in the absolute mortality rate [18]. Kevin Volppe and colleagues examined the outcomes of 318,636 patients at teaching hospitals in Veterans Affairs (VA) system and found a significant relative improvement in mortality in common medical conditions, but no change in surgical patients [19]. Another study by Amy Rosen and colleagues analyzed outcomes from over 14 million VA and Medicare patients and found that patient safety indicators did not change after the ACGME 2003 reforms [20].

Several controlled trials of different work patterns have failed to demonstrate that limiting doctors' work hours benefits patients. Sanjay Desai randomly assigned four medical house staff teams to care for patients under different work-hour models [21]. They found that interns who were on call less often or used a night float system slept more, but there were "deteriorations in educational opportunities, continuity of patient care, and perceived quality of care." The quality of care under the night float system was perceived to be so poor that it was terminated before the study ended. Karl Bilimoria and colleagues randomized 117 general surgery residencies to adhere to the ACGME work rules or to waive them, allowing residents to work longer hours. They analyzed outcomes from 138,691 patients, and found no difference in their outcome. There was also no difference in the residents' satisfaction with their education and overall well-being [22]. In response to these studies, the ACGME relaxed its rules in 2016 to allow residents to work 24-hour shifts (with another 4 hours to perform non-patient care duties), up from 16 hours.

There are several possible explanations for these inconclusive findings. The first is that compliance with the ACGME work regulations may be less than perfect. Residents are periodically asked about their work hours, and several prominent programs, such as Yale and Johns Hopkins, faced disciplinary action for work-hour violations [23]. As such penalties will negatively impact their own training and careers, there is a strong disincentive for many residents to honestly report work-hour violations. In one study of 253 neurosurgery residents, 60% reported that they had underreported duty hours at least once, and almost 25% reported doing it consistently [24]. At times, I lied about the number of hours I worked during residency. Telling the truth would have only invited unwanted attention and scorn.

Additionally, limiting clinicians' work hours may reduce clinician fatigue, but it creates other problems. In today's hospitals, patients may be transitioned from one clinician to another several times per day. As a result, no one single clinician may feel "ownership" of a patient's care. As neurosurgeon Larry Schlachter said, "Things have evolved now to the point where doctors are shift workers. They don't care as much. They don't feel that responsibility as much." Moreover, these transitions of care create multiple opportunities for communication breakdowns with potentially devastating consequences for patients. As a result of handoff-related errors, the ACGME mandated formal handoff training in 2010. A study by Amy Starmer and colleagues showed that with the use of standardized handoffs, the medical-error rate decreased by 23% and the rate of preventable adverse events decreased by 30% compared to the pre-intervention period.

While the impact of clinician fatigue on patients has received the most attention, equally worrisome are the effects on the clinicians themselves. This includes depression, burn-out, and the tragic fact that accidents are not uncommon among tired clinicians. For example, Ronak Patel, a trainee anesthesiologist, died at age 33 after working three consecutive night shifts [25]. He was singing with his wife on the phone, trying to stay awake, when he hit an oncoming truck. In a study by Laura McClelland and colleagues of 2,155 anesthetist trainees, nearly 90% used caffeinated drinks to stay awake and 57% reported have being involved in an accident or near miss after a long shift [26]. As Dr. McClelland said, "These are very worrying findings. Junior doctors are putting their lives at risk due to fatigue resulting from their shift work and the lack of rest facilities at their hospitals both during and after shifts" [27]. Another survey of 2,737 interns found that every extended work shift per month increased the monthly risk of a motor vehicle crash by 9% overall and by 16.2% during the commute home from work [28]. Recognizing that even seemingly small amount of sleep deprivation can be quite dangerous, traffic safety expert Jake Nelson said, "If you have not slept seven or more hours in a given 24-hour period, you really shouldn't be behind the wheel of a car" [29]. Sleep deprivation is also linked to chronic diseases such as obesity, diabetes, and cardiovascular disease.

Depression and burnout are also unfortunately very common in exhausted, overworked clinicians. As Daniel Barron, a psychiatrist, wrote:

Medical trainees are not depressed or suicidal because they are disgruntled (though for some this may be the case). They are depressed—5.7% are suicidal—because they have been pushed beyond their human, physiological limit by chronic stress and sleep deprivation; because in the intensive care unit or on the medical floors they've stared disease and death in the face; because despite courageous efforts, they have watched patients' fragile lives slip away [30].

One doctor quoted by Dr. Wible said:

I was struck down with a very severe depression in the context of emotional conflicts and severe sleep deprivation, after doing a surgical rotation with every other night call and lots of degrading comments from the surgeons recommending that I go into nursing or teaching instead since those were "good professions for women." This was 1983. I was supported in the sense that I missed six weeks of medical school without censure while I was too debilitated to move physically. I spent those weeks mainly sitting in a corner of my apartment, crying, and seeing my psychiatrist once/week for therapy and meds [31].

Again, studies confirm these anecdotes. In 2016, Lisa Totenstein and colleagues published a meta-analysis of over 120,000 medical students from around the world. They found that 27% had depression or depressive symptoms, that 11% reported suicidal ideation, and 15.7% sought psychiatric treatment [32]. All of these were higher than the general population. A study of over 2,000 medical interns by Constance Guille and colleagues found that depression was significantly more common in females than males [33]. They found that work-family conflict best explained this discrepancy and that prior to starting their internship, depression rates were similar between males and females.

Unfortunately, a denial of depression and a refusal to seek help for it is common in doctors in particular. As Dr. Wibble wrote:

Medical training teaches us to "suck it up," so help-seeking is not a well-honed skill among doctors. Many lack self-awareness that they are suffering from depression. Because the majority of doctors are overworked, exhausted, and discontent, they don't necessarily see themselves as outliers. They've normalized their misery and pretend that it's not as bad as it seems. Distraction, avoidance, and denial are popular tactics among depressed doctors. I believe that most physicians do not seek the appropriate care that they would recommend for their own depressed patients [34].

Unfortunately, not all clinicians' reluctance to seek help for mental health concerns is due to stubborn denial. In some states, clinicians are explicitly asked about their mental health when obtaining a license. A survey by Liselotte Dyrbye and colleagues found that, "Nearly 40% of physicians (2,323 of 5,829) reported that they would be reluctant to seek formal medical care for treatment of a mental health condition because of concerns about repercussions to their medical licensure" [35]. In a similar survey by Tait Shanafelt and colleagues, 6.3% of surgeons reported having suicidal thoughts in the past year [36]. Only a minority of them sought psychiatric or psychological treatment, and 60% were reluctant to do so for fears that it might affect their medical license.

The consequences of this can be lethal for doctors and medical students. Unfortunately, suicides are not rare events for this population. As of December 2017, Dr. Wible has studied 723 doctor suicides [37]. She correctly calls this a public health crisis, one that has almost been completely ignored by the medical community.

Finally, when clinicians are depressed, burnt-out, and miserable, they are unlikely to give their patients optimal care. A study by Jennifer Haas and colleagues asked 2,620 patients and 166 doctors about their level of satisfaction. It found that, "The patients of physicians who have higher professional satisfaction may themselves be more satisfied with their care" [38]. In the same way that no patient would want to be care for be a sleep-deprived clinician, no patient would want to be cared for by a clinician that hated his job.

Conclusion

Decision fatigue occurs when people make suboptimal decisions because they are exhausted and worn out from having made multiple previous decisions. Healthcare is a 24/7, 365 enterprise. As such, there are times when all clinicians will have to work while tired or hungry. While there has been increased awareness devoted to the impact of sleep deprivation and overall wellness on clinician performance in recent years, historically a tired clinician was thought to be a weak one. Still today large swaths of medicine, especially the surgical specialties, do not reward clinicians who admit to being impaired due to fatigue or hunger. As Dr. Landrigan said, "Doctors think they're a special class and not subject to normal limitations of physiology" [39].

Clinicians are human. As such, they should strive to recognize when they are impaired by basic human needs. Minimizing patient care during these times is a sign of strength, not weakness. A clinician who continues to care for patients while fatigued is scarcely different from a surgeon who operates with an injured hand. Clinicians should be encouraged to take naps and breaks if they feel their performance might be impaired. Similarly, they should be taught to recognize signs of fatigue and burnout in their peers, encouraging them to rest if they feel they are unable to safely care for patients.

References

1. Danziger S, Levav J, Avnaim-Pesso L. Extraneous factors in judicial decisions. Proc Natl Acad Sci. 2011;108(17):6889–92. https://doi.org/10.1073/pnas.1018033108.
2. Baer D. (2015, April 28). The scientific reason why Barack Obama and Mark Zuckerberg wear the same outfit every day. Business Insider. Retrieved from https://www.businessinsider.com/barack-obama-mark-zuckerberg-wear-the-same-outfit-2015-4.
3. Linder JA, Doctor JN, Friedberg MW, Nieva HR, Birks C, Meeker D, Fox CR. Time of day and the decision to prescribe antibiotics. JAMA Intern Med. 2014;174(12):2029–31. https://doi.org/10.1001/jamainternmed.2014.5225.

4. Bakalar N. (2014, Oct 27). Doctors and decision fatigue [Blog post]. The New York Times. Retrieved from https://well.blogs.nytimes.com/2014/10/27/doctors-and-decision-fatigue/.

5. Chan MY, Cohen H, Spiegel BMR. Fewer polyps detected by colonoscopy as the day progresses at a Veteran's Administration teaching hospital. Clin Gastroenterol Hepatol. 2009;7(11):1217–23. https://doi.org/10.1016/j.cgh.2009.07.013.

6. Almadi MA, Sewitch M, Barkun AN, Martel M, Joseph L. Adenoma detection rates decline with increasing procedural hours in an endoscopist's workload. Clin Gastroenterol Hepatol. 2015;29(6):304–8. https://doi.org/10.1155/2015/789038.

7. Wible P. (2017, Mar 12). The secret horrors of sleep-deprived doctors [Blog post]. KevinMD. com. Retrieved from https://www.kevinmd.com/blog/2017/03/secret-horrors-sleep-deprived-doctors.html.

8. Friedman RC, Bigger T, Kornfeld DS. The intern and sleep loss. N Engl J Med. 1971;285(4):201–3. https://doi.org/10.1056/NEJM197107222850405.

9. Gander P, Purnell H, Garden A, Woodward A. Work patterns and fatigue-related risk among junior doctors. Occup Environ Med. 2007;64(11):733–8. https://doi.org/10.1136/oem.2006.030916.

10. Barger LK, Ayas NT, Cade BE, Cronin JW, Rosner B, Speizer FE, Czeisler CA. Impact of extended-duration shifts on medical errors, adverse events, and attentional failures. PLoS Med. 2006;3(12):e487. https://doi.org/10.1371/journal.pmed.0030487.

11. Landrigan CP, Rothschild JM, Cronin JW, Kaushal R, Burdick E, Katz JT, Lilly CM, Stone PH, Lockley SW, Bates DW, Czeisler CA. Effect of reducing interns' work hours on serious medical errors in intensive care units. N Engl J Med. 2004;351(18):1838–48. https://doi.org/10.1056/NEJMoa041406.

12. Lockley SW, Cronin JW, Evans EE, Cade BE, Lee CJ, Landrigan CP, Rothschild JM, Katz JT, Lilly CM, Stone PH, Aeschbach D, Czeisler CA. Effect of reducing interns' weekly work hours on sleep and attentional failures. N Engl J Med. 2004;351(18):1829–37. https://doi.org/10.1056/NEJMoa041404.

13. Van Boven L, Loewenstein G, Dunning D, Nordgren LF. Chapter three – changing places: a dual judgment model of empathy gaps in emotional perspective taking. Adv Exp Soc Psychol. 2013;48:117–71. https://doi.org/10.1016/B978-0-12-407188-9.00003-X.

14. Read D, Loewenstein G. Enduring pain for money: decisions based on the perception and memory of pain. J Behav Decis Mak. 1999;12(1):1–17. https://doi.org/10.1002/(SICI)1099-0771(199903)12:1<1::AID-BDM310>3.0.CO;2-V.

15. A blog posted photos shaming a doctor for sleeping on the job and it started a social media movement. (2015, May 20). Sunny Skyz. Retrieved 15 Sept 2018 from https://www.sunny-skyz.com/good-news/1165/A-Blog-Posted-Photos-Shaming-A-Doctor-For-Sleeping-On-The-Job-And-It-Started-A-Social-Media-Movement.

16. Dovas. (n.d.). Doctors post pics where they sleep at work to defend med resident caught asleep. Retrieved 15 Sept 2018 from https://www.boredpanda.com/medical-resident-sleeping-overworked-doctors-mexico-yo-tambien-mi-dormi/.

17. Lerner BH. (2006, Nov 28). A case that shook medicine. The Washington Post. Retrieved from http://www.washingtonpost.com/wp-dyn/content/article/2006/11/24/AR2006112400985.html.

18. Shetty KD, Bhattacharya J. Changes in hospital mortality associated with residency work-hour regulations. Ann Intern Med. 2007;147(2):73–80. https://doi.org/10.7326/0003-4819-147-2-200707170-00161.

19. Volpp KG, Rosen AK, Rosenbaum PR, Romano PS, Even-Shoshan O, Canamucio A, Bellini L, Behringer T, Silber JH. Mortality among patients in VA Hospitals in the first 2 years following ACGME resident duty hour reform. JAMA. 2007;298(9):984–92. https://doi.org/10.1001/jama.298.9.984.

20. Rosen AK, Loveland SA, Romano PS, Itani KMF, Silber JH, Even-Shoshan OO, Halenar MJ, Teng Y, Zhu J, Volpp KG. Effects of resident duty hour reform on surgical and procedural patient safety indicators among hospitalized Veterans Health Administration and Medicare patients. Med Care. 2009;47(7):723–31. https://doi.org/10.1097/MLR.0b013e31819a588f.

21. Desai SV, Feldman L, Brown L, Dezube R, Yeh HC, Punjabi N, Afshar K, Grunwald MR, Harrington C, Naik R, Cofrancesco J. Effect of the 2011 vs 2003 duty hour regulation-compliant models on sleep duration, trainee education, and continuity of patient care among internal medicine house staff: a randomized trial. JAMA Intern Med. 2013;173(8):649–55. https://doi.org/10.1001/jamainternmed.2013.2973.

22. Bilimoria KY, Chung JW, Hedges LV, Dahlke AR, Love R, Cohen ME, Hoyt DB, Yang AD, Tarpley JL, Mellinger JD, Mahvi DM, Kelz RR, Ko CY, Odell DD, Stulberg JJ, Lewis FR. National cluster-randomized trial of duty-hour flexibility in surgical training. N Engl J Med. 2016;374(8):713–27. https://doi.org/10.1056/NEJMoa1515724.
23. Miller ED. (2004). Times of trouble. Johns Hopkins Medicine News. Retrieved 15 Sept 2018 from https://www.hopkinsmedicine.org/mediaII/Enews/PostOp.html.
24. Fargen KM, Dow J, Tomei KL, Friedman WA. Follow-up on a national survey: American neurosurgery resident opinions on the 2011 accreditation council for graduate medical education-implemented duty hours. World Neurosurg. 2014;81(1):15–21. https://doi.org/10.1016/j.wneu.2013.08.015.
25. Dr Ronak Patel 'had been singing to stay awake' before fatal crash. (2016, July 12). BBC News. Retrieved from https://www.bbc.com/news/uk-england-suffolk-36767868.
26. McClelland L, Holland J, Lomas JP, Redfern N, Plunkett E. A national survey of the effects of fatigue on trainees in anaesthesia in the UK. Anaesthesia. 2017;72(9):1069–77. https://doi.org/10.1111/anae.13965.
27. Campbell D. (2017, July 6). Half of junior doctors having accidents or near misses after night shifts. The Guardian. Retrieved from https://www.theguardian.com/society/2017/jul/06/half-of-junior-doctors-having-accidents-or-near-misses-after-night-shifts.
28. Barger LK, Cade BE, Ayas NT, Cronin JW, Rosner B, Speizer FE, Czeisler CA. Extended work shifts and the risk of motor vehicle crashes among interns. N Engl J Med. 2005;352(2):125–34. https://doi.org/10.1056/NEJMoa041401.
29. Aubrey A. (2016, Dec 6). Drivers beware: crash rate spikes with every hour of lost sleep. National Public Radio. Retrieved from https://www.npr.org/sections/health-shots/2016/12/06/504448639/drivers-beware-crash-rate-spikes-with-every-hour-of-lost-sleep.
30. Barron D. (2016, Dec 19). Should we let doctors-in-training be more sleep-deprived? [Blog post]. Scientific American. Retrieved from https://blogs.scientificamerican.com/mind-guest-blog/should-we-let-doctors-in-training-be-more-sleep-deprived/.
31. Wible P. (2017, Mar 12). The secret horrors of sleep-deprived doctors [Blog post]. KevinMD.com. Retrieved 15 Sept 2018 from http://www.kevinmd.com/blog/2017/03/secret-horrors-sleep-deprived-doctors.html.
32. Rotenstein LS, Ramos MA, Torre M, Segal JB, Peluso MJ, Guille C, Sen S, Mata DA. Prevalence of depression, depressive symptoms, and suicidal ideation among medical students: a systematic review and meta-analysis. JAMA. 2016;316(21):2214–36. https://doi.org/10.1001/jama.2016.17324.
33. Guille C, Frank E, Zhao Z, Kalmbach DA, Nietert PJ, Mata DA, Sen S. Work-family conflict and the sex difference in depression among training physicians. JAMA Intern Med. 2017;177(12):1766–72. https://doi.org/10.1001/jamainternmed.2017.5138.
34. Wible P. (2017, May 11). Doctors and depression: suffering in silence. Medscape. Retrieved from https://www.medscape.com/viewarticle/879379_2.
35. Dyrbye LN, West CP, Sinsky CA, Goeders LE, Satele DV, Shanafelt TD. Medical licensure questions and physician reluctance to seek care for mental health conditions. Mayo Clin Proc. 2017;92(10):1486–93. https://doi.org/10.1016/j.mayocp.2017.06.020.
36. Shanafelt TD, Balch CM, Dyrbye L, Bechamps G, Russell T, Satele D, Rummans T, Swartz K, Novotny PJ, Sloan J, Oreskovich MR. Special report: suicidal ideation among American surgeons. Arch Surg. 2011;146(1):54–62. https://doi.org/10.1001/archsurg.2010.292.
37. Wible P. (2017, Oct 28). What I've learned from 1,013 doctor suicides. Pamela Wible MD. Retrieved from http://www.idealmedicalcare.org/ive-learned-547-doctor-suicides/.
38. Haas JS, Cook EF, Puopolo AL, Burstin HR, Cleary PD, Brennan TA. Is the professional satisfaction of general internists associated with patient satisfaction. J Gen Intern Med. 2000;15(2):122–8. https://doi.org/10.1046/j.1525-1497.2000.02219.x.
39. Sanghavi D. (2011, Aug 5). The phantom menace of sleep-deprived doctors. The New York Times. Retrieved from https://www.nytimes.com/2011/08/07/magazine/the-phantom-menace-of-sleep-deprived-doctors.html.

Case

Tracy was a 24-year-old woman who presented with two weeks of numbness in her legs and hands and weakness in her legs. An MRI of the cervical spine revealed a large lesion shown in Fig. 7.1. A brain MRI was normal.

The radiologist read the lesion as a spinal cord tumor as shown below.

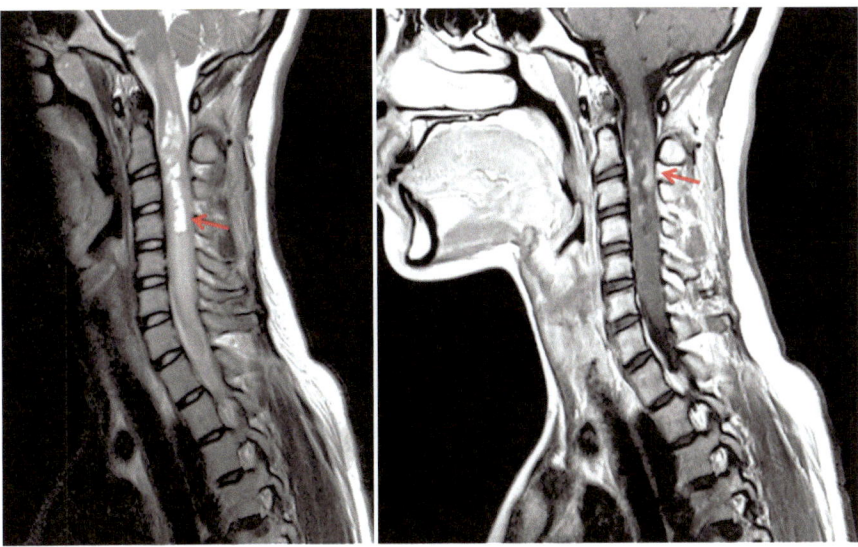

Fig. 7.1 A sagittal STIR and post-contrast T1-weighted MRI show a large, actively inflamed lesion in the cervical spine (red arrows)

© Springer International Publishing AG, part of Springer Nature 2019
J. Howard, *Cognitive Errors and Diagnostic Mistakes*,
https://doi.org/10.1007/978-3-319-93224-8_7

Impression:
Normal MRI appearance of the brain with and without contrast. Extensive intramedullary cord signal abnormality and expansion from the cervicomedullary junction to the upper thoracic spine with patchy areas of enhancement and suggestion of segmental central canal dilatation.
Primary differential considerations include infiltrative intramedullary mass such as astrocytoma less likely ependymoma.

Based on the radiologist's suspicion of a tumor, Tracy was sent for a spinal cord biopsy. The biopsy revealed demyelinating disease, and based on subsequent tests, she was diagnosed with neuromyelitis optica (NMO). NMO is an uncommon, inflammatory condition that presents with acute episodes of visual loss, weakness in the extremities, or brainstem syndromes that present with nausea, vomiting, and hiccups. It is diagnosed with a blood test, and there is no role for a biopsy in such patients. The radiologist had read several MRIs of the spine in a similar manner before a neurologist informed him that these cases had turned out to be NMO.

What Dr. Sheploh Was Thinking
I was obviously not thrilled that I misread the initial scan as a spinal cord tumor when it turned out to be NMO. However, learning that I had made the mistake several times previously was really disturbing. I work at an independent MRI facility, and we receive referrals from several neurological practices throughout the city. As such, we almost never have interactions with the referring doctors. When a radiologist makes an error, the consequences are almost never immediate, and in my defense, no one ever told me the outcome of these cases. So it was not really possible for me to know that I was making this mistake.

We have since instituted dinners twice per year where we invite referring doctors to give us honest feedback on any mistakes we may have made and to discuss diagnostic mysteries. We also make it clear on our reports that the referring doctor should contact us if they feel our reports are not adequate or erroneous in any way. I also try to follow-up with a phone call to the referring doctor to learn more about ambiguous cases. Ultimately, it is my responsibility to follow-up on such cases and improve my skills, not that of the referring doctor.

I should also note that NMO was not a disease that was really discussed much in my training. Although historical descriptions of it exist, the blood test used to diagnose it was only discovered in 2004. This was not something that was on my radar as much as it should have been. While it is not a common disease, I have since made the diagnosis perhaps five times in the past few years. So learning about my mistake was definitely worth it.

Discussion
Feedback sanction is a form of ignorance trap and time-delay trap. Making an error may carry no immediate consequences, as considerable time may elapse before the error is discovered, if it is discovered at all. Additionally, poor system feedback

processes may prevent important information from getting back to the decision maker. The particular error that failed the patient persists because of these temporal and systemic sanctions. Pat Croskerry summarized the problem by saying:

> *The following features have been identified as obstructive to optimal feedback operation: incomplete awareness of the significance of the problem, excessive time and work pressures, case infrequency, deficiencies in specialty follow-up, communication failures, deficient reporting systems for near-misses, error, and adverse events, biases in case review processes, shift changeover times, and shiftwork* [1].

In many cases, the consequences of an error are clear and immediate. If a surgeon nicks an artery, the problem will be immediate and obvious. In other instances, however, the connection between an intervention and a negative outcome might be so distant that only careful scientific studies can uncover the relationship. For example, diethylstilbestrol (DES) is a synthetic estrogen that was given to pregnant women from 1940 to 1971 to prevent miscarriages and premature labor. It was only discovered many years later that women whose mothers took DES during pregnancy were at much higher risk of developing clear cell adenocarcinoma of the vagina as well as fertility problems themselves. A similar situation occurred more recently with the pain medication rofecoxib (Vioxx™), which was withdrawn from the market after it was found to increase the risk of heart attacks and strokes. The situation with rofecoxib was worse in that the drug manufacturer withheld evidence of its dangers.

Of course, it would not be fair to say that a clinician made an "error" by using a medication that was found to cause a problem many years later. By definition, knowledge of long-term side effects emerges only after a drug has been on the market for many years, sometimes decades. Additionally, a medication often needs to be taken by large numbers of people before rare side effects are identified. If clinicians were to restrict their use of medications to those that have been available for decades, they would just now begin to use treatments approved in the 1990s. I use several medications to treat multiple sclerosis (MS) that are less than five years old. There are not decades of safety data on these medications.

This shows the importance of phase IV trials in minimizing feedback sanction. These studies are carried out after a medication is in general use to gather information on side effects due to long-term use or rare side effects that might not have emerged during earlier trials. Such trials are usually relatively small and of short duration. Indeed significant side effects have been elucidated in some of these medications after their approval. In the phase III trials of the MS medication natalizumab, there were two cases of a serious, even fatal, brain infection, progressive multifocal leukoencephalopathy (PML). In the 13 years since its approval, there have been over 750 cases, and information has emerged that allows clinicians to better determine a patient's risk of this infection. With two other drugs for MS, fingolimod and dimethyl fumarate, there were no cases of PML in the phase III clinical trials. Since their approval, there have been nearly 30 cases with these medications, a relatively small number, but not zero. To their credit, the pharmaceutical companies that make these medications have been active in information on these cases and sending updates to clinicians several times per year.

Potential long-term harms are not just limited to medications. In most hospitals, whenever a patient presents with head trauma, however minor, they are often sent for a CT scan to evaluate for intracranial bleeding. In hospitalized patients who fall, it is essentially a given that they will be sent for a CT. The pressure to order a scan "just to make sure" is large. Clinicians who use their clinical acumen to determine when head CTs are unnecessary are unlikely to be rewarded for their judicious use of this test. However, CTs are not benign. They are a source of radiation, and especially in patients who have received multiple CT scans, the cumulative risk of cancer is small, but not negligible. Any cancer resulting from such radiation will occur many years or even decades after the scan was done.

Feedback sanction occurs not only when there is a long temporal lag between the action and bad outcome, but also if the bad outcome doesn't reach the responsible clinician. Too often there is no mechanism for clinicians to learn about their errors. Formal mentoring is virtually unheard of in medicine once training ends. After employing a coach to observe him in the operating room, Atul Gawande commented that many of his peers found this unusual. However, he wrote:

> The stranger thing, it occurred to me, was that no senior colleague had come to observe me in the eight years since I'd established my surgical practice. Like most work, medical practice is largely unseen by anyone who might raise one's sights. I'd had no outside ears and eyes [2].

Even when errors are observed, many people are too timid to speak out. At times, a failure to speak out against an error can have devastating consequences. For example, the former Secretary of State, Colin Powell, famously gave a speech to the United Nations in 2003, in which he used faulty intelligence to describe nonexistent Iraqi weapons programs. This helped lead to the Iraq war and will remain a major stain on his record. He later said about the intelligence failures that, "There were some people in the intelligence community who knew at that time that some of these sources were not good, and shouldn't be relied upon, and they didn't speak up. That devastated me" [3].

Silence is often a problem in medicine as well. In my experience, except for egregious mistakes, it is not common for clinicians to inform each other when an error has been made. Though I don't purport to catch too many errors from my colleagues, other than pointing a missed finding to a radiologist, I can't remember the last time I've done it. This is not something to be proud of.

My reluctance to discuss errors with my colleagues does not make me unique. Thomas Gallagher and colleagues identified several reasons why clinicians may be reluctant to discuss errors with each other [4]. These include:

- Clinicians may not feel they know everything about a case if they were not directly involved in it.
- Clinicians may not want to gain an unfavorable reputation with their colleagues.
- Junior clinicians may have trouble challenging more senior clinicians.

- Clinicians may not want their colleagues to face malpractice claims or formal sanction. They may be worried about becoming embroiled in such proceedings themselves if they report an error.
- Clinicians may depend on each other for business.
- Clinicians may expect retaliation if they report a colleague's error. As Brant Mittler, a cardiologist who became a medical malpractice attorney said, "There's not a culture where people care about feedback. You figure that if you make them mad they'll come after you in peer review and quality assurance. They'll figure out a way to get back at you" [5].
- Clinicians face time constraints and coordinating meetings with multiple clinicians and administrators.
- Clinicians may be loath to damage a relationship between a patient and their clinician when there is an ongoing relationship.

However, as John Meagher, a family and ER doctor wrote, "Giving and receiving negative feedback is a duty of all healthcare professionals" [6]. Moreover, as Dr. Croskerry has pointed out, not giving negative feedback can be interpreted as positive feedback. Though it requires some courage and tact, clinicians should not be afraid to notify their colleagues if they feel they have made an error, especially if it is one that is likely to reoccur. In the same way that clinicians are mandated reporters when they suspect child abuse, certain hospitals require clinicians to report all errors, even if no patients were harmed [5].

The duty of clinicians to give negative feedback implies that clinicians should be open-minded when receiving criticism from other clinicians, as well as from patients and their families. Most people's instinct when criticized is to reject the criticism as quickly and forcefully as possible. Clearly, this is a mistake, as the best source for identifying bias in oneself is almost always feedback from others.

Additionally, clinicians should strive to seek information on patients who were only temporarily in their care, though their ability to do so may be limited by regulations that protect patient privacy. ER clinicians, for example, may only learn whether they made proper decisions if they make the effort to follow-up on at least some patients after their shifts have ended. Even on hospital wards, treatment teams usually change every few weeks, and clinicians who don't follow-up on patients may be unaware that an error was made.

Feedback sanction can be mitigated through formal mechanisms, such as peer-review committees and morbidity and mortality (M&M) conferences. M&Ms are periodic conferences where poor patient outcomes are reviewed. The conference is confidential and not designed to be punitive, but rather to identify problems and propose potential solutions. In this way, clinicians may become aware of errors that might have otherwise escaped their notice. Many hospitals also have committees that perform a root cause analysis when patients have poor outcomes.

Conclusion
Many errors go unnoticed because there is a large time lag between the error and its consequences or because there are inadequate mechanisms for clinicians to learn

about these errors. For many medical treatments or tests, long-term harms can only be revealed by diligent scientific investigations.

Medicine is generally a self-regulating profession. Currently, there are few feedback mechanisms by which clinicians can learn about anything other than their most obvious errors. However, patients are best served when there is culture where clinicians both receive and ask for feedback. In the words of Dr. Gallagher, clinicians should adopt an "explore, don't ignore" attitude towards potential errors. This exploration needs be done in the spirit of identifying problems and improving patient care, not primarily as a punitive measure. Peer-review committees and formal M&M conferences are crucial for this reason.

References

1. Croskerry P. The feedback sanction. Acad Emerg Med. 2000;7(11):1232–8. https://doi.org/10.1111/j.1553-2712.2000.tb00468.x.
2. Gawande A (2011, Oct 3). Top athletes and singers have coaches. Should you? The New Yorker. Retrieved from https://www.newyorker.com/magazine/2011/10/03/personal-best.
3. Weisman SR. (2005, Sept 9). Powell calls his U.N. speech a lasting blot on his record. The New York Times. Retrieved from https://www.nytimes.com/2005/09/09/politics/powell-calls-his-un-speech-a-lasting-blot-on-his-record.html.
4. Gallagher TH, Mello MM, Levinson W, Wynia MK, Sachdeva AK, Sulmasy LS, Truog RD, Conway J, Mazor K, Lembitz A, Bell SK, Sokol-Hessner L, Shapiro J, Puopolo AL, Arnold R. Talking with patients about other clinicians' errors. N Engl J Med. 2013;369(18):1752–7. https://doi.org/10.1056/NEJMsb1303119.
5. Allen M. (2013, Nov 8). Why doctors stay mum about mistakes their colleagues make. ProPublica. Retrieved from https://www.propublica.org/article/why-doctors-stay-mum-about-mistakes-their-colleagues-make.
6. Meagher J. (2015, Sept 11). Giving negative feedback is a duty. FewerErrors. Retrieved from http://www.fewererrors.com/2015/09/11/giving-negative-feedback-a-duty/.

Financial Bias

Case

Eric was a 56-year-old man who presented with trouble walking and weakness in his legs for eight months. An MRI revealed several herniated discs in his cervical spine with compression of his spinal cord. As he had no insurance, he consulted a neurosurgeon at a local public hospital who said that no operation was indicated and suggested a course of physical therapy. Eric never tried physical therapy. He returned four weeks later, with his insurance re-instated, and saw the same neurosurgeon, though in his private office. The neurosurgeon did not remember Eric from his previous visit. During this appointment, the doctor suggested that Eric schedule an operation the next week.

What Dr. Marcola Was Thinking

If you had told me that I operated on patients primarily for money, I would have vigorously denied the accusation, and I would have been incredibly offended. Yet, this case made it clear how difficult it is to separate my clinical decision-making from the financial incentives. In my private office, when I decide not to operate on a patient, I get paid a few hundred dollars for the consultation. When I operate on a patient, however, I get thousands of dollars. In contrast, at the public hospital, I get paid a flat salary. I get paid the same amount if I operate on 100 patients or no one at all. With spine surgery, there are a lot of borderline cases where it's not always clear who will benefit from surgery and who won't. I guess I was more inclined to operate on patients when I would get paid for doing so.

Discussion

The financial bias occurs when clinicians are influenced by financial compensation rather than the interests of their patients. It is formally known as physician-induced demand, which broadly describes any time a clinician makes a decision that is in their own best interest, not the best interest of their patient [1]. Jack Hadley and colleagues defined physician-induced demand as follows [2]:

© Springer International Publishing AG, part of Springer Nature 2019   109
J. Howard, *Cognitive Errors and Diagnostic Mistakes*,
https://doi.org/10.1007/978-3-319-93224-8_8

The concept of physician-created demand or demand-inducement refers to the physician's alleged ability to shift patients' demand for medical care at a given price, that is, to convince patients to increase their use of medical care without lowering the price charged.

Physician-induced demand is possible because there is a market failure, known as asymmetric information, where the clinician generally knows more about the illness and its treatments than the patient. A clinician who acts a "perfect agent" would make the same decisions that the patient themselves would make if they had the same knowledge as the clinician [3].

The financial bias can occur when clinicians consciously overtreat patients, chose a more lucrative treatment amongst several options, or increase the volume of patients they see in order to earn more money. It can also occur unconsciously, when a clinician is swayed towards the most remunerative tests and treatments option. Acknowledging this bias recognizes that a clinician's judgment, like anyone else's, is not immune to financial considerations. As author Upton Sinclair said, "It is difficult to get a man to understand something, when his salary depends on his not understanding it."

Clinicians who practice under a fee-for-service model, where they are paid based on the services they perform, have a direct financial incentive to perform more tests and procedures. There is ample evidence that clinicians directly respond to financial incentives. Erin Johnson and M. Marit Rehavi examined births in California and Texas, comparing physician to non-physician mothers [4]. In the same way that a real estate agent is less likely to be overcharged when she purchases a new home, a knowledgeable physician mother may be less likely to receive overtreatment. They found that physician mothers were approximately 10% less likely to receive a cesarean section (C-section). The difference occurred only with unscheduled C-sections, where a quick decision has to be made to perform the surgery or try to proceed with vaginal birth. As the difference occurred only in this scenario, the obstetricians did not seem to be consciously performing more procedures to boost their incomes. Rather, when there was a borderline case, they were more likely to perform a C-section on non-physician mothers. As C-sections are generally more profitable than vaginal births, these findings are consistent with the physician-induced demand hypothesis. The authors conclude, "financial incentives have a large effect on a non-physician's probability of receiving a C-section: in hospitals where there is a financial incentive to perform C-sections, they have much higher C-section rates."

The difference between physician and non-physician mothers was reversed at hospitals where obstetricians were paid a flat salary and therefore lacked a financial incentive to perform C-sections. In this environment, physician mothers had a *higher* C-section rate than non-physician mothers. As such, salaried obstetricians may have underperformed C-sections on non-physician mothers. Perhaps most importantly, physician mothers and their babies had less morbidity compared to non-physician mothers, though this may be due to multiple factors other than the decisions of obstetricians. Overall, a study by Darren Grant found that for every $1,000 increase in the reimbursement for a C-section, there is about one percentage point increase in the cesarean delivery rates [5]. While this may appear to be relatively small increase, given that there are about 1,300,000 C-sections annually in the US, the population level effect is quite large [6].

These findings are not isolated to C-sections. Gianfranco Domenighetti and colleagues similarly compared the rates of seven common surgeries in physicians and non-physicians [7]. They found that, except for appendectomies, "doctors have much lower rates of surgery than does the general population" and "in a fee-for-services health care market without financial barriers to medical care, less-informed patients are greater consumers of common surgical procedures."

Other researchers have taken advantage of changes in reimbursement rates to investigate changes in clinicians' behavior. Predictably, clinicians' practices often change dramatically in response to changes in reimbursements rates. When reimbursement for a treatment goes down, clinicians either abandon it in favor of more lucrative treatments, or perform it more often to avoid losing money. Winnie Yip, a professor of health policy, took advantage of a reduction in Medicare payments to thoracic surgeons to investigate how it changed their behavior. She found that surgeons who were most affected by this reduction increased their surgical volume to maintain their incomes [8]. Similarly, a study by Mireille Jacobson and colleagues found that oncologists increased their use of chemotherapy drugs when faced with Medicare payment cuts and changed their practice habits to favor the use of high-margin medications while decreasing the use of less-profitable ones [9].

When I was in medical school, it seemed like every older patient was sent for coronary artery catheterization and ended up with a stent or two to open a blocked artery. While this made intuitive sense, the financial rewards could not be ignored; each procedure cost $30,000–50,000. As David Brown, a cardiologist, wrote:

> In many hospitals, the cardiac service line generates 40% of the total hospital revenue, so there's incredible pressure to do more procedures. When you put in a stent, everyone is happy— the hospital is making more money, the doctor is making more money—everybody is happier except the health care system as a whole, which is paying more money for no better results [10].

Of course, the patients might not be happier, especially if they knew that such stents were often of no benefit to them. Despite their popularity, clinical trials failed to demonstrate any benefit from coronary artery stent in patients with stable coronary artery disease. In response, Medicare began to stop paying for unnecessary procedures, leading to a decline in their number.

As the number of coronary stents fell, clinicians looked outside the heart and began performing lucrative stenting procedures to open narrowed vessels in the arms and legs. Though professional societies say that such procedures should only be performed in patients with severe vascular disease, from 2005 to 2013 the number of stenting procedures for vessels outside the heart soared by almost 70%, according to the Advisory Board Company, which analyzes Medicare payment information. A clinician who can earn $12,000 for performing a short, outpatient procedure may find it easy to justify the treatment in a large number of patients. Indeed, doctors who perform many of these procedures can earn millions of dollars per year. One such physician, who earned over four million dollars in one year, argued that there are too few of these procedures done, saying "these patients are grossly undertreated" [11]. He may be right, but it is hard to imagine that his perspective would be the same if the reimbursement for these procedures dropped dramatically.

The financial bias occurs with more than just surgeries and procedures. Ben Paxton and colleagues reviewed the charts of 500 patients who received MRIs of their lumbar spine [12]. Patients referred by clinicians who had a financial interest in the MRI had significantly more normal scans than those referred by clinicians who did not have a conflict. There was an 86% increase in normal scans (42% versus 23%), when the ordering clinician owned the MRI. In contrast, there was no difference in number of positive lesions per scan. This showed there was not a fundamental difference in the patient populations between clinicians who did and did not own the MRI. Rather, clinicians had a lower threshold to order an MRI when it earned them money. With regards to his findings, Dr. Paxton said, "It is important for patients to be aware of the problem of self-referral and to understand the conflict of interest that exists when their doctor orders an imaging exam and then collects money on that imaging exam" [13].

The financial bias also likely affects clinicians who don't take insurance, instead accepting only cash for their services. I can imagine it must be very difficult for such clinicians to disentangle their financial interests from the interests of their patients. Imagine a psychiatrist who charges $800 per session and sees a patient three times per week. If the patient begins to improve, the psychiatrist has a powerful disincentive to tell the patient that frequent visits are no longer necessary. In contrast, a psychiatrist who receives an annual salary can decrease the frequency of the patient's visit without having to worry that this will affect her income.

Personally, I have worked under two different payment models. In one payment model, I got paid per unit of time worked (either per hour or per year) regardless of how many patients I saw. In this instance, a patient who missed their visit did not affect my income at all and often meant I could catch up on notes from earlier in the day. In the other payment model, I got paid for doing one-time psychiatric evaluations. As long as the patient showed up, I got paid the same amount regardless of how long their visit took. In this instance, a patient who missed their visit meant that I lost money. While I hope that I treated every patient the same during their visits, I would be deceiving myself if I were to pretend I had the same attitude towards patients who missed their visits.

The issue of how to fairly compensate clinicians while maximizing patient care is a complex one. Not surprisingly, a fee-for-service model leads to more, but not necessarily better, care. Jonathan Bergman and colleagues examined data from by the Centers for Medicare and Medicaid Service in 2012 [14]. They found that in Medicare's fee-for-service system, the clinicians who made the most money were the ones who ordered the most tests, not those who saw the most patients or whose patients had the best outcome. Dr. Bergman suggested that, "Perhaps it would make more sense to reimburse clinicians for providing high-quality care, or for treating more patients. There probably shouldn't be such wide variation in services for patients being treated for the same conditions" [15].

Many hospitals have decided to make their clinicians salaried employees, removing any potential conflicts of interest. Steven Nissen, chairman of cardiovascular medicine at the Cleveland Clinic, said "I have a dozen or so cardiologists, and they get the exact same salary whether they put in a stent or don't, and I think that's made a difference and kept our rates of unnecessary procedures low" [16]. I have no doubt he's right. However, making clinicians salaried employees comes with trade-offs. In contrast to fee-for-service doctors, salaried doctors have less incentive to work above and beyond what they will be paid for and may undertreat patients as a result. If an ill patient arrives at the end of the day, a salaried clinician will earn no extra money by staying late to treat them. It may be easy for this clinician to convince themselves the patient's problem can wait until tomorrow, though perhaps this is not the case.

On exceptional occasions, clinicians can be guilty of outright fraud for financial gain. Mark Midei, for example, was paid "millions in salary and perks" according to *The New York Times* for "putting more stents in more patients than almost any other cardiologist in Baltimore" [17]. When his practices were scrutinized, he was found to have violated guidelines by placing stents in arteries that that were only minimally occluded, though his operative reports did not reflect this. A Senate investigation found he overtreated almost 600 patients, charging $6.6 million. After he lost his hospital privileges, Abbott Labs hired Dr. Midei to promote stents in several Asian countries [18]. "It's the right thing to do because he helped us so many times over the years," an Abbott executive wrote in an e-mail. Dr. Midei's hospital ended up paying a $22 million fine to settle charges.

Sadly, Dr. Midei is not an isolated case. In 2017, Jerrold Rosenberg, a physiatrist, pled guilty to healthcare fraud and to taking kickbacks, in the form of speaker's fees, for prescriptions for Subsys, a fast-acting, dangerous, and highly-addictive opioid [19]. In 2009, Mehmood Patel, an interventional cardiologist in Louisiana, was found guilty of 51 counts of billing insurers for unnecessary stent placement. He was sentenced to 10 years in federal prison for healthcare fraud [20]. Another horrific example of fraud is the oncologist Farid Fata, who gave $35 million in needless chemotherapy to over 500 patients. Perhaps most troublingly, not all of his patients even had cancer. Dr. Fata received a 45-year prison term for his crime. In 2017, the Department of Justice charged 412 physicians, nurses, pharmacists and other medical professionals with defrauding the government of $1.3 billion, the largest such scandal to date [21]. Fifty-six of these people were doctors, and one-third of the arrests were related to opioid prescriptions. According to the acting director of the F.B.I., Andrew McCabe, some individual doctors wrote more prescriptions for controlled substances than entire hospitals. According to one news account:

> In one case, a group of six Michigan doctors allegedly operated a scheme to provide patients with unnecessary opioid prescriptions and later billed Medicare for $164 million in false claims. Some of the those prescribed painkillers, authorities said, were resold on the street to addicts [22].

Given the potential for conflicts of interest, patients often feel it is important to know how their clinicians are compensated. Many are rightly suspicious that their clinicians have financial motives independent of their own health. This is fueled by complementary and alternative medicine (CAM) practitioners, whose livelihoods depend on fostering a climate of mistrust between mainstream clinicians and their patients. The alternative medicine site Natural News, for example, publicized the findings of Dr. Bergman by writing an article titled *Top-Earning Doctors Milk Their Patients for Every Dollar Possible, Research Shows* [23]. Natural News also

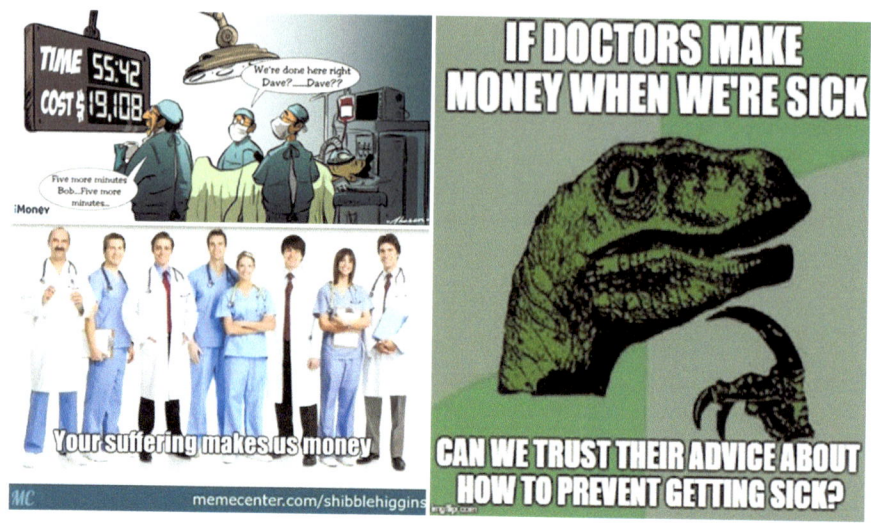

Fig. 8.1 Anti-doctor memes show how the perceived greed of doctors erodes the public's trust in them. (DocWatchDog Admin. A picture paints a thousand words [Blog post, Image files]. DocWatchdog. 2016. Retrieved from http://www.docwatchdog.net/2016/02/a-picture-paints-thousand-words.html.)

gleefully celebrated the scandal of Dr. Fata and used his crimes to further mistrust of mainstream medicine. They even used his case to smear honest clinicians who merely worked in the same building as him, writing an article titled, *Vaccine Propagandist David Gorski Worked Alongside Cancer Fraud Doctor Farid Fata* (Figs. 8.1 and 8.2) [24].

Patients who know how their clinicians are being compensated may have greater trust in them. Steven Pearson and colleagues studied 8,000 adult patients at two multispecialty group practices. They found that a single disclosure letter from the physician "was associated with improved knowledge of physicians' compensation models. Patients' trust in their physicians was unharmed, and their loyalty to their physician group was strengthened" [25].

Additionally, the current method of paying clinicians creates incentives for medical students that do not align with those of society at large. A report by the Institute of Medicine in 2009 found that:

> *higher levels of reimbursement for procedures (e.g., surgeries, invasive procedures, diagnostic imaging, and chemotherapy) compared with the level of reimbursement for non-procedure-related services (e.g., history taking, medical evaluations, and counseling) have contributed to an escalation in the use of procedures and to the shift in the performance of certain lucrative procedural services from hospitals to physicians' offices* [26].

This payment system has created an unfortunate incentive for medical students to choose procedural-based specialties over primary care. A clinician who treats a heart attack with a coronary artery stent can earn thousands of dollars. In contrast, a clinician who prevents a heart attack by counselling a patient on a healthy lifestyle will earn a small fraction of this. According to the Medscape Physician Compensation

Fig. 8.2 The stereotype of the greedy doctor is an old one. In this lithograph from the early 1800s, a doctor, straddled by a skeleton, holds a full purse in his hands, signifying that he lives well off others' deaths. Two pall-bearers are walking in the bottom right-hand corner. The script in the skeleton's hand says "ordonnance," signifying the collusion of the doctor with the call of death. (Wellcome Collection Gallery. A doctor, straddled by a skeleton, holds a full purse in his hands [Image file]. In: Wikimedia commons. 2014. Retrieved from https://commons.wikimedia.org/wiki/Category:Caricatures_of_physicians#/media/File:A_doctor,_straddled_by_a_skeleton,_holds_a_full_purse_in_his_Wellcome_V0011675.jpg.)

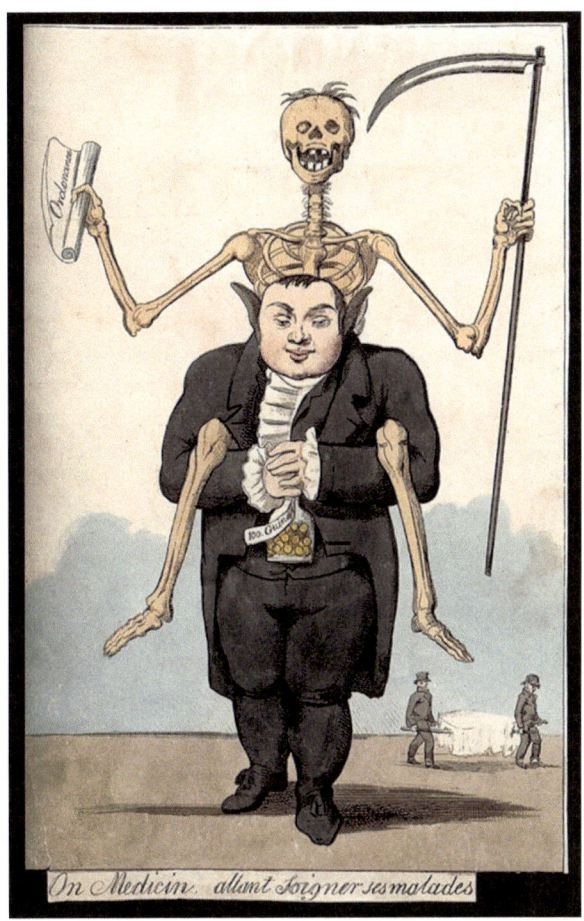

Report in 2016, cardiologists make $410,000 annually, more than twice the salary of pediatricians [27]. Is it any wonder that cardiology is a more competitive specialty for medical students than pediatrics? The Association of American Medical Colleges estimated that the US will have a shortage of 12,000–31,000 primary care physicians by 2025 [28]. The lack of primary care clinicians is a looming crisis for the American healthcare system and might best be solved by eliminating this gross inequity in payment.

Finally, the financial bias is certain to occur with CAM practitioners, many of whom sell supplements and a wide variety of other products, such as mattresses and saunas that purportedly treat autism and Lyme disease [29]. Though CAM practitioners pretend that supplements are categorically different than pharmaceutical drugs, they are wrong. At a fundamental level, supplements and drugs are the same; they are chemicals designed to treat and prevent illnesses or relieve suffering. The distinction between supplements and drugs is only in how they are regulated and how much scientific evidence supports their use. As neurologist Steven Novella wrote:

First and foremost, herbs and plants that are used for medicinal purposes are drugs – they are as much drugs as any manufactured pharmaceutical. A drug is any chemical or combination of chemicals that has biological activity within the body above and beyond their purely nutritional value. Herbs have little to no nutritional value, but they do contain various chemicals, some with biological activity. Herbs are drugs. The distinction between herbs and pharmaceuticals is therefore a false dichotomy [30].

The difference between supplement and pharmaceutical companies in fundamentally a legal and regulatory one, not a medical one. Currently, CAM practitioners benefit from a double standard where they can market supplements that are not tested for efficacy or safety. Importantly, supplements often have the potential to harm patients. A study by Ziv Harel and colleagues found that, "From January 1, 2004, through December 19, 2012, 465 drugs were subject to a class I recall in the US. Just over one-half (237 [51%]) were classified as dietary supplements as opposed to pharmaceutical products" [31]. Some supplements have led to severe liver injuries and even death at a higher rate than medications that at least have a legitimate purpose [32].

Despite their tendency to bash "Big Pharma," selling supplements to patients (as well as household products and beauty supplies) is the norm for CAM practitioners. The supplement industry is worth $36 billion annually, a number that is growing rapidly each year [33]. A survey published in 2010 by the trade publication *Nutrition Business Journal* of 600 medical doctors, naturopathic physicians, chiropractors, nutritionists, and other practitioners found that 76% sold supplements in their office (Fig. 8.3) [34].

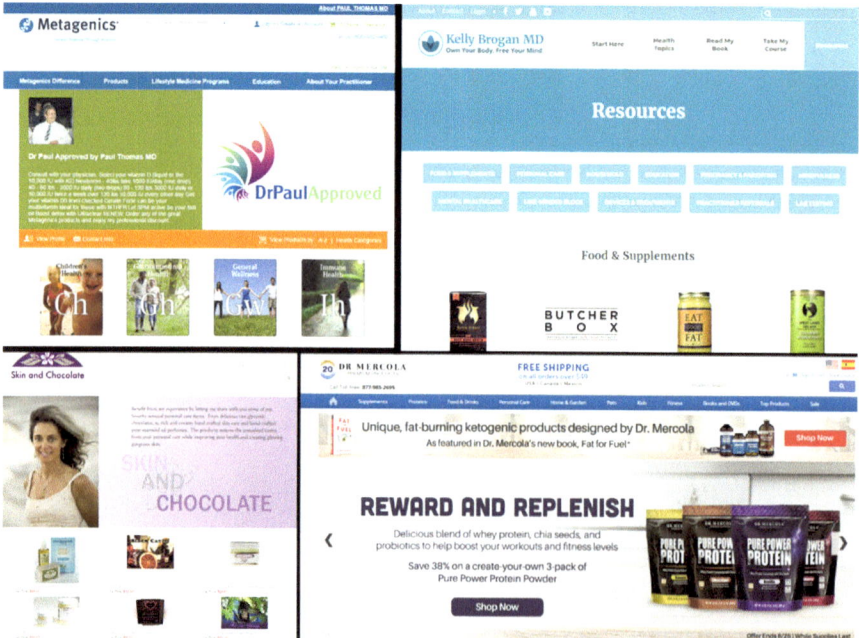

Fig. 8.3 The online stores of anti-vaccine doctors Paul Thomas, Kelly Brogan, Toni Bark, and Joseph Mercola. (Clockwise from upper left: Dr. Paul Thomas, DrPaulApproved.com; Dr. Kelly Brogan, KellyBroganMD.com; Dr. Joseph Mercola, Mercola.com; Dr. Toni Bark, Disease-Reversal.com.)

One doctor who participated in the *Nutrition Business Journal* survey said, "My patients want supplements, and I want to give them high-quality professional supplements that I know and trust. Selling supplements also helps augment my income" [34]. Perhaps this doctor has convinced himself that he is doing the best thing for his patients while helping his bottom line at the same time. However, selling supplements and other products to patients is grossly unethical in my opinion. It encourages clinicians to see their patients as customers, completely distorting the clinician-patient relationship.

A number of seemingly mainstream clinicians peddle supplements as well. Amos Grunebaum, an obstetrician and gynecologist at Cornell University, sells FertilAid® supplements for both men and women. They are backed almost exclusively by "success stories" on his website. Scientific evidence that they actually help couples conceive a baby is sparse. Even Brenda Fitzgerald, the current director of the CDC, described herself as an "anti-aging specialist," and peddled untested supplements on her website [35]. Moreover, some CAM practitioners profit by positing medically dubious diagnoses and then selling the cure. This is common with Lyme disease, which unquestionably is a real illness, at least in the acute form. However, some "Lyme literate" practitioners blame the disease in its supposed "chronic" form for innumerable symptoms and profit handsomely from its treatment. As Paul Auwaerter, an infectious disease specialist, wrote:

> I have a less charitable view of the so-called "Lyme literate medical physicians" who diagnose patients with tick-borne illness and treat them long-term. These physicians are in private practices and often do not accept insurance and charge substantial sums for care and purchase of supplies from their offices [36].

Certainly, most CAM practitioners and their patients would be rightly outraged to learn that a mainstream doctor received kickbacks from a pharmaceutical company as sometimes happens. Supplement-selling clinicians would lose their license and risk jail time if they sold pharmaceutical products the same way they sell supplements. Indeed, in 2016, psychiatrist Michael Reinstein was sentenced to nine months in federal prison and fined nearly $600,000 for accepting hundreds of thousands of dollars in kickbacks from the pharmaceutical industry [37].

Yet, clinicians who sell supplements to their patients are different from this psychiatrist only in that they eliminate the middleman. While pharmaceutical companies can legally pay clinicians to speak or consult on their behalf, at least these payments are publicly available through the Sunshine Act (www.cms.gov/open-payments/). In contrast, money that clinicians earn from selling supplements and other products via their online stores is hidden. It is a clear conflict of interest for clinicians to own facilities to which they refer patients. Clinician self-referral is illegal under the "Stark laws," which prohibit clinicians or their immediate family members from referring patients for health services to an entity with which they have a "financial relationship." It is not clear to me why the online stores of CAM practitioners are seemingly exempt from these laws (Fig. 8.4).

Even worse is that many CAM practitioners peddle products not only to their own patients, but also to strangers via online stores, though they have no knowledge of these individuals' condition or medical history. It is even more ethically dubious

Fig. 8.4 I agree. (The Logic of Science. [Facebook status update]. 2016. Retrieved from https://www.facebook. com/thelogicofscience/ posts/1743103342587728.)

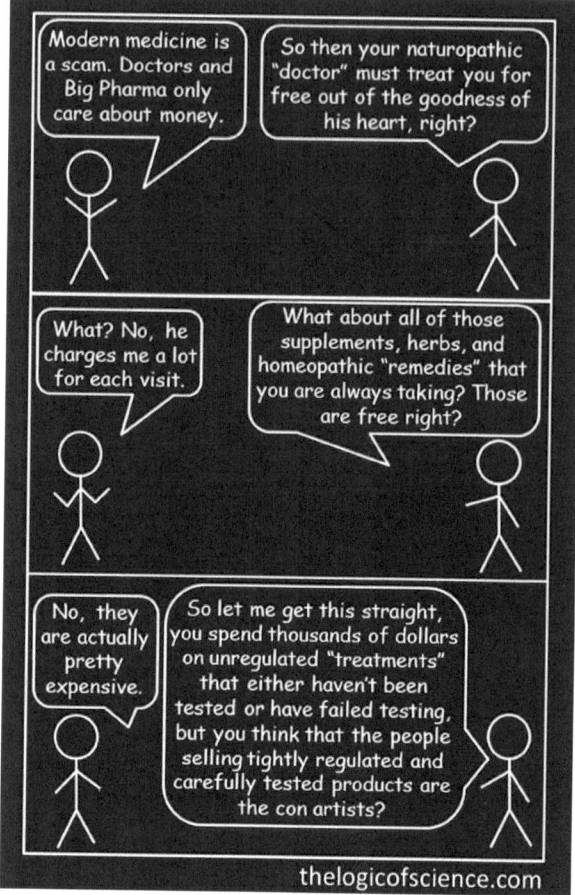

to sell products online to strangers whom the clinician has not examined. Yet, as long as the credit card payment goes through, CAM practitioners are perfectly willing to accept their money and ship them their product.

Ironically, some of these supplements sold by CAM practitioners contain ingredients that they disparage as extremely dangerous when they are found in products such as vaccines. For example, science writer Mark Aslip made the following points about CAM practitioner, psychiatrist Kelly Brogan [38].

- Kelly Brogan, M.D. claims aluminum is toxic to all life forms and falsely links it to a plethora of diseases.
- Brogan's fearmongering re: aluminum includes steering patients away from life-saving vaccines that contain small amounts of the element.
- Via her online store, the doctor sells aluminum via a health supplement, in amounts that equal or exceed the aluminum found in the vaccines she wrongly vilifies.

Fig. 8.5 Turning patients into customers and then into billboards. (Brogan K. (Kelly Brogan MD). Vital mind Monday [Facebook status update]. 2017. Retrieved from https://www.facebook.com/KellyBroganMD/posts/773355096204674.)

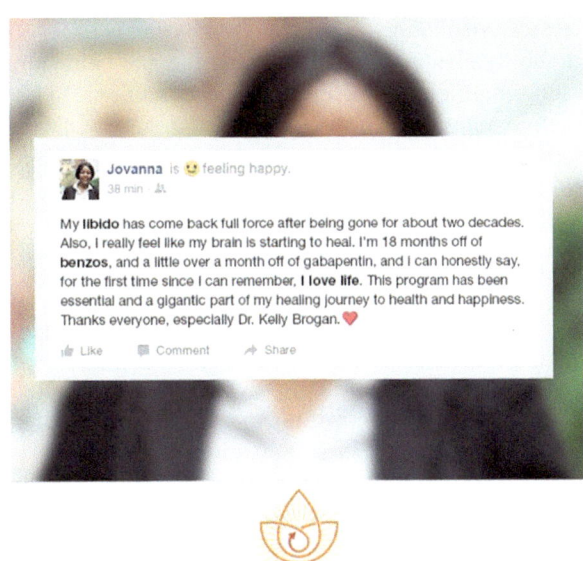

Jovanna is 😊 feeling happy.
38 min

My **libido** has come back full force after being gone for about two decades. Also, I really feel like my brain is starting to heal. I'm 18 months off of **benzos**, and a little over a month off of gabapentin, and I can honestly say, for the first time since I can remember, **I love life**. This program has been essential and a gigantic part of my healing journey to health and happiness. Thanks everyone, especially Dr. Kelly Brogan. ♥

👍 Like   💬 Comment   ➤ Share

VITAL MIND RESET

While selling supplements and other products to patients and strangers alike may seem like the pinnacle of unprofessional behavior, some CAM practitioners exploit people in even worse ways. At times, they will use their patients as "success stories," publishing their information online. While I am sure this is done with patients' consent, this turns patients not just into customers, but into billboards and advertisements for the CAM practitioner (Fig. 8.5).

Some CAM practitioners have found other unethical ways to profit. In June 2015, after a large measles outbreak that started at Disneyland, California enacted Senate Bill 277 (SB277), which mandated that all school children had to be vaccinated unless they had a medical exemption. According to an investigation by the *Los Angeles Times*, the year before the bill passed, 991 kindergartners received a medical exemption, while the next year that number increased to 2,850 [39]. At some schools, 20% of children received a medical exemption. According to James Cherry, an expert in pediatric infectious disease, "This idea of 20% having medical exemptions is nonsense, and certain doctors buy into that, but it's wrong." Another study found that in the two years after the passage of SB277, the rate of medical exemptions for kindergartners tripled [40]. In certain schools, 30–40% of the children received a medical exemption [41].

What explains this? Unfortunately, some doctors were eager to profit by selling medical exemptions to vaccine-hesitant parents. For example, Tara Zandvliet, an anti-vaccine pediatrician board certified in "integrative" medicine, wrote on her website, "After you are pre-approved and documented by email you will have a group appointment, $120 for each person receiving an exemption" [42]. Anti-vaccine pediatrician Bob Sears, listed multiple scientifically invalid reasons to obtain vaccine exemptions on his Facebook page [43]. These included a family history of allergies, learning and behavioral disorders, autism, genetic abnormalities, or "severe medical conditions." Others charged for seminars to help parents learn how to circumvent the law. During such a seminar, Dr. Sears confirmed that he would be willing to see children for a one-time visit in order to issue them a vaccine exemption. According to science blogger and surgeon David Gorski:

> He (Dr. Sears) also confirmed that a one-time medical exemption visit is $180 and that he'd be willing to issue such an exemption and send the child back to his primary pediatrician. When asked whether that was a conflict of interest, Dr. Bob was taken aback, reacting with genuine surprise and answering, "Do you expect me to see them for free?" [44].

Clinicians who are willing to sell fraudulent medical exemptions to vaccines are violating the oath of their profession. As Richard Pan (D-Sacramento), a physician who co-authored SB277 said, "It would be very unfortunate if there were physicians who've shirked their professionalism, and basically are trying to monetize their professional license by putting children at risk and betraying public health" [39].

The financial bias is also the primary reason many of the most prestigious medical centers in the US have set up "integrative" medical centers, which offer pseudo-scientific treatments such as reiki, homeopathy, and acupuncture. Hospitals can charge thousands of dollars for "wellness" memberships, and patients are willing to pay. Many of these centers sell supplements directly to patients and over-promise the potential results. For example, a seminar at an integrative medicine conference at the University of Florida asked, "Can herbs affect the course of dementia?" [45] (No, they can't.) Once a patient is affiliated with an integrative medical center, they are also more likely to use it for more lucrative procedures.

While the clinicians who work at the centers often do their best to portray their work as evidence-based, when pressed they acknowledge that the evidence behind most of their treatments is sorely lacking or completely absent. According to an article on *Stat News*, the "Cleveland Clinic struggled to find anyone on its staff to defend the hospital's energy medicine program, ultimately issuing a statement that it's 'responding to the needs of our patients and patient demand'." It's rare for hospitals to admit they offer services merely because patients will pay. Yet, this is what integrative medical centers are all about. As bioethicist Arthur Caplan said, "The people running the hospitals are doctors, but they also have MBAs. They talk of patients as customers. Customers have demands. Your job is to sell them what they want" [46].

Having said this, financial incentives can be harnessed to improve healthcare outcomes as well. Several insurance companies offer incentives to clinicians who promote healthy behaviors such as smoking cessation, vaccination, recommended cancer screenings, and multiple other evidence-based practices [47]. Clinicians who deviate from accepted practices, by ordering unnecessary imaging tests or antibiotics may face penalties. In 2006, the Massachusetts General Physicians Organization began a quality incentive program that successfully "facilitated the adoption of an electronic health record, improved hand hygiene compliance, increased efficiency in radiology and the cancer center, and decreased emergency department use" [48]. Financial incentives may be useful for patients as well. One study found financial incentives helped motivate patients to lose weight [49]. Another study found that taking money away from patients if they did not meet daily physical activity goals motivated them to be more active [50]. There is also an app that provides financial incentives to patients who properly adhere to their medications [51].

Lastly, clinicians should be aware that their salaries affect not only their relationship with their patients, but also their own attitude and enjoyment of medicine. A psychological phenomenon known as the overjustification effect posits that external incentives decrease the intrinsic motivation to perform a task, thus lowering its overall enjoyment. Clinicians who make career decisions primarily based on financial considerations are less likely to derive personal satisfaction from their work. They may also be less likely to do anything for which they are not paid. Moreover, if payment is stopped, people may refuse to resume the activity until the reward returns.

Paying people to perform an activity changes their entire outlook, such that pleasurable activities can be perceived as a chore. In one experiment, children who were promised a reward for playing with markers later played with them less during optional play-time compared to children who got an unexpected reward or received no reward at all [52]. The overjustification effect helps explain why professional athletes sometimes seem to play with less passion than amateurs, who play only for their love of sport. In medicine, a student who is initially enthusiastic about volunteering in the ER may enjoy it less and put in less effort if she gets paid for it.

Conversely, when people are not given a reward to perform a task, they justify their actions by citing intrinsic factors. In other words, they will say they enjoy it and derive personal satisfaction from it. People may be more willing to do a task for free rather than for a small payment. Every year I happily talk to patients at MS Society events for free because I like it and enjoy helping people. However, if they offered to pay me $20, I might decline, feeling that such a small payment is not worth my effort. People are also more willing to do tasks that are perceived as recreational, rather than work. This is well-illustrated in Mark Twain's novel *The Adventures of Tom Sawyer*. In one scene, Tom is made to whitewash a fence as punishment for skipping school. By pretending that this chore is in fact an honor, he cleverly persuades several friends not only to do the work, but to pay him for the privilege. As Twain wrote:

> *If he had been a great and wise philosopher, like the writer of this book, he would now have comprehended that Work consists of whatever a body is obliged to do, and that Play consists of whatever a body is not obliged to do…. There are wealthy gentlemen in England who drive four-horse passenger-coaches twenty or thirty miles on a daily line, in the summer, because the privilege costs them considerable money; but if they were offered wages for the service, that would turn it into work and then they would resign* [53].

Conclusion

Beneficence is one of the four core principles of medical ethics. It states that clinicians should strive to always do the most good for their patients. Clinicians who view their patients as an ATM machine by performing unnecessary procedures and tests or selling supplements to them are violating this principle. Their primary duty, the health of their patients, becomes intertwined with the potential for increased income.

Clinicians should not pretend they are immune from unconsciously responding to financial incentives. Jamie Koufman, an otolaryngologist, wrote:

> Though they would vigorously deny it, entrepreneurial doctors often treat each patient as an opportunity to make money. Research shows that physicians quickly adapt their treatment choices if the fees they get paid change. But the current payment incentives do more than drive up costs—they can kill people [54].

He's right. When clinicians get paid on a fee-for-service model, they are incentivized to perform tests and procedures, some of which may be unnecessary and even potentially harmful patients. Additionally, ethical clinicians do not sell supplements or other products to their patients. As Orly Avitzur, a neurologist, wrote:

> Selling supplements might yield a handsome profit for some doctors. But having a financial stake in promoting any health product to patients represents a serious conflict of interest. It subverts the responsibility of physicians to place their patients' interests before their own opportunity for financial gain. It also places undue pressure on the patient, especially if the pitch is aggressive. And it can erode trust in the doctor [55].

Clinicians will give the best care when the advice they give their patients is separated from financial considerations as much as possible. Despite this, few people would argue that clinicians should be paupers or that they should feel guilty for wanting a decent salary. I have never turned down a raise and can't imagine I ever will. Additionally, because of the overjustification effect, clinicians who chose their specialty based on money are unlikely to be happy doing it. I chose my medical specialty because I find the brain fascinating, not because it is the most lucrative field.

Mere Exposure Effect and Norm of Reciprocity

Case

James was 25-year-old man who presented for a routine evaluation after having a seizure. The neurologist gave him a sample of pregabalin (Lyrica™) and wrote a prescription for this medication. James refused to take it after seeing several pens and notebooks with "Lyrica" emblazoned on them and learning the neurologist had been paid thousands of dollars by its manufacturer to speak about it to other doctors.

What Dr. Daniels Was Thinking

Pregabalin was a perfectly reasonable medication to start with James. I tried to convince James that my decision to prescribe pregabalin was based only on my belief that this was the best medication for him. I told him—correctly—that I was not being paid to prescribe the drug and that I would not speak for it unless I was convinced of its efficacy. There was no way, I thought, that my prescribing practices could be influenced by trinkets like this or by the lunches the pharmaceutical representative used to buy for our office. Yet, James's reluctance piqued my curiosity. In researching this issue, I came across a doctor who wrote, "I think as long as we continue to prescribe what is best for our patients, no amount of drug samples, informational lunches, anatomical models, or a well-paid consultantships can influence our desire to provide the best care for our patients" [56]. Certainly this was how I felt at the time.

Yet, drug companies are not stupid. Pregabalin was the 13th best-selling medication in 2015, with nearly $5 billion in sales. Is it *really* that much better than older medications that cost significantly less money? I don't think so. My eyes were opened when I read a complaint by a pharma whistleblower. He was reportedly told by a pharmaceutical executive in 1996:

> *I want you out there every day selling Neurontin.... We all know Neurontin's not growing for adjunctive therapy, besides that's not where the money is. Pain management, now that's money. Monotherapy [for epilepsy], that's money.... We can't wait for [physicians] to ask, we need [to] get out there and tell them up front. Dinner programs, CME programs, consultantships all work great but don't forget the one-on-one. That's where we need to be, holding their hand and whispering in their ear, Neurontin for pain, Neurontin for monotherapy, Neurontin for bipolar, Neurontin for everything. I don't want to see a single patient coming off Neurontin before they've been up to at least 4800 mg/day. I don't want to hear that safety crap either, have you tried Neurontin, every one of you should take one just to see there is nothing, it's a great drug* [57].

After reading this and other accounts about how the pharmaceutical industry tries to influence doctors, I decided that pharmaceutical representatives would not be allowed in my office, and I would no longer accept gifts from them. I now concede it was possible that even small gifts, often given to me by friendly, attractive representatives, may have unconsciously influenced my prescribing habits. I also stopped speaking for pharmaceutical companies and attending their dinners. Interestingly my prescribing practices changed. I guess I was being subtly influenced all along. I lost some free lunches, speaker's fees, and some relationships that were actually genuine (or seemed that way), but I regained my independence and integrity.

Discussion
The mere exposure effect, also known as the familiarity principle, occurs when people develop a preference for something simply because they are familiar with it. Familiarity doesn't breed contempt. It creates fondness. As such, clinicians may be motivated to use a drug, device, or test simply because they are familiar with it. Pharmaceutical companies know this. The job of pharmaceutical companies and their representatives is to make their products familiar, and therefore attractive, to both patients and clinicians. They know that exposing clinicians to their drug, even in seemingly trivial ways, will increase the likelihood it will be prescribed.

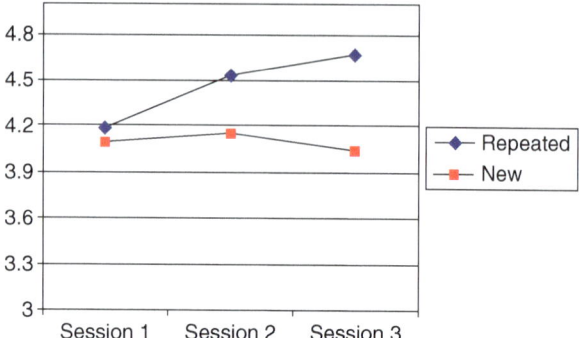

Fig. 8.6 Statements repeated across three sessions were deemed to be more plausible

Related to this is a phenomenon known as the illusory truth effect. It occurs as people are more likely to believe statements are true merely because they have heard them repeatedly. Myths, such as the notion that people use only 10% of their brain, persist simply because they are repeated so often. Lynn Hasher and colleagues demonstrated this by giving study subjects 60 plausible statements on three occasions, separated by two weeks [58]. On each occasion, the subjects were asked to rate how confident they were that the statements were true. Twenty statements of the statements were repeated across the three sessions, and by the third session, those statements were rated as more truthful than the first session. The illusory truth effect explains the value of simple messages and slogans in selling medications to both clinicians and the general public (Fig. 8.6) [59].

Pharmaceutical representatives also count on the norm of reciprocity in their relationships with clinicians. Reciprocity is the unwritten, though powerful, social norm that people are obligated to repay gifts and favors that others have done for them. It is well known to salesmen, who may give someone a "free sample," knowing that this then triggers feelings of obligation to return the favor and buy their product. While reciprocity is normally a healthy way for individuals to function in a group, it is of dubious merit when a third party is introduced into the clinician-patient relationship.

Pharmaceutical companies provided clinicians with trinkets, such as pens and mugs (a practice now banned), to take advantage of the mere exposure effect and norm of reciprocity. They know that small gifts can unconsciously trigger clinicians to feel in debt to the pharmaceutical representative; a debt that can be repaid by prescribing their product. As L. Lewis Wall and Douglas Brown wrote, "Even small gifts produce in their recipients a disproportionately powerful willingness to reciprocate in some manner. The simple act of providing food has been shown to make any message more palatable and more likely to be favorably received" [60].

Pharmaceutical companies also take advantage of the mere exposure effect by having their representatives call on clinicians' offices frequently and establish relationships with them. In studies of interpersonal attraction, people appear more attractive, likeable, and trustworthy if they are seen more frequently. They also take advantage of the affective bias by hiring representatives who are affable and physically attractive. According an article in *The New York Times*, many pharmaceutical representatives were cheerleaders in their youth, their outgoing personality and attractiveness making them natural fits for the job [61]. Bioethicist Carl Eliot wrote about this as well:

> *Drug reps are still easy to spot in a clinic or hospital, but for slightly different reasons. The most obvious is their appearance. It is probably fair to say that doctors, pharmacists, and medical-school professors are not generally admired for their good looks and fashion sense. Against this backdrop, the average drug rep looks like a supermodel, or maybe an A-list movie star. Drug reps today are often young, well groomed, and strikingly good-looking. Many are women. They are usually affable and sometimes very smart. Many give off a kind of glow, as if they had just emerged from a spa or salon. And they are always, hands down, the best-dressed people in the hospital* [62].

I am sure that most clinicians would agree that pharmaceutical representatives are mostly honest people who believe in their products. They are friendly and outgoing, hoping to make clinicians like them and therefore like their product. However, on several occasions, I have seen them switch companies. Witnessing a representative extol the benefits of one drug one day and its competitor the next serves as a reminder that despite the smiles and questions about how my family is doing, they are salesmen whose salaries depend on manipulating clinicians like me.

Drug samples play a similar role in influencing clinicians' and patients' judgment. They allow pharmaceutical representatives to gain access to clinicians' offices and expose them to the medication. Such samples engage feelings of reciprocity in clinicians, their staff, and patients. Drug companies give away billions of dollars of free samples to clinicians each year [63]. These samples are almost always the newest, most expensive drugs, and they rarely go to needy patients who otherwise can't afford them [64]. Much like a restaurant trying to entice customers by handing out free samples, medication samples are a marketing tool and nothing else.

The mere exposure effect, the illusory truth effect, and norm of reciprocity are also the main reasons clinicians are invited to speak at pharmaceutical company programs. Pharmaceutical companies often recruit clinicians respected by their peers to speak at dinners, billed as "educational" events, on behalf of their product. When clinicians speak about a drug, even if everything in their talk is completely accurate and fair, that drug is then embedded in the mind of the speaker and listener alike. This gives it an edge over less familiar, and possibly much cheaper, yet equally effective competitors. While it may seem that these speakers are there to influence other clinicians attending the talk, this is not necessarily the case. Shahram Ahari is a former pharmaceutical sales representative who revealed many of the practices representatives use to influence clinicians [65]. He said about such drug dinners, "the main target of these gatherings is the speaker, whose appreciation may be reflected in increased prescribing of a company's product." Mr. Ahari had no illusions that his job was anything other than to manipulate clinicians. He explained:

> *It's my job to figure out what a physician's price is. For some it's dinner at the finest restaurants, for others it's enough convincing data to let them prescribe confidently and for others it's my attention and friendship…but at the most basic level, everything is for sale and everything is an exchange* [65].

Additionally, much of the behavior of pharmaceutical companies is designed to stoke the egos of clinicians, who are called thought leaders or key opinion leaders (KOLs.) As Erick Turner, a psychiatrist, said, "It strokes your narcissism. You get to hobnob with these mega-thought leaders and these aspiring thought leaders. They make you feel like you're special." He further described the process of helping a drug company launch a new drug by saying:

> The first thing they do is ferry you to a really nice hotel. And sometimes they pick you up in a limo, and you feel very important, and they have really, really good food. And they make you sign a confidentiality agreement and say you need to sign this if you want to get paid [66].

Carl Elliot elaborated on this further by writing:

> There is the money, of course, which is no small matter. Some high-level KOL's make more money consulting for the pharmaceutical industry than they get from their academic institutions. But the real appeal of being a KOL is that of being acknowledged as important. That feeling of importance comes not so much from the pharmaceutical companies themselves, but from associating with other academic luminaries that the companies have recruited. Academic physicians talk about the experience of being a KOL the way others might talk about being admitted to a selective fraternity or an exclusive New York dance club. No longer are you standing outside the rope trying to catch the doorman's eye, waiting hungrily to be admitted. You are one of the chosen.

Pharmaceutical companies certainly devote a lot of effort to recruiting clinicians and monitoring their prescribing habits. Psychiatrist Daniel Carlat described his experience as a speaker for the antidepressant Effexor™ in *The New York Times* [67]. He wrote:

> As the reps became comfortable with me, they began to see me more as a sales colleague. I received faxes before talks preparing me for particular doctors. Naïve as I was, I found myself astonished at the level of detail that drug companies were able to acquire about doctors' prescribing habits. I asked my reps about it; they told me that they received printouts tracking local doctors' prescriptions every week.

The fact that some clinicians receive hundreds of thousands of dollars for their efforts speaks to the value pharmaceutical companies feel they derive from such talks. Figure 8.7, for example, shows the payments from a neurologist who received 158 payments, totaling $169,238 in 2015 from pharmaceutical companies who make drugs for multiple sclerosis. Some physicians make much more than this, exceeding their compensation from their clinical and academic work.

I have little doubt that this neurologist honestly believes these payments do not influence her prescribing habits. However, I think that it is exceedingly unlikely that these payments, which total almost $500 per day, have not affected her in any way. In hopes of avoiding such influence, one doctor I knew used to consciously avoid prescribing any drug he spoke about for several weeks after he was paid to speak about it. But this was not in the interests of his patients either. Perhaps a drug he recently spoke about would have been the best option for one of his patients, but he refused to use it to avoid the perception of a conflict of interest.

Nature of Payment	Total Payments	Total Amount	Total Amount (%)
Compensation for services other than consulting, including serving as faculty or as a speaker at a venue other than a continuing education program ❶	35	$106,880.00	63.2%
Consulting Fee ❶	8	$46,170.00	27.3%
Travel and Lodging ❶	49	$12,776.00	7.5%
Food and Beverage ❶	65	$3,406.01	2.0%
Education ❶	1	$6.00	0.0%

Fig. 8.7 The payments a neurologist received in 2015

Despite most clinicians' perception that their judgment is independent of financial considerations, studies have shown clinicians' judgment can be influenced by money. For example, Daniel Murrie and colleagues studied 108 forensic psychologists and psychiatrists and asked them to review the case of an offender [68]. Those who thought they were working for the prosecution assigned higher risk scores to the offender, while those who thought they were working for the defense assigned a lower risk score.

There is copious evidence that pharmaceutical and device companies get a good return on their investment in marketing to clinicians. A study published in 2016 by ProPublica found "doctors who receive payments from the medical industry do indeed tend to prescribe drugs differently than their colleagues who don't. And the more money they receive, on average, the more brand-name medications they prescribe" [69]. A study by Thomas Schwartz and colleagues found that "psychiatric residents preferentially start companies' medications shortly after sales visits. Furthermore, as sales visits increase in frequency, more of their medications may be started in newly admitted psychiatric outpatients" [70]. A study by Colette DeJong and colleagues examined 279,669 physicians who received a total of 63,524 payments. They examined four medications (Crestor™, Bystolic™, Benicar™ and Pristiq™) for which there are cheaper, equally effective alternatives [71]. They found that "Receipt of industry-sponsored meals was associated with an increased rate of prescribing the brand-name medication that was being promoted." For one of the drugs, meals alone were enough to increase the prescribing rate fivefold, and even one meal was enough to change a doctor's prescribing pattern. Another study by James Yeh and colleagues examined 2,444 doctors in Massachusetts [72]. It found that "industry payments to physicians are associated with higher rates of prescribing brand-name statins." In a meta-analysis by Hneine Brax and colleagues of 19 studies, "15 found a consistent association between interactions promoting a medication, and inappropriately increased prescribing rates, lower prescribing quality, and/or increased prescription costs" [73].

Unfortunately, the influence of the pharmaceutical industry can be detected early in a clinician's training. A survey by Kirsten Austad and colleagues of 1,601 residents and medical students found that trainees who reported high levels of involvement in pharmaceutical marketing were the least likely to provide evidence-based answers concerning appropriate drug choices [74]. They were the most likely to select brand-name drugs, though they were not the ideal treatment. This was confirmed in another study, where residents who correctly answered questions about evidence-based medications were about 30% less likely to have gone to lectures sponsored by the pharmaceutical industry [75].

Payments to clinicians are not just influential, they are also common. According to data collected in 2015 by Propublica, "Companies made about $2 billion in general payments to 618,000 physicians each year, in addition to another $600 million a year to teaching hospitals. General payments cover promotional speaking, consulting, meals, travel, gifts and royalties, but not research" [76]. A survey by Genevieve Pham-Kanter and colleagues found that approximately 65% of patients had visited a doctor within the last year who had received payments or gifts, though only 5% of patients were aware of this relationship [77]. Dr. Pham-Kanter said about her results:

> These findings tell us that if you thought that your doctor was not receiving any money from industry, you're most likely mistaken. Patients should be aware of the incentives that their physicians face that may lead them to not always act in their patients' best interest. And the more informed patients are about their providers and options for care, the better decisions they can make.

Not surprisingly, complementary and alternative medicine (CAM) advocates exploit data like this to discredit mainstream medicine. In addition to articles spreading conspiracy theories about vaccines, the website Natural News, for example, wrote an article celebrating Dr. Pham-Kanter's findings titled, *65% of Doctors Are Getting Cash 'Kickbacks' From Big Pharma* (Fig. 8.8) [78].

At times, payments to prominent clinicians and various regulatory agencies may impact enormous swaths of medicine with potentially devastating consequences. Shortly after the approval of powerful, addicting opioid medications such as Oxycontin™ in 1995, the American Pain Society introduced a campaign making pain the "5th Vital Sign." Clinicians were instructed to ask every patient about their level of pain during every visit and patients' "Bill of Rights" stressed their right to pain relief. Patients were asked about their pain during nearly every clinical encounter, and clinicians were rated by their patients' responses. Hospitals paid attention too. The Veterans Health Administration (VHA) produced a 57-page "Pain as the 5th Vital Sign Toolkit" in 2000 [79]. Medications that were formerly reserved for terminal cancer patients were now offered to patients with chronic pain from a variety of causes.

Additionally, the risks of opioid medications were downplayed. A small paper of 38 patients with non-cancer pain by pain-management specialists, Russell Portenoy and Kathleen Foley, found that only two had issues with addiction to the opioids [80]. Moreover, those two patients were said to have previous issues with drug

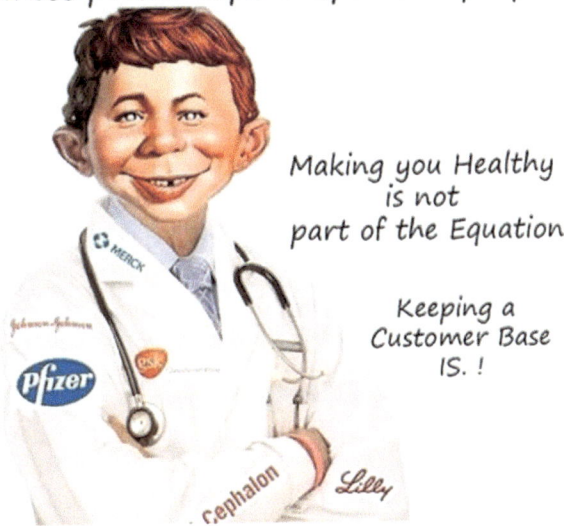

TRUTH

Mainstream "Doctors" are simply Big Pharma Sales Reps in White Coats. Pushers for a Cartel whose profits depend upon sick people.

Making you Healthy is not part of the Equation

Keeping a Customer Base IS. !

abuse. Their paper concluded that "opioid maintenance therapy can be a safe, salutary and more humane alternative to the options of surgery or no treatment in those patients with intractable non-malignant pain and no history of drug abuse."

Treating pain became a crusade. A guideline produced by the Joint Commission declared, "Some clinicians have inaccurate and exaggerated concerns about addiction, tolerance and risk of death. This attitude prevails despite the fact there is no evidence that addiction is a significant issue when persons are given opioids for pain control" [81]. The VHA toolkit only mentioned addiction as a "bias" that might prevent clinicians from prescribing pain medications to their patients. Clinicians who were reluctant to prescribe opioids were said to suffer from "opiophobia" [82]. In 1998, the Federation of State Medical Boards formulated a policy that clinicians would not face disciplinary action for prescribing large amounts of opioids for their patients, and in 2004 it suggested that state medical boards make the under-treatment of pain a punishable offense.

Despite the seemingly well-intentioned movement to relieve the suffering of people in pain, financial motives were at play as well. Influential leaders of the American Pain Society, such as Dr. Portenoy, had financial relationships with the pharmaceutical companies that sold opioids; though, of course, they denied that this influenced their thinking on the subject. The Joint Commission pain guideline was, in fact, sponsored by Purdue Pharma, the manufacturer of Oxycontin™ [83]. Similarly, according to *The Wall Street Journal*, a book published by the Federation of State Medical Boards "outlining the opioid policy was funded by opioid makers including Purdue Pharma, Endo Health Solutions Inc. and others, with proceeds totaling $280,000 going to the federation" [81].

The consequences of the overuse of opioids are now manifest by addiction and tens of thousands of deaths from overdoses annually. Studies also found that making pain the 5th vital sign did not improve the quality of pain management that patients received [84]. In 2009, The Joint Commission eliminated its standard to ask all patients about their pain. In 2016, the American Medical Association pushed to eliminate pain as the 5th vital sign. In the face of hundreds of thousands of deaths due to opioid overdoses, Dr. Portenoy largely backtracked on his endorsement of the widespread use of opiates for patients with chronic pain.

Not surprisingly, many clinicians remain unaware of how they might be influenced by pharmaceutical companies. In an interview with *The New York Times*, an obstetrician reflected the conventional wisdom regarding small gifts by saying, "It's hard for me to believe it influences what you prescribe." In another article, a dermatologist wrote:

> *I think as long as we continue to prescribe what is best for our patients, no amount of drug samples, informational lunches, anatomical models, or a well-paid consultantships can influence our desire to provide the best care for our patients* [85].

A meta-analysis of 15 articles from 10 countries by Shahrzad Salmasi and colleagues confirmed these anecdotes, finding "that most physicians believed that their prescribing would not be influenced by pharmaceutical representatives" [86].

This shows that clinicians, like everyone else, are vulnerable to a phenomenon known as the third-person effect. It describes the tendency of people to believe they are immune to advertising and mass media messages while others are vulnerable to them. It was first described by W. Phillips Davison who wrote, "Each individual reasons: 'I will not be influenced, but they (the third persons) may well be persuaded'." The third-person effect has been demonstrated experimentally many times. In a typical study, Douglas McLeod and colleagues found that when violent or misogynistic rap lyrics were played to students, they felt they were immune to their effects, but youths in New York or Los Angeles would be influenced by them [81]. A review by Daniella Zipkin and Michael Steinman on the role of the pharmaceutical industry in residency programs showed that most clinicians believe themselves immune to the influence from gifts and contacts with pharmaceutical representatives [87]. They found that "A minority felt that their own prescribing could be influenced by contact or gifts, but were more likely to believe that others' prescribing could be influenced." As psychologist Erin McCormick wrote:

> *When physicians receive gifts from pharmaceutical companies, they may claim that the gifts do not affect their decisions about what medicine to prescribe because they have no memory of the gifts biasing their prescriptions. However, if you ask them whether a gift might unconsciously bias the decisions of other physicians, most will agree that other physicians are unconsciously biased by the gifts, while continuing to believe that their own decisions are not. This disparity is the bias blind spot, and occurs for everyone, for many different types of judgments and decisions* [88].

Like most biases, the third-person effect can be difficult or impossible to detect in oneself, but easy to spot in others. Do you feel other people can be swayed to vote for a political candidate or buy a product simply because of an emotional TV ad or a "free" sample? Probably you do. What about yourself? Do mass marketing campaigns and small gifts have any substantial influence on you? Of course not! If you think that you're an individual who thinks for yourself and is immune from marketing, you're probably wrong, but you're not alone. Almost everyone feels this way about themselves. My office used to have a weekly breakfast hosted by a rotating group of pharmaceutical companies. From 2012 to 2015, I received a total of $700 in these meals. However, this was stopped, correctly I believe, to avoid any subtle, unconscious effect on our prescribing patterns and to eliminate perceived conflicts of interest. I certainly didn't think these meals influenced me. I hope I was right.

Clinicians should be aware that their patients view gifts differently, and probably more accurately, than they do. A study by Robert Gibbons and colleagues found "that patients consider pharmaceutical gifts more influential and less appropriate than do their physicians." This includes small gifts such as a "pen, textbooks, and meals associated with educational conferences" [89]. A study by Michael Green and colleagues of 192 clinic patients found that between 50% and 60% of patients would trust their clinician less if they accepted gifts greater than $100 or went on industry-sponsored trips or sporting events. Twenty-five percent said they would be less likely to take a medication if their clinician had received a gift in exchange for hearing a sales pitch from a pharmaceutical representative [90]. Avoiding a sense of reciprocity is also why clinicians should avoid accepting anything but trivial gifts from patients. It may be hard for a clinician to decline a patient's request for an inappropriate treatment if that patient has previously given them an expensive gift.

Certainly a number of improvements have occurred in recent years to minimize conflicts of interest between clinicians and the pharmaceutical industry. Organizations such as the American Medical Student Association (AMSA) have a "PharmFree campaign." They believe that:

> Information used by physicians in making clinical decisions should be comprehensive, transparent in its methodology and results, and independent from institutions and individuals with a financial interest in physician prescribing. Physicians should not seek education from industry marketing efforts, whether they are in the form of advertisements, sales pitches from representatives, or sponsored lectures by paid physicians [91].

Many medical schools have rules forbidding interactions between students and pharmaceutical representatives. Since 2007, AMSA has released a scorecard grading medical schools on their conflict of information policies. In 2016, the results were generally positive. Out of 173 US medical schools, 42 received "A"s (24%), 76 "B"s (44%), 28 "C"s (16%), and 28 Incompletes (16%) [92]. Unfortunately, there is evidence the benefits of these medical school policies are short-lived, and once they become residents, students who attended medical schools with restrictive policies were just as likely to engage with the pharmaceutical industry [75].

Additionally, in response to a backlash against its practices, the Pharmaceutical Research and Manufacturers of America created a voluntary code for pharmaceutical representatives. The practice of giving of clinicians expensive tickets or paying for trips to resorts is over. This code was further strengthened in 2008 to eliminate branded trinkets such as pens and notepads. Despite this, pharmaceutical companies still pay clinicians large fees to speak at expensive dinners or serve as consultants.

Fortunately, all pharmaceutical industry payments to clinicians are public through the Sunshine Act (www.cms.gov/openpayments/).

This is not to say all contact between clinicians and the pharmaceutical industry is inappropriate. Pharmaceutical companies have employees called medical science liaisons (MSLs), who typically have advanced scientific degrees and can provide unique information about their products to clinicians. I rely on MSLs to keep me informed on side effects of their medications that come to their attention through reporting systems that are not publicly available. Moreover, many academic physicians partner with pharmaceutical companies to carry out valuable research that neither organization could do alone. Pharmaceutical companies have the money, and academic physicians have the patients. However, this research is likely to be devalued if the clinician is on the payroll of the company, and certainly the practice of having companies "ghostwrite" articles for clinicians should be strongly discouraged.

Direct-to-consumer advertising is another tactic the pharmaceutical industry uses to increase its profits, though it is currently only legal in the USA and New Zealand. Such advertising has been criticized for medicalizing the normal human experience, such as decreased sexual dysfunction in older men, and for encouraging patients to ask their clinicians for expensive treatments when a cheaper alternative might suffice. Formal evidence that such advertising is effective is mixed. However, given the ubiquity and volume of drug commercials, pharmaceutical companies seem to believe they are getting a good return on their investment [93].

The mere exposure effect can influence clinicians in other ways as well. Alexander Serenko and Nick Bontis surveyed 233 active researchers in the field of knowledge management and intellectual capital [94]. They found that those who previously published in a particular journal or served as a reviewer or editor rated that journal higher than those who had not. There is some rationale for this. A prestigious and familiar journal is likely to have high standards for publication and rigorous peer-review. In contrast, "predatory publishers" are pseudo-journals that charge publication fees to authors without any significant oversight or quality control.

Finally, the mere exposure effect can be used in positive ways. Specifically, it can be used to overcome potentially harmful biases, particularly with regards to stereotypes about race, culture, sexual orientation, and gender. Leslie Zebrowitz and colleagues found that "White participants' familiarity with an other-race facial prototype through exposure to Korean or Black faces increased the likeability of a different set of Korean or Black faces" [95]. This suggests that certain types of bias are, in part, due to lack of familiarity with other races, and that this can be diminished with exposure, a phenomenon termed passive tolerance [96].

Conclusion

Pharmaceutical companies use the mere exposure effect and norm of reciprocity to manipulate clinicians into prescribing their products. While many clinicians believe they are immune to these influences, this is not the case. As Jason Dana and George Loewenstein point out, "because even small gifts can subtly bias how arguments are evaluated, they can be surprisingly influential. The sheer ubiquity of trinkets given by pharmaceutical companies is evidence of their effectiveness; why else would profit-minded companies continue to provide them?" [97]

When clinicians are influenced by the pharmaceutical industry, it clouds their judgment, makes patients suspicious of clinicians' motives, and gives CAM practitioners an avenue to attack mainstream medicine and peddle their own lucrative pseudoscientific treatments.

In order to avoid conflicts with the pharmaceutical and medical device companies, the Institute of Medicine made the following suggestions in 2009 [98]. Clinicians, wherever their site of clinical practice, should:

- Not accept items of material value from pharmaceutical, medical device, and biotechnology companies, except when a transaction involves payment at fair market value for a legitimate service.
- Not make educational presentations or publish scientific articles that are controlled by industry or contain substantial portions written by someone who is not identified as an author or who is not properly acknowledged.
- Not enter into consulting arrangements unless they are based on written contracts for expert services to be paid for at fair market value.
- Not meet with pharmaceutical and medical device sales representatives except by documented appointment and at the physician's express invitation; and
- Not accept drug samples except in specified situations for patients who lack financial access to medications.

The mere exposure effect and reciprocity are somewhat unique in that, unlike other biases, knowledge of the bias can drastically reduce its influence. When pharmaceutical representatives ask for a minute of a clinician's time, the clinician can completely avoid their influence by politely but firmly telling them "no." As Wall and Brown wrote, "physician prescribing habits should be based upon careful consideration of what medication is really in the patient's best clinical interests, not on who most recently provided the doctor with a free lunch" [60]. This is exactly right.

References

1. Johnson EM. Physician-induced demand. Encyclopedia of Health Economics. 2014;3:77–82. https://doi.org/10.1016/B978-0-12-375678-7.00805-1
2. Hadley J, Holahan J, Scanlon W. Can fee-for-service reimbursement coexist with demand creation? Inquiry. 1979;16(3):247–58.
3. Folland S, Goodman AC, Stano M. The economics of health and health care. 7th ed. Boston, MA: Pearson; 2012. p. 305–8.
4. Johnson EM, Rehavi MM. Physicians treating physicians: information and incentives in childbirth. Am Econ J Econ Pol. 2016;8(1):115–41. https://doi.org/10.1257/pol.20140160.
5. Grant D. Physician financial incentives and cesarean delivery: new conclusions from the healthcare cost and utilization project. J Health Econ. 2009;28(1):244–50. https://doi.org/10.1016/j.jhealeco.2008.09.005.

6. Centers for Disease Control and Prevention. (2017). Births – method of delivery. Retrieved 15 Sept 2018 from https://www.cdc.gov/nchs/fastats/delivery.htm.
7. Domenighetti G, Casabianca A, Gutzwiller F, Martinoli S. Revisiting the most informed consumer of surgical services: the physician-patient. Int J Technol Assess Health Care. 1993;9(4):505–13. https://doi.org/10.1017/S0266462300005420.
8. Yip WC. Physician response to Medicare fee reductions: changes in the volume of coronary artery bypass graft (CABG) surgeries in the Medicare and private sectors. J Health Econ. 1998;17(6):675–99. Retrieved from https://doi.org/10.1016/S0167-6296(98)00024-1.
9. Jacobson M, Earle CC, Price M, Newhouse JP. How Medicare's payment cuts for cancer chemotherapy drugs changed patterns of treatment. Health Aff. 2010;29(7):1391–9. https://doi.org/10.1377/hlthaff.2009.0563.
10. Bakalar N. (2012, Feb 27). No extra benefits are seen in stents for coronary artery disease. The New York Times. Retrieved from https://www.nytimes.com/2012/02/28/health/stents-show-no-extra-benefits-for-coronary-artery-disease.html.
11. Creswell J, Abelson R. (2015, Jan 29). Medicare payments surge for stents to unblock blood vessels in limbs. The New York Times. Retrieved from https://www.nytimes.com/2015/01/30/business/medicare-payments-surge-for-stents-to-unblock-blood-vessels-in-limbs.html.
12. Paxton B, Lungren M, Jung S, Kranz P, Kilani R. (2011). A case study in lumbar spine MRI and physician self-referral of imaging. Radiological Society of North America 2011 Scientific Assembly and Annual Meeting, November 26 – December 2, 2011 ,Chicago IL. Retrieved 15 Sept 2018 from http://archive.rsna.org/2011/11009567.html.
13. Harmon K. (2011, Nov 30). Patients get more unnecessary scans from doctors who own equipment [Blog post]. Scientific American. Retrieved 15 Sept 2018 from https://blogs.scientificamerican.com/observations/patients-get-more-unnecessary-scans-from-doctors-who-own-equipment/.
14. Bergman J, Saigal CS, Litwin MS. Service intensity and physician income conclusions from Medicare's physician data release. JAMA Intern Med. 2015;175(2):297–9. https://doi.org/10.1001/jamainternmed.2014.6397.
15. Irwin K. (2014, Dec 11). Higher-earning physicians make more money by ordering more procedures per patient. UCLA Newsroom. Retrieved from http://newsroom.ucla.edu/releases/higher-earing-physicians-make-more-money-by-ordering-more-procedures-per-patient-says-ucla-report.
16. Epstein D. (2017, Feb 22). When evidence says no, but doctors say yes. ProPublica. Retrieved https://www.propublica.org/article/when-evidence-says-no-but-doctors-say-yes.
17. Harris G. (2010, Dec 5). Doctor faces suits over cardiac stents. The New York Times. Retrieved from https://www.nytimes.com/2010/12/06/health/06stent.html.
18. JDWolverton. (2010, Dec 8). The curious case of Dr. Midei - Medical over-utilization or fraud? [Blog post]. Daily Kos. Retrieved from https://www.dailykos.com/stories/2010/12/08/926435/-The-Curious-Case-of-Dr-Midei-Medical-Over-Utilization-or-Fraud/.
19. Sullivan M. (2017, Oct 25). Jamestown doc pleads guilty to healthcare fraud. Newport Patch. Retrieved from https://patch.com/rhode-island/newport/jamestown-doc-pleads-guilty-healthcare-fraud.
20. O'Riordan M. (2009, June 26). Cardiologist gets 10 years for performing unnecessary interventions. Medscape. Retrieved from https://www.medscape.com/viewarticle/705029.
21. Ruiz RR. (2017, July 13). U.S. charges 412, including doctors, in $1.3 billion health fraud. The New York Times. Retrieved from https://www.nytimes.com/2017/07/13/us/politics/health-care-fraud.html.
22. Johnson K. (2017, July 13). Jeff Sessions: 400 medical professionals charged in largest health care fraud takedown. USA Today. Retrieved 2017 from https://www.usatoday.com/story/news/politics/2017/07/13/jeff-sessions-authorities-charge-400-people-health-care-fraud/475089001/.
23. Lilley J. (2014, Dec 30). Top-earning doctors milk their patients for every dollar possible, research shows. Natural News. Retrieved from https://www.naturalnews.com/048150_doctors_medical_fraud_healthcare_fees.html.
24. Benson J. (2016, May 10). Vaccine propagandist David Gorski worked alongside cancer fraud doctor Farid Fata. Natural News. Retrieved from https://www.naturalnews.com/053958_David_Gorski_Farid_Fata_cancer_fraud.html.

25. Pearson SD, Kleinman K, Rusinak D, Levinson W. A trial of disclosing physicians' financial incentives to patients. Arch Intern Med. 2006;166(6):623–8. https://doi.org/10.1001/archinte.166.6.623.
26. Lo B, Field MJ. (Eds.). Chapter 6. In: Conflicts of interest in medical research, education, and practice. Washington, DC: The National Academies Press; 2009.
27. Peckham C. (2016, Apr 1). Medscape physician compensation report 2016. Medscape. Retrieved from https://www.medscape.com/features/slideshow/compensation/2016/public/overview.
28. Association of American Medical Colleges. (2016, Apr 5). New research confirms looming physician shortage. Retrieved from https://www.aamc.org/newsroom/newsreleases/458074/2016_workforce_projections_04052016.html.
29. Brogan K. (n.d.). Resources. Kelly Brogan MD. Retrieved 15 Sept 2018 from https://kellybroganmd.com.
30. Novella S. (2008, Jan 2). The plant vs pharmaceutical false dichotomy. Science-Based Medicine. Retrieved from https://sciencebasedmedicine.org/the-plant-vs-pharmaceutical-false-dichotomy/.
31. Harel Z, Harel S, Wald R, Mamdani M, Bell CM. The frequency and characteristics of dietary supplement recalls in the United States. JAMA Intern Med. 2013;173(10):929–30. https://doi.org/10.1001/jamainternmed.2013.379.
32. Navarro VJ, Barnhart H, Bonkovsky HL, Davern T, Fontana RJ, Grant L, Vuppalanchi R. Liver injury from herbals and dietary supplements in the U.S. Drug-Induced Liver Injury Network. Hepatology. 2014;60(4):1399–408. https://doi.org/10.1002/hep.27317.
33. Statista: The Statistics Portal. (n.d.). Retail sales of vitamins & nutritional supplements in the United States from 2000 to 2017 (in billion U.S. dollars). Retrieved 15 Sept 2018 from https://www.statista.com/statistics/235801/retail-sales-of-vitamins-and-nutritional-supplements-in-the-us/.
34. NBJ survey: health professionals value revenue-generating potential of selling supplements [Blog post]. (2010, Apr 20). New Hope Network: NBJ Blog. Retrieved from https://www.newhope.com/blog/njb-survey-health-professionals-value-revenue-generating-potential-selling-supplements.
35. Rubin R. (2017, July 9). New CDC head Fitzgerald peddled controversial 'anti-aging medicine' before leaving private practice. Forbes. Retrieved from https://www.forbes.com/sites/ritarubin/2017/07/09/new-cdc-head-fitzgerald-peddled-controversial-anti-aging-medicine-before-leaving-private-practice/amp/.
36. Summers D. (2014, Sept 9). Predator doctors take advantage of patients with 'chronic Lyme' scam. Daily Beast. Retrieved from https://www.thedailybeast.com/predator-doctors-take-advantage-of-patients-with-chronic-lyme-scam.
37. Department of Justice. Offices of the United States Attorneys: Northern District of Illinois. (2016, Mar 11). Chicago psychiatrist who took kickbacks to prescribe mental health medication sentenced to nine months in federal prison. Retrieved from https://www.justice.gov/usao-ndil/pr/chicago-psychiatrist-who-took-kickbacks-prescribe-mental-health-medication-sentenced.
38. Alsip M. (2017, Dec 18). Kelly Brogan, MD: a-salt with a "Deadly" weapon (Part one). Bad Science Debunked. Retrieved from https://badsciencedebunked.com/2017/12/18/kelly-brogan-md-a-salt-with-a-deadly-weapon-part-one/.
39. Karlamangla S, Poindexter S. (2017, Aug 13). Despite California's strict new law, hundreds of schools still don't have enough vaccinated kids. Los Angeles Times. Retrieved from http://www.latimes.com/health/la-me-kindergarten-vaccination-20170813-htmlstory.html.
40. Delamater PL, Leslie TF, Yang T. Change in medical exemptions from immunization in California after elimination of personal belief exemptions. JAMA. 2017;318(9):863–4. https://doi.org/10.1001/jama.2017.9242.
41. Nix J. (2018, Jan/Feb). There is a whole cottage industry of doctors helping parents skip their kids' vaccines. Mother Jones. Retrieved from https://www.motherjones.com/politics/2018/01/there-is-a-whole-cottage-industry-of-doctors-helping-parents-skip-their-kids-vaccines/.
42. Zandvliet T. (n.d.) Medical exemptions for California vaccinations. Retrieved 15 Sept 2018 from http://www.southparkdoctor.com/vaccine_exemption.php.

43. Sears B. [Dr. Bob] (2015, July 3). Dr. Bob's daily: navigating the new vaccine law in California [Facebook status update]. Retrieved from https://www.facebook.com/permalink.php?story_fbid=914575131914305&id=116317855073374.
44. Orac. (2015, July 22). After SB 277, medical exemptions to vaccine mandates for sale, courtesy of Dr. Bob Sears [Blog post]. ScienceBlogs. Retrieved from http://scienceblogs.com/insolence/2015/07/22/after-sb-277-medical-exemptions-to-vaccine-mandates-for-sale-courtesy-of-dr-bob-sears/.
45. University of Florida. (2018). About the UF Health Integrative Medicine 5th Annual Conference on April 21, 2018. Retrieved 15 Sept 2018 from https://integrativemed.cme.ufl.edu/about/.
46. Ross C, Blau M, Sheridan K. (2017, Mar 7). Medicine with a side of mysticism: Top hospitals promote unproven therapies. STAT. Retrieved from https://www.statnews.com/2017/03/07/alternative-medicine-hospitals-promote/.
47. VaccinesWorkBlog. (2016, Aug 19). Do doctors get paid to vaccinate? [Blog post]. VaccinesWorkBlog. Retrieved from https://vaccinesworkblog.wordpress.com/2016/08/19/do-doctors-get-paid-to-vaccinate/.
48. Torchiana DF, Colton DG, Rao SK, Lenz SK, Meyer GS, Ferris TG. Massachusetts General Physicians Organization's quality incentive program produces encouraging results. Health Aff. 2013;32(10):1748–56. https://doi.org/10.1377/hlthaff.2013.0377.
49. Volpp KG, John LK, Troxel AB, Norton L, Fassbender J, Loewenstein G. Financial incentive–based approaches for weight loss: a randomized clinical trial. JAMA. 2008;300(22):2631–7. https://doi.org/10.1001/jama.2008.804.
50. Patel MS, Asch DA, Rosin R, Small DS, Bellamy SL, Heuer J, Sproat S, Hyson C, Haff N, Lee SM, Wesby L, Hoffer K, Shuttleworth D, Taylor DH, Hilbert V, Zhu J, Yang L, Wang X, Volpp KG. Framing financial incentives to increase physical activity among overweight and obese adults: a randomized, controlled trial. Ann Intern Med. 2016;164(6):385–94. https://doi.org/10.7326/M15-1635.
51. Wellth. (n.d.). Home. Wellthapp.com. Retrieved from https://wellthapp.com/home.
52. Lepper MR, Greene D, Nisbett RE. Undermining children's intrinsic interest with extrinsic reward: a test of the "overjustification" hypothesis. J Pers Soc Psychol. 1973;28(1):129–37. https://doi.org/10.1037/h0035519.
53. Twain M. The adventures of Tom Sawyer [Google Books version]. Hartford: The American Publishing Company; 1881.
54. Koufman J. (2017, June 3). The specialists' stranglehold on medicine. The New York Times. Retrieved from https://www.nytimes.com/2017/06/03/opinion/sunday/the-specialists-stranglehold-on-medicine.html.
55. Avitzur O. (2011, April). Your doctor as salesman. Consumer Reports. Retrieved from https://www.consumerreports.org/cro/2012/05/your-doctor-as-salesman/index.htm.
56. Goldenberg G. (2008, Sept 4). Pharma influence: does it affect physician prescribing practices? The Dermatologist. Retrieved from https://www.the-dermatologist.com/article/7308.
57. Landefeld CS, Steinman MA. The neurontin legacy — marketing through misinformation and manipulation. N Engl J Med. 2009;360(2):103–6. https://doi.org/10.1056/NEJMp0808659.
58. Hasher L, Goldstein D, Toppino T. Frequency and the conference of referential validity. J Verbal Learn Verbal Behav. 1977;16(1):107–12. https://doi.org/10.1016/S0022-5371(77)80012-1.
59. It took a brilliant marketing campaign to create the best-selling drug of all time. (2011, Dec 28). Business Insider. Retrieved from https://www.businessinsider.com/lipitor-the-best-selling-drug-in-the-history-of-pharmaceuticals-2011-12.
60. Wall LL, Brown D. The high cost of free lunch. Obstet Gynecol. 2007;110(1):169–73. https://doi.org/10.1097/01.AOG.0000268800.46677.14.
61. Saul S. (2005, Nov 28). Gimme an rx! Cheerleaders pep up drug sales. The New York Times. Retrieved from https://www.nytimes.com/2005/11/28/business/gimme-an-rx-cheerleaders-pep-up-drug-sales.html.
62. Elliot C. (2006, April). The drug pushers. The Atlantic. Retrieved from https://www.theatlantic.com/magazine/archive/2006/04/the-drug-pushers/304714/.
63. Howard M. (2009, June 10). Just say no to free drug samples. Tufts Journal. Retrieved from http://tuftsjournal.tufts.edu/2009/06_1/features/03/.

64. Chimonas S. No more free drug samples? PLoS Med. 2009;6(5):e1000074. https://doi.org/10.1371/journal.pmed.1000074.
65. Fugh-Berman A, Ahari S. Following the script: how drug reps make friends and influence doctors. PLoS Med. 2007;4(4):e150. https://doi.org/10.1371/journal.pmed.0040150.
66. Elliot C. (2010, Sept 12). The secret lives of big pharma's 'thought leaders'. The Chronicle of Higher Education. Retrieved from https://www.chronicle.com/article/The-Secret-Lives-of-Big/124335.
67. Carlat D. (2007, Nov 24). Confessions of a drug rep with an M.D. in the drug-marketing juggernaut. The New York Times. Retrieved from https://www.nytimes.com/2007/11/23/your-money-23iht-wbdrug.1.8445704.html.
68. Murrie DC, Boccaccini MT, Guarnera LA, Rufino KA. Are forensic experts biased by the side that retained them? Psychol Sci. 2013;24(10):1889–97. https://doi.org/10.1177/0956797613481812.
69. Ornstein C, Tigas M, Jones RG. (2016, Mar 17). Now there's proof: docs who get company cash tend to prescribe more brand-name meds. ProPublica. Retrieved from https://www.propublica.org/article/doctors-who-take-company-cash-tend-to-prescribe-more-brand-name-drugs.
70. Schwartz TL, Kuhles DJ II, Wade M, Masand PS. Newly admitted psychiatric patient prescriptions and pharmaceutical sales visits. Ann Clin Psychiatry. 2001;13(3):159–62. https://doi.org/10.3109/10401230109148963.
71. DeJong C, Aguilar T, Tseng C, Lin GA, Boscardin J, Dudley A. Pharmaceutical industry-sponsored meals and physician prescribing patterns for Medicare beneficiaries. JAMA Intern Med. 2016;176(8):1114–22. https://doi.org/10.1001/jamainternmed.2016.2765.
72. Yeh JS, Franklin JM, Avorn J, Landon J, Kesselheim AS. Association of industry payments to physicians with the prescribing of brand-name statins in Massachusetts. JAMA Intern Med. 2016;176(6):763–8. https://doi.org/10.1001/jamainternmed.2016.1709.
73. Brax H, Fadlallah R, Al-Khaled L, Kahale LA, Nas H, El-Jardali F, Akl EA. Association between physicians' interaction with pharmaceutical companies and their clinical practices: a systematic review and meta-analysis. PLoS One. 2017;12(4):e0175493. https://doi.org/10.1371/journal.pone.0175493.
74. Austad KE, Avorn J, Franklin JM, Campbell EG, Kesselheim AS. Association of marketing interactions with medical trainee's knowledge about evidence-based prescribing: results from a national survey. JAMA Intern Med. 2014;174(8):1283–9. https://doi.org/10.1001/jamainternmed.2014.2202.
75. Yeh JS, Austad KE, Franklin JM, Chimonas S, Campbell EG, Avorn J, Kesselheim AS. Medical schools' industry interaction policies not associated with trainees' self-reported behavior as residents: results of a national survey. J Grad Med Educ. 2015;7(4):595–602. https://doi.org/10.4300/JGME-D-15-00029.1.
76. Jones RG, Ornstein C, Tigas M. (2016, Dec 13). We've updated dollars for docs. Here's what's new. ProPublica. Retrieved from https://www.propublica.org/article/updated-dollars-for-docs-heres-whats-new.
77. Drexel University. (2017, Mar 6). Two-thirds of Americans see docs who got paid by drug companies. ScienceDaily. Retrieved from https://www.sciencedaily.com/releases/2017/03/170306114211.htm.
78. Dishaw T. (2017, Mar 8). 65% of doctors are getting cash "kickbacks" from big pharma. Natural News. Retrieved from https://www.naturalnews.com/2017-03-08-65-of-doctors-are-getting-cash-kickbacks-from-big-pharma.html.
79. Department of Veterans Affairs. (2000, Oct). Pain as the 5Th Vital Sign Toolkit [PDF file]. Retrieved from https://www.va.gov/PAINMANAGEMENT/docs/TOOLKIT.pdf.
80. Portenoy RK, Foley KM. Chronic use of opioid analgesics in non-malignant pain: report of 38 cases. Pain. 1986;25(2):171–86. https://doi.org/10.1016/0304-3959(86)90091-6.
81. Catan T, Perez E. (2012, Dec 17). A pain-drug champion has second thoughts. The Wall Street Journal. Retrieved from https://www.wsj.com/articles/SB10001424127887324478304578173342657044604.
82. Opiophobia. (n.d.). In: Pain & Policy Studies Group: glossary. Retrieved from http://www.painpolicy.wisc.edu/glossary/opiophobia.

83. Moghe S. (2016, Oct 14). Opioid history: from 'wonder drug' to abuse epidemic. CNN. Retrieved 15 Sept 2018 from https://www.cnn.com/2016/05/12/health/opioid-addiction-history/.

84. Mularski RA, White-Chu F, Overbay D, Miller L, Asch SM, Ganzini L. Measuring pain as the 5th vital sign does not improve quality of pain management. J Gen Intern Med. 2006;21(6):607–12. https://doi.org/10.1111/j.1525-1497.2006.00415.x.

85. Singer N. (2008, Dec 30). No mug? Drug makers cut out goodies for doctors. The New York Times. Retrieved from https://www.nytimes.com/2008/12/31/business/31drug.html.

86. Salmasi S, Ming LC, Khan TM. Interaction and medical inducement between pharmaceutical representatives and physicians: a meta-synthesis. J Pharm Policy Pract. 2016;9(37):1–12. https://doi.org/10.1186/s40545-016-0089-z.

87. Zipkin DA, Steinman MA. Interactions between pharmaceutical representatives and doctors in training: a thematic review. J Gen Intern Med. 2005;20(8):777–86. https://doi.org/10.1111/j.1525-1497.2005.0134.x.

88. Rea S. (2015, June 8). Researchers find everyone has a bias blind spot. Carnegie Mellon University News. Retrieved from https://www.cmu.edu/news/stories/archives/2015/june/bias-blind-spot.html.

89. Gibbons RV, Landry FJ, Blouch DL, Jones DL, Williams FK, Lucey CR, Kroenke K. A comparison of physicians' and patients' attitudes toward pharmaceutical industry gifts. J Gen Intern Med. 1998;13(3):151–4. https://doi.org/10.1046/j.1525-1497.1998.00048.x.

90. Green MJ, Master R, James B, Simmons B, Lehman E. Do gifts from the pharmaceutical industry affect trust in physicians? Fam Med. 2012;44(5):325–31.

91. American Medical Student Association. (n.d.). The campaign. Retrieved 15 Sept 2018 from http://www.pharmfree.org/campaign/.

92. American Medical Student Association. (2016, Oct 24). Executive summary: AMSA Scorecard 2018. Retrieved 15 Sept 2018 from https://amsascorecard.org/executive-summary/.

93. Ventola CL. Direct-to-consumer pharmaceutical advertising: therapeutic or toxic? Pharm Ther. 2011;36(10):669–84.

94. Serenko A, Bontis N. What's familiar is excellent: the impact of exposure effect on perceived journal quality. J Informet. 2011;5(1):219–23. https://doi.org/10.1016/j.joi.2010.07.005.

95. Zebrowitz LA, White B, Wieneke K. Mere exposure and racial prejudice: Exposure to other-race faces increases liking for strangers of that race. Soc Cogn. 2008;26(3):259–75. https://doi.org/10.1521/soco.2008.26.3.259.

96. Bunting M. (2014, Mar 16). If you don't think multiculturalism is working, look at your street corner. The Guardian. Retrieved from https://www.theguardian.com/commentisfree/2014/mar/16/passive-tolerance-beacon-hope-diverse-communities.

97. Dana J, Loewenstein G. A social science perspective on gifts to physicians from industry. JAMA. 2009;290(2):252–5. https://doi.org/10.1001/jama.290.2.252.

98. Lo B, Field MJ, editors. Conflicts of interest in medical research, education, and practice. Washington, DC: The National Academies Press; 2009.

Case

Evie was a 45-year-old woman who presented with a panoply of symptoms, which included fatigue, weight gain, "brain fog," decreased libido, loss of energy, difficulty falling asleep, joint pains, poor concentration, and anxiety. She had seen multiple different clinicians who had ordered a large number of tests and images, none of which had revealed the cause of her symptoms. A friend of hers suggested she take an online test for "adrenal fatigue." She found that she had "nearly every symptom." She contacted the clinician who designed the test, and the clinician confirmed the diagnosis after an in-person consultation.

What Dr. Grater Was Thinking

Adrenal fatigue is both common and undiagnosed. I had reviewed the results of Evie's survey prior to her arrival. She matched most of the symptoms perfectly. Of course, I ruled out common mimics of adrenal fatigue, such as thyroid disorders and low vitamin B12. Once Evie's blood work came back normal, the diagnosis was pretty clear. We worked hard on minimizing stress in her life, making sure she got enough sleep and exercise. We made a lot of changes to her diet and started her on rosemary essential oils, vitamin supplementation, magnesium, and adaptogenic herbs such as ashwagandha, rhodiola rosea, schisandra, and holy basil. Within two months she was feeling much better.

Discussion

The Forer effect is a psychological phenomenon in which people feel that vague, nonspecific descriptions of their personality are, in fact, highly specific to them. These statements are called "Barnum statements" after the circus entertainer P. T. Barnum, who reportedly said that "we have something for everybody." The Forer effect is named after the psychologist Bertram Forer, who gave his students a test called the

"Diagnostic Interest Blank" [1]. They were then given a supposedly personalized description of their personality and asked to rate how well it described them. It consisted of the following 12 descriptors:

1. You have a great need for other people to like and admire you.
2. You have a tendency to be critical of yourself.
3. You have a great deal of unused capacity, which you have not turned to your advantage.
4. While you have some personality weaknesses, you are generally able to compensate for them.
5. Disciplined and self-controlled outside, you tend to be worrisome and insecure inside.
6. At times you have serious doubts as to whether you have made the right decision or done the right thing.
7. You prefer a certain amount of change and variety and become dissatisfied when hemmed in by restrictions and limitations.
8. You pride yourself as an independent thinker and do not accept others' statements without satisfactory proof.
9. You have found it unwise to be too frank in revealing yourself to others.
10. At times you are extroverted, affable, sociable, while at other times you are introverted, wary, reserved.
11. Some of your aspirations tend to be pretty unrealistic.
12. Security is one of your major goals in life.

Unbeknownst to the students, these items were taken from the astrology section of a newspaper, and each person received the same list. Despite this, most students felt it applied to them very well, rating it a 4.26 out of 5. Many others have repeated Forer's initial experiment, and the results have been very similar in their studies. The journalist John Stossel has an amusing video where a group of people receive a horoscope that was supposedly selected specifically for them based on their birthdate and birthplace and prepared by a qualified astrologer. They were amazed at how well it described their personality, until the truth is revealed—it was actually based on the horoscope of a serial killer [2].

The Forer effect exists because Barnum statements are highly generalized, but people perceive them to be highly specific and unique to them. People are eager to take vague statements and apply them to their own lives, especially when the statements are positive, felt to be specifically for them, and provided to them by a trusted source. As philosopher Robert T. Carroll wrote:

> People tend to accept claims about themselves in proportion to their _desire_ that the claims be true rather than in proportion to the empirical accuracy of the claims as measured by some non-subjective standard. We tend to accept questionable, even false statements about ourselves, if we deem them positive or flattering enough [3].

The Forer effect largely explains the ability of psychics, fortune tellers, horoscopes, and online personality tests to convince people something unique about them is being revealed, when in fact they are only receiving vague, generic statements about their life and personality. Many psychics employ a technique called cold reading, in which the psychic makes general statements that can apply to almost everyone. For example, I predict that you, the reader, are an open-minded person who is willing to consider an idea, but may quickly become impatient with sloppy, lazy thinking. (The trick of describing a person with one personality trait, and its opposite, is called the "rainbow ruse"). I predict you sometimes have spent a large sum of money on something you didn't need. I predict you generally like your job, but sometimes wonder if it's *really* what you want to do for the rest of your life. The Forer effect is so powerful that there are even some instances where initially skeptical people convinced themselves they had genuine psychic abilities because of the positive response they received after providing people with vague statements such as these.

When applied to medicine, the Forer effect is a form of the selection bias where patients fill out a survey (often online), and indeed discover they have the condition tested by the survey. To see how this might work, let's consider a very prevalent and serious condition known as Howard's Syndrome (HS). It occurs in people who don't eat donuts every day. If you have at least four of the following symptoms, you may suffer from HS!

1. You don't have as much energy as you used to. You often feel "run down."
2. You cannot exercise as vigorously as in the past.
3. You have trouble losing weight.
4. At times, you have trouble falling asleep. At other times, you wake up too early and have trouble falling back asleep.
5. You sometimes get a dull headache or pain in your lower back.
6. Certain foods upset your stomach.
7. Sometimes you feel sad, anxious, or irritable for no particular reason.
8. You have unexplained muscle and joint pains.
9. Your sex drive is not the same as it was when you were younger.
10. Your vision is not as sharp as it used to be.

How well do these descriptions fit you? I imagine if you gave this list of symptoms to a group of busy adults, most would check off at least a few symptoms, and some would check of most of them. Voila! They have HS and must rush to the bakery to eat as many gluten-laden donuts as possible. However, like the vague personality statements in the Forer effect, seemingly specific symptoms are actually vague and general.

Though they are likely unaware of doing so, some clinicians employ a version of the Forer effect to convince people that they have diseases of dubious validity. Complementary and alternative medicine (CAM) practitioners are particularly noted to employ this method. As I did with HS, they use vague symptom "checklists" and online questionnaires that could apply to many people coping with the aches and pain of normal aging and the stressors of the modern world. Consider, for example, the following list from the website healthynaturalwellness.com, which proposes that Candida infections are responsible for a large panoply of symptoms affecting multiple organ systems [4]. (Not surprisingly, they also seem to be selling the cure in the form of probiotics).

Symptoms and Diseases Caused by Candida

Numerous symptoms and diseases are caused by Candida ranging from allergies to autoimmune diseases to cancer. Here is a partial list of issues:

Acne	Eye Floaters	Laryngitis
Allergies	Fatigue	Low Sex Drive
Anxiety Attacks	Feeling Spaced Out	Low Temperature
Appetite Loss	Flu-Like Symptoms	Memory Loss
Arthritis	Food Cravings	Menstruation Problems
Asthma	Gas	Mood Swings
Athlete's Foot	Glands Swollen/Blocked	Muscle Problems
Bloating	Hair Loss	Nail/Skin Fungus
Body Odor	Hashimoto's Disease	Nasal Congestion
Brain Fog	Headaches/Migraines	Nightmares
Canker Sores	Heart Palpitations	Numbness
Colic	Heartburn	Painful Intercourse
Constipation	Hemorrhoids	Panic Attacks
Cough	Hiatal Hernia	PMS
Cysts	Hives	Prostitis
Depression	Hypoglycemia	Psoriasis
Diabetes	Hypothyroidism	Rashes
Diaper Rash	Impotence	Rectal Itching
Diarrhea	Inability To Concentrate	Ringworm
Difficulty Urinating	Indigestion	Sore Throat
Digestive Problems	Infections (Various)	Thrush
Dizziness	Infertility	Ulcers
Ear Infections	Insomnia	Urinary Issues
Eczema	Irritability	Vaginal Itching/Burning
Endometriosis	Itching Skin	Vaginitis
Epstein Barr	Jock Itch	Vomiting

Almost identical symptom checklists can be found for chronic Lyme disease, multiple chemical sensitivity, adrenal fatigue, bartonella infections, leaky gut syndrome, gluten intolerance, fluoride toxicity, and perceived injuries from vaccines. Articles such as "10 Signs You Have a Leaky Gut—and How to Heal It" abound on the internet [5]. I suspect that if only the name of the disease being discussed were changed from leaky gut syndrome to gluten sensitivity, the article would work just as well.

These checklists and articles are most likely to be encountered by frustrated people with undefined illnesses for whom mainstream medicine has offered no diagnosis or treatment. As such, finding a checklist that explains their symptoms and provides a diagnostic label is likely to be very reassuring. In questioning the existence of these diagnoses, I am by no means minimizing the suffering of the patients who have been diagnosed with these disorders. However, these diagnoses are essentially unfalsifiable, meaning there is no way to rule them out. What test could be performed to definitively tell a person they *don't* have leaky gut syndrome, adrenal fatigue, or gluten sensitivity? Even when tests exist, such as for Lyme disease, CAM practitioners often claim those tests are insensitive, and instead use unvalidated tests performed by unaccredited laboratories.

Patients are likely not the only ones fooled by these checklists. The existence of questionable diseases is reinforced for the CAM practitioner who routinely encounters people whose symptoms are largely matched by their checklist. In this way, they are like a phony psychic who inadvertently becomes convinced of his own powers after consistently receiving positive feedback from his readings.

It is undeniably true that similar symptom checklists exist for diseases of unquestioned validity, such as multiple sclerosis (MS). Consistent with the Forer effect, many patients convince themselves they have the disease after reading these lists online. It is quite common for patients to come to my office certain they have MS as they have "every symptom." However, unlike the conditions theorized by CAM practitioners, responsible clinicians do not create these lists to suggest the diagnosis to potential patients. Moreover, MS can almost always be definitively ruled out with imaging and a spinal tap, though even when these results are normal, some patients continue to insist they have the disease.

The Forer effect also explains the value of asking open-ended questions while taking a patient's history. A simple request that patients describe their symptoms, combined with thoughtful, targeted follow-up questions, is most likely to yield accurate information. In contrast, leading questions may suggest symptoms to the patient. Like those who marvel at the accuracy of their horoscope, patients may feel that a clinician's leading questions are specifically for them, yielding false positive results.

Conclusion

The Forer effect uses vague, nonspecific statements to convince people that a specific truth about them is being revealed. When given vague statements, especially positive ones that are perceived as specifically for them, people easily connect these statements to their life. Psychics use the Forer effect to produce cold readings, convincing people they know amazing details of their lives, when in fact they know only platitudes that apply to most of us in one way or another.

In medicine, online symptoms checklists are commonly employed by CAM practitioners. This technique replicates the cognitive trick of the Forer effect. People with multiple symptoms that lack a unifying diagnosis may easily be made to feel that their correct diagnosis has been miraculously revealed. Similarly, CAM practitioners may genuinely come to believe their diagnostic criteria can reveal diagnoses that eluded their close-minded, conventional colleagues (Fig. 9.1).

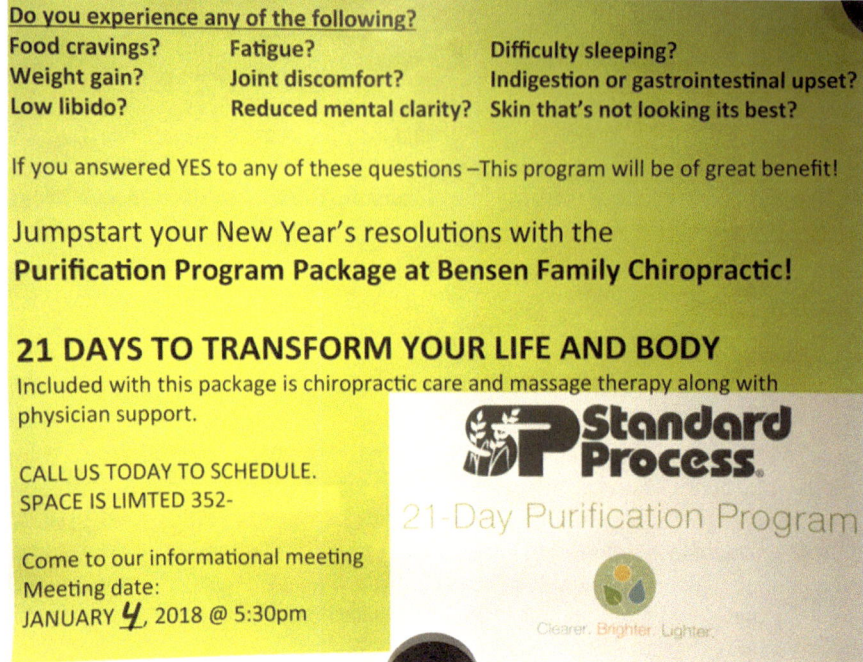

Fig. 9.1 Marketing a purification package using the Forer effect. (Standard Process. 2018. Advertising flyer distributed at various locations [Personal image].)

However, no responsible clinician solicits prospective patients with a long laundry list of vague, common symptoms only to invariably diagnosis them with the "disease" they treat based on their responses. Rather, clinicians should ask patients what symptoms they have, order appropriate diagnostic tests, and render a diagnosis in combination with the history, exam, and supportive evidence.

References

1. Forer BR. The fallacy of personal validation: a classroom demonstration of gullibility. J Abnorm Soc Psychol. 1949;44(1):118–23.
2. Gardiner B. (2014, Aug 25). Amusing demo of the Forer Effect in astrology [Video file]. Retrieved from https://www.youtube.com/watch?v=Vba2ZHMjxBc.
3. Carroll RT. (2003). Forer effect. In: The skeptic's dictionary. Retrieved from http://skepdic.com/forer.html.
4. Symptoms and diseases caused by candida. (n.d.). In: WaybackMachine. Retrieved from https://web.archive.org/web/20160606172940/http://healthynaturalwellness.com/wp-content/uploads/2015/06/symptoms-and-diseases-causes-by-candida.png.
5. Walravens SP. (n.d.). 10 signs you have a leaky gut – and how to heal it [Blog post]. Healthy women. Retrieved from https://www.healthywomen.org/content/blog-entry/10-signs-you-have-leaky-gut%E2%80%94and-how-heal-it.

Framing Effect and Loss Aversion

Case

Claire was a 57-year-old woman who presented with the acute onset of right-sided weakness and word-finding difficulties. She arrived to the ER within 60 minutes and a head CT was normal. She was diagnosed with an acute ischemic stroke. The doctor, Dr. Jones, was prepared to treat her with tissue plasminogen activator (tPA). It helps break down blood clots and had been approved several months prior for the treatment of acute strokes. However, Dr. Jones was dissuaded from doing so when the nurse told her, "don't you know that 6% of patients who get that medicine bleed in their brains?"

What Dr. Jones Was Thinking

Tissue plasminogen activator was a relatively new medication when Claire came to the ER, though it is now the standard of care. I knew the basic data fairly well, and Claire was a textbook candidate to receive it. The nurse was right when he reminded me that 6% of patients can have a symptomatic hemorrhage and that these can have catastrophic effects. This frightened me into not giving a medication that would likely have benefitted the patient. However, another way to present the data would be to say that "94% of the patients who get the medicine don't bleed, and some of these will be helped significantly." Had the nurse said this to me, I almost certainly would have given tPA to Claire. This would have been the correct decision.

Discussion

How people view the risks and benefits of a treatment or test largely depends on the way the risks and benefits are framed. The perceptions of a test or treatment are strongly influenced by whether the outcome is expressed in terms of the possibility that the patient may be harmed or that they might benefit. We are all used to contemplating whether a glass is half empty or half full. However, the implications of this question are more than theoretical. People feel differently about a treatment when

J. Howard, *Cognitive Errors and Diagnostic Mistakes*,
https://doi.org/10.1007/978-3-319-93224-8_10

they are told it succeeds 90% of the time than when they are told it fails 10% of the time. A product that costs $1 per day is viewed more favorably than one that costs $365 per year.

Daniel Kahneman and Amos Tversky demonstrated how changing the frame of an outcome affects how it is perceived and the resultant decisions people make [1]. They presented a hypothetical disease outbreak affecting 600 people and asked subjects which treatment they would use. Treatment A would definitely save one-third of the people while the rest would die. With treatment B, there was a one-third chance that no one would die, but a two-thirds chance that everyone would die. These choice were then presented as how many people would live (positive framing), or how many people would die (negative framing).

Frame	Treatment A	Treatment B
Positive	200 people will be saved	There is a 1/3 chance of saving all 600 people and a 2/3 chance of saving no one.
Negative	400 people will die	There is 1/3 chance that no people will die, and a 2/3 chance that all 600 will die.

In both frames, treatment A and B lead to the same potential outcomes. Yet, in the positive frame, program A was chosen by 72% of participants, while in the negative frame, program B was chosen by 78% of participants. This shows the tendency to be more risk-taking to avoid losses and more risk-averse to achieve rewards. In other words, in the positive frame, people didn't want to lose the "200 people will be saved" by taking a risk on program B. However, in the negative frame they wanted to avoid "400 people will die" by taking a risk on program B.

In a similar experiment, subjects were given $50 and asked to choose one of the following options [2].

1. Keep $30.
2. Take a 50/50 chance of keeping or losing the entire $50.

In this frame the first option is described as a gain, and 57% of subjects decided to keep the $30, acting in a risk-averse way.

Then the experimenters changed the secure option. They asked participants to choose between the following options:

1. Lose $20.
2. Take a 50/50 chance of keeping or losing the entire $50.

In this frame, the first option is described as a loss, and only 39% of subjects acted in a risk-averse way and chose to lose the $20.

To see how framing might affect a clinician's judgment, imagine you are in the middle of an epidemic and have to choose one of two treatment options [3].

In the following scenario, choose A or B:

A. 80% chance to save 1,000 people, 20% chance to save 0.
B. Save 700 for sure.

This choice is a high chance of significant gains. Most people will favor a risk adverse strategy and choose B, even though the expected value of A is higher.

In the following scenario, choose A or B:

A. 80% chance to kill 1,000 people, 20% chance to kill 0.
B. Kill 700 for sure.

This is framed in terms high risk of significant loss. Most people will favor a risk seeking strategy and choose A, even though the expected value of B is higher.

Kahneman and Tversky called this pattern of decision-making "prospect theory" [4]. It posits that losses and gains are perceived differently and that people make choices based more on perceived gains than perceived losses. If a person has to choose between two equal options, they are more likely to choose the one that is framed as a gain over one that is framed as a loss. A key concept related to this is that of loss aversion, which refers to people's tendency to prefer avoiding losses over obtaining equivalent gains. The pain of losing $100, for example, will out-weigh the pleasure of gaining $100. Their work showed that psychologically, losses are twice as powerful as equivalent gains. The tennis player Jimmy Connors expressed loss aversion perfectly by saying, "I hate to lose more than I love to win."

The concept of loss aversion is easy to illustrate with the following thought experiment. Imagine walking down the street and finding two $100 bills. You'd be thrilled. Now imagine if someone else saw them at the same time and grabbed one of them, leaving you with only $100. You would be much less happy than if you just found one $100 bill and got to keep it. In each case, you'd walk away with $100, but in the first scenario, the pain of knowing that you "lost" $100 by not being a bit faster would significantly lessen your pleasure (Fig. 10.1).

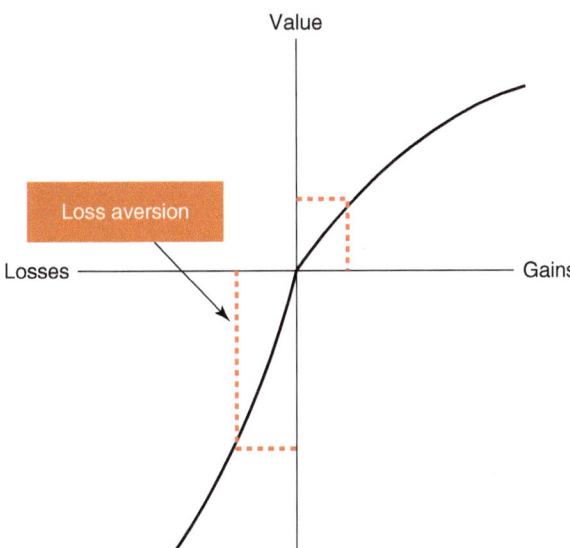

Fig. 10.1 Loss aversion. The pain of a loss is felt more than the joy of a gain

	Significant gain	**Significant loss**
High probability	**Risk adverse** (Under-weigh potential benefit) Patients undervalue favorable practices in favor of status quo. They fear disappointment and become risk averse. Patients who feel well may refuse to quit smoking and refuse interventions such as cancer screening and vaccines.	**Risk seeking** (Under-weigh potential harm) Risky practices will likely be sought in an unlikely attempt to rid oneself of certain loss. Patients who are ill will be prone to engage in risky, unproven treatments such as stem cells and "detox."
Low probability	**Risk seeking** (Over-weigh potential benefit) Patients embrace dubious treatments thinking "what's the harm?" and hoping for a miraculous benefit.	**Risk adverse** (Under-weigh potential harm) Patients embrace unwarranted diagnostic tests, such as total-body MRI scans for healthy people "just to be sure."

Fig. 10. 2 Fourfold pattern for the predictions of prospect theory

Loss aversion and the framing effect have obvious implications for how people inter-pret gains and loses. A salesman trying to sell more fuel-efficient cars would be more effective in his sales pitch if he said, "you're losing money with your current car" than by saying "you will save money if you get this new car." Similarly, people will feel very differently if they are told that a treatment has a 90% chance of saving their life than if they are told a treatment 10% chance of failure, resulting in death. Kahneman described a "fourfold pattern" for the predictions of prospect theory, which was adapted to medi-cine by John Byrne [3]. This has implications for clinicians and patients alike (Fig. 10.2).

Not surprisingly, pharmaceutical companies are aware of the framing effect. To present a real-life example, consider the multiple sclerosis medication terifluni-mode, which can lead to hair loss. How do you think the company framed this side effect on the website? [5].

1. "Hair thinning or hair loss was a side effect of AUBAGIO reported in clinical trials. 13% of patients on AUBAGIO 14 mg and 10% of patients on AUBAGIO 7 mg reported hair thinning or hair loss."
2. "Hair thinning or hair loss was a side effect of AUBAGIO reported in clinical trials. 87% of patients on AUBAGIO 14 mg and 90% of patients on AUBAGIO 7 mg did not report hair thinning or hair loss."

If you guessed #2, give yourself a cookie.

Additionally, people have an interesting cognitive flaw related to the framing effect when making comparisons between two items. Namely, they might prefer item A to item B when they are presented separately, but item B to item A when they are presented simultaneously. Christopher Hsee coined the term the "less-is-better effect," demonstrating that people's preferences largely depend on how their choices are framed. He performed studies showing that:

> *(1) a person giving a $45 scarf as a gift was perceived to be more generous than one giving a $55 coat; (2) an overfilled ice cream serving with 7 oz of ice cream was valued more than an under-filled serving with 8 oz of ice cream; (3) a dinnerware set with 24 intact pieces was judged more favorably than one with 31 intact pieces (including the same 24) plus a few broken ones* [6].

Importantly, he noted that this effect was noted "only when the options were evaluated separately, and reversed itself when the options were juxtaposed." His general observation was that when people judge the value of an item, they do so by comparing it to other items in the same category.

Even when numbers are not involved, framing the same question with different words can change the response. Eldar Shafir demonstrated this using a fictional child custody case [7]. Subjects read that Parent A was moderately suitable to have custody. Parent B had a mixture of positive and negative qualities: a close relationship with the child, but a job that would frequently separate the two for lengthy periods (Fig. 10.3).

When asked, "Which parent should be awarded custody of the child?" 64% of subjects looked for positive attributes and gave custody to Parent B. However, when asked, "Which parent should be denied custody of the child?" they looked for negative attributes and 55% felt Parent B should be denied custody. This shows that when opting *for* something, we look for its positive attributes. However, when opting *against* something, we look for its negative attributes. Pollsters know this phenomenon and are cognizant that subtle changes in how questions are framed can lead to large changes in the answers they receive. Several experiments have demonstrated that how a question is framed dramatically influences how people answer it. For example, a poll from 2010 found that most people were open to gay men and women serving in the military, but opposed to homosexuals doing so [8].

Finally, clinicians should be aware that how they communicate with patients and their caregivers is also affected by the framing affect. Lucas Zier and colleagues found that family members of ill patients were often able to correctly interpret a positive prognosis when told a patient had "a 90% chance of surviving" [9].

Parent A	Parent B
Average income	Above-average income
Average health	Very close relationship with the child
Average working hours	
Reasonable rapport with the child	Extremely active social life
	Lots of work-related travel
Relatively stable social life	Minor health problems

Fig. 10. 3 Who should get custody, parent A or B?

However, they fared poorly when asked to interpret a pessimistic one, "a 5% chance." In interviews with the patient surrogates, they felt that "attributes unknown to the physician would lead to better-than-predicted outcomes," a form of the optimism bias.

In another study, Katherine Berry and colleagues surveyed 539 subjects to determine if the way a skin condition, actinic keratosis, was framed would influence their willingness to receive treatment for it. The found that when it was presented as "precancer," 92% of subjects opted for treatment. When it was not described this way, the number of subjects opting for treatment fell to about 60% [10]. Steven Feldman, a dermatologist, commented:

> What is remarkable about this study is that it raises a general issue of tremendous importance to patient care: that how we frame issues has dramatic effects on how patients interpret those issues. Humans assess things very subjectively. That's the way our minds work. How we present something to a patient will certainly affect his or her willingness to agree and adhere to treatment. If we tell patients, "Actinic keratoses can turn into cancers," they would be very likely to accept treatment, while if we say, "99 out of 100 of these actinic keratoses are likely not to turn into anything bad," they would be much less likely to want to treat. Both of these statements are accurate and in no way in conflict, but they would be perceived very differently by patients [11].

Conclusion

Clinicians, like everyone else, are not perfectly rational decision-makers. Our decisions depend largely on how our options are framed. We think in terms of wins and losses and, because of the psychological phenomenon of loss aversion, we feel the pain of losses more than we feel the joy of gains. This distorts rational analysis. We overvalue probability when thinking in terms of loss (risk seeking) and we undervalue probability when thinking in terms of gains (risk averse). Patients may be highly influenced by the framing effect and loss aversion. How clinicians frame risks to patients will also affect their willingness to undergo a particular treatment. Even a subtle twist in the way a risk is framed can have a dramatic impact on how it is perceive by patients.

Sunk Costs, Endowment Effect, Choice-Supportive Bias

Case

Luisa was a 50-year-old woman who initially presented with dizziness, vertigo, nausea, and vomiting, which had begun upon awakening. On examination, she was clearly uncomfortable and had an unsteady, wide-based gait and nystagmus (jerky eye movements) when looking to the left. On review of symptoms, she reported "blurry vision" at times and "brain fog." She reported a prior episode of double vision in her twenties, but had trouble remembering the details. She had quit smoking several years prior and had mild hypertension, but was otherwise healthy. A brain MRI in the ER showed "extensive bilateral white matter lesions which are consistent with demyelinating disease, vasculitis, microvascular disease, migraines, post-infectious, or vasculitis." Based on Luisa's current symptoms, her reports of previous neurological symptoms, and the MRI findings, she was diagnosed with relapsing-remitting MS and told to follow-up with Dr. Morris, a neurologist. She was started on interferon-beta, an injectable medication to prevent relapses.

Luisa continued this medication for nearly 10 years. Over that time, she had no new attacks and no new lesions on her MRI. She then moved to a different state where a second neurologist questioned the diagnosis. He ordered a spinal tap to look for oligoclonal bands, a marker of inflammation present in over 90% of patients with MS. When this finding was absent, the second neurologist informed the patient that she had been misdiagnosed with MS. Instead, it was felt that her imaging findings were likely due to microvascular disease, which is present on the MRI of many patients over the age of 50, especially smokers and those with other medical comorbidities.

What Dr. Morris Was Thinking

I first met Luisa after she was discharged from the ER. She told me that she had been diagnosed with MS, and I had little reason to doubt the diagnosis. Looking back, there were a few red flags that should have alerted me that this diagnosis was unlikely. She was older, though still within the range patients can be diagnosed with MS. Her exam was normal when I first met her, which would be unusual for a patient with MS and the degree of white matter disease on her MRI. However, the real mistake was not to re-evaluate her diagnosis over the course of a decade. She would usually come to my office and tell me that she was feeling well, though the injections made her feel miserable. At other times, she complained of vague findings that were not specific for MS, such as back pain or word-finding difficulties. However, her lack of clinical progression and the overall stability of her MRI should have led me to reconsider the diagnosis, or at least suggest additional diagnostic tests, such as a spinal tap.

Had I retracted her MS diagnosis, it would have been a significant blow to her self-identity. She had become active in the MS community and was the leader of the local support group. She also would likely have been quite angry. She had been on a medication which was safe, but expensive and quite unpleasant for her to take. By the time another neurologist reversed her diagnosis, her insurance company had spent hundreds of thousands of dollars on the medication. Additionally, she had stopped working and had gone on disability because of her diagnosis. So "undiagnosing" her MS could have threatened her financial well-being in a very serious way.

Finally, it would have been difficult for me personally to have admitted I was incorrect. Don't get me wrong, if I were convinced that she did not have MS, I would have told her. But my ego and protecting myself against her potential anger were probably unconscious reasons I never revisited her diagnosis. The correct diagnosis was made only when someone who had no history with her was able to view her case with fresh, unbiased eyes.

Discussion

A sunk cost refers to a cost that has already been incurred and cannot be recovered. The sunk cost error is the tendency to continue a suboptimal course of action because substantial resources have already been devoted to it. Imagine a woman who bought a ticket to musical that then received horrible reviews. The musical now sounds so awful she is no longer sure if she wants to see the performance. Since she has already purchased the ticket and cannot get her money back, its cost should not factor into her decision-making. Rationally, if she thinks she will not like the show, she shouldn't go. Yet, people will often feel obligated to use something they have purchased based on the faulty reasoning that they don't want to "waste" the money they have already spent. "Losing" money this way hurts. Similarly, businesses that have invested heavily in a losing strategy may be hesitant to abandon it once they have devoted substantial resources to it. Sunk costs need not be monetary. It started raining during my walk home recently. I was about a mile away from home and got sick of the walk about half way home. Rather than do the reasonable thing and get a taxi, I continued to walk home, foolishly reasoning that I should do so since I had already walked a long distance.

The sunk cost error largely occurs because of loss aversion, which posits that from a psychological perspective, the pain of losing is more powerful than the joy of winning. Tversky and Kahneman have shown that losses are generally twice as powerful as equivalent gains. In a classic study, they demonstrated how the sunk cost error and loss aversion can lead to irrational decision-making [12]. They presented study subjects with the following scenarios:

Case 1: Imagine that you have decided to see a play and paid the admission price of $10 per ticket. As you enter the theater, you discover that you have lost the ticket. The seat was not marked, and the ticket cannot be recovered. Would you buy another ticket?

In this case, 46% said "Yes," and 54% said "No."

Case 2: Imagine that you have decided to see a play and paid the admission price of $10 per ticket. As you enter the theater, you discover that you have lost a $10 bill. Would you buy another ticket?

In the second case, 88% said, "Yes," and only 12% said "No."

Yet, the cases are no different. In each case, $10 has been lost, and the decision about whether the play is worth that price should be independent of a loss that preceded it. But that's not how people feel.

Under the right circumstances, the sunk cost error and loss aversion can lead people to make horribly irrational decisions. One striking example of this is known as the dollar auction. In this game, designed by economist Martin Shubik, a dollar bill is presented for auction to a group of people. There are two rules.

1. Bids must increase in $1 increments.
2. Both the winner and the runner-up must pay their last bid.

The winner must pay his bid and will get the dollar. Though the second-place finisher must also pay, she will get nothing. So, what happens when this game is played in real life?

As Max Bazerman, a business professor who often runs this experiment with a $20 bill, explained, "The pattern is always the same. The bidding starts out fast and furious until it reaches the $12 to $16 range" [13]. Invariably, two students start to compete against each other, paying more than $20 to get $20. Once students start paying more than $20, they are not playing to win, they are playing not to lose, and Bazerman said that students have paid a record of $204 for that $20 bill.

Another important concept related to the sunk cost error and loss aversion is a phenomenon known as the endowment effect, a term coined by the economist Richard Thaler. It posits that once someone has acquired an item, this ownership alone increases its value in their eyes. People are willing to pay more to retain something they own, than to obtain something new, even if the objects in question are of equal value. Someone who might not pay $10 for an object, for example, might not sell the same object for $20. It is a version of the status quo bias, where people believe the current state of affairs is ideal. Kahneman and colleagues demonstrated the endowment effect in a simple experiment in which participants were given a coffee mug and then given the opportunity to sell or trade it for pens [14]. They found that people demanded a higher price for a mug that had been given to them, but put a lower price on one they did not yet own. The endowment effect is likely to be especially powerful for an expensive item or one that required a great deal of effort to obtain. With such purchases, people will work hard to justify it to themselves and others.

To complicate the pictures even further, our memories are faulty in a way that increases our vulnerability to the sunk cost error. Once a decision has been made, the chosen option is recalled as more positive and the rejected alternatives as more negative, a phenomenon known as the choice-supportive bias. Did you buy an expensive new phone? You are likely to bask in its virtues, while degrading its competitors. Did you vote for Donald Trump for president? You are more likely to extol his perceived accomplishments, while magnifying the imperfections of Hillary Clinton, saying how much worse things would be had she won the presidency. As Lottie Brown and colleagues wrote, "irreversible decision-making increases the accessibility of the positive aspects of the chosen and the negative aspects of the rejected alternatives" [15].

In one experiment demonstrating the choice-supportive bias, Mara Mather and colleagues asked subjects to choose between two job candidates, each with four positive and four negative traits. Later, the subjects remembered more positive traits of the candidate they chose and more negative traits of the one they rejected [16]. As Mather and Marcia Johnson wrote [17]:

Many studies … have demonstrated that after making a choice, people shift their attitudes to be more consistent with the decision they made. People also seem to remember their choices in a regret-minimizing fashion…. These choice-supportive asymmetries presumably reflect the constructive-reconstructive processes that are a key aspect of remembering. In

*particular, people may have the implicit theory that because one of the options was selected
over the other, it probably had more positive features and fewer negative features than the
other option.*

The choice-supportive bias may affect clinicians who have invested a large
amount of time or effort in a particular diagnosis or treatment. A clinician who
chooses a treatment for a patient and continues with it for many years is going to be
emotionally invested in its success. As such, they are more likely to remember the
treatment's successes than its failures, and they will therefore be able to more easily
justify their decision-making.

A study by Jennifer Braverman and J.S. Blumenthal-Barby examined 389 clinicians by providing them with several clinical cases that varied based on the source and
type of prior investment [18]. They found that only 11% of subjects suggested continuing an ineffective treatment, and many clinicians demonstrated a significant tendency to over-compensate for the previous use of an ineffective treatment. Similarly,
Brian Bernstein and colleagues surveyed internal medicine and family practice residents and also found no evidence of a sunk cost effect in their decision-making when
presented with hypothetical scenarios [19]. Both of these studies suffer from the same
limitation of using hypothetical scenarios, rather than studying clinicians who had
actually devoted their time and energy to an ineffective treatment in real patients.

Perhaps the best demonstration of the sunk cost effect in medicine can be seen in
how clinicians react when a key treatment of theirs is found to be ineffective. Not
surprisingly, when coronary artery stenting was shown to not benefit patients with
stable angina, many cardiologists did not eagerly embrace these findings. Instead,
many spun negative results as best they could in an attempt to continue to justify the
procedure [20]. Similarly, interventional radiologists generally did not celebrate
when studies showed that vertebroplasty was ineffective for vertebral compression
fractures. These clinicians had devoted much of their careers to (and derived much
of their income from) treatments that did not work, and showing the sunk cost
effect, they did not rush to abandon these procedures even in the face of powerful
evidence they should do so [21].

Patients are also susceptible to these same biases. A patient who has paid a large
amount of money for a treatment or suffered through a painful procedure is likely
to recount aspects of this treatment that cast their decision in a favorable light. As
such, they may over-report the benefit of a treatment if it is expensive or if they
invested a large amount of time and emotional capital in its success. Someone who
traveled 100 miles and paid $2,000 for a turmeric detox is likely to do whatever they
can to justify the cost to themselves and others, attributing significant benefits to it
rather than admit to themselves they were swindled. This shows the importance of
judging the efficacy of treatments in formal scientific studies, not anecdotes.

Conclusion

The sunk cost error is the tendency to continue an ineffective treatment because
time, money, and emotional capital have already been devoted to it. Clinicians
who have spent significant resources as well as their sense of professional

capability in diagnosing and treating a patient will come to "own" their decisions. They will be less likely to reconsider their treatment than a clinician who has not made a similar investment. Retracting a diagnosis or reconsidering a treatment is more difficult once time and resources have been invested in it than at the treatment's inception. However, just because time and money have been spent in a wrong diagnosis or suboptimal treatment, this is not a reason to continue that treatment plan.

While recognizing the sunk cost error can be relatively easy in financial transactions, it can be difficult to recognize in medicine. Is a clinician who continues with a treatment that does not seem to be working persistent or stubborn? Will their perseverance be rewarded, or are they losing valuable time due to the sunk cost error? The answer may only be known in hindsight.

When seeing a well-known patient, clinicians should periodically pause and think to themselves, "If I were meeting this patient for the first time, would I make the same diagnosis and would I start the treatment I am currently using?" If the answer to either of these question is "no," then the clinician should abandon their current treatment, no matter what resources have been devoted to it. Businesses are advised not to throw good money after bad. This applies to clinicians as well.

Anchoring Effect

Case
Luke was a 35-year-old man who was diagnosed with MS after he developed double vision. His neurologist presented him with several treatment options, including glatiramer acetate and fingolimod. She told Luke that glatiramer acetate was a completely safe medication, and that while fingolimod had a risk of a serious brain infection, the overall risk was low. The neurologist felt fingolimod was the best treatment option, as it is more effective than glatiramer acetate and Luke's disease was quite active. However, upon hearing that fingolimod came with some serious risks, while glatiramer acetate did not, Luke rejected the advice to start fingolimod. He said, "Why would I take a medication that had some serious risks, when I could take one that is perfectly safe?" Luke had several more relapses while on glatiramer acetate and agreed to change to fingolimod, but only after he started using a cane to walk.

What Dr. Torrence Was Thinking
I commonly present my patients with a choice between glatiramer acetate, fingolimod, and natalizumab. Glatiramer acetate is extremely safe, but not particularly effective. In contrast fingolimod and natalizumab are more effective, but they come with a risk of a very serious, potentially fatal infection: progressive multifocal leukoencephalopathy (PML). The risk of this infection with fingolimod is about one in 6,000 and there have been 13 cases of PML due to this medication. Undoubtedly there will be more. The risk of this infection with natalizumab is much higher.

In certain patients, the risk can be as high as one in 100, and there have been nearly 800 cases due to this medication.

I have learned that how patients perceive the risk of these treatments depends on the order in which I present them. If I present the risk of glatiramer acetate first, for example, the risk posed by fingolimod is perceived as high. However, if I present the risk of natalizumab first, the risk posed by fingolimod is perceived as low. My job is to present patients with an honest appraisal of their treatment options, but also to make a recommendation. I do not want a patient to choose a medication that is not strong enough to control their disease, nor do I want to expose them to unnecessary risk by having patients with milder disease take an unsafe medication.

I am not saying Luke necessarily made an unreasonable choice. For some patients, the fear of a medication side-effect can be overwhelming. If he did not want even the slightest risk of a serious infection, then he made the right choice. However, it is not clear that the way I presented the medications helped him make the best decision. By presenting a medication with a real, but very low, risk after presenting a medication with a zero risk, I heightened the risk of that medication in his mind. He was unable to perceive the risk of fingolimod in an objective way, but only how it compared to a completely safe medication.

I now know that the first number I present to patients has powerful implications for how they perceive risk. Certainly, I must present the risks of a medication to the patient in a completely honest way. However, my job is not just to present the raw data, but also do my best to help patients think about risk in a rational way. I now tailor my discussion to help patients take a medication that offers the best benefit to risk ratio, in my opinion. For example, I tell my patients that the risk posed by fingolimod is statistically less than their risk of death from "excessive natural heat." I am aware that patients perceive the risk of a medication based not only on the risk that medication poses, but also compared to the risks of the alternatives I discuss before or after.

Discussion

The anchoring bias occurs when an initial data point, the "anchor," serves as a reference point that subsequently influence all other decisions. At a perceptual level, how we perceive objects is influenced by what surrounds them. This is the basis for many optical illusions. In Fig. 10.4, for example, the orange circles are the same size, though they certainly do not appear that way (Ebbinghaus illusion).

Our perception of numbers is vulnerable to a similar cognitive error. In medicine, the anchoring bias occurs when the risk or benefit of a treatment is perceived as low or high because it is presented after an initial number that serves as the anchor. The anchoring bias can also lead to diagnostic errors when an initial piece of information serves as a lens through which the patient's entire case is viewed. (This type of error is discussed in the section on premature closure, Chapter 23).

Amos Tversky and Daniel Kahneman demonstrated the power of the anchoring bias in several classic experiments, showing the first numbers we encounter have a powerful effect on our perception of subsequent numbers. In one study, they spun a wheel with 100 numbers that was rigged to stop at either 10 or 65 [22]. They then

Fig. 10. 4 The Ebbinghaus illusion. (Ebbinghaus illusion. [Image file]. In Wikipedia. 2018. Retrieved from https://en.wikipedia.org/wiki/Ebbinghaus_illusion#/media/File:Mond-vergleich.svg.)

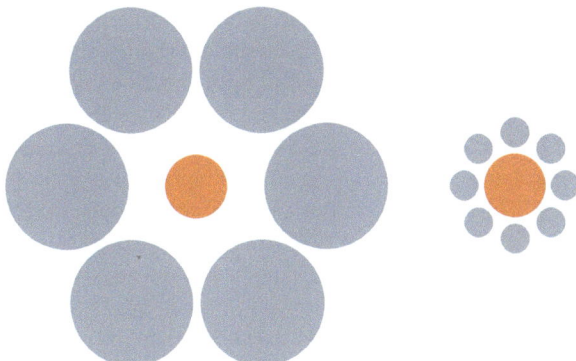

asked subjects whether the percentage of African nations in the United Nations was smaller or larger or smaller than the number on the wheel. They then asked them to estimate the correct number. Those who spun the wheel to a 10 guessed 25%, while those who spun the wheel to 65 guessed 45%.

In another experiment, subjects were given 5 seconds to calculate the product of the numbers one through eight. Some subjects were shown them arranged lowest to highest ($1 \times 2 \times 3 \times 4 \times 5 \times 6 \times 7 \times 8$). For these subjects, the average estimate was 512. Other subjects were shown them arranged highest to lowest ($8 \times 7 \times 6 \times 5 \times 4 \times 3 \times 2 \times 1$). For these subjects, the average estimate was four times as large, 2,250 [22].

Tversky and Kahneman also demonstrated how the anchoring bias can influence professionals. In one experiment, they showed real estate agents a house priced either substantially too high or low [23]. They asked the agents to ignore this number and estimate a reasonable price for the house, something the real estate agents felt they could do. However, the price difference between the two groups was 41%. In yet another experiment, they rolled a pair of dice for judges. The dice were rigged to total either three or nine. They then presented them with the case of a woman who had been caught shoplifting and asked them to determine an appropriate sentence. Judges who rolled a nine averaged a sentence of eight months, while those who rolled a three gave her five months [23]. Even purposefully absurd anchors can influence our judgment. One study asked subjects to estimate the year Albert Einstein first came to the US. Anchors of 1215 and 1992 affected subjects' responses as much as plausible answers such as 1905 and 1939 [24].

Dan Ariely wrote in *Predictably Irrational* about an experiment he conducted also demonstrating the impact of random numbers on people's perception [25]. He first asked students to write down the last two digits of their Social Security number. He then asked them how much they would be willing to pay for several items: a fancy bottle of wine, an average bottle of wine, a book, or a box of chocolates. Those students whose Social Security numbers ended in the highest digits were willing to pay the most money, while those with the lowest digits were willing to pay the least. The difference was large. Those with the highest digits were willing to pay three times more than those in the lowest digits for the same objects. As expected, the students denied that their Social Security number had an influence over their decision. This shows how even completely arbitrary numbers can serve as an unconscious anchor, influencing our judgment in important ways.

Examinations of real-world prices have demonstrated that the anchoring bias influences how items are priced and sold. Grace Bucchianeri and Julia Minson analyzed 14,000 real estate transactions and found that after controlling for other variables, higher asking prices were associated with higher sales prices [26]. Overpricing a property by 10–20% lead to an increase in sales price. Though the effect was rather modest, earning the seller an additional $117 to $163, it was consistent with the anchoring effect.

Predictably, advertisers and salesmen are well aware of how the anchoring bias influences potential customers. People will be more likely to buy a $100 bottle of wine if they are first presented with the option to buy a $250 bottle than a $20 bottle. Similarly, in perhaps the oldest trick around, a "discounted" item is perceived as less expensive if the "full' price is presented first. During a recent trip to the aquarium, I was offered the opportunity to buy two plush animals for $30. This was meant to seem like a great deal, considering that it was a $40 value, or so I was meant to think. It's difficult to go to a large store without seeing "special offers" like this (Fig. 10.5).

Stores also try to anchor customers with ploys such as limiting the number of items a customer can purchase. Given that stores presumably want to sell as much as they can, what is the rationale for policies that limit the number of items customers can purchase? This also sets an anchor, suggesting to the shopper that 12 is an appropriate number of items for them to purchase, and indeed research has shown it does tend to get customers to purchase more items (Fig. 10.6).

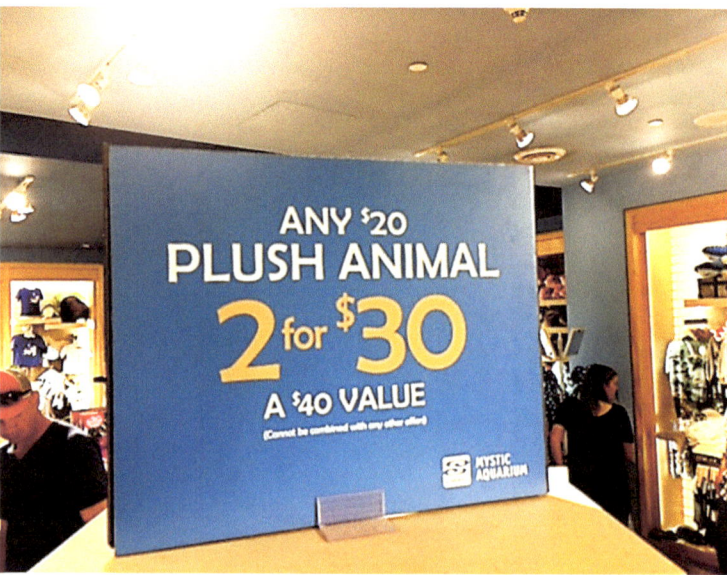

Fig. 10. 5 An advertisement taking advantage of the anchoring bias

SPECIAL BUY NO. 2 OF 5

UP TO 54% OFF SELECT OUTDOOR POWER

Homelite 14 in. 10 Amp Electric Dethatcher
Internet# 205481730

★★★★★ (7)   Learn More

~~$149.00~~   WAS

-$50.00   SPECIAL BUY
          SAVINGS
_____
$99.00   YOUR NEW
          PRICE

ADD TO CART

Limit 5 per customer

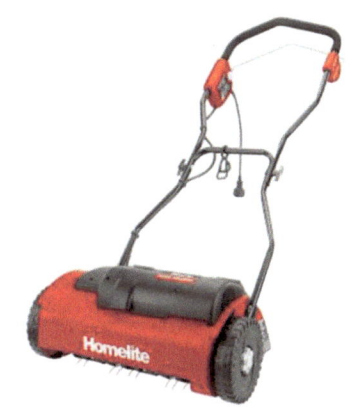

Fig. 10. 6 An advertisement taking advantage of the anchoring bias both by showing a "discount," and also having a limit of five per customer. (Home Depot: Save up to 54% on power tools for yard & home. [Image file]. In: The coupon project. 2016. Retrieved from http://thecouponproject.com/home-depot-save-up-to-54-on-power-tools-for-yard-home-215-only/.)

Sometimes, more sophisticated ploys are used. Dan Ariely showed how an advertisement for *The Economist* magazine used the anchoring bias to potentially boost its sales [27]. It initially presented the following subscription options:

Economist.com Subscription....................$59
(On-line access to all articles for 1 year)

Print and Web Subscription.....................$125
(1-year subscription to the printed edition and full on-line access)

Given these two options, only 32% of people purchased the $125 product. They then added a "decoy" product to the advertisement above.

Economist.com Subscription....................$59
(On-line access to all articles for 1 year)

Print Subscription...................................$125
(1-year subscription to the printed edition)

Print and Web Subscription.....................$125
(1-year subscription to the printed edition and full on-line access)

In this case, 84% purchased the $125 product. Potential buyers compared the two $125 products, and obviously, one was much better than the other. This contrast blinded them to a comparison between the $59 and $125 products. Robert Levine told of a cable company that was raising its prices, but used the anchoring bias to try to convince their customers they should feel happy about this. They told them:

It's not often you get good news instead of a bill, but we've got some for you. If you've heard all those rumors about your basic cable rate going up $10 or more a month, you can relax: it's not going happen! The great news is...the rate for basic cable is only increasing by $2 a month [28].

In medicine, the risks and benefits of treatments are similarly vulnerable to the anchoring bias. A procedure with a complication rate of 5% might seem safe if compared with alternative with a complication rate of 25%. The same 5% complication rate might seem unacceptable if compared with alternative with a complication rate of 1%. However, a procedure with a complication rate of 5% has a complication rate of 5%, independent of the safety of alternative procedures.

Let's do a thought experiment. Your patient has meningitis. A powerful antibiotic can cure this infection, but can also lead to serious bleeding, which has been fatal to several patients, including one at your hospital. Based on a genetic marker, it is possible to divide patients into a high-risk group, which has a one in 10 chance of bleeding and a low-risk group, which has a one in 100 chance of bleeding. Your patient, happily, is in the low-risk group. Would you use this medication for your patient?

Now, consider the same case, but let's alter the numbers. Again, your patient has meningitis. Based on a genetic marker you can divide patients into a low-risk group, which has a one in 1,000 chance of bleeding, and a high-risk group, which has a one in 100 chance of bleeding. Your patient, unfortunately, is in the high-risk group. Now, how do you feel about the use of this medication for your patient?

In each of the scenarios above, your patient has a 1% chance of bleeding. Therefore, it is rational not to care whether your patient is in the low or high-risk group. You should be willing to use this medication (or not) equally in both scenarios. However, by presenting the patient in the "high" and "low" risk groups, the same risk is perceived differently. In the first case, the one in 10 risk is presented first and serves as an anchor for the one in 100 risk, perhaps making it seem low. In the second case, the one in 1,000 risk is presented first and serves as an anchor for the one in 100 risk, perhaps making it seem high.

The anchoring bias has important implications for how clinicians should discuss risk with patients. Almost every day, I discuss medications for MS that can lead to PML a serious and potentially fatal infection. One medication comes with a one in 100 risk of PML in susceptible patients, another comes with a one in 6,000 risk, while several others carry no risk at all. Unfortunately, the medications with the highest benefit tend to carry the greatest risk. I have learned that many patients will perceive the one in 6,000 risk as acceptably low if I first present the medication with the one in 100 risk. Conversely, most will perceive the one in 6,000 risk as unacceptably high, if I first discuss the medications with zero risk. Obviously, a medication with a one in 6,000 risk does not become safer or more dangerous simply because other medications carry a lesser or greater risk.

However, once an "anchor" is introduced, it is difficult, if not impossible, for patients (and clinicians) to perceive that risk in isolation. I am often faced with patients who are, in my opinion, excessively scared of a medication that is likely to be of significant benefit to them. With these patients, I use the anchoring bias to hopefully reassure them by comparing the risk of the medication with common risks they may be taking already, such as driving or smoking. Even staying at home and doing nothing is potentially more dangerous than some of the medications that cause my patients great anxiety. After all, exposure to fire, flames, or smoke is the cause of death in one out of 1,498 Americans according to the National Safety Council [29]. Compared to this, a medication that carries a one in 6,000 risk of a serious side effect doesn't sound so bad.

Note also that people are more strongly influenced by the percentage change in value, rather that the absolute change in value. With regards to perceptual stimuli, this is known as the Weber–Fechner law. In Fig. 10.7, the bottom boxes contain ten more dots than the top boxes. This difference is more easily perceived when the number of dots increases from 10 to 20 than from 110 to 120.

How we think about numbers is vulnerable to a similar distortion. For example, a $100 discount on a $20,000 car will not seem like a big deal. If you were buying a car and heard that another dealer across town was selling the same

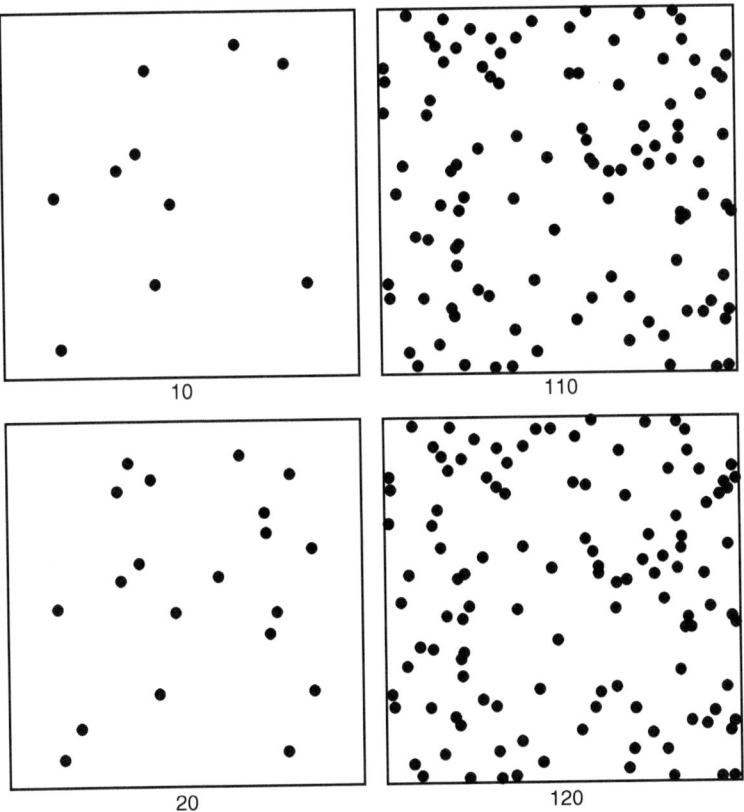

Fig. 10. 7 The Weber–Fechner law. It is much easier to notice an increase of ten dots when the starting point is low. (MrPomidor. An illustration of the Weber-Fechner law [Image file]. In: Wikipedia. 2017. Retrieved from https://en.wikipedia.org/wiki/Weber%E2%80%93Fechner_law#/media/File:Weber-Fechner_law_demo_-_dots.png.)

car for $19,900, you'd probably think travelling across town wasn't worth the effort. In contrast, a $100 discount on a pair of shoes that costs $200 seems amazing. You'd definitely make the crosstown trip to get the shoes at another store. However, in each case you'd be saving $100. In a demonstration of this, Kahneman and Tversky asked subjects if they would be willing to drive 20 minutes across town to save $5 on a $15 calculator. Sixty-eight percent of subjects said they would make the trip. However, only 29% of subjects would drive across town to save $5 on a $125 coat [1]. Similarly, a medication that increases the risk of a serious infection from 1% to 6% will be perceived as much more dangerous than a medication that increases the risk from 65% to 70%. Yet, in each case the risk of a serious infection increases by 5% (Fig. 10.8).

A particular variation of the anchoring bias is known as the zero-risk bias. It occurs as people have a natural tendency to prefer an option that removes all risk, even over an option that represents a greater reduction in overall risk. A guarantee of a small benefit may be preferred to a larger benefit of less certainty. In one study, people were asked to select one of three plans to clean up two hazardous waste sites [30]. One site caused eight cases of cancer per year while the other caused four. Two plans reduced the number of cancer cases by six. A third plan decreased the number of cases by five, but completely eliminated cancer cases coming from the less-dangerous site. Although this plan had the lowest total number of cancer cases eliminated, it was nonetheless chosen by 42% of subjects.

Our Encounter Programs are sure to make a splash!

Year round	Non-Members	Members
PAINT WITH A STINGRAY	$50	$40
PENGUIN ENCOUNTER	$79	$69
PENGUINS UP CLOSE	$119	$109
Seasonal		
MARINE THEATER GUEST STAR	$79	$69
WHALES UP CLOSE	$99	$89
SEALS UP CLOSE	$119	$109
PAINT WITH A WHALE	$139	$129
BELUGA ENCOUNTER	$179	$169
TRAINER FOR A DAY	$389	$379

Become a member today and get free admission all year!

Fig. 10. 8 For each of the following aquatic experiences, members save $10. However, for the expensive experiences, $10 feels like a trivial discount

I see the zero-risk bias often. My patients with MS face a threat from the disease itself and from the medications used to treat it. Some of them choose a medication that has minimal impact on their disease but also carries zero risk of serious side effects over a medication that can substantially slow down their disease, but comes with a small, but non-zero risk of serious side effects. Even though, for many patients, their disease poses an overall greater risk to their health, I believe the opportunity to completely avoid a risk caused by a medication is preferable to them. Some patients chose not to take any medication at all, the clearest example of the zero-risk bias.

Conclusion
In offering treatment choices to patients, all that matters is the risk/benefit ratio. Different people can have different opinions on what constitutes an acceptable risk or benefit. However, clinicians should make all efforts to view the risks and benefits of any treatment independently. The safety and efficacy of a given treatment does not change merely because it is compared with another treatment. When presented with a treatment, clinicians should do their best to be aware if their perception of its risks and benefits have been distorted by a frame or anchor. Similarly, when presenting options to patients, clinicians should be aware that how they frame the risks and benefits will have a profound effect on how the patient perceives that treatment.

Contrast Effect

Case
Maxwell was an 18-year-old man who presented to the ER after he was found trying to sneak into the bedroom of his college professor. He was convinced that she was in love with him, and was surprised when she called 911 instead. He was agitated on exam and said that he had barely slept the week prior. He was diagnosed with bipolar disorder and was admitted to the hospital, where he was treated with an antipsychotic, (olanzapine) and a mood stabilizer (valproic acid). He improved over the next two weeks and was discharged home. When seen in follow-up the next month, he continued to do well from a psychiatric standpoint, but had gained 12 pounds, much to his distress. He had read that both of his medications could cause weight gain, and had discontinued olanzapine on his own. He requested his psychiatrist change his valproic acid to another mood stabilizer, either lithium or lamotrigine, but she refused, fearing more serious complications from the alternatives. Maxwell discontinued the valproic acid after he gained another 10 pounds. He was brought to the ER two months later, this time under arrest, after he again tried to enter his professor's house.

What Dr. Sloan Was Thinking
All of medicine is judging the risks and benefits. Lamotrigine can cause a skin disease known as Stevens-Johnson syndrome, a rare, but potentially very serious, even fatal complication. I saw it once as a medical student—in the hospital burn ward. Lithium is a fine medication, but can cause kidney failure over the long run, and is not a medication I like to use initially. So to me, the fact that Maxwell gained 12

pounds was no big deal in the scheme of things. Yet, it was a big deal to him, enough so that he stopped his medication. Had I considered his weight gain on its own, not just in relation to the potential side effects of other medications, I likely would recognized its severity and come up with an alternative plan.

Case

Larry was a 75-year-old man who presented with the acute onset of numbness on the left side of his body. An MRI revealed a small, ischemic stroke in his right thalamus in an area that contains the sensory pathway. Investigations of his carotid arteries and heart were normal. In an encounter that took less than 10 minutes, the neurologist told him that his symptoms were due to his uncontrolled hypertension. He was started on an anti-hypertensive medication, a cholesterol-lowering medication, and aspirin. He was discharged the next day. Larry felt that the neurologist dismissed his condition and he didn't grasp the importance of taking three new medications. Additionally, he received no counseling on the importance of dietary modification and exercise. He returned several months later with another stroke, having taken his medications for only two weeks.

What Dr. Charles Was Thinking

There were several other patients on the neurology service besides Larry, and his case was the most mundane and benign. He had only some mild sensory loss, and there is nothing exceptional about an older guy with hypertension having a small stroke (called a lacunar stroke). The patient I saw before him was a 35-year-old mother with an aggressive brain tumor, and the patient I saw after him was a young guy in respiratory distress due to myasthenia gravis. There was another man in his 60s who had a huge left-sided stroke that left him unable to say much more than his name. Another older woman had a tremor and rapidly-progressive cognitive changes. We had no clue what was wrong with her, and spent a long time every day at her bedside and discussing her case during rounds. So Larry was probably the healthiest and most routine of any patient on the neurology service that week. The advice I gave him was sound; he needed medications to control his high blood pressure and cholesterol, as well as take a daily aspirin. No one reviewing his chart would be able to find any flaw in my management.

But I failed to acknowledge how devastating his stroke was to him. While Larry was extremely upset by his stroke, it was honestly a rather mundane matter to me. As a result, I failed to emphasize how important it was for him to take his medications, and I didn't speak to him about the lifestyle modifications he could make to reduce the risk of a subsequent stroke. I spent much less time with him that with my other patients. Had the service consisted of patients with less severe disorders, Larry probably would have received the attention he needed. Also, Larry was one of the patients for whom I could have done the most good. There is every expectation that his second stroke could have been prevented. It's sad to say, but there was little I could do for the woman with brain tumor, for example.

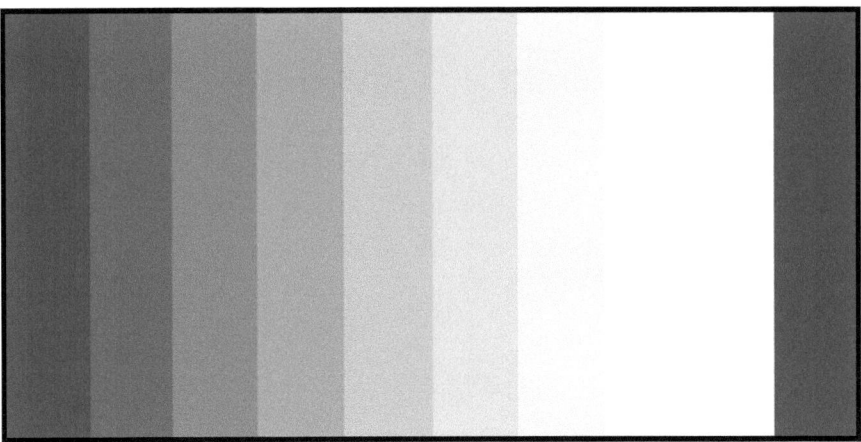

Fig. 10. 9 The grey bars on the outer edges in this figure are the same color

Discussion

The contrast effect occurs when the value of information or the severity of a case is enhanced or diminished through juxtaposition to other information of greater or lesser value. It is a form of the anchoring bias, where an initial piece of information influences how we perceive subsequent events. We rarely perceive things in isolation, but rather in comparison to similar items that surround them. A positive contrast effect occurs when the perception of something is enhanced through comparison with something worse. A negative contrast effect occurs when the perception of something is diminished through comparison with something better.

The contrast effect is very easy to demonstrate on a perceptual level, and it explains many simple optical illusions. The grey bars on the outer edges in the Fig. 10.9 are the same color. Yet, the bar on the right appears darker than the bar on the left because it borders a white bar.

A related demonstration is to put one hand into hot water and the other in cold water. If both are then placed in lukewarm water, the hot hand will feel cold and the cold hand will feel hot. Muzafer Sherif and Daniel Taub demonstrated that subjects who lifted a heavy object then underestimated the weight of lighter object they subsequently lifted [31].

On a perceptual level, the contrast effect and similar optical illusions have implications for radiologists and pathologists. However, our cognition and emotions are similarly vulnerable to the contrast effect. An intelligent person may seem dim in a room of Nobel Prize winners. The worst player in the NBA seems to be a horrible basketball player, but only because he is compared to the world's best. An otherwise attractive person may appear average in a room of supermodels. In medical school, my grades suffered when I rotated with the geniuses in my class. Compared to them, I appeared not-so-bright, something which my evaluators explicitly noted on occasion (Fig. 10.10).

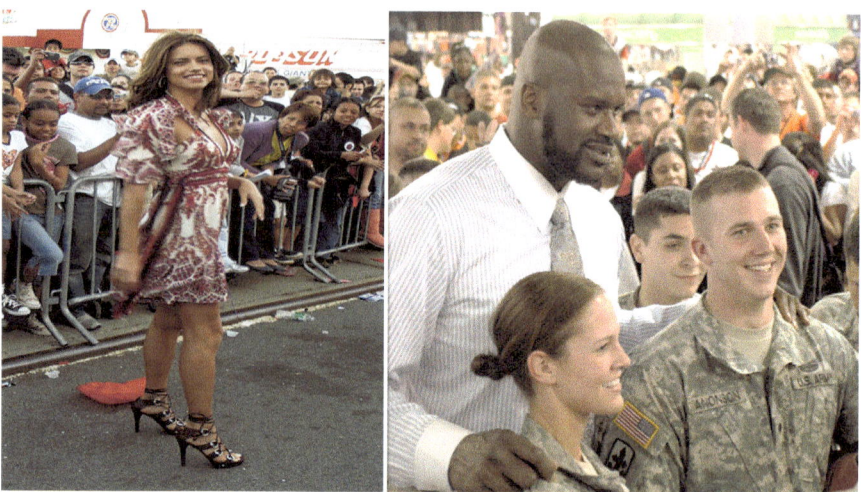

Fig. 10.10 Regular people appear especially regular when compared to a glamorous supermodel, and people of average height appear extremely short when compared to someone of great stature. (**Left**: Shankbone D. (David). Adriana Lima [Image file]. In: Wikimedia commons. 2007. Retrieved from   https://commons.wikimedia.org/wiki/Adriana_Lima#/media/File:Adriana_Lima_by_ David_Shankbone.jpg; **Right**: Walz A. (Angela). Army National Guard members Staff Sgt. Maygen Matson, left, and Spc. Taylor Anonson pose for a photo with National Basketball Association superstar Shaquille O'Neal during NBA All-Star weekend [Image file]. In: Wikimedia commons. 2009. Retrieved from https://commons.wikimedia.org/wiki/Shaquille_O%27Neal#/ media/File:Shaq_@NBA_All_star_game.jpg.)

The contrast effect can influence clinicians in several ways. A patient with a significant but non-disabling illness may be perceived as having a relatively mild condition if they find themselves on a hospital ward full of extremely sick people. For example, clinicians may unconsciously minimize the suffering of a patient with migraines if the other patients under their care have fatal conditions, such as brain cancer or amyotrophic lateral sclerosis. While migraines are indeed not as serious as these conditions, they can be horribly disabling. A patient with a migraine should not get short thrift merely because her roommate has a more severe condition. In my clinic, for example, I routinely see devastated, wheelchair-bound young people with multiple sclerosis. It can be difficult after seeing such a patient to validate the symptoms of an older, ambulatory patient who has had a milder disease course, but suffers nonetheless.

Additionally, a patient with a common disease might receive minimal attention compared to a patient with a rare, fascinating disease. Even if their symptoms are mild, patients with rare diseases may receive more thought and attention than patients with significant impairment from more common conditions. For example, a patient with mild symptoms from a rare disease, such as lymphocytic adenohypophysitis, may receive more concern and care than a patient disabled by a common condition, such as low back pain due to a herniated disc.

Finally, a medication side effect, such as stomach upset, may appear to be a "nuisance" to the clinician when compared with more significant side effects, such as fatal infections. However, these seemingly trivial side effects may be devastating to patients and should not be minimized simply because other, more serious side effects are possible.

Conclusion

Clinicians should do their best to view each patient's condition individually, not merely in comparison to other patients. A patient might be incorrectly perceived as having a mild condition if their neighbor has a serious or fascinating illness.

References

1. Tversky A, Kahneman D. The framing of decisions and the psychology of choice. Science. 1981;211(4481):453–8. https://doi.org/10.1126/science.7455683.
2. De Martino B, Kumaran D, Seymour B, Dolan RJ. Frames, biases, and rational decision-making in the human brain. Science. 2006;313(5787):684–7. https://doi.org/10.1126/science.1128356.
3. Byrne J. (n.d.). Poor decisions and prospect theory. Skeptical Medicine. Retrieved 15 Sept 2018 from https://sites.google.com/site/skepticalmedicine/poor-decisions-and-prospect-theory.
4. Tversky A, Kahneman D. Advances in prospect theory: cumulative representation of uncertainty. J Risk Uncertain. 1992;5(4):297–323. https://doi.org/10.1007/BF00122574.
5. Genzyme S. (n.d.). Aubagio FAQs. Aubagio.com. Retrieved 15 Sept 2018 from https://www.aubagio.com/aubagio-faqs.
6. Hsee CK. Less is better: when low-value options are valued more highly than high-value options. J Behav Decis Mak. 1998;11(2):107–21. https://doi.org/10.1002/(SICI)1099-0771(199806)11:2<107::AID-BDM292>3.0.CO;2-Y.
7. Shafir E. Choosing versus rejecting: why some options are both better and worse than others. Mem Cogn. 1993;21(4):546–56. https://doi.org/10.3758/BF03197186.
8. Sussman D. (2010, Feb 11). New poll shows support for repeal of 'Don't Ask, Don't Tell' [Blog post]. The New York Times: The Caucus. Retrieved from https://thecaucus.blogs.nytimes.com/2010/02/11/new-poll-shows-support-for-repeal-of-dont-ask-dont-tell/.
9. Zier LS, Sottile PD, Hong SY, Weissfield LA, White DB. Surrogate decision makers' interpretation of prognostic information: a mixed-methods study. Ann Intern Med. 2012;156(5):360–6. https://doi.org/10.7326/0003-4819-156-5-201203060-00008.
10. Berry K, Butt M, Kirby JS. Influence of information framing in patient decisions to treat actinic keratosis. JAMA Dermatol. 2017;153(5):421–6. https://doi.org/10.1001/jamadermatol.2016.5245.
11. Draelos ZD. (2017, Dec 16). Parabens and phthalates: what patients may want to know. MedPage Today. Retrieved from https://www.medpagetoday.com/resource-centers/advances-in-dermatology/medpage-today-news-parabens-and-phthalates-patients-may-want-know/1750.
12. Kahneman D, Tversky A. Choices, values, and frames. Am Psychol. 1984;39(4):341–50. https://doi.org/10.1037/0003-066X.39.4.341.
13. Kane E. (2011, July 2). $20 and a Harvard MBA. Highland Park Patch. Retrieved from https://patch.com/illinois/highlandpark/bp%2D%2D20-and-a-havard-mba.
14. Kahneman D, Knetsch JL, Thaler RH. Experimental tests of the endowment effect and the Coase theorem. J Polit Econ. 1990;98(6):1325–48. https://doi.org/10.1086/261737.
15. Bullens L, van Harreveld F, Forster J, van der Pligt J. Reversible decisions: the grass isn't merely greener on the other side; it's also very brown over here. J Exp Soc Psychol. 2013;49(6):1093–9. https://doi.org/10.1016/j.jesp.2013.07.011.
16. Mather M, Shafir E, Johnson MK. Misremembrance of options past: source monitoring and choice. Psychol Sci. 2000;11(2):132–8. https://doi.org/10.1111/1467-9280.00228.

17. Mather M, Johnson MK. Choice-supportive source monitoring: do our decisions seem better to us as we age? Psychol Aging. 2000;15(4):596–606. https://doi.org/10.1037/0882-7974.15.4.596.
18. Braverman JA, Blumenthal-Barby JS. Assessment of the sunk-cost effect in clinical decision-making. Soc Sci Med. 2012;75(1):186–92. https://doi.org/10.1016/j.socscimed.2012.03.006.
19. Bornstein BH, Emler AC, Chapman GB. Rationality in medical treatment decisions: is there a sunk-cost effect? Soc Sci Med. 1999;49(2):215–22. https://doi.org/10.1016/S0277-9536(99)00117-3.
20. Wendling P. (2017, Nov 3). ORBITA: sham comparison casts doubt on PCI for stable angina. Medscape News. Retrieved from https://www.medscape.com/viewarticle/888011.
21. Gorski D. (2017, Nov 6). ORBITA: another clinical trial demonstrating the need for sham controls in surgical trials. Science-Based Medicine. Retrieved from https://sciencebasedmedicine.org/orbita-another-clinical-trial-demonstrating-the-need-for-sham-controls-in-surgical-trials/.
22. Tversky A, Kahneman D. Judgment under uncertainty: heuristics and biases. Science. 1974;185(4157):1124–31. https://doi.org/10.1126/science.185.4157.1124.
23. Kahneman D. Thinking, fast and slow. New York: Farrar, Straus and Giroux; 2011.
24. Yudkowsky E. Cognitive biases potentially affecting judgment of global risks. In: Bostrom N, Ćirković MM, editors. Global catastrophic risks. New York: Oxford University Press; 2008. p. 91–9.
25. Ariely D. The fallacy of supply and demand. In: Predictably irrational: the hidden forces that shape our decisions (Chapter 2). New York: HarperCollins; 2008.
26. Bucchianeri GW, Minson J. A homeowner's dilemma: anchoring in residential real estate transactions. J Econ Behav Organ. 2013;89:76–92. https://doi.org/10.1016/j.jebo.2013.01.010.
27. The Economist. (2009, May 22). The importance of irrelevant alternatives [Blog post]. The Economist. Retrieved from https://www.economist.com/democracy-in-america/2009/05/22/the-importance-of-irrelevant-alternatives.
28. Levine R. The power of persuasion—how we're bought and sold. Hoboken: John Wiley & Sons; 2003. p. 100–1.
29. National Safety Council. (n.d.). What are the odds of dying from. Retrieved 15 Sept 2018 from https://www.nsc.org/work-safety/tools-resources/injury-facts/chart.
30. Baron J, Gowda R, Kunreuther H. Attitudes toward managing hazardous waste: what should be cleaned up and who should pay for it? Risk Anal. 1993;13:183–92. https://doi.org/10.1111/j.1539-6924.1993.tb01068.x.
31. Sherif M, Taub D, Hovland CI. Assimilation and contrast effects of anchoring stimuli on judgments. J Exp Psychol. 1958;55(2):150–5. https://doi.org/10.1037/h0048784.

Affective Error

11

Case

Paul was a 58-year-old man who presented to a neurosurgeon's office with difficulty walking for six months. He had been sent there by a neurologist who diagnosed him with spinal cord compression from multiple herniated discs. The neurologist also warned the neurosurgeon that Paul had been verbally abusive and inappropriate with staff members. Paul arrived 30 minutes late to his first appointment and swore at the receptionist when she told him he could not be seen that day. During his second visit, he demanded that his spine be operated on the following week. He refused to provide anything other than a basic history saying, "It's in the record." On exam, he was weak in his legs and needed a cane to walk. An MRI showed narrowing of his cervical spine with compression of his spinal cord. Despite this, the neurosurgeon refused to operate, saying that he would be a "poor operative candidate." Paul found another neurosurgeon who was willing to operate on him, with excellent results.

What Dr. Warren Was Thinking

Let me be honest, I didn't like Paul. He was nasty and inappropriate. By refusing to operate on him, I assured that he would not become my patient. I wouldn't have to see him in the hospital or for post-operative visits, nor would I have to deal with him had his surgery not gone well. Patients often have unrealistic expectations from spine surgery. I knew that Paul was the kind of guy who would have been a horror to deal with had there been any problem after the operation. My staff was also pleased when I decided not to operate on him. They were happy knowing they would probably never see him again. Despite this, Paul had bad spinal cord compression, and as another neurosurgeon proved, he benefitted significantly from an operation. Although I would not have admitted this at the time, I didn't operate on Paul because I didn't like him, and I didn't want to see him again.

Case

Larry, pictured below, was a 60-year-old man who arrived by ambulance after he fell down a flight of stairs while intoxicated. He was malodorous, dirty, and was

© Springer International Publishing AG, part of Springer Nature 2019
J. Howard, *Cognitive Errors and Diagnostic Mistakes*,
https://doi.org/10.1007/978-3-319-93224-8_11

Fig. 11.1 Larry. (Rinald E. (Eva). Terry, homeless in Sydney, Australia [Image file]. In: Wikimedia commons. 2011. Retrieved from https://commons.wikimedia.org/w/index. php?title=Category:Homeless_ people&filefrom=Teenage+Dr ug+Addicts.jpg#/media/ File:Homeless_male_in_ Sydney.jpg.)

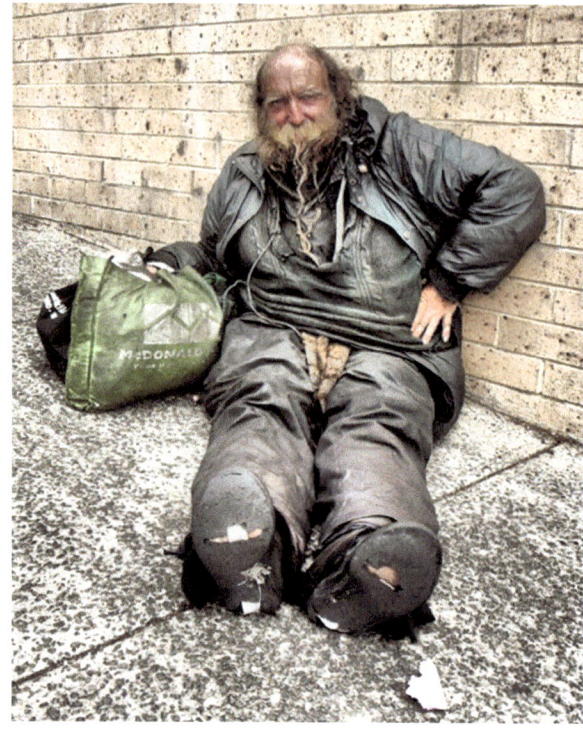

covered in feces and bedbugs. Basic labs were drawn, and were normal other than mild anemia and an alcohol level of 356 mg/dL. A head CT showed only mild atrophy and cervical spine CT was normal. Larry said he felt "fine" and was able to move all of his extremities. He was placed in a corner of the ER and allowed to "sleep it off" for 4 hours. Upon re-evaluation, he was found to be hypotensive and complained of severe abdominal pain. Repeat labs revealed worsening anemia and an abdominal CT scan revealed a ruptured spleen with internal bleeding. He was then taken for emergency surgery (Fig. 11.1).

What Dr. Moya Was Thinking

This is tough for me to admit, but Larry disgusted me. I had treated him several times previously, and he actually was a generally happy guy who didn't give us a hard time. Yet, going near him triggered an automatic reaction that literally made me want to throw up. He smelled just awful, and I didn't want to go anywhere near him. This was completely inappropriate. I couldn't control my visceral reaction to him, but this was no excuse not to examine him. When he was finally undressed and examined, it was obvious he had sustained significant abdominal trauma.

Fig. 11.2 Deena. (Shankbone D. (David). A young unidentified woman, who modelled for many photographers. [Image file]. In: Wikimedia commons. 2008. Retrieved from https://commons. wikimedia.org/wiki/ File:Young_woman_-unidentified_model_at_ Mercedes-Benz_Fashion_ Week.jpg.)

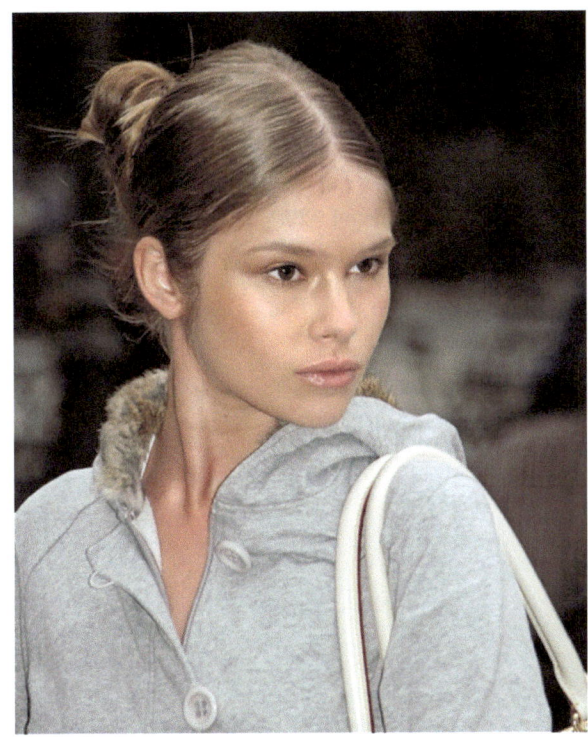

Case

Deena above was a 21-year-old medical student who presented with anxiety in multiple situations (Fig. 11.2). She said she had trouble participating in small group discussions, something that her school required several times per week. She said that she had never taken medications, but that her mother had benefitted from taking Xanax™, a potentially addictive benzodiazepine. She was given a prescription for Xanax™ and reported significant success in controlling her anxiety. She returned every six weeks for a refill of her medications and said that she was generally doing well. On several visits, she requested more medications than usual, as she had "a big test" or an "important presentation." Six months later, Deena presented to the ER having had a withdrawal seizure. She later admitted that she had been getting multiple prescriptions from different doctors and taking much higher doses of Xanax™ than anyone knew.

What Dr. Blakeson Was Thinking:

I really liked Deena a lot. She was smart, funny, and interested in being a psychiatrist like me. We talked a lot about the difficulties of being a first-year medical student, and being only a few years older than her, I could really relate to what she was going through. And let me be honest, Deena was pretty. I was always happy to see that she was on my schedule. I didn't think twice about giving her Xanax™. Had she been some random person who walked off the street asking for Xanax™, I never would have given it to her on the first visit. Similarly, I would have done screens to make sure she was not taking other drugs and also to make sure she actually was taking the Xanax™ and not selling it. I also would have checked our state database for controlled substances and probably discovered that she was getting prescriptions from other doctors. I always treated Deena professionally, but the fact that I liked her and could relate to her as a medical professional blinded me to the fact that she had a substance abuse problem.

Case

Jane was a 48-year-old woman with multiple sclerosis (MS) who had developed a close relationship with her doctor, whom she had known for nearly a decade. They often ran into each other at the gym, and their husbands had known each other since high school. After several relapses of her MS, she was started on natalizumab, a highly effective treatment for MS, but one that carries with it a substantial risk of progressive multifocal leukoencephalopathy (PML), a potentially fatal viral infection of the brain.

Jane did well on the medication for four years, without clinical relapses or disease progression. However, after this, she started "bumping into things" and reported difficulty seeing out of her right eye. An MRI revealed a new lesion in her left occipital lobe, and neurological examination revealed a right visual field deficit. She was treated with steroids for a presumed MS relapse. Jane worsened over the next two weeks and was again treated with steroids. Per her request, she received another infusion of natalizumab during this time. Jane continued to deteriorate and eventually developed severe cognitive deficits and weakness of her right side. The diagnosis of PML was first considered two months after the onset of her initial symptoms and was confirmed with a spinal tap.

What Dr. Anthony Was Thinking

I was aware that PML is a risk of treatment with natalizumab, and I could have easily quoted the risk factors for contracting PML. However, when confronted with one of my own patients who had PML, I missed it. I had known Jane for some time and felt quite close to her. I worked hard to convince her to start natalizumab, and both of us were pleased at how well it controlled her disease. When she developed symptoms of PML, in retrospect, I missed it initially because I didn't *want* it to be true. The disease can be fatal, and I didn't want to worry her or subject her to painful tests, such as a spinal tap. I am pretty confident that had I met her for the first time the day she developed symptoms of PML, it would have been easy to diagnose, or at least consider. However, because I felt close to her, I put an upsetting diagnosis in the back of my mind, to her detriment.

Discussion

An affective error occurs when clinicians allow their personal feelings towards patients, called countertransference in psychiatric parlance, to affect their care. Clinicians are human, and they will naturally like some patients and dislike others. As such, countertransference is normal and unavoidable. Importantly, it is not necessarily counter-therapeutic and something to always be avoided. If a patient elicits certain emotions in a clinician and their staff, they are likely to elicit similar emotions in others around them. This can be important information for psychiatrists and other mental health professions. Yet, in many settings, a clinician's personal feelings towards a patient can interfere with their care.

Examples of "difficult" patient behaviors include:

- Manipulative, angry, or threatening patients.
- Deceptive patients.
- Patients with multiple, vague symptoms who have already seen multiple doctors previously.
- "Frequent fliers" who come to the hospital on a regular basis.
- Patients who do not respect a clinician's time by coming late or staying significantly beyond their appointment time.
- Patients who seemingly do not care for their own health.
- Overtly racist or sexist patients.

In a classic essay titled *Taking Care of the Hateful Patient*, James Groves grouped such patients into four categories [1]:

1. **Dependent clingers:** Patients evoke aversion. Their care requires limits on expectations for an intense doctor-patient relationship.
2. **Entitled demanders:** Patients evoke a wish to counterattack. Such patients need to have their feelings of total entitlement rechanneled into a partnership that acknowledges their entitlement—not to unrealistic demands but to good medical care.
3. **Manipulative help-rejecters**: Patients evoke depression. "Sharing" their pessimism diminishes their notion that losing the symptom implies losing the doctor.
4. **Self-destructive deniers:** Patients evoke feeling of malice. Their management requires the physician to lower Faustian expectations of delivering perfect care.

Clinicians may consciously or unconsciously avoid giving proper care to patients they do not like or those that disgust them. They may not schedule appropriate follow-up visits and might spend minimal time rounding on them in the hospital. Seeking to minimize time spent with difficult patients, clinicians may fail to elicit an important piece of information or may overlook an important exam finding. They also may avoid giving patients information that is likely to trigger an unpleasant reaction. It may be easier to give in to a difficult patient's inappropriate demands for pain medication, for example, than to provoke a nasty confrontation. It may be challenging to inform difficult patients that an error has been made, that a diagnosis remains elusive, or that a treatment is not working. Clinicians may not fully examine disheveled, malodorous patients whose condition repulses them.

Clinicians may also feel uncomfortable discussing sensitive subjects with patients from a different religion or culture. A Christian, male doctor from Mexico may feel uncomfortable taking a sexual history from a young, orthodox Jewish woman from Israel who only speaks Hebrew. However, it is not difficult to imagine a scenario in which this information is vital to caring for her health. Patients with linguistic barriers may also trigger a negative reaction from clinicians. Busy clinicians may resent the added time and effort it takes to use translator services to communicate with the patient.

Clinicians routinely have to care for difficult patients. It is just part of the job. According to one survey of 500 adults presenting to a primary care walk-in clinic, doctors rated 15% of patient encounters as difficult [2]. Patients rated as difficult were more likely to have depression and/or anxiety, more than five somatic symptoms, and more severe symptoms. In a Medscape survey in 2016, 62% of doctors identified "emotional problems" as the main trigger for their own affective bias [3]. When queried further, patient behaviors that were most likely to trigger a negative reaction included drug-seeking and substance abuse, followed by "malingering, entitled, and noncompliant patients." Besides emotional problems, other patient characteristics likely to trigger negative countertransference included obesity, low-intelligence, language differences, and a lack of insurance coverage. At other times, clinicians have an involuntary disgust reaction to patients who can be covered in all manner of bodily fluids or parasites.

Importantly, our judgments of other people can be extremely rapid, and these first judgments may be long-lasting. Judgments made in a short time are not necessarily inaccurate, and psychologists have demonstrated that judgments people make about others based on very brief exposures can be as accurate as the judgments they make based on longer exposures. In one sense this is obvious, we can instantly distinguish a businessman getting out of a limousine from a homeless person on the street and likely accurately infer important aspects of their life. However, it can take an extremely brief amount of time for people to make such unconscious judgments in less extreme situations.

This phenomenon is known as thin-slicing, a term coined by Nalini Ambady and Robert Rosenthal [4]. They demonstrated its presence in an experiment that showed subjects videos of teachers, lasting only 2–10 seconds. The subjects were then asked to rate the teachers on various attributes, such as their honesty, empathy, and competence. They found that subjects shown even these extremely brief clips rated those teachers very similarly to students who had completed their entire course [5]. They even found that sound was not necessary. Subjects shown 30-second clips of teachers with the sound off rated them similarly to students who had worked with them for months.

In a related study, Dr. Ambady and colleagues provided subjects with audio records from 114 surgeon-patient interviews [6]. The recordings were only two, 10-second sound clips per surgeon, and one had been edited so that only the tone of a surgeon's voice was discernible, but not the content of what they were saying. Subjects were asked to rate the surgeon on characteristics such as warmth, hostility, dominance, and anxiety. Armed only with this brief information, subjects were able to use a surgeon's tone of voice to predict their malpractice claims history. As Dr. Ambady said:

> We were really amazed because we found that with just 20 seconds of each doctor's voice, you could postdict malpractice claims. For instance, surgeons who sounded more unfeeling or dominant were more likely to have been sued in the past. This is very interesting, because it feeds into lay stereotypes about surgeons as being cold and uninterested in people—and it turns out that doctors who fit that stereotype are more likely to be sued [7].

In another study by Christopher Olivola and Alexander Todorov, subjects shown faces of political candidates for as little as 100 ms made strong impression about their competence that reliably predicted voting decisions and the outcomes of elections [8]. They concluded that "first impressions based on appearances are remarkably influential, frustratingly difficult to overcome, and occur with astonishing speed." Additionally, they said that:

> getting people to overcome the influence of first impressions will not be an easy task. The speed, automaticity, and implicit nature of appearance-based trait inferences make them particularly hard to correct. Moreover, often people don't even recognize that they are forming judgments about others from their appearances.

Building on this thin-slicing, Brad Verhuls and colleagues found that even preconscious judgments, specifically familiarity and attractiveness, exert downstream effects on conscious judgments of competence [9]. Clinicians are not immune to this, of course, and should be aware that their first glimpse of a patient may exert a powerful impact over the entire clinical encounter.

Interestingly, how clinicians feel about a patient may depend, on how well the clinician treated that patient, a phenomenon known as the Benjamin Franklin effect. It posits that when we do something kind for someone, we end up liking them more. A person who performs a favor for someone may feel the need to justify their behavior to themselves, concluding they did the favor because they liked the other person. It takes its name from how Mr. Franklin manipulated one of his biggest political opponents, turning him into a lifelong supporter, by requesting a favor. As he wrote in his autobiography:

> Having heard that he had in his library a certain very scarce and curious book, I wrote a note to him, expressing my desire of perusing that book, and requesting he would do me the favour of lending it to me for a few days. He sent it immediately, and I return'd it in about a week with another note, expressing strongly my sense of the favour. When we next met in the House, he spoke to me (which he had never done before), and with great civility; and he ever after manifested a readiness to serve me on all occasions, so that we became great friends, and our friendship continued to his death.

Jon Jecker and David Landy designed an experiment, titled *Liking a Person as a Function of Doing Him a Favour*, that demonstrated the Benjamin Franklin effect [10]. Subjects were enrolled in a study where they were allowed to win money. The study was run by an actor who pretended to be a rude, obnoxious researcher. At the end of the study:

- 1/3 were approached by the researcher and asked to return money who said he had been using his own money and was running out.
- 1/3 were approached by a secretary and asked to return money who said it was from the psychology department and was running out.
- 1/3 were not approached.

All of the subjects agreed to return the money and were then asked the opinion of the researcher. Those who were asked by the researcher to return the money rated him the most favorably, while those asked by the secretary to return the money rated him the least favorably. A corollary to this is that a person may come to loathe someone they injured, allowing them to justify the harm they did. As science writer David McRaney wrote:

> *Jailers come to look down on inmates; camp guards come to dehumanize their captives; soldiers create derogatory terms for their enemies. It's difficult to hurt someone you admire. It's even more difficult to kill a fellow human being. Seeing the casualties you create as something less than you, something deserving of damage, makes it possible to continue seeing yourself as a good and honest person, to continue being sane* [11].

In a medical setting, clinicians may be prone to like patients whom they have helped. A clinician who worked throughout the night to fix a patient's broken leg may feel proud of their work and view that patient more favorably. Conversely, a clinician who misses a diagnosis may dislike the patient, finding a way to blame the patient for the error.

One clinician's negative reaction to a patient can also influence other healthcare workers as well. Patients can be very easily labeled as "difficult," impacting the care they receive from nearly everyone they meet. As much as the facts they share, the tone of voice in which clinicians communicate, their body language, or subtle verbal cues (*"Sigh, the same alcoholic who always comes in with chest pain is back for the third day in a row!"*) also have the potential to add significant bias. As such, clinicians, especially those with leadership roles, must be mindful of how they speak about difficult patients in the presence of students and younger clinicians. Their actions invariably create a culture and template upon which trainees model their own attitudes and behavior. This is sometimes called the "hidden curriculum" of medical school. Though it is not formalized, it is at least as important as learning the anatomy of the cranial nerves and the coagulation pathway.

Unfortunately, much of medical school training results in a loss of empathy. A survey of 11 medical students by Hanne-Lise Eikeland and colleagues found that this loss of empathy occurred most commonly in the third year of medical school, when students make the transition from the classroom to the hospital wards and clinics [12]. While the factors behind this are complex and not fully understood, the practice of referring to some patients, such as those with addiction or mental illness, in dehumanizing terms certainly plays an important role.

There is some evidence that difficult patients receive worse care. Brian Birdwell and colleagues performed a study showing how a patient's personality-style can dramatically affect they care they receive [13]. They showed 44 internists video of a 40-year-old actress reporting chest pain. Half of the doctors saw her report these symptoms in a businesslike style. Fifty percent of these doctors suspected a cardiac cause for her symptoms, and 93% suggested a cardiac evaluation. The other half saw her report these symptoms in a histrionic manner. Only 13% of these doctors suspected a cardiac cause for her symptoms and only 53% suggested a cardiac evaluation.

Silvia Mamede and colleagues studied 74 internal medicine residents who were given eight clinical vignettes [14]. They vignettes were identical, except some patients' behavior was neutral, while other patients' behavior was difficult. Difficult behaviors included: (1) "frequent demander"; (2) an aggressive patient; (3) a patient who questions his doctor's competence; (4) a patient who ignores his doctor's advice; (5) a patient who has low expectations of his doctor's support; (6) a patient who presents herself as utterly helpless; (7) a patient who threatens the doctor; and (8) a patient who accuses the doctor of discrimination. They found that diagnostic accuracy scores decreased by 10% when the patient was difficult. The authors conclude that "difficult patients' behaviors induce doctors to make diagnostic errors, apparently because doctors spend part of their mental resources on dealing with the difficult patients' behaviors, impeding adequate processing of clinical findings."

In a related study, Henk Schmidt and colleagues studied 63 family practice residents and found that the likelihood of misdiagnosis rose by 42% when the doctors were challenged with a difficult patient exhibiting a set of complex symptoms, compared to a polite patient with identical symptoms [15]. There is little doubt that faced with a patient actually threatening or humiliating a doctor in the real world, not in a study, a clinician's ability to properly gather and synthesize information would be impaired to an even greater degree. Dr. Mamede recognized this, saying:

> *The most likely is that the effect of behaviors displayed by real patients is stronger. In real settings, physicians need to determine which information needs to be gathered and search for it themselves, which tends to make reasoning more demanding and therefore more prone to flaws* [16].

Clinician characteristics also play an important role in the clinician-patient dynamic. Sharon Hull and Karen Broquet identified several traits of clinicians; angry or defensive, fatigued or harried, and dogmatic or arrogant, which make them more prone to have negative encounters with difficult patients [17]. In another study, clinicians with poorer psychosocial attitudes as measured by the Physician's Belief Scale were more likely to perceive patients as difficult [18]. Additionally, situational factors, such as a loud and chaotic ER or having to deliver bad news, can also contribute to difficult clinician-patient interactions. Indeed, in the Medscape survey, emergency clinicians were the most likely to report bias (62%) and to report that it influenced their care (14%) [3].

While empathy is a buzzword in medical education today, does it really affect patient care? Several studies have documented that an empathetic physician can improve patient outcomes. A study of 20,000 patients with diabetes found that those treated by clinicians with high empathy scores had a significantly lower rate of acute metabolic complications, while another study of nearly 900 diabetic patients found that patients treated by clinicians with high empathy scores were significantly more likely to have lower blood sugar levels and lower cholesterol levels [19, 20]. Another study of 710 patients with cancer found that empathic clinicians were associated with improvement in patient-reported outcomes of depression and quality of life [21]. Even patients with the common cold reported less severe and shorter-lasting symptoms when treated by clinicians whom they rated as having perfect empathy scores compared to those treated by clinicians with imperfect scores [22]. In cases where having an empathetic physician is unlikely to improve outcomes, there is no reason for a doctor not to try to be kind. As Danielle Ofri pointed out in her book *How Doctors Feel*, "so far, there haven't been any documented 'adverse outcomes' in patients treated by highly empathetic doctors" [23].

Fortunately, the importance of humanism is becoming increasing recognized in the medical community. The Gold Foundation, for example, sponsors a Humanism Honor Society that "recognizes students, residents and faculty who are exemplars of compassionate patient care and who serve as role models, mentors, and leaders in medicine" [24]. Medical students and residents are publically acknowledged for their kindness and care at graduation ceremonies.

Advocating for patience and empathy is easy while comfortably sitting at home, well-rested and well-fed. It's not so easy when you're hungry and exhausted, on your 20th hour at work, and a belligerent patient spits at you and threatens to punch you if you don't give her methadone. Anecdotes of abused clinicians abound. After describing a typically abusive, threatening patient, Ahmad Yousef an internal medicine physician wrote:

> Health care professionals deal with patients like the one above every day. The verbal abuse and physical threats are so common that we have settled in to just trying to find some humor in them. This type of abuse is not unique to the health care field, but the difference is that you cannot just stop treating your abuser. You have to make sure he or she gets better. You cannot fire a patient in an ER who would die in the street if you kicked him out. Every doc or nurse has an anecdote in which they have been spit on, urinated on, cursed at, assaulted, or threatened [25].

Similarly, Jenny Hartsock, a hospitalist working in an Ohio city ravaged by the opioid epidemic wrote:

> What you will see throughout the city is a community exhausted by opiate abuse. Our job is to take care of all patients, but you can clearly see over time a degradation of empathy and willingness to keep endlessly helping drug abusers. When day after day you are

constantly verbally abused and threatened, sometimes physically as well, it is very hard
to maintain any kind of positive outlook and caring bedside demeanor. It wears on us to
be abused and mistreated by our patients and to even fear for our safety in caring for
them [26].

Statistics support clinicians' perception that they are frequent targets of patients' inappropriate behavior, including violence. A survey of 822 doctors found that 59% had been insulted by patients based on their age, race, gender, weight, or ethnicity. Not surprisingly, African-American and Asian-American doctors as well as women were the most likely to receive prejudicial complaints [27]. According to Bureau of Labor Statistics data from 2015, health care workers face an average of 146 attacks for every 10,000 workers, compared to seven assaults per 10,000 workers across the entire US labor force [28]. Patients occasionally do extremely dangerous things. One patient of mine, upset at the hospital for unknown reasons, managed to sneak around after hours and light a number of trash cans on fire. Several floors filled with smoke, but thankfully no one was hurt. During another incident in the ER, an upset patient sprayed mace on myself and several of my colleagues. In exceptional cases, angry patients have murdered clinicians. Orthopedist Todd Graham, for example, was shot to death by the husband of a patient for whom he had refused to prescribe opioid pain medications [28].

These facts raise difficult questions. What should clinicians do when patients behave horribly, when patients are threatening, racist, sexist, or manipulative and dishonest? Should clinicians just sit there and take it with a feigned smile? Can they refuse to treat certain patients? Internist Sachin Jain shared his experience with a patient who made racist slurs towards him, telling him to "go back to India." He responded by asking the patient to "leave our [expletive] hospital" Upon reflection, he did not regret his action, writing, "Even as I had chosen a profession that calls on me to serve, there are clear limits to that service that I am unwilling to compromise" [29]. In their principles on medical ethics, the American Medical Association (AMA) largely supports his decision, saying that clinicians can "terminate the patient-physician relationship with a patient who uses derogatory language or acts in a prejudicial manner only if the patient will not modify the conduct. In such cases, the physician should arrange to transfer the patient's care" [30].

I certainly forgive any clinician who lashes out at a vulgar, racist patient in the heat of the moment. I will not argue that clinicians need be silent in the face of hateful patients. I have and will continue to tell patients when their behavior is inappropriate. However, I do not believe that a patient's racist behavior allows a clinician on duty to step out of their professional role and into the shoes of a citizen on the street. There is no evidence Dr. Jain abandoned this patient in an emergency. Perhaps this is easy for me to say as a white, American male, but it is my belief that as long as they are not imminently threatening, then clinicians must be willing to treat even the most vile, racist patients. After all, we are willing to treat patients who have literally murdered children, something I have done on multiple occasions. Additionally, my colleagues at Bellevue Hospital have provided care to several terrorists, one of whom murdered eight pedestrians by running them over with a truck.

Esther Choo, an Asian-American emergency room physician, reported similar experiences in dealing with racist patients. She has what seems to me to be a thoughtful approach to such patients, writing on Twitter:

> *The conversation usually goes like this. Me: 'I understand your viewpoint. I trained at elite institutions & have been practicing for 15 years. You are welcome to refuse care under my hands, but I feel confident that I am the most qualified to care for you. Especially since the alternative is an intern.' And they invariably pick the intern, as long as they are white. Or they leave. I used to cycle through disbelief, shame, anger. Now I just show compassion and move on"* [31].

Amanda Emerson, a nurse who works with prisoners, told me about the challenge she faces working with people who have done horrible things and how she works to see the humanity in all of her patients. She wrote:

> *A particular patient of mine had been sexually abused as a child, and he was my patient in the jail because he'd been found guilty of possession of child porn. And part of you wants to say, "Nope, child porn is over the line, this guy is scum, no hope he will ever recover from that."*

> *But then you start thinking about how he was abused. About how we know that the statistics say he would also be an abuser, how it's a pathological response to the trauma of the abuse to be attracted to children. And most of all talking to this guy. He was in my infirmary because he was attempting suicide by starvation. Not for attention. He wanted me to leave him alone and let him die because he hated himself so much. The self-loathing was heartbreaking. He was yellow and hollow looking from the prolonged starvation. I needed him to eat because he was losing consciousness from dehydration. So I sat him down and talked to him, told him he didn't deserve to die. Told him he'd get through it. He responded, "I do deserve to die. Don't you know what I'm here for? What I've done? I hate myself more than anyone else ever could, and I just want the pain to end." And I couldn't help thinking of the small child inside, the boy who was abused, and how heartbreaking it was for him and his victims what he'd become.*

Sami Saba, a neurologist, relayed a story of how a clinician's care may have helped transform a patient's racism, writing:

> *When I was a medical intern a few years ago, I helped take care of a man in his early 40s who had developed severe heart failure, which caused him to become severely fatigued and short of breath after walking just a short distance. To make things even worse, he had fallen on hard times and was homeless, going in and out of shelters, which made it even more difficult for him to adequately address his medical needs.*

> *His cardiologist, who had been treating him for about two years, was extremely dedicated to all of his patients, including this man. The patient told me on more than one occasion how he owed his life to this doctor, that every day he lives and every breath he takes is a testament to his dedication and support.*

> *I had noticed early on several mysterious tattoos on the patient's arms – an eagle, a cross, some vague symbols whose significance I didn't perceive. Then, one day I was called to his room because the patient was short of breath, but now without even having exerted himself. I listened to his heart, as I usually did, by pulling down his shirt and putting my stethoscope over his right upper chest. A minute later the cardiologist came in, but opened the patient's shirt completely to get better access to the lower part of the chest. For the first time, I saw what was tattooed there, that made clear the significance of all of the other tattoos – a*

swastika. The cardiologist must have seen my look of surprise and revulsion, because he gave me a knowing look and a half-nod as he put his stethoscope to his chest, just inches from the tattoo; at that angle, his kippah was just visible on the crown of his head.

The patient survived that day, and later told me about how he used to be a much different person, a person of whom he had grown to be ashamed. He told me (again) that he owed his life to this cardiologist; he also told me that every day he wished he had the money to remove the symbols of hate that were displayed on his body. The cardiologist, on the other hand, never said a word; it seemed like he took it for granted that he would treat this patient the same as he did any other. Months later, I called the patient to see how he was doing; someone else picked up the phone and told me he had recently passed away.

Having said this, unless there is an emergency, clinicians do not have an obligation to treat all patients. Simply because someone is registered in the hospital computer system and is given the title of "patient," they are not exempt from expectations of basic human decency. If someone were to threaten or attack me on the street, this would be unacceptable, even criminal behavior. Assuming the person is mentally competent, this behavior should not be excused merely because it occurs in the hospital.

As long as appropriate alternatives are provided, clinicians may terminate relationships with patients who are violent, threatening, or who violate core aspects of the doctor-patient relationship. The AMA recognizes that patients have responsibilities as well, writing that patients contribute to their own care when they [30]:

1. Are truthful and forthcoming with their physicians and strive to express their concerns clearly.
2. Provide as complete a medical history as they can.
3. Cooperate with agreed-on treatment plans.
4. Accept care from medical students, residents, and other trainees under appropriate supervision.
5. Meet their financial responsibilities with regard to medical care or discuss financial hardships with their physicians.
6. Recognize that a healthy lifestyle can often prevent or mitigate illness and take responsibility to follow preventive measures and adopt health-enhancing behaviors.
7. Be aware of and refrain from behavior that unreasonably places the health of others at risk. They should ask about what they can do to prevent transmission of infectious disease.
8. Refrain from being disruptive in the clinical setting.
9. Not knowingly initiate or participate in medical fraud.
10. Report illegal or unethical behavior by physicians or other health care professionals.

Some hospital systems refuse to honor patient's requests for a different clinician when that request is perceived to be based on prejudice alone [32]. In an essay on dealing with racist patients, Kimani Paul-Emile and colleagues do recognize some exceptional situations, such as emergencies, demented or psychotic patients, or special cases, such as a war veteran not wishing to be treated by a clinician whose ethnicity matches that of his former combatants [33].

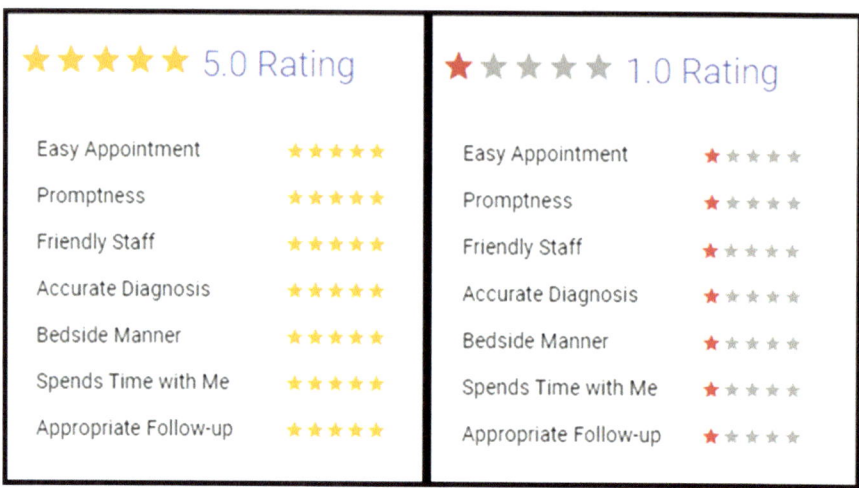

Fig. 11.3 Consistent with the halo effect a doctor who was rated well or poorly on some aspect of their care is likely to be similarly rated on all aspects of their care, even those out of their control

Additionally, it is not inappropriate for clinicians to communicate to one another that a particular patient is difficult. In fact, it is essential for clinicians to warn their colleagues if a patient is likely to behave in a hostile or aggressive manner. However, care must be taken not to bias them into thinking that the patient is not worth taking care of.

While the problems that may arise from treating difficult patients are clear, having positive feelings towards a patient also may adversely impact patient care, though in a less obvious way. An important factor to consider when discussing positive countertransference is known as the halo effect, a term coined by the psychologist Edward Thorndike. It is a variant of the affective error in which a single, positive attribute determines how a person's entire character is perceived. Thorndike first noticed the halo effect after observing that commanding officers in the military had a quirk when evaluating the soldiers under their command. A soldier who scored high on several attributes was likely to be highly rated on multiple, unrelated attributes. A soldier who was physically strong was also likely to be perceived as intelligent and having leadership qualities. Thorndike concluded that a soldier's attributes became aggregated into a positive or negative global impression, their halo. I have noticed a similar effect with online doctor reviews. A reviewer who rates a doctor poorly for their "accurate diagnosis" and "bedside manner" almost always rates them poorly for unrelated items, such as "friendly staff" and "easy appointment" (Fig. 11.3).

The halo effect is especially prominent with regards to physical appearance. Physically attractive people are more likely to be thought of as honest, intelligent, and hard-working as well. This has been well-demonstrated in politics where attractive candidates are judged to be more competent. Marketers are well-aware of the halo effect, and this explains why they are so eager to have their brand associated with successful, attractive celebrities.

When a clinician develops a positive halo around a patient, they may be less willing to consider serious diseases, share bad news, subject them to unpleasant procedures, or refuse inappropriate requests for tests or medications. Positive countertransference may lead clinicians to make inappropriate assumptions about certain patients, finding it difficult to believe that a friendly or attractive person could engage in social stigmatized behaviors, such as drug abuse or promiscuous sex. Ordering an HIV test and drug screen on a sex worker may be easy. Ordering these tests on the child of a prominent member of the community may be difficult. Refusing to give a belligerent, homeless patient an addictive medication may be easy. Refusing this to a friendly, attractive, well-educated patient may be difficult. As a result, except for emergencies and trivial ailments, clinicians should avoid treating family members and close friends to avoid emotional biases. They should certainly avoid treating themselves. As Sir William Osler, one of the founders of Johns Hopkins Hospital, famously said, "the doctor who treats himself has a fool for a patient."

Conclusion

In the past, and all too often today, clinicians were taught that it was wrong for them to have feelings towards their patients. Such feelings were seen as a sign of weakness and unprofessionalism. This was a mistake, and clinicians should not deny it or feel guilty when they have strong feelings towards their patients. Liking certain patients while finding others unpleasant or even odious, is not the sign of a poor or unprofessional clinician. I certainly don't pretend to like every patient. Some annoy me and several even horrify me. There is one man who has threatened to attack me on several occasions because I have not admitted him to the hospital. He is big, scary, and awful to care for. If I ever see him outside the relatively protected confines of the ER, I will run the other direction. While I certainly dread seeing him, I am obligated to give him the best care I can when he comes, as difficult as that may be.

While it is not inappropriate for clinicians to have feelings towards their patients, it is inappropriate for clinicians to deny or ignore these feelings. Clinicians should acknowledge their emotions and do their best to recognize how they might impact the care they provide. It is inappropriate for clinicians to let their feelings, either positive or negative, significantly impact how they treat patients. Sometimes a quick break from the exam room might be all a clinician needs to regain their composure when faced with a challenging patient. Ultimately, if a clinician feels they cannot provide proper care for a patient due to their emotions, they should refer them to another provider. There is also an important lesson for patients: you are likely to get better care if you are nice to your clinician.

Attribution Biases: The Fundamental Attribution Error and Self-Serving Bias

Case

George, pictured below, was a 49-year-old man who presented with the acute onset of left-sided numbness (Fig. 11.4). An MRI revealed a small stroke in his thalamus on the right. He smoked one pack of cigarettes daily and was morbidly obese. He

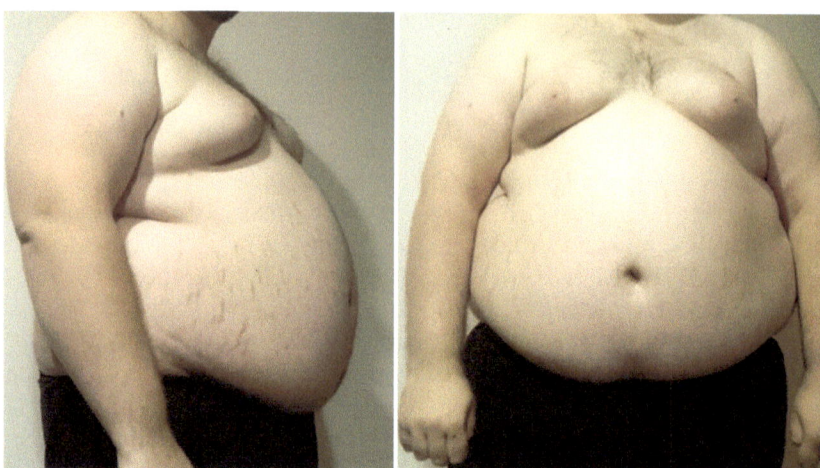

Fig. 11.4 George. (**Left**: FatM1ke. Side-on photo of an obese man [Image file]. In: Wikimedia commons. 2015. Retrieved from https://commons.wikimedia.org/wiki/File:ObeseManSideView. jpg; **Right**: FatM1ke. Front-on view of an obese man [Image file]. In Wikimedia commons. 2015. Retrieved from https://commons.wikimedia.org/wiki/File:ObeseManFrontView.jpg.)

was started on an aspirin and medications to control his cholesterol and high blood pressure. The stroke neurologist, Dr. Broder, spent five minutes with him the day of discharge, telling him, "You need to stop smoking and eating so much. You're really overweight and you can expect more strokes if you don't change your life around. Even with my busy schedule, I find time to exercise a minimum of four times per week, and you need to do the same."

George was next seen in follow-up by his primary care doctor two months later. Since his stroke, he had gained 15 pounds and was smoking even more. He said he was depressed and only intermittently took his medications as he felt "nothing I do really matters." His primary care doctor reinforced the neurologist's advice that his stroke risk factors were modifiable. She empathized with his inability to make lifestyle adjustments and told him to concentrate on making one or two improvements at a time. She prescribed an anti-smoking medication and referred him to a smoking cessation clinic and a weight loss center. One year later, he had quit smoking and lost 50 pounds.

What Dr. Broder Was Thinking

No one reviewing the chart would recognize I did anything wrong with George. I ordered all the appropriate tests and treatments. I exercise often, I eat right, and I don't smoke. So it frustrates me that people like George don't seem to do anything to care for their health. Although I would have denied it, my attitude towards patients like George was essentially "what do you expect?"

I later learned that George was a single father with two children ages eight and ten. Along with his sister, he also helped care for his elderly mother. He worked 12 hours per day, days per week as a bus driver, and was largely living paycheck to paycheck. He had no time to go the gym or prepare healthy meals. George was not a lazy guy who didn't care for his health. He was actually working harder and had more on his plate than just about anyone I knew.

My admonishments that he needed to lose weight and stop smoking were not inappropriate. However, I was a complete jerk. My telling him in essence "you're a fat, lazy, smoker who caused your stroke" was the opposite of helpful. He knew that he was obese and he knew that smoking was unhealthy for him. Had I simply been kind and understanding and spent a few more minutes trying to get to know George and learn about his life, I would have understood some of the challenges he was facing. I could have worked harder to set him up with resources outside the hospital that would have maximized his chances of making positive changes in his life. Instead, I shoved a bunch of prescriptions at him and walked out of his room. When he met a caring primary care doctor, she was able to really sit down with him and help him make small, incremental changes that yielded large, positive results.

I don't want to overstate the power a clinician has. Some patients will continue to smoke, eat an unhealthy diet, and not exercise no matter what we say. But judging them, withholding compassion, and not searching for resources to help them doesn't benefit anyone.

Case

Janice was a 26-year-old woman who presented having made a laceration to her forearm requiring sutures and antibiotics. She denied that she was suicidal, and a psychiatric evaluation found no evidence of mental illness. On her second day in the hospital, she removed her sutures, requiring them to be redone. She was placed on direct observation in the hospital and discharged two days later. She returned weeks later, again having cut her arm. During her second hospitalization, a medical student spent an hour with her and discovered that she had been beaten several times and had been forced into prostitution. With Janice's permission, a social worker notified the police, and she was discharged to a secure, domestic violence shelter. She did not return to the hospital.

What Dr. Malloy Was Thinking

Cutters are, unfortunately, pretty common, and they are frustrating to take care of. I was sure that Janice had problems in her life, but I felt my job was to suture her arm and make sure it didn't get infected. In my mind, she was someone who was inappropriately using and manipulating the hospital system for one reason or another. I never stopped to try to find out what that reason was. During her first hospitalization, no one really tried to find out why she had cut herself. We all thought that she was just crazy or attention-seeking. Some people really seem to enjoy being cared for in the hospital.

Once a medical student took the time to find out about the abuse she was suffering, her actions seemed fairly logical. Her world of sexual abuse is completely alien to me, but to the extent I can put myself in her shoes, I might have done something to try to enter the hospital as well. It's beyond a clinician's powers to solve the ills of society, as I feel we are sometimes asked to do. I could not help the fact that

Janice was homeless and that she was a target of abuse. But, even if I didn't have the time to talk with her like the medical student, I could have made more appropriate referrals to social workers and our victim outreach team. I could have been kinder. Instead, I was angry with Janice. While I cared for her wounds, that's all I cared for, and that was wrong. I'm far from perfect, but whenever I get angry at a patient I try to remember what Socrates said: "Be nicer than necessary to everyone you meet. Everyone is fighting some kind of battle."

Discussion

Attribution is defined by psychologists as the process of inferring the causes of behaviors and events. The act of attribution is an automatic process that everyone performs multiple times daily, both with our own actions and those of other people. Two attribution biases will be discussed here; the fundamental attribution error and the self-serving bias.

The fundamental attribution error (also called the correspondence bias) is the tendency to believe other people's behavior is driven primarily by their character and personality traits (dispositional attribution) rather than their circumstances (situational attribution). It leads us to assume unwarranted purposefulness or inappropriateness in the behavior of others, without consideration of factors in their life that may be influencing their behavior. At times, the fundamental attribution error leads people to assume positive characteristics about others. Movie stars are often felt to be wise, brave, or heroic like the characters they play on screen. Because it is easy to confuse with actor with the characters they play, they are bathed in undeserved adulation. Why else would anyone pay $66 to Gwyneth Paltrow for a rock designed to be inserted into one's vagina? [34] At other times, the fundamental attribution error leads people to assume negative characteristics about others. At its worst, it is a form of blaming the victim, where sick people and those in unfortunate circumstances are held responsible for whatever fate befalls them. In particular, patients with psychiatric conditions and other marginalized groups tend to suffer from this bias.

Edward Jones and Victor Harris demonstrated how hard it can be to account for a person's situation when explaining their behavior [35]. In their study, subjects read essays either supporting or objecting to Fidel Castro. They were told that the writer's position was determined by a coin toss. Despite this, study subjects still rated those who wrote pro-Castro essays as having a more positive attitude towards him compared to those who wrote essays opposing him. Even though they were intellectually aware of the situational constraints placed upon the writers, they could not refrain from attributing sincere beliefs to them. Imagine how you would feel if you were read an essay defending a position you found abhorrent, perhaps one titled *10 Reason to Eat the Family Pet* or *Why it Makes Sense to Marry Your Sister*. Even if you found out the author of those essays was forced to write them, I suspect you would still view them a bit differently. Similarly, writing those essays would make you uncomfortable, even if you were forced to do it. Psychologist Lisa Feldman wrote about this phenomenon in *The New York Times*. She challenged her students to debate eugenics, hoping that they would learn about someone else's odious views

Fig. 11.5 Is someone rude or are we committing the fundamental attribution error? (Not sure if troll. [Image file]. In: Meme generator. (n.d.). Retrieved from https://memegenerator.net/Not-Sure-If-Troll.)

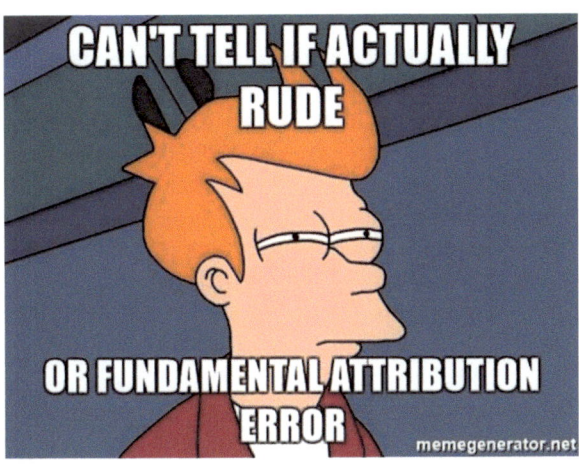

by pretending to argue for it. Though obviously being assigned to argue a viewpoint does not mean one agrees with it, the students nonetheless refused. "No one was willing to argue, even as part of a classroom exercise, that certain races were genetically superior to others," she wrote [36].

In contrast to the fundamental attribution error, when explaining our own behaviors, we are subject to the self-serving bias. This refers to the tendency to attribute our accomplishments to our internal, positive traits, while believing our failures are instead due to external circumstances beyond our control. A student who aces an exam might attribute this success to their intellect and hard work. In contrast, a student who fails an exam might blame an incompetent teacher or claim the exam was unfair.

How might attribution biases distort our perceptions? Let's say someone skipped ahead of me in line to grab the last spot on a crowded hospital elevator. I might assume this person was a selfish jerk, rotten to his core. If I were to encounter this person again, I might interpret their every action in this light. This would be an example of the fundamental attribution error. In reality, perhaps this person is rushing to say goodbye to a dying relative and proper elevator etiquette was the last thing on their mind (Fig. 11.5).

However, if someone were to point out a time when I skipped to the front of an elevator line, I would likely say it was because I was distractedly thinking about a sick patient, innocently lost in my own thoughts. Certainly I am not a selfish jerk. This is an example of the self-serving bias. When a clinician makes a challenging diagnosis, they may view themselves (perhaps correctly) as intelligent and hardworking. However, if they fail to make a diagnosis, they are unlikely to consider themselves incompetent. Rather, they may blame factors outside of their control, such as a patient withholding a crucial piece of information or a test result not being reported correctly.

Attribution biases exist for several reasons. Firstly, attribution is a mechanism to support and protect one's self-esteem. Our ego is bolstered when we take credit for our successes, and it is protected when we blame external factors for our failures.

Secondly, while we can readily access information about our own lives, often we can only speculate about the internal state and motivations of others, a phenomenon known as actor-observer asymmetry. As a result, when people evaluate their own actions, they are likely to attribute their behavior to situational factors. For example, if I were up all night with a sick child, I know why I am short-tempered the next day. In contrast, when observing the behavior of others, their behavior will likely be attributed their fundamental disposition rather than their circumstances. If someone were short-tempered with me, unless I know about some stressor in their life, I might assume that this represented their core personality. There is less actor-observer asymmetry with people we know well and with those whose situations we understand. As such we are less likely to make the fundamental attribution error with our family and close friends than with strangers.

Additionally, a person's underlying cognitive disposition, namely a concept known as locus of control, plays a strong role in how they attribute both their own behavior and the behavior of others. The locus of control refers to the degree to which people believe they control events in their own lives compared to external forces out of their control. People with a strong internal locus of control feel their own actions and beliefs are responsible for events in their life. They believe their successes are due to their own positive attributes. In contrast, those with a strong external locus of control credit or blame external factors for most aspects of their life. They believe their failures are because life is stacked against them. Interestingly, attribution biases tend occur less often in depressed people, who are likely to blame themselves for their failures. Attribution biases are also more common in Western cultures, where individualism is highly valued.

It is my informal observation that doctors and medical students tend to have a strong internal locus of control when judging themselves and their colleagues. As such, they may be particularly vulnerable to attribution biases. They pride themselves on their work ethic and ability to delay gratification, spending the prime of their life studying and working difficult overnight shifts. They are high-achievers who are used to attributing their successes to their intelligence and drive. They hold each other to very high standards and can be unforgiving of each other when a mistake is made. It may be difficult to rapidly switch from the high standards expected during doctors' rounds, to be empathetic and nonjudgmental at a patient's bedside. Additionally, doctors and medical students are, for the most part, healthier and wealthier than the average person. From this privileged vantage point, it may be difficult for them to understand the myriad of challenges their less fortunate patients often face.

Awareness of the fundamental attribution error has grown in medicine. Peter Attia, a general surgeon, gave a TED talk in which he discussed a fundamental attribution error he made while dealing with an obese woman with type 2 diabetes who required an urgent foot amputation [37]. He admitted that he quietly blamed her, feeling that if she had eaten less, exercised more, and taken better care of her health, her fate could have been avoided. "As a doctor, I delivered the best clinical care I could, but as a human being, I let you down," he said. "You didn't need my judgment and my contempt. You needed my empathy and compassion." As he told *The New York Times*:

> *I probably spent a lot of my time in medicine judging people who I thought brought conditions on themselves. Maybe I need to walk a mile in that*

person's shoes. There's probably a reason this person lived the life that they did, and maybe I have a privilege that they didn't have.

Dr. Attia, who himself was later diagnosed with diabetes, reported receiving many messages from other doctors who expressed similar regret towards patients they inappropriately judged or mistreated. A comment in *The New York Times* article about Dr. Attia speaks to this point:

> *I have a friend who was a medical student at Duke a few years ago. She once complained to me of the overweight people, smokers, who came to the emergency room. Exasperated, she asked me "Why don't they take better care of themselves? Why don't they stop smoking, why don't they lose weight?" I tried to explain to her that her life was very different from their lives. She was brilliant, starting on a rewarding career with financial and intellectual rewards. She had everything to look forward to, but those people she complained about had to go back to their minimum wage jobs as fry cooks and dishwashers at the Waffle House. They had to go home to cheap apartments every night with no hope to really do any better - ever. My friend got rewards from her life and her work, but these people got none. And now she wanted them to give up cigarettes and ice cream too? I'm sorry to say that my young friend just didn't get it* [37].

She's right. Many people lead challenging lives and making changes that require sustained effort can be exceedingly difficult.

Several studies have demonstrated that attribution biases can negatively affect patients. People who are felt to have caused their illness are judged more negatively than seemingly innocent victims of random diseases. Conversely, unpleasant patients are more likely to be blamed for their illness. Gisela Steins and Bernard Weiner investigated the attitudes of 134 Germans and 171 Americans towards a fictional person (K.C.) who was infected with HIV [38]. Several different scenarios were provided, one in which K.C. was an antisocial criminal and one in which K.C. was a kind nurse. Different scenarios of HIV infection were provided, with different levels of responsibility (low, medium, or high) for the infection, ranging from an accidental needle stick, to unsafe sex, to intravenous heroin use. They found that "The more responsible the target was, the more likely the participants were to evaluate the target as negative. Conversely, the more negative the target was, the higher was the perceived responsibility." Furthermore, as K.C.'s responsibility increased, participants' pity for K.C. decreased, and their anger increased. A similar study by Jill Borchert and Cheryl Rickabaugh found that "People who contracted HIV through IV drug use were held more accountable for their illness, and evoked more negative affect and less willingness to help than people who it contracted it through unprotected heterosexual sex" [39]. Similarly, Jessie Gruman and Peter Sloan found that college students presented with stories of ill people held derogatory views of them, and that, except for cancer patients, derogation increased with increasing illness severity [40]. People suffering from a disease (such as a heart attack) that was felt to be preventable were derogated more than those with a disease deemed unpreventable (such as stomach cancer) [41].

An important aspect to attribution biases is known as the just-world hypothesis, a term coined by the psychologist Melvin Lerner. This hypothesis refers to the innate belief that our natural sense of justice and the way we feel the world *should* be is the actual way the world is. It is characterized by the adages "what goes around comes around," "chickens come home to roost," and "you reap what you sow." It is comforting to believe in a world where "everything happens for a reason," and people generally get what they deserve. A smoker who gets lung cancer fits in well with our sense of justice. "He deserved it," we might think.

In contrast, our sense of justice is offended when a person who leads an ostensibly healthy lifestyle is felled by a devastating illness. "They must have done *something*," we may think to ourselves. There is evidence that those who believe highly in the just-world hypothesis are more likely to succumb to attribution biases and have negative attitudes to patients with certain diseases. A study by Adrian Furnham and Eddie Proctor in 1992 found that "high believers in just worlds will have negative attitudes to AIDS victims" [42]. They conclude that believing AIDS victims "deserve their fate" allows people "to put their own fears to rest because in a just world, AIDS is something which strikes those 'who ask for it.' Thus, the Just World Hypothesis not only explains why people get AIDS, but also why other people do not."

The most extreme version of the just-world hypothesis is known as the law of attraction. This is the magical belief that thoughts are composed of "pure energy" and that positive or negative thoughts have a direct influence on health, relationships, and money. It is based on the idea that "like attracts like," such that people who think positively will have positive things happen to them. This was popularized in the best-selling self-help book, *The Secret*, by Rhonda Byrne, published in 2006. Such wishful thinking is especially prominent in the world of complementary and alternative medicine (CAM). Consider this statement from CAM practitioner Christiane Northrup: "Fear and anger are present in all diseases. This is because emotions, such as fear and anger, when held too long, create chemical reactions in your body that do not support your health" (Fig. 11.6) [43].

This is not some metaphor or a comment on the uncontroversial finding that extreme stress over long periods of time can have deleterious health effects. According to this worldview, sick people literally cause their illness because of unreleased negative thoughts and emotions. Perhaps Dr. Northrup, who practices astrology and consults guardian angels, has access to some knowledge I do not. However, I challenge her to enter a pediatric oncology ward and spread this belief to the patient's and their families.

Perhaps the most egregious example of blaming the victim can be found in the book *You Can Heal Your Life* by Louise Hay. She believed that essentially every illness or symptom is an expression of negative emotions, and as such, "If we are willing to do the mental work, almost anything can be healed" [44]. She acquired this belief after she apparently cured her own cancer. Below is a small excerpt from a long list of conditions with their punitive associated mental deficiencies as determined by Ms. Hays [45]:

- **Malaria**: Out of balance with nature and with life.
- **Menopause Problems**: Fear of no longer being wanted. Fear of aging. Self-rejection. Not feeling good enough.
- **Menstrual Problems**: Rejection of one's femininity. Guilt, fear. Belief that the genitals are sinful or dirty.
- **Migraine Headaches**: Dislike of being driven. Resisting the flow of life. Sexual fears.

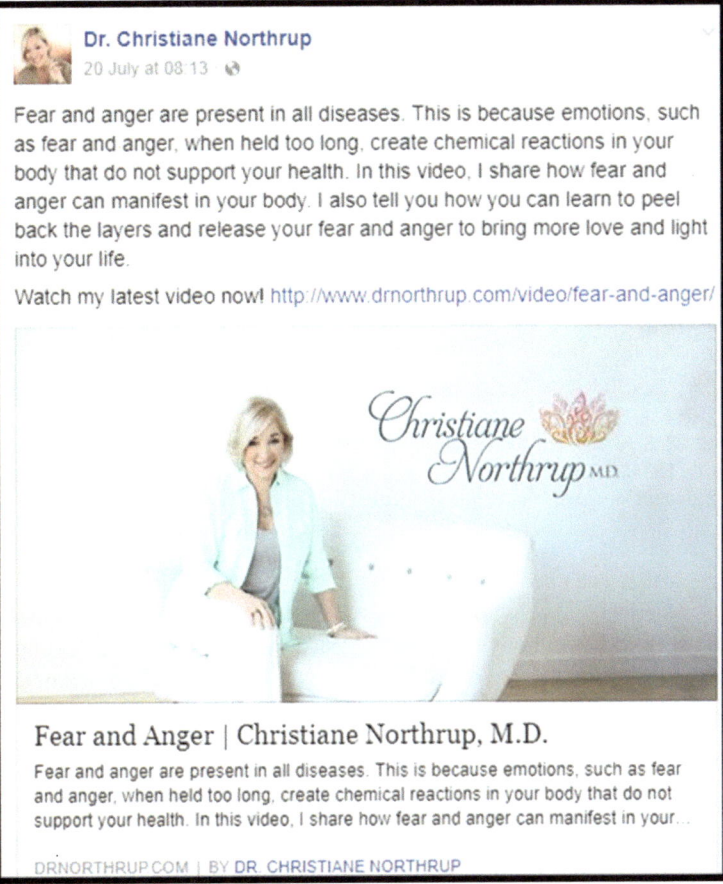

Fig. 11.6 Dr. Christiane Northrup blaming "fear and anger" for all diseases. (Northrup C. (Dr. Christiane). [Facebook status update]. 2017. Retrieved from https://www.facebook.com/DrChristianeNorthrup/posts/10159054573250029.)

- **Miscarriage**: Fear of the future. Inappropriate timing.
- **Mononucleosis**: Anger at not receiving love and appreciation. No longer caring for the self.
- **Motion Sickness**: Fear. Bondage. Feeling of being trapped.
- **Mouth**: Represents taking in of new ideas and nourishment. Set opinions. Closed mind. Incapacity to take in new ideas.
- **Multiple Sclerosis**: Mental hardness, hard-heartedness, iron will, inflexibility.
- **Muscles**: Resistance to new experiences. Muscles represent our ability to move in life.
- **Muscular Dystrophy**: "It's not worth growing up."

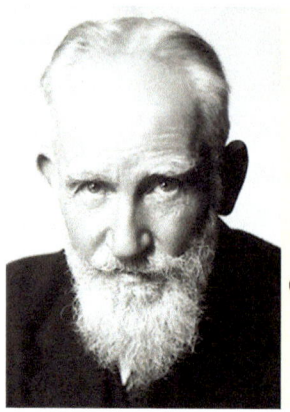

The fact that a believer is happier than a skeptic is no more to the point than the fact that a drunken man is happier than a sober one. The happiness of credulity is a cheap and dangerous quality of happiness, and by no means a necessity of life.

George Bernard Shaw

Fig. 11.7 George Bernard Shaw gets it right. (Nobel Foundation. Shaw in 1925, from Nobel Foundation [Image file]. In: Wikimedia commons. (n.d.). Retrieved from https://commons.wiki-media.org/wiki/George_Bernard_Shaw#/media/File:George_Bernard_Shaw_1925.jpg.)

She felt that even accidents were due to an "Inability to speak up for the self. Rebellion against authority. Belief in violence."

The belief that our thoughts alone can ensure good health is appealing to many people. It gives them a sense of control. However, as it is false, clinicians should not engage in wishful thinking, even if they find the thought comforting (Fig. 11.7).

For many such CAM practitioners, the idea that genetics and other factors outside a person's control, influences the risk for many diseases is an anathema that absolves people of responsibility for the illnesses that befall them. Consider the decision by the actress Angelina Jolie to have her ovaries and fallopian tubes prophylactically removed due to a genetic mutation that placed her at high risk of cancer. Her own mother died at age 56 after a nearly eight-year battle with ovarian and breast cancer. Jolie's doctors estimated that she had an 87% risk of breast cancer and a 50% risk of ovarian cancer. Through surgery, she lowered her breast cancer risk to less than 5%. She was vocal in explaining her decision, writing about it in *The New York Times* in an attempt to educate other women who may be in a similar predicament.

Her exceedingly difficult choice became a particular point of ire for CAM advocates, who themselves will never be in a position to actually treat women like Ms. Jolie. In an essay titled *Beware of Organ Removal for 'Cancer Prevention' Jolie's Precautionary Tale*, Sayer Ji, the founder of the CAM website Greenmedinfo, proclaimed, "the idea that genes play a dominant role in determining biological destiny and cancer risk is proliferating in the mainstream media and popular consciousness uncontrollably like a cancer" [46]. In a separate essay titled *Did Angelina Jolie Make A Mistake By Acting On The 'Breast Cancer Gene' Theory?* he wrote:

> The central dogma of molecular biology – that our DNA controls protein expression, and therefore disease risk – was disproved. Our genome was found to contain roughly 20,000 genetic instructions – not even enough to account for the 100,000 proteins in the human body! As a result, we must now accept that factors beyond the control of the gene, known as

epigenetic factors, and largely determined by a combination of nutrition, psychospiritual states that feed back into our physiology, lifestyle factors, and environmental exposures, constitute as high as 95% of what determines any disease risk [47].

Mr. Ji was not alone. In an essay titled "Angelina Jolie Duped Into Self Mutilation for Breast Cancer She Never Had," Mike Adams, the founder of the CAM website Natural News, wrote:

Cancer is not a disease you just "get" like being randomly struck by lightning. It's some-thing you must "manage" or "prevent" day by day, meal by meal, through a lifestyle choice that involves vitamin D supplementation, nutrition, superfoods, vegetable juices and avoid-ance of cancer-causing chemicals and radiation [48].

Similarly, psychiatrist and CAM practitioner Kelly Brogan wrote in an essay titled *The Game-Changing Science of Epigenetics* that:

One of the most powerful examples of the relevance of epigenetics is the lore of the "breast cancer gene." Jolie, and many other women have succumbed to the hex or the belief that they are cursed by their genes, doomed to develop diseased breasts, ovaries, and uteruses if they just go on living with them in their bodies [49].

Consistent with the philosophy that cancer is caused primarily by unhealthy attitudes, Dr. Brogan suggests in her essay "What Is Your Greatest Cancer Risk?" that cancer can largely prevented with positive thinking, writing, "True preven-tion looks more like dedicated self love…prevention can start with exhibiting a deep regard for yourself, every day. Send your body, mind, and spirit a signal of safety from multiple directions" [50]. CAM doctor Joseph Mercola expressed a similar belief that thoughts alone can alter genetic conditions by writing, "You actually have a tremendous amount of control over how your genetic traits are expressed, by changing your thoughts and altering your diet and your environ-ment" [51].

While obviously diet and other environmental factors can contribute to the risk of some cancers, the idea that the fundamental expression of genetic traits can be altered through "thoughts" and food is nonsense. Women who inherit the BRCA mutation are going to have a greatly elevated risk for breast and ovarian cancers no matter what they do. I have a simple challenge for any CAM practitioner who dis-agrees with this: change your eye color with your thoughts and lifestyle modifica-tions. Eye color is controlled by a few genes and altering it should be an easy, yet powerful, demonstration of the control they have over their genes.

A natural consequence of the belief that people can completely control illnesses with positive thoughts and healthy behaviors is that patients are blamed when they get sick or if their illness does not resolve. The idea of a random world, where ter-rible illnesses befall innocent people is difficult to accept for many people. As such, many patients inappropriately blame themselves for their illnesses. I see this all the time with my multiple sclerosis patients. Many hold themselves responsible for contracting the disease in the first place or for suffering an exacerbation. Too many feel that if only they had exercised more or avoided eating some junk food their health would have been fine.

Even worse, some patients get blamed by their clinicians for their illness or failure to improve. This is a common practice amongst CAM practitioners who seem constitutionally unable to doubt the efficacy of their treatment under any circumstances. As Dr. Brogan puts it in her essay "Holistic Medicine: Do You Believe?":

I want to help the patients who want to be helped. Who truly want to be guided back to themselves. Because some people need to be sick and want to be sick even when this isn't conscious. Others harbor so much fear that I could never wrest their attention from the conventional model's rhetoric [52].

When patients improve under her care, her treatment regimen gets the credit. In contrast, when patients fail to improve, they are blamed. They either do not *want* to get better or are too fearful. It is hard to think of a better example of the fundamental attribution error and self-serving biases than this.Undoubtedly, there are some patients who revel in the sick role. Rarely, patients have Munchausen syndrome, where they injure themselves or create an illness to gain sympathy, attention, and other benefits of being ill. However, such cases are dwarfed by the number of patients who want to get better, but have a disease that is difficult to treat. As such, clinicians must be very careful before blaming patients for their illness or for failing to improve. As psychiatrist Richard Friedman wrote, "Chronically ill, treatment-resistant patients can challenge the confidence of therapists themselves, who may be reluctant to question their treatment; it's easier — and less painful — to view the patient as intentionally or unconsciously resistant" [53].

It is potentially very damaging to suggest that patients are responsible for their illness and can will themselves to health by thinking positively. First of all, it is scientifically wrong. There is no evidence a negative attitude predisposes people to cancer, nor is there evidence that once a patient has been diagnosed with cancer, a positive attitude can extend their life. One study examined almost 60,000 people, who were tracked for at least 30 years [54]. It found no connection between personality traits and cancer risk or cancer survival. Second of all, telling patients that they must "think positive thoughts" can extract a significant emotion toll, forcing patients to suppress negative feelings and to feel guilty about experiencing completely legitimate, natural emotions.

Cancer survivor and author Barbara Ehrenreich discussed her negative experience with positive thinking by writing:

Breast cancer, I can now report, did not make me prettier or stronger, more feminine or spiritual. What it gave me, if you want to call this a "gift," was a very personal, agonizing encounter with an ideological force in American culture that I had not been aware of before – one that encourages us to deny reality, submit cheerfully to misfortune and blame only ourselves for our fate [55].

Clinicians who tell patients that diseases like cancer can be prevented or treated by "changing your thoughts" are deceiving them and placing an undue burden on them. A friend of mine, Amanda, underwent a double-mastectomy after being diagnosed with breast cancer at the age of 30. She was found to carry the BRCA mutation and will soon have her ovaries removed. She had this to say about being blamed for her illness. She wrote:

> *I think it's simply ridiculous and mind-boggling that people buy into this junk "science." It's actually offensive to those of us who have faced our mortality by no fault of our own. Victim-blaming makes unaffected people feel safe. The family history of those of us with BRCA mutations is filled with generations of mothers and daughters lost too young. We are cursed by our genes, but not in the way Dr. Brogan believes. Jolie has given us a quick and concise way to convey our situation to those who are (or were) oblivious to what a BRCA mutation is.*

While everyone but the most devoted practitioners of CAM can at least intellectually accept that illness may randomly befall people who live healthy lifestyles, it can be challenging for clinicians to treat the not insubstantial number of people who seem indifferent to the consequences of their behaviors or even directly cause their own illnesses. Every clinician will treat patients who smoke, drink excessively, overeat, have unprotected sex, don't exercise, and engage in all manners of unhealthy behaviors. It is not easy to care for a patient in alcohol withdrawal who has had multiple prior admissions and will likely drink the moment he leaves the hospital, only to be readmitted within a few days. Often, it seems that a clinician may care more about a patient's health than the patient themselves. Treating people who purposely injure themselves poses an even greater challenge. Clinicians should not attempt to suppress or deny their feelings towards these patients. Rather, they should strive to be aware of how any negative emotions they experience may inappropriately influence their care.

Importantly, we are often very poor judges of what motivates our own behavior, and as such, should exercise great caution when attempting to explain the behavior of others. As implausible as it seems, our own introspections are often unreliable. The workings of our own minds are often as inaccessible to us as the workings of our pancreas. People incorrectly think they have direct and accurate access into the causes of their beliefs and mental states, while the introspections of others cannot be trusted. We overestimate our ability to understand not only the motivations of others, but also the reasons behind our own behavior and choices. When assessing our behaviors, we may search our own thoughts and feelings for biased motives. Since biases are unconscious, however, our introspections are often misleading in ways to which we are blind. People wrongly treat introspections as a reliable indication that they are immune to bias, unlike others. In contrast, when people decide that another person is biased, they use their observable behavior. This phenomenon is known as the introspection illusion, a term coined by psychologist Emily Pronin [56]. She describes the illusion as having four components:

1. People give a strong weighting to introspective evidence when assessing themselves.
2. They do not give such a strong weight when assessing others.
3. People disregard their own behavior when assessing themselves, but not others.

4. Own introspections are more highly weighted than others. It is not just that people lack access to each other's introspections: they regard only their own as reliable.

Psychologists Richard Nisbett and Timothy Wilson conducted several experiments demonstrating we often don't know what we want [57]. In one experiment, researchers presented female college students with five posters: a Monet, a van Gogh, and three silly cat posters [58]. The subjects were then asked to rate each poster on a scale from one to nine. Half of the subjects, the "reasoners," were also asked to fill out a questionnaire asking them to explain their preferences. The results were quite different. 64% of the "reasoners" chose an art poster, while 95% of the control group did. At the end of the experiment, the students got to take home their favorite poster. Subjects preferred art when asked to go with their gut, but cat posters when asked to explicitly state the reason behind their choice. After all, it's easy to put into words what's attractive about a cute cat poster, but virtually impossible to do so with abstract art. When they were surveyed several weeks later, the "reasoners" were much less satisfied with their poster than the control group. Seventy five percent of the "reasoners" regretted their choice, while no students in the control group did so. As author Jonah Lehrer explained:

> The women who listened to their emotions ended up making much better decisions than the women who relied on their reasoning powers. The more people thought about which posters they wanted, the more misleading their thoughts became. Self-analysis resulted in less self-awareness [59].

In another experiment by Peter Johansson and colleagues, subjects were shown two small photographs and asked to choose the more attractive person [60]. They were then handed a larger picture of the person they supposedly chose and asked to explain their decision. In a trick in the experiment, they were actually handed a photograph of a different person, though few people noticed. Despite this, people nonetheless provided reasons for their "decision." However, these reasons were confabulated, given that they had not chosen the person in the photograph. This phenomenon, called choice blindness, has been replicated in other ways. In a twist on this experiment, Lars Hall and colleagues set up a jam and tea tasting booth at a supermarket [61]. After asking subjects which jam and tea they preferred, they secretly switched the containers, and asked the subject to taste the product they chose and explain why. Fewer than 20% of the subjects noticed the change. Those who did not notice confabulated reasons for their "decision." This occurred despite the fact that some of the jams tasted were remarkably different from each other.

These and similar studies show that the act of introspection is not a simple matter of accessing our inner mental world and motivations. Rather, often we look at our choices and actions after the fact and then confabulate an explanation for our behavior that makes sense to ourselves and others. The implications for attributional biases are clear: if we lack insight into the reasons behind our own decisions, how can we hope to know what motivates others?

Closely related to this is a phenomenon known as the illusion of asymmetric insight, also elucidated by Dr. Pronin and colleagues [62]. It occurs as people believe their knowledge of others exceeds other people's knowledge of them. How well do you feel understand the core essence of your partner, sibling, or best friend? You probably think that you know them very well. Now consider the reverse. How well do you think these people *really* understand you? Probably you think that there are core aspects to your personality that only you understand well. We tend to think that choices a person makes on word-completion tasks, for example, reveals fundamental aspects of their personality. In contrast, we feel our choices on the same tasks reveal nothing about ourselves.

The same is true at a group level. Liberals feels they understand conservative beliefs better than conservatives themselves. Similarly, they feel conservatives don't understand their position at all. This can lead to conflict and misunderstanding. As science writer David McRaney stated:

In a political debate you feel like the other side just doesn't get your point of view, and if they could only see things with your clarity, they would understand and fall naturally in line with what you believe. They must not understand, because if they did they wouldn't think the things they think. By contrast, you believe you totally get their point of view and you reject it. You see it in all its detail and understand it for what it is – stupid. You don't need to hear them elaborate. So, each side believes they understand the other side better than the other side understands both their opponents and themselves [63].

In attempting to avoid attribution biases, this does not mean clinicians should consider patients to be helpless victims of their circumstances and genetics, unable to make changes to improve their health. This would be paternalistic and completely untrue. In their statement on patient responsibilities, the AMA states that patients should "Recognize that a healthy lifestyle can often prevent or mitigate illness and take responsibility to follow preventive measures and adopt health-enhancing behaviors" [30].

Nor does avoiding attribution biases mean clinicians should avoid counselling patients regarding their unhealthy behaviors due to a fear of sounding judgmental. Smokers must be told about how this behavior endangers their health and must be encouraged to quit. Sedentary people must be encouraged to exercise. It is appropriate to tell overweight patients (who may not be sedentary), about the risk obesity poses to their health. However, all of this must be done in a supportive, non-judgmental manner. The goal is to improve the patient's health, not to allow the clinician to vent their frustrations or feel superior to their patients.

Simply telling people to lose weight and stop smoking, without additional support and resources, is unlikely to be effective. In fact, there is evidence that shaming people, particularly with regards to obesity, can actually backfire, leading to increased weight gain. Sarah Jackson and colleagues studied 2,944 people and found that individuals who experienced weight discrimination ended up gaining more weight [64]. They concluded, that "rather than encouraging people to lose weight, weight discrimination promotes weight gain and the onset of obesity." In another study of 6,157 people, Angelina Sutin and Antonio Terracciano found that:

Those who experienced weight discrimination were approximately 2.5 times more likely to become obese by follow-up and participants who were obese at baseline were three times more likely to remain obese at follow up than those who had not experienced such discrimination [65].

Additionally, in avoiding the fundamental attribution error, clinicians need not dispense with morality. A person who injures themselves while driving drunk was behaving unethically. It may not be the job of a clinician to sermonize to a patient, but they are not required to excuse unethical behavior. Nor does recognizing how external forces influence a patient's actions require that a clinician dispense with their agency. A prisoner who swallows razor blades is responsible for complications that arise from this. To suggest otherwise would be to infantilize patients. However, clinicians should at least consider a reasonable explanation for this prisoner's behavior. Perhaps he was surrounded by rival gang members who might viscously attack him and swallowing razors to spend a few days in the hospital was, to him, a rational decision.

Moreover, just because we naturally explain our achievements as products of our own positive attributes, this does not mean internal factors should be minimized in times of success. A medical student who aces a test may explain this happy result by referencing their hard work and intelligence, and they are likely correct. It is true that many clinicians may come from relatively privileged backgrounds. However this does not negate the enormous amount of hard work they put in to studying medicine. Clinicians have every right to take pride in their accomplishments.

Finally, when there is a bad outcome, clinicians themselves may be victims of the fundamental attribution error. Anthony Artino and colleagues argue that over-reliance on clinician characteristics may obscure other factors than can lead to errors, such as patient characteristics and the practice environment [66]. They write:

The success of any clinical encounter is often framed solely in terms of physician quality. That is, patients and other stakeholders assume that clinical quality is synonymous with physician quality. Physicians are labeled as knowledgeable, efficient, empathetic, or incompetent, as if the events that unfold in a clinical encounter emerge entirely from the personal qualities….When thinking about clinical quality, one naturally assumes that the characteristics of the physician are solely causal to both good and bad outcomes. After all, doctors largely direct most clinical encounters, and so it seems reasonable to assume that physicians' clinical behaviors result from their underlying personal characteristics, such as their knowledge, communication skills, and attitudes. In making this fundamental attribution error, we forget that clinical practice occurs in many different and complex environments, ranging from busy ambulatory clinics and emergency rooms to stressful inpatient wards and operating rooms. This is not to say that the physician is not partially responsible for good and bad outcomes; however, we would argue that the physician is only one of several factors leading to such outcomes.

Conclusion

Every clinician will at some point treat patients who are responsible, to varying degrees, for their illness. This can range from people who smoke to people who intentionally injure themselves. Such patients tend to elicit less sympathy and care than patients who are perceived as having had no role in their disease, such as innocent trauma victims or patients with sporadic diseases. While clinicians should not minimize the responsibility patients have for their own health, they must also be very careful before blaming them for their illness. Given that we cannot adequately assess our own motivations, how can we reliably do so for others? Even when it is clear that a patient is largely responsible for their illness, clinicians should do their best to recognize there may be unknown factors that led to a patient's behavior.

But on a fundamental level, it doesn't matter. It is not a clinician's job to judge their patients. Their job is to treat disease and relieve suffering, no matter the cause. A mechanic fixing a damaged car is unlikely to do their job differently based on whether the car belonged to a drunk-driver or a sober one. While the analogy isn't perfect, clinicians should largely take this approach with their patients. Certainly, patients should be counseled on unhealthy behaviors. Yet, a patient who contracted lung cancer due to smoking is no less deserving of care than a patient who got cancer due to a genetic mutation. A patient who fractures their leg while driving drunk should be treated exactly the same as an innocent person whom the drunk driver injured.

Finally, patients should not be blamed when they don't improve. Only in exceptionally rare cases do patients aim to be sick. To again quote Richard Friedman, "a vast majority of patients want to feel better, and for them the burden of illness is painful enough. Let's keep the blame on the disease, not the patient" [53]. Exactly.

References

1. Groves JE. Taking care of the hateful patient. N Engl J Med. 1978;298(16):883–7. Retrieved from https://doi.org/10.1056/NEJM197804202981605.
2. Jackson JL, Kroenke K. Difficult patient encounters in the ambulatory clinic: clinical predictors and outcomes. JAMA Intern Med. 1999;159(10):1069–75. https://doi.org/10.1001/archinte.159.10.1069.
3. Cornwall L. (2016, Jan 25). Physician bias: trends from the 2016 Medscape Lifestyle Report. CompHealth. Retrieved from https://comphealth.com/resources/physician-bias-trends-from-the-2016-medscape-lifestyle-report/.
4. Ambady N, Rosenthal R. Thin slices of expressive behavior as predictors of interpersonal consequences: a meta-analysis. Psychol Bull. 1992;111(2):256–74. https://doi.org/10.1037/0033-2909.111.2.256.
5. Ambady N, Rosenthal R. Half a minute: predicting teacher evaluations from thin slices of nonverbal behavior and physical attractiveness [PDF file]. J Pers Soc Psychol. 1993;64(3):431–41. Retrieved from https://ambadylab.stanford.edu/pubs/1993Ambady.pdf.
6. Ambady N, Laplante D, Nguyen T, Rosenthal R, Chaumeton N, Levinson W. Surgeons' tone of voice: a clue to malpractice history. Surgery. 2002;132(1):5–9. Retrieved from https://doi.org/10.1067/msy.2002.124733.
7. Hodder HF. (2001, July 1). Snap judgments work! Harvard Magazine. Retrieved from https://harvardmagazine.com/2001/07/snap-judgments-work.html.
8. Olivola CY, Todorov A. Elected in 100 milliseconds: appearance-based trait inferences and voting. J Nonverbal Behav. 2010;34(2):83–110. https://doi.org/10.1007/s10919-009-0082-1.
9. Verhulst B, Lodge M, Lavine H. The attractiveness halo: why some candidates are perceived more favorably than others. J Nonverbal Behav. 2010;34(2):111–7. https://doi.org/10.1007/s10919-009-0084-z.
10. Jecker J, Landy D. Liking a person as a function of doing him a favour. Hum Relat. 1969;22:371–8.

11. McRaney D. (2011, Oct 5). The Benjamin Franklin effect. You Are Not So Smart. Retrieved from https://youarenotsosmart.com/2011/10/05/the-benjamin-franklin-effect/.
12. Eikeland HL, Ørnes K, Finset A, Pedersen R. The physician's role and empathy–a qualitative study of third year medical students. BMC Med Educ. 2014;14(165):1–8. https://doi.org/10.1186/1472-6920-14-165.
13. Birdwell BG, Herbers JE, Kroenke K. Evaluating chest pain: the patient's presentation style alters the physician's diagnostic approach. Arch Intern Med. 1993;153(17):1991–5. https://doi.org/10.1001/archinte.1993.00410170065006.
14. Mamede S, Van Gog T, Schuit SC, Van den Berge K, Van Daele PL, Bueving H, Van der Zee T, Van den Broek WW, Van Saase JL, Schmidt HG. Why patients' disruptive behaviours impair diagnostic reasoning: a randomised experiment. BMJ Qual Saf. 2016;26:13–8. https://doi.org/10.1136/bmjqs-2015-005065.
15. Schmidt HG, Van Gog T, Schuit SC, Van den Berge K, Van Daele PL, Bueving H, Van der Zee T, Van den Broek WW, Van Saase JL, Mamede S. Do patients' disruptive behaviours influence the accuracy of a doctor's diagnosis? a randomised experiment. BMJ Qual Saf. 2017;26:19–23. https://doi.org/10.1136/bmjqs-2015-004109.
16. Milmo C. (2016, Mar 15). Doctors 'more likely to misdiagnose patients' if they are 'difficult'. The Independent. Retrieved from https://www.independent.co.uk/life-style/health-and-families/health-news/doctors-more-likely-to-misdiagnose-patients-if-they-are-difficult-a6930781.html.
17. Hull SK, Broquet K. How to manage difficult patient encounters. Fam Pract Manag. 2007;14(6):30–4.
18. Jackson JL, Kroenke K. Difficult patient encounters in the ambulatory clinic: clinical predictors and outcomes. Arch Intern Med. 1999;159(10):1069–75. https://doi.org/10.1001/archinte.159.10.1069.
19. Hojat M, Louis DZ, Markham FW, Wender R, Rabinowitz C, Gonnella JS. Physicians' empathy and clinical outcomes for diabetic patients. Acad Med. 2011;86(3):359–64. https://doi.org/10.1097/ACM.0b013e3182086fe1.
20. Del Canale S, Louis DZ, Maio V, Wang X, Rossi G, Hojat M, Gonnella JS. The relationship between physician empathy and disease complications: an empirical study of primary care physicians and their diabetic patients in Parma, Italy. Acad Med. 2012;87(9):1243–9. https://doi.org/10.1097/ACM.0b013e3182628fbf.
21. Neumann M, Wirtz M, Bollschweiler E, Mercer SW, Warm M, Wolf J, Pfaff H. Determinants and patient-reported long-term outcomes of physician empathy in oncology: a structural equation modelling approach. Patient Educ Couns. 2007;69(1–3):63–75. https://doi.org/10.1016/j.pec.2007.07.003.
22. Rakel D, Barrett B, Zhang Z, Hoeft T, Chewning B, Marchand L, Scheder J. Perception of empathy in the therapeutic encounter: effects on the common cold. Patient Educ Couns. 2011;85(3):390–7. https://doi.org/10.1016/j.pec.2011.01.009.
23. Ofri D. What doctors feel: how emotions affect the practice of medicine. Boston: Beacon Press; 2013.
24. Gold Foundation Contributors. (n.d.). Gold humanism honor society. Retrieved 15 Sept 2018 from https://www.gold-foundation.org/programs/ghhs/.
25. Yousaf A. (2016, May 22). With doctors losing respect, perhaps it's time to expose medicine's dark side [Blog post]. KevinMD.com. Retrieved from https://www.kevinmd.com/blog/2016/05/with-doctors-losing-respect-perhaps-its-time-to-expose-medicines-dark-side.html.
26. Hartsock J. (2017, July 19). What it's like to be a doctor in the heroin capitol of the U.S [Blog post]. KevinMD.com. Retrieved from https://www.kevinmd.com/2017/07/like-doctor-heroin-capital-u-s.html.
27. WebMD News Staff. (2017, Oct 18). Patient prejudice survey results. WebMD. Retrieved 15 Sept 2018 from https://www.webmd.com/a-to-z-guides/news/20171018/patient-prejudice-survey-results?ecd=stat.
28. Thielking M. (2017, Aug 8). A doctor's murder over an opioid prescription leaves an Indiana city with no easy answers. STAT. Retrieved from https://www.statnews.com/2017/08/08/indiana-doctor-murdered-opioids/.

29. Jain SH. The racist patient. Ann Intern Med. 2013, April 16;158(8):632. https://doi.org/10.7326/0003-4819-158-8-201304160-00010.

30. American Medical Association. (2016). Chapter 1: opinions on patient-physician relationships [PDF file]. AMA Journal of Ethics. Retrieved 15 Sept 2018 from https://www.ama-assn.org/sites/default/files/media-browser/code-of-medical-ethics-chapter-1.pdf.

31. King A. (2017, Aug 20). Asian-American doctor says white nationalists refuse her care. CNN Newsroom. Retrieved from https://www.cnn.com/2017/08/19/us/asian-american-doctor-white-nationalists-crace-cnnt/index.html.

32. Tedeschi B. (2017, Oct 18). 6 in 10 doctors report abusive remarks from patients, and many get little help coping with the wounds. STAT. Retrieved from https://www.statnews.com/2017/10/18/patient-prejudice-wounds-doctors/.

33. Paul-Emile K, Smith AK, Lo B, Fernández A. Dealing with racist patients. N Engl J Med. 2016;374(8):708–11. https://doi.org/10.1056/NEJMp1514939.

34. Egg J. (n.d.). In: goop. Retrieved on 15 Sept 2018 from https://shop.goop.com/shop/products/jade-egg?irgwc=1&utm_campaign=10079_Online%20.

35. Jones EE, Harris VA. The attribution of attitudes. J Exp Soc Psychol. 1967;3(1):1–24. https://doi.org/10.1016/0022-1031(67)90034-0.

36. Barrett LF. (2017, July 14). When is speech violence? The New York Times. Retrieved from https://www.nytimes.com/2017/07/14/opinion/sunday/when-is-speech-violence.html.

37. O'Connor, A. (2013, July 12). Blaming the patient, then asking forgiveness [Blog post]. The New York Times. Retrieved from https://well.blogs.nytimes.com/2013/07/12/blaming-the-patient-then-asking-forgiveness/.

38. Steins G, Weiner B. The influence of perceived responsibility and personality characteristics on the emotional and behavioral reactions to people with AIDS. J Soc Psychol. 1999;139(4):487–795. https://doi.org/10.1080/00224549909598408.

39. Borchert J, Rickabaugh CA. When illness is perceived as controllable: the effects of gender and mode of transmission on AIDS-related stigma. Sex Roles. 1995;33(9–10):657–68. https://doi.org/10.1007/BF01547723.

40. Gruman JC, Sloan RP. Disease as justice: perceptions of the victims of physical illness. Basic Appl Soc Psychol. 1983;4(1):39–46. https://doi.org/10.1207/s15324834basp0401_4.

41. Sloan RP, Gruman JC. Beliefs about cancer, heart disease, and their victims. Psychol Rep. 1983;52:415–24. https://doi.org/10.2466/pr0.1983.52.2.415.

42. Furnham A, Procter E. Sphere-specific just world beliefs and attitudes to AIDS. Hum Relat. 1992;45(3):265–80. https://doi.org/10.1177/001872679204500303.

43. Northrup C. (2017). Fear and anger. Dr. Christiane Northup. [Video file]. Retrieved from https://www.drnorthrup.com/video/fear-and-anger/.

44. Hay L. You can heal your life. Carlsbad: Hay House; 1984.

45. Afshar F. (2013, Dec 15). Causes of symptoms according to Louise Hay. The Alchemy of Healing. Retrieved from http://alchemyofhealing.com/causes-of-symptoms-according-to-louise-hay/.

46. Ji S. (2015, Mar 24). Beware of organ removal for "cancer prevention": Jolie's precautionary tale [Blog post]. GreenMedInfo. Retrieved from http://www.greenmedinfo.com/blog/beware-organ-removal-cancer-prevention-jolies-precautionary-tale-2.

47. Ji S. (2013, May 14). Did Angelina Jolie make a mistake by acting on the 'breast cancer gene' theory? [Blog post]. GreenMedInfo. Retrieved from http://www.greenmedinfo.com/blog/did-angelina-jolie-make-mistake-acting-breast-cancer-gene-theory.

48. How Angelina Jolie was duped by cancer doctors into self mutilation for breast cancer she never had. (n.d.). RealFarmacy.com. Retrieved 15 Sept 2018 from https://realfarmacy.com/how-angelina-jolie-was-duped-by-cancer-doctors-into-self-mulilation-for-breast-cancer-she-never-had/.

49. Brogan K. (n.d.). The game-changing science of epigenetics. Kelly Brogan MD. Retrieved 15 Sept 2018 from https://kellybroganmd.com/gamechanging-science/.

50. Brogan K. (n.d.). What is your greatest cancer risk? Kelly Brogan MD. Retrieved 15 Sept 2018 from https://kellybroganmd.com/what-is-your-greatest-cancer-risk/.

51. Falling for this myth could give you cancer. (2012, April 11). Mercola. Retrieved 15 Sept 2018 from https://articles.mercola.com/sites/articles/archive/2012/04/11/epigenetic-vs-determinism.aspx.

52. Brogan K. (n.d.). Holistic medicine: do you believe? [Blog post]. Kelly Brogan MD. Retrieved 15 Sept 2018 from https://kellybroganmd.com/do-you-believe.
53. Friedman RA. (2008, Oct 20). When all else fails, blaming the patient often comes next. The New York Times. Retrieved from https://www.nytimes.com/2008/10/21/health/21mind.html.
54. Nakaya N, Bidstrup PE, Saito-Nakaya K, Frederiksen K, Koskenvuo M, Pukkala E, Kaprio J, Floderus B, Uchitomi Y, Johansen C. Personality traits and cancer risk and survival based on Finnish and Swedish registry data. Am J Epidemiol. 2010;172(4):377–85. https://doi.org/10.1093/aje/kwq046.
55. Ehrenreich B. (2010, Jan 1). Smile! You've got cancer. The Guardian. Retrieved from https://www.theguardian.com/lifeandstyle/2010/jan/02/cancer-positive-thinking-barbara-ehrenreich.
56. Pronin E. The introspection illusion. Adv Exp Soc Psychol. 2009;41:1–67. https://doi.org/10.1016/S0065-2601(08)00401-2.
57. Nisbett RE, Wilson TD. Telling more than we can know: verbal reports on mental processes. Psychol Rev. 1977;84(3):231–59. https://doi.org/10.1037/0033-295X.84.3.231.
58. Wilson TD, Lisle DJ, Schooler JW, Hodges SD, Klaaren KJ, LaFleur SJ. Introspecting about reasons can reduce post-choice satisfaction. Personal Soc Psychol Bull. 1993;19(3):331–9. https://doi.org/10.1177/0146167293193010.
59. Lehrer J. How we decide. Boston: Houghton Mifflin; 2009. p. 144.
60. Johansson P, Hall L, Sikström S, Tärning B, Lind A. How something can be said about telling more than we can know: on choice blindness and introspection. Conscious Cogn. 2006;15(4):673–92. https://doi.org/10.1016/j.concog.2006.09.004.
61. Hall L, Johansson P, Tärning B, Sikström S, Deutgen T. Magic at the marketplace: choice blindness for the taste of jam and the smell of tea. Cognition. 2010;117(1):54–61. https://doi.org/10.1016/j.cognition.2010.06.010.
62. Pronin E, Kruger J, Savtisky K, Ross L. You don't know me, but I know you: the illusion of asymmetric insight. J Pers Soc Psychol. 2001;81(4):639–56.
63. McRaney D. (2011, Aug 21). The illusion of asymmetric insight. You Are Not So Smart. Retrieved from https://youarenotsosmart.com/2011/08/21/the-illusion-of-asymmetric-insight/.
64. Jackson SE, Beeken RJ, Wardle J. Perceived weight discrimination and changes in weight, waist circumference, and weight status. Obesity. 2014;22(12):2485–8. https://doi.org/10.1002/oby.20891.
65. Phelan SM, Burgess DJ, Yeazel MW, Hellerstedt WL, Griffin JM, van Ryn M. Impact of weight bias and stigma on quality of care and outcomes for patients with obesity. Obes Rev. 2015;16(4):319–26. https://doi.org/10.1111/obr.12266.
66. Artino AR, Durning SJ, Waechter DM, Leary KL, Gilliland WR. Broadening our understanding of clinical quality: from attribution error to situated cognition. Clin Pharmacol Ther. 2012;91(2):167–9. https://doi.org/10.1038/clpt.2011.229.

Case

Simone was a 23-year-old woman who had been acting oddly for the past week, fearful that her neighbors were spying on her. She had left home two days prior, and her mother had not seen her since. She was brought to the hospital after she tried to enter City Hall to warn the mayor about an upcoming invasion. She was admitted to the psychiatric unit where she was diagnosed with an "acute psychotic disorder." Her mother heard from hospital staff that two women on the unit had been recently diagnosed with limbic encephalitis, an autoimmune disorder that presents with memory loss, personality changes, psychiatric symptoms, involuntary movements, and seizures. She insisted that her daughter be evaluated for this disorder, though the psychiatrist declined. On her fifth day in the hospital, she had a seizure and was transferred to the neurology service where an MRI showed abnormalities of the temporal lobes consistent with limbic encephalitis.

What Dr. Patricia Was Thinking

I had already seen two cases of limbic encephalitis that month. Perhaps it is more common than we recognized, but I was taught this was a rare diagnosis in medical school—the kind of thing a doctor might see once or twice in their career. As such, when Simone arrived, I discounted the possibility that she might have this rare disease. The odds that I would see this disease at all were not that high. The odds that I would see it twice in a week were extremely low. The odds that I would see it three times in a week were essentially zero, or so I thought. I didn't want to be seen as one of those doctors who did a "million-dollar" work-up on everyone. Yet, Simone's case was independent of the two cases that preceded her, and the fact that two people presented with the disease before her didn't protect her in any way.

Case

Lewis was a 22-year-old man who presented with confusion and altered mental status. His girlfriend brought him in after he called her that afternoon "not making sense." On examination, he did not know the date and had trouble remembering

© Springer International Publishing AG, part of Springer Nature 2019
J. Howard, *Cognitive Errors and Diagnostic Mistakes*,
https://doi.org/10.1007/978-3-319-93224-8_12

why he was in the hospital. He accused the hospital staff of trying to hurt him, became agitated, and tried to leave the ER. Hospital police were called, and Lewis was sedated to prevent him from leaving. The doctor in the ER attributed his symptoms to the use of K2, a form of synthetic marijuana known to cause agitation and psychosis. His girlfriend said that he had smoked marijuana several times in college, but hadn't done so for several months. Lewis was observed for several hours and discharged home when the sedation wore off. He returned the next day after having a seizure. A CT scan at that time revealed hemorrhage in the left temporal lobe. He was immediately started on acyclovir, an anti-viral agent used in the treatment of herpes encephalitis. Further studies on his spinal fluid confirmed the diagnosis.

What Dr. Xiang Was Thinking
The use of K2 was a pretty common cause of psychosis and altered mental status, unfortunately. There had been several "outbreaks" of people smoking it, and it had led to multiple similar ER visits. At times, up to 10 people would come in completely altered, having smoked it. It would not have been possible to have obtained a CT scan on every patient who presented with such altered mental status. Additionally, CT scans are a source of radiation, which pose a small but real risk of increased cancer. So, while we order them all the time in the ER, we also have to be judicious. When I saw Lewis, I was ending my shift and had seen three other cases like him that night. I simply assumed that he was the fourth. There is little doubt that had I not seen the three patients who were clearly under the influence of K2 prior to seeing Lewis, that I would have listened to his girlfriend, who seriously doubted his use of K2. Almost certainly, I would have ordered the tests that would have made the diagnosis.

Case
Nicole was a 46-year-old woman presented to a neurologist's office for an evaluation of multiple sclerosis (MS). She had multiple complaints that she had listed on a piece of paper. Her main complaints were fatigue and "brain fog," which had been significant over the past year. She also complained of headaches, blurry vision, word-finding difficulties, tingling in her hands and feet, stomach upset, palpitations, and pain during sex. She was felt not to put forth full effort on examination of her muscles, but neurological examination was otherwise normal. She had an extensive laboratory work-up, which was unrevealing. An MRI of her brain revealed approximately 10 small lesions, which prompted the evaluation for MS. The neurologist did not feel that the overall presentation was consistent with MS.

Nicole reluctantly accepted that she did not have MS, but remained frustrated with the inability of her neurologist to correctly diagnosis her condition. She returned to the neurologist's office several times per year for evaluations. During each visit she listed a number of bothersome symptoms, and each time was reassured about them. On her sixth visit, she complained of shortness of breath and a "racing heart." She had a heart rate of 110 bpm, and was sent home with an anti-anxiety medication. She returned to the ER that night where she was diagnosed with a pulmonary embolism, which is a potentially fatal condition due to a blood clot in the one of the arteries in the lung.

What Dr. Gonzalez Was Thinking

I had seen Nicole on several occasions and concluded that she did not have MS. It is quite common for patients to present with a large panoply of symptoms and a few, nonspecific white matter lesions on their brain MRI. I felt that she had somatic symptom disorder, which is characterized by multiple physical symptoms that that are characteristic of physical illness, but for which no explanation is found. Although I am an MS specialist, I continue to see these patients, as I hope I can prevent them from receiving unnecessary treatment for a disease they do not have. Nicole was labeled in my mind as someone who somaticizes, meaning they turn anxiety and depression into physical symptoms. As such, when she presented with classic symptoms of a pulmonary embolism, my guard was down. I am not saying that I could have diagnosed a pulmonary embolism then and there in my office. However, there were certainly enough clues that something potentially serious was wrong, and I should have sent her to the ER. With patients like this, there is a constant tension between not doing a "million dollar" work-up for every complaint, and ignoring complaints and missing real diseases. I was fooled by Nicole's case, but her "streak" of false complaints unconsciously made me think nothing could ever be wrong with her. Of course, the fact that she had multiple unexplained somatic complaints in the past didn't mean she was protected from life-threatening diseases in the future.

Case

Juliette was a 56-year-old woman who developed the acute onset of right-sided weakness and trouble "getting out the right words." She was eating lunch with a friend at the time and 911 was called. The patient arrived to the ER within 90 minutes, and a head CT was normal. Though the neurologist felt a stroke was the most likely diagnosis, she decided against giving tissue plasminogen activator (tPA), a medication used to help break up blood clots in acute strokes. The neurologist declined to give the medication, in part because several patients to whom she had recently given the medication had significant hemorrhages.

What Dr. Mirsky Was Thinking

Prior to Juliette coming to the hospital, the last three patients to whom I gave tPA had intracerebral hemorrhages. One patient died. Each case was reviewed by a hospital safety panel, and there was no question I did the right thing. There is about a 6% risk of serious bleeding with this medication, and I was unlucky enough to have it happen three times in a row. This was just bad luck. I certainly didn't consciously decide not to use tPA again. But I felt kind of cursed. I had seen too many bad outcomes recently and didn't want that bad streak to continue.

Discussion

In Bayesian statistics, the prior probability of an event is the original probability that reflects established knowledge before new information is uncovered. Once new evidence emerges, more accurate probabilities can be estimated, termed posterior probabilities. For example, the prior probability that a patient with a headache has a tumor may be low until we learn that she is a 65-year-old woman who smoked for 50 years and has a mass on her chest X-ray. At this point, the probability that she has metastatic cancer to her brain increases significantly.

The posterior probability error occurs when the estimate for the likelihood of an event is inappropriately influenced by prior, unrelated or minimally related events. In medicine, a clinician may overestimate or underestimate the probability of a disease based on prior encounters with either that patient or other similar patients. Thus, the pretest probability that a patient will have a particular diagnosis might be unduly colored by preceding, but independent events. Additionally, a clinician's perception of a treatment may be inappropriately influenced by a streak of successes or failures with it. Specific examples of the posterior probability error are the gambler's fallacy and the hot hand fallacy.

The gambler's fallacy is the belief that a streak of some sort will be broken. If something occurs more often than normal, victims of the gambler's fallacy will presume the event will happen less often in the future. For example, if a roulette ball lands on red ten times in a row, some people will believe the 11th spin of the wheel will have a greater chance of landing on black, even though a fair wheel has no memory. It is also called the Monte Carlo fallacy after the following unpredictable event:

> On August 18, 1913, at the casino in Monte Carlo, black came up a record twenty-six times in succession [in roulette]. … [There] was a near-panicky rush to bet on red, beginning about the time black had come up a phenomenal fifteen times. In application of the maturity [of chances] doctrine [the gambler's fallacy], players doubled and tripled their stakes, this doctrine leading them to believe after black came up the twentieth time that there was not a chance in a million of another repeat. In the end the unusual run enriched the Casino by some millions of francs [1].

Other instances of the gambler's fallacy include:

- Many people erroneously believe that someone who has gone on 10,000 plane trips is more likely to crash on their next flight than someone going on their first trip.
- Sports broadcasters commonly say that a good baseball player who has gone multiple at bats without getting a hit, is "due" to get one.
- In Venice, the number 53 failed to appear in the lottery from 2003–2005. Many people bet their life savings away, feeling that the number was bound to come up soon. Several players killed themselves and family members due to their debts [2].

- An early instance of the gambler's fallacy was described in 1796 by Pierre-Simon Laplace. He wrote how expectant fathers used recent births in the community to help determine the sex of the own child. Laplace wrote:

    I have seen men, ardently desirous of having a son, who could learn only with anxiety of the births of boys in the month when they expected to become fathers. Imagining that the ratio of these births to those of girls ought to be the same at the end of each month, they judged that the boys already born would render more probable the births next of girls [3].

In medicine, the gambler's fallacy may affect a clinician who sees several cases in a row of a particular condition and as a result, lowers the probability of this diagnosis for a subsequent patient. Consider, for example, a clinician who sees a series of patients with headaches and correctly diagnoses them all with a sinus venous thrombosis. As this is a rare diagnosis, she might assume the sequence is unlikely to continue, and this diagnosis might be prematurely dismissed for the next patient with a headache.

Psychologists Amos Tversky and Daniel Kahneman felt that the gambler's fallacy is a variant of the representativeness heuristic, which posits that people evaluate the probability of an event by evaluating how similar it is to events that they have experienced before. A roulette wheel with a smattering of black and red outcomes is familiar to us, whereas a wheel that lands on red ten times in a row is not. As such, Tversky and Kahneman wrote, "after observing a long run of red on the roulette wheel, for example, most people erroneously believe that black will result in a more representative sequence than the occurrence of an additional red" [4]. The gambler's fallacy occurs because people sense that small samples are representative of the larger population (the law of small numbers). People intuitively believe that a small sequence of random outcomes should be similar to larger sequences and that deviations from average should naturally be balanced. James Sundali and Rachel Croson have suggested that people who have a strong internal locus of control are more vulnerable to the gambler's fallacy, as they may have a hard time appreciating that randomness can sometimes govern their fate [5].

In contrast, the hot hand fallacy is the belief that an unusual streak of some sort will continue. Like the gambler's fallacy, it often occurs in sports. It has been most commonly applied to basketball and was first described in a 1985 paper, *The Hot Hand in Basketball: On The Misperception Of Random Sequences*, by psychologist Thomas Gilovich and colleagues [6]. They examined the common belief that a player who has made several shots in a row is more likely to make the next one and found this was not the case. They concluded that a "hot hand" is a myth, and that it is simply the product of expected variation. After all, if a fair coin is tossed five times in a row, the odds are 1/32 that there will be five heads in a row. Therefore, it is not surprising that in almost every basketball game, one player will make five shots in a row based on chance alone. This player will then seem to have a hot hand.

Fig. 12.1 Stores often try
to entice patrons to buy
lottery tickets, using the
hot hand fallacy

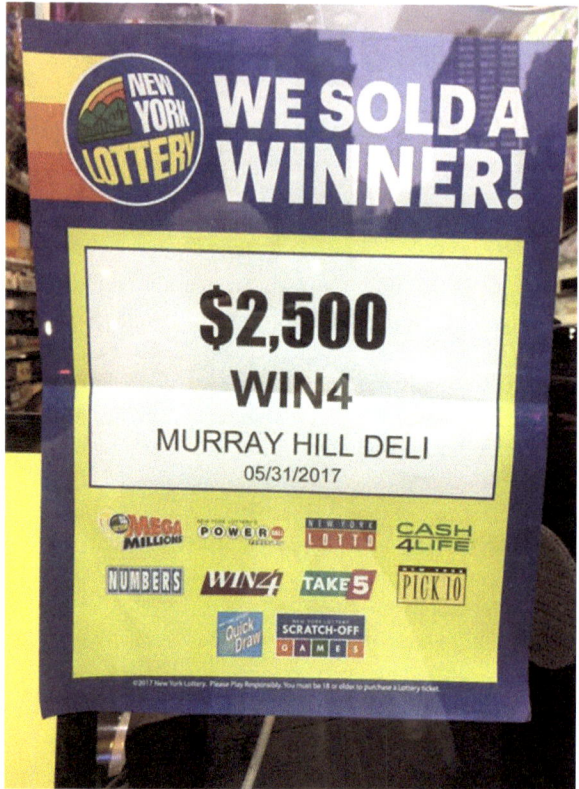

Though Gilovic's paper was thought to have debunked the hot hand phenomenon, by analyzing large data samples, such as 300,000 free throws over five seasons and 2,000,000 baseball at-bats over 12 years, statisticians have uncovered evidence that the hot hand phenomenon does exist, though not nearly to the extent enthusiastic sportscasters make it seem [7]. Moreover, Joshua Miller and Adam Sanjurjo found that the original paper by Gilovich made flawed statistical assumptions rendering its findings more questionable [8].

While the hot hand phenomenon does seem to exist to a very small degree in non-random events such as shooting free throws, people can still detect a hot hand "pattern" where none exists. Stores routinely post when they sell a winning lottery ticket, hoping to entice statistically ignorant customers who believe the streak of good luck will continue (Fig. 12.1).

At times, peoples' ability to see streaks of good fortune where there is only randomness can impact entire professions. Daniel Kahneman the performance of 25 wealth advisers for eight years in a row [9]. They were given a bonus at the end of the year based on their performance, and he wanted to determine whether or not a manager who did well one year was likely to do so the next year. He found that there was no correlation from one year to the next. Their performance was what would be predicted if they made decisions completely at random, though no one at the firm was aware of this. As Kahneman said:

> *No one in the firm seemed to be aware of the nature of the game that its stock pickers were playing. The advisers themselves felt they were competent professionals performing a task that was difficult but not impossible, and their superiors agreed.*

He reported this finding to the directors of the firm, and predictably it was dismissed. "Facts that challenge such basic assumptions — and thereby threaten people's livelihood and self-esteem — are simply not absorbed. The mind does not digest them," he wrote.

The hot hand fallacy can occur in several ways in medicine. Individual patients may seem to have "streaks." Clinicians cannot help but be influenced by the previous presentation of a given patient. Of course, patients are not random coin tosses or lottery numbers. It is not possible to approach each subsequent encounter with a patient as a fresh visit, nor would this be wise. A basketball player who makes 100 shots in a row is more likely to make the next shot than a player who hasn't made a single shot. Some players are simply a lot better than others. Similarly, if a patient has presented with chest pain due to a panic attack nine times in a row, it is not unreasonable to assume that the same will be true on the tenth visit. Making predictions about the future based on past performance is not necessarily an error. However, just because a patient has had nine episodes of panic-induced chest pain, this does not mean they are protected from other, more serious conditions during their tenth visit.

Similarly, the hot hand fallacy can also occur from one patient to the next. For example, if nine patients in a row are diagnosed with a migraine after presenting with a headache, there may be a tendency to diagnose the tenth as having a migraine as well. This is closely related to availability bias. However, that tenth patient may have a stroke, tumor, or other life-threatening condition. Considering previous patients' cases also is not necessarily an error, as certain conditions such as infections or the use of substances of abuse often cluster together. However, just because an influenza outbreak is responsible for a fever in nine consecutive patients, this does not necessarily mean it is to blame for the tenth febrile patient.

Lastly, a clinician who has had success with a treatment for several patients in a row may have unwarranted optimism about its future use. It is very common in medicine for a clinician to extol a treatment based on several recent successes. Yet, a medication that works 60% of the time, will continue to work 60% of the time, even if it has worked for ten consecutive patients for one fortunate clinician.

Interestingly, people who fall prey to the gambler's fallacy are also more likely to succumb to hot-hand phenomenon, showing that randomness is a difficult phenomenon for some people to grasp [10].

Conclusion

The human mind is extraordinarily good at finding meaning in unexpected streaks and patterns where only random variation exists. Unexpected streaks may violate our sense of how the world should work, and we may expect that unexpected streaks will soon be broken (the gambler's fallacy). Conversely, we may feel that an unexpected streak is likely to continue (the hot hand fallacy). Certain conditions, such as outbreaks of infectious diseases and drug overdoses, can cluster together. Yet, even in such instances, each patient should be treated independently of the preceding case. Just because the last three patients with altered mental status have taken a drug doesn't mean the streak will continue, nor does it mean it will be broken.

References

1. Huff D, Geis I. How to take a chance. New York: W. W. Norton & Company; 1959. p. 28–9.
2. Arie S. (2005, Feb 10). No 53 puts Italy out of its lottery agony. The guardian. Retrieved from https://www.theguardian.com/world/2005/feb/11/italy.sophiearie.
3. Barron G, Leider S. The role of experience in the Gambler's fallacy. J Behav Decis Mak. 2010;23(1):117–29. https://doi.org/10.1002/bdm.676.
4. Tversky A, Kahneman D. Judgment under uncertainty: heuristics and biases. Science. 1974;185(4157):1124–31. https://doi.org/10.1126/science.185.4157.1124.
5. Sundali J, Croson R. Biases in casino betting: the hot hand and the gambler's fallacy. Judgm Decis Mak. 2006;1(1):1–12.
6. Gilovich T, Vallone R, Tversky A. The hot hand in basketball: on the misperception of random sequences. Cogn Psychol. 1985;17(3):295–314. https://doi.org/10.1016/0010-0285(85)90010-6.
7. Andrews EL. (2014, March 25). Jeffrey Zwiebel: why the "hot hand" may be real after all. Stanford business. Retrieved from https://www.gsb.stanford.edu/jeffrey-zwiebel-why-hot-hand-may-be-real-after-all.
8. Miller J, Sanjurjo A. (2017, March 26). Momentum isn't magic – vindicating the hot hand with the mathematics of streaks. The Conversation. Retrieved from https://theconversation.com/momentum-isnt-magic-vindicating-the-hot-hand-with-the-mathematics-of-streaks-74786.
9. Kahneman D. (2011, Oct 19). Don't blink! The hazards of confidence. The New York Times Magazine. Retrieved from https://www.nytimes.com/2011/10/23/magazine/dont-blink-the-hazards-of-confidence.html.
10. Sundali J, Croson R. Biases in casino betting: the hot hand and the gambler's fallacy. Judgm Decis Mak. 2006;1(1):1–12.

Hasty Generalization, Survival Bias, Special Pleading, and Burden of Proof

Case

Laura was a 56-year-old woman who was diagnosed with multiple sclerosis (MS) at the age of 25 when she developed double vision. She had deteriorated to the point where she needed a wheelchair outside and a walker in the house. She sought treatment with a doctor who claimed to be able to reverse progressive MS. She was advised to eat only meals that the doctor sold through an affiliate program from an internet "paleo" food supplier. She was also advised to do periodic "detoxes" and stop taking many pharmaceutical medications. After three months, Laura reported feeling more energetic, however her family noticed no difference in her condition and objective tests of her strength and gait were unchanged.

What Dr. Walls Was Thinking

I was quite pleased with Laura's improvement, and I have seen multiple patients like this. Sadly, conventional medicine is a one-size-fits-all model. But individuals shouldn't be viewed as a cookie cutter problem, and they shouldn't be offered cookie cutter solutions. It's more complex than that. No two people are alike. We are all unique in our genes, lifestyles, and physiology. What leads to illness in one person is not the same for another, and the treatment for each will be different. I know this from my vast clinical and personal experience. I strive to practice personalized medicine. I aim to solve the root cause of a patient's disease, not simply cover up its symptoms. I have a collection of compelling testimonials on my website demonstrating the efficacy of my protocol.

I have come under some criticism for not doing any trials of my treatment. However, it is simply not possible to do a randomized, controlled trial of the diet and lifestyle changes that are part of my program. The pharmaceutical industry doesn't want these studies done, and the model of medicine that worships the randomized, double-blind, placebo study just isn't capable of evaluating a treatment like mine. I invite anyone skeptical of my treatment to meet Laura and other patients like her. No one can deny the improvement they made.

© Springer International Publishing AG, part of Springer Nature 2019
J. Howard, *Cognitive Errors and Diagnostic Mistakes*,
https://doi.org/10.1007/978-3-319-93224-8_13

Discussion

Anecdotal evidence is evidence obtained in a casual or informal manner, relying primarily or completely on personal testimonies. As such, it is inherently subjective, lacking any and all scientific controls. Using anecdotes to make decisions is an informal logical fallacy known as hasty generalization or the law of small numbers. This occurs when a person uses a small number of data points to draw a broad conclusion. For example, if a subway rider in New York City refused to give up their seat for a pregnant woman, it would be inappropriate to then conclude that all New Yorkers are rude.

In medicine, anecdotes all too easily become fodder for the availability heuristic, where clinicians use "it worked for my patients" to guide treatment decisions. Importantly, anecdotes are how most of us understand the world. Telling ourselves a story is the primary way in which our brains manage to grasp the world around us and make sense of our experiences. When our brains put together all the bits and pieces, the sights and the sounds, the feelings and the facts, and our relationship to them, the end result is an extrapolation that takes the form of who, what, where, when, and why. Anecdotes are part of the very cognition that allows us to derive meaning from experiences and turn noise into signal. Our brain, seeking to be efficient, is particular about what it will spend its energy on. Somewhere in a part of our brain that we are helpless to influence, evolution mandated that anecdotes are worthy of attention.

Anecdotes are incredibly powerful from an emotional standpoint. They capture our imagination and attention in a way numbers and facts cannot. There is a reason why each chapter of this book begins with an anecdote. I have sat through innumerable lectures, full of dry statistics. Just when we are all starting to fall asleep, the lecturer presents a patient case. All of a sudden, everyone starts to pay attention. We are being told a story. A compelling story of a treatment's success or failure is often more impactful than a formal clinical trial, even for clinicians who pride themselves on dispassionate, rational thought. There is a reason for the saying that goes "The death of one person is a tragedy, the death of one million is a statistic." (Fig. 13.1).

Anecdotes have the power to persuade, but this means they also have the power to deceive or mislead. When our brains encounter these stories, they don't like to leave gaps. This means they tend to fill in the holes and connect the dots in a way that feels comfortable and consistent with other stories we've told ourselves. This takes place unconsciously, so not only are we unaware of all the factors and conditions left out of the story, we can't be sure that what made it into the story is at all accurate. The only thing we do know for sure is that the story is biased. Even worse, not only were these stories told using heuristics and biases, but clinicians listening to them brought their own biases along as well. Merely having an abundance of anecdotes available to the clinician facilitates the proliferation of biases, and clinicians who rely heavily on anecdotal evidence often fall prey to them. These most commonly include the self-serving bias, the tendency to claim more responsibility for successes than for failures, and the survivor bias, the fallacy of only paying attention to the survivors, while neglecting the drop-outs and victims (Fig. 13.2).

Anecdotal evidence reliable? One man says "yes".

A STUDY CONDUCTED YESTERDAY by a man on himself concluded that self-reported anecdotal evidence is, in fact, both reliable and relevant.

The landmark study, conducted by Mark Mattingly of Virginia Beach in his apartment, concluded with 100% accuracy that data collected from personal experience can disprove other data conducted by reputable scientific institutions, thereby proving once and for all that "statistics can't be trusted".

In a press release Mr. Mattingly took aim at his detractors saying that "...this study shows what I've been telling people on the internet for years: all your fancy evidence and statistics don't mean nothing in the real world.".

A frequenter of internet forums, comment sections, and social media, Mr. Mattingly recounts that he was inspired to undertake the study when someone reportedly kept insisting that he provide evidence for his claims. "I think everyone's entitled to an opinion, and that my opinion is worth just as much as anyone else's" Mr. Mattingly said.

Academic types have criticised the study, and papers who are publishing it, saying that it lacks everything and makes no sense. When shown the study, Emeritus Professor James Albrecht of Carnegie Mellon University looked all confused and hopeless before making pining, guttural sounds.

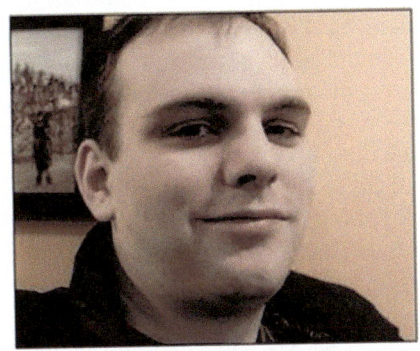

Mr. Mattingly in his apartment looking all smug.

Mr. Mattingly has responded saying that this is just the first of many studies he intends to conduct, and that a meta-analysis of people who have opinions and anecdotal experiences independent of controls, methodological rigor, blinding and peer review are soon to be published, adding further weight to his initial findings.

Published Saturday 22 February 2014 by yourlogicalfallacyis.com/anecdotal   *Photo: Weasello*

Fig. 13.1 Is anecdotal evidence reliable? One man says "yes." (HastyUsernameChoice. Anecdotal evidence reliable? One man says "yes" [Image file, Reddit post]. (ca. 2014). Retrieved from https://www.reddit.com/r/atheism/comments/1ylp32/anecdotal_evidence_reliable_one_man_says_yes/.)

Fig. 13.2 The limits of anecdotes. (The Logic of Science. Only Colbert could so simply and perfectly illustrate why your personal experiences are irrelevant to large scale trends [Facebook status update]. 2015. Retrieved from https://www.facebook.com/thelogicof-science/photos/a.1618699508361446/1631888767042520/?type=3.)

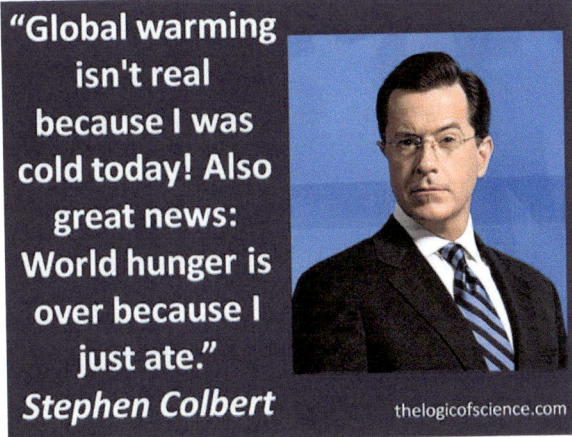

"Global warming isn't real because I was cold today! Also great news: World hunger is over because I just ate."
Stephen Colbert

thelogicofscience.com

Having said this, anecdotes can be an important *starting* point for formal investigations. Numerous seminal discoveries in medicine have occurred simply because someone paid attention to a few anecdotes. For example, the first cases of the AIDS epidemic appeared when the CDC published a report of five young, previously healthy, gay men in Los Angeles who developed a rare lung infection [1]. Perhaps the most important medical treatment in history, vaccination, was discovered because people paid attention to anecdotes that milkmaids infected with cowpox were then immune to smallpox. For decades before Edward Jenner performed his seminal studies on vaccines, such milkmaids were known to be able to care for smallpox victims without risk of contracting the disease.

Given this potential, anecdotal evidence is common in medicine. Reports of single patients are called case reports, and reports of groups of patient are called case series. Though they are nothing more than carefully reported anecdotes, occasionally they can be of great value. As described, new treatments and diseases may be first described as anecdotes. Moreover, there are many rare conditions for which there is simply not evidence from large clinical trials to guide treatment. As such, anecdotal evidence, hopefully collected from a large number of patients in a careful and systematic manner, is often the best and only evidence. Additionally, there are many situations where it would be unethical to study a treatment in a prospective clinical trial. It would unethical to conduct a trial of a new medication in certain populations, such as pregnant women, for example. It would similarly be unethical to purposefully expose people to a potential harm, such as cigarettes, to see what happens.

In order to justify a clinical trial, there must be clinical equipoise, meaning that there is genuine uncertainty among medical experts over whether a treatment is beneficial or not. For example, as there is no disagreement amongst experts, it would be unethical to conduct a trial of whether intravenous fluids are beneficial in patients with massive blood loss from trauma. A parody in the *British Medical Journal* titled *Parachute Use to Prevent Death and Major Trauma Related to Gravitational Challenge: Systematic Review of Randomised Controlled Trials* made this point well. It concluded:

> As with many interventions intended to prevent ill health, the effectiveness of parachutes has not been subjected to rigorous evaluation by using randomised controlled trials. Advocates of evidence based medicine have criticised the adoption of interventions evaluated by using only observational data. We think that everyone might benefit if the most radical protagonists of evidence based medicine organised and participated in a double blind, randomised, placebo controlled, crossover trial of the parachute [2].

Despite their potential, anecdotes are never an appropriate *ending* point in medicine. Responsible clinicians should know that anecdotal evidence is the weakest form of evidence, and with the exceptions mentioned above, "it worked for my patients" is not a valid criterion for judging any medical intervention. However, even when anecdotal evidence is the best and only evidence, an honest clinician will acknowledge this limitation both to their patients and themselves. Most crucially, they will be willing to change their practice if compelling new evidence emerges that contradicts their anecdotal experiences. The history of medicine is full of treatments that *really* seemed to work based on anecdotes, but failed when tested in formal clinical trials.

Importantly, not all anecdotal evidence is equal. Anecdotes that are consistent with preexisting medical and scientific knowledge carry a greater weight than anecdotes implying large swaths of such knowledge are wrong or incomplete. For example, anecdotes that patients with a neuro-inflammatory disorder improve when placed on an anti-inflammatory treatment provide a rationale for using this treatment in the absence of evidence from formal clinical trials. In contrast, as there is an enormous amount of evidence to the contrary, anecdotes that vaccines cause autism should be met with great skepticism. Similarly, the magnitude of the anecdotal evidence must be considered. Anecdotal claims of modest benefit are more plausible than grandiose claims. If someone purports to have achieved an astonishing cure of a devastating disease, anecdotal evidence alone should not be convincing. Anecdotes that both overturn existing medical knowledge and make a grandiose claim, such as anecdotes that coffee enemas cure cancer by removing toxins, can almost always be rejected outright (Fig. 13.3).

Not surprisingly, anecdotal evidence is the lifeblood of complementary and alternative medicine (CAM) practitioners. Patient testimonials have long been used by

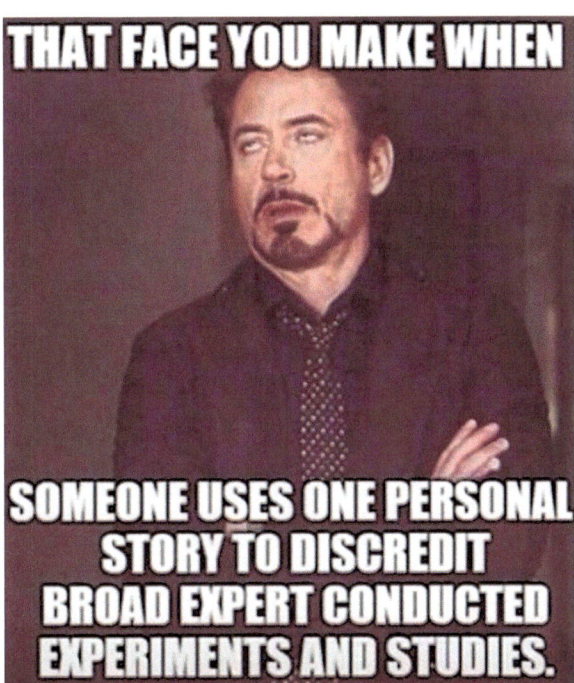

Fig. 13.3 The proper reaction to most anecdotal evidence

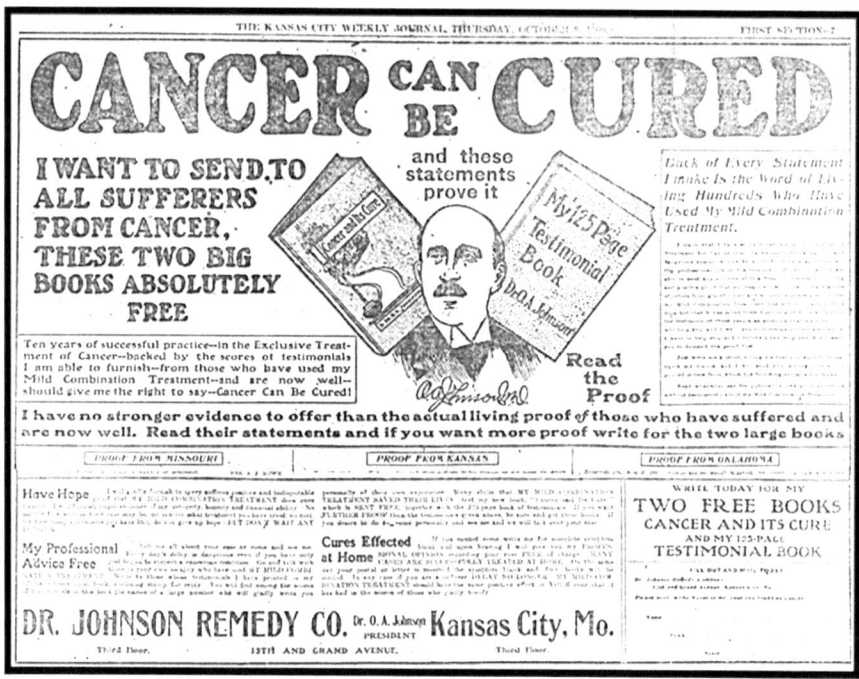

Fig. 13.4 Anecdotal evidence is nothing new. (Janssen WF. Cancer quackery: past and present [Image file]. FDA Consumer, 1977(July-August). 1977. Retrieved from https://www.cancertreat-mentwatch.org/q/janssen.shtml.)

CAM practitioners and snake oil salesmen to market their supposed "miracle cures." As the advertisement for Dr. Johnson from 1908 states, "Cancer can be cured and these statements prove it…I have no stronger evidence to offer than the actual living proof of those who have suffered and are now well." (Fig. 13.4) [3].

Another advertisement featured in the 1921 book *Nostrums and Quackery* similarly boasts of "testimonials of thousands cured at home." Another has multiple testimonials from patients cured with "Adkin Vitaopathic Treatment." Yet another declares that "every testimonial is a sworn statement!" (Fig. 13.5).

While it is easy to detect and scoff at the quackery of bygone times, our era is no different. Terry Wahls, an internist, is a contemporary example of a CAM practitioner who uses anecdotal evidence to make similarly extraordinary claims. Specifically, she claims to have not just halted the progression of MS, but actually *reversed* disability with a "paleo" diet and "neuromuscular electrical stimulation." The evidence she uses for this claim is something highly available to her: her own experience. According to her website, "In December 2007, I began the Wahls Protocol™. The results stunned my physician, my family, and me: within a year, I was able to walk through the hospital without a cane and even complete an 18-mile bicycle tour." As evidence for this claim, she has "before-and-after" pictures of herself posted on her website [4]. In the "before" picture, she is seated in a wheelchair, frowning, bathed

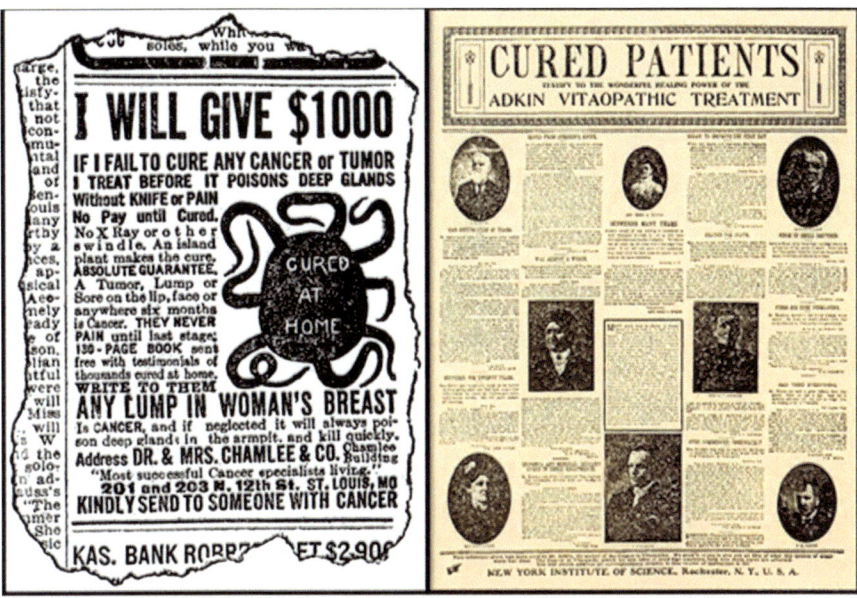

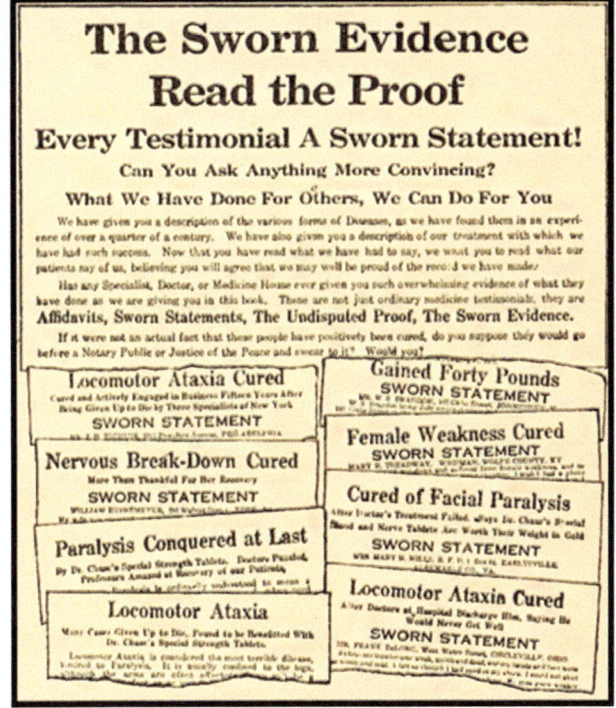

Fig. 13.5 Patient testimonials from the past. (**Upper left**: Wellcome images. Quack advert for the cure of cancer [Image file]. In: Wikimedia commons. 2018. Retrieved from https://commons.wikimedia.org/wiki/File:Quack_advert_for_the_cure_of_cancer_Wellcome_M0014464.jpg.)

in the fluorescent light of a drab hospital hallway. In the "after" picture, taken just one year later, she is smiling outside on a sunny day, standing on her bike, with green trees and grass in the background. In yet another picture, she is smiling, her fist raised triumphantly in the air as she stands next to a wheelchair. Her website also features several patient testimonials she calls "Wahls Warriors." These testimonials are different from the cancer cures of 100 years ago only in that they appear on a modern-day website.

Does she have any evidence for her claim beyond her anecdotes? Were Dr. Wahls to convincingly demonstrate that her treatment reversed the symptoms of MS, there is no doubt she would win a Nobel Prize and would be forever remembered as having made one of the most important discoveries in the history of medicine. The largest and most rigorous study of her treatment was titled *Randomized Control Trial Evaluation of a Modified Paleolithic Dietary Intervention in the Treatment of Relapsing-Remitting Multiple Sclerosis: A Pilot Study* [5]. It randomized 17 patients to a "paleo" diet and 17 patients to maintain their usual diet. At the end of the study, which lasted 3.5 months, only eight patients remained in the "paleo" arm, while only nine patients remained in the standard diet arm. The study found that subjects in the "paleo" arm reported improved fatigue, and they had slightly improved motor function in their hand. Another study of 26 patients found that a modified "paleo" diet, neuromuscular electrical stimulation, exercise, and stress management techniques such as meditation and self-massage led to improved mood and cognitive symptoms in patients with MS [6]. Another study of 10 patients investigated the effects of a paleo diet, exercise, meditation, massage, and supplementation. It found that the six subjects who finished the year-long study had less fatigue than when they started [7]. Yet one more study of 20 patients investigated the Wahls Protocol at three, six, nine, and 12 month intervals. It found that, "The entire cohort did not show significant changes in any of the assessments over 12 months except higher speed of walking toward the 10 feet mark during timed up and go test at six months compared with baseline" [8]. The authors properly conclude, "We did not find significant changes in gait and balance outcomes in our study cohort following a multimodal intervention for 12 months."

There is nothing inherently wrong with these studies, and the authors acknowledge their many limitations. However, the findings are not revolutionary. Who would be surprised to learn that exercise and stress reduction techniques make patients feel better? At best, these are small, preliminary studies that suggest a modest benefit to lifestyle interventions in MS. At worst, they show that her protocol has no effect and is incredibly difficult to follow. Before they can considered meaningful, however, these findings would need to be replicated by independent researchers with larger numbers of patients. By comparison, the most recently approved medication for MS, ocrelizumab, had three separate phase III trials, involving over 2,300 subjects recruited from multiple different locations.

But we now have an answer: there is not a scintilla of scientific evidence supporting Dr. Wahls' claim that she can reverse disability in patients with progressive MS. She has no evidence to suggest a "paleo" diet will allow wheelchair-bound patients to leap up and start biking 18-miles within one year. She has no evidence

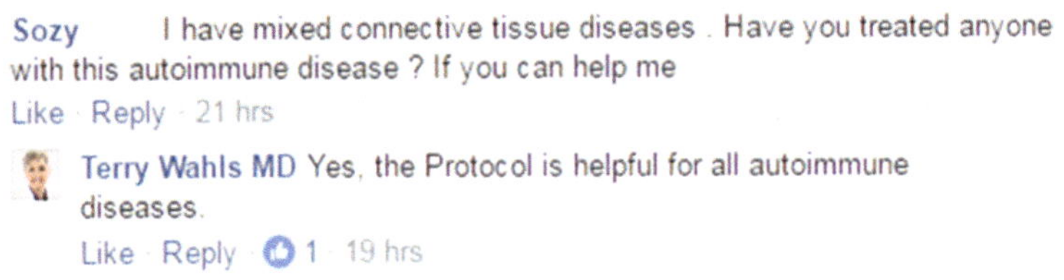

Sozy   I have mixed connective tissue diseases . Have you treated anyone with this autoimmune disease ? If you can help me
Like · Reply · 21 hrs

Terry Wahls MD Yes, the Protocol is helpful for all autoimmune diseases.
Like · Reply · 1 · 19 hrs

Fig. 13.6 Dr. Wahls claiming her treatment works for all autoimmune conditions. (Wahls T. (Terry Wahls MD). Response to a Facebook comment [redacted for privacy].)

that her protocol is "helpful for all autoimmune diseases," though this hasn't stopped her from making that claim on social media (Fig. 13.6). One critic of Dr. Wahls made the following wise point on a Reditt Ask Me Anything (AMA) forum:

> You cannot say that it saved your life, so far all you can say is that you used these treatments and coincidentally your symptoms went into remission. It is a great coincidence, and I am happy that you are better today than you were in 2005, but to write an entire book about how this "saved your life" doesn't equate to medical opinion but rather to a belief you hold [9].

In fact, from the small studies she has published thus far, one could reasonably conclude that her protocol is unlikely to be effective in most patients. Her largest study screened 82 patients and enrolled 71 of them, but for various reasons, only 17 were included in the final analysis. Over half of patients randomized to the "paleo" arm failed to complete her relatively brief study. In another study of 13 patients, only six of them were able to adhere to her protocol for 12 months. This dropout rate is especially concerning given that most patients who enter clinical trials are highly motivated individuals who may be poorly representative of the general population. On a common sense level, we can be reasonably sure that if her treatment worked as advertised, stories of wheelchair-bound patients biking many miles within one year of adopting her protocol would be commonplace by now. Sadly, they are not.

Unfortunately, the lack of evidence does not deter Dr. Wahls from promoting her story and similar anecdotes, on social media, in speeches, and on her website. I am sure it will shock few readers to learn that her website is mostly a store where she sells multiple items, including menus for $204 and annual memberships to her site for $187. She also holds seminars that cost $1,984 to teach her protocol to health professionals. At the end of the seminar, attendees can pay $597 to take a certification exam. Surprisingly, given the large number of products she sells, Dr. Wahls declared in her study that she had "no conflicts of interest in this work" (Fig. 13.7).

At times, CAM practitioners may use anecdotal evidence not just to posit new treatments, like Dr. Wahls, but to actually contradict large, properly controlled studies. Consider the following statement from pediatrician Paul Thomas, who routinely spreads fear and misinformation about vaccines: "Data from my own practice shows that those infants who got the rotavirus vaccines were four times more likely to have gastroenteritis and diarrheal illnesses than those who did not get the vaccine" [10]. Dr. Thomas believes his own "data," which does not seem to be published in the peer-reviewed medical literature, supersedes multiple clinical studies involving tens of thousands of children.

However his "data" is nothing more than anecdotes, packaged in a book he is selling.

In exceptional instances, CAM practitioners extol the perceived virtues of anecdotes over controlled scientific studies. Kelly Brogan, a psychiatrist and CAM practitioner, wrote in an essay titled *Why Detox*:

> *Like everything else in our reframing of the human experience, we are* de-standardizing *health. We are bringing medicine back into the realm of the 'N of 1' or the 'study of You'. You are not a randomized clinical trial. You are a* specific *symphony of information.*

While of course patients are not randomized clinical trials, the advice clinicians provide them should be made based on the best available evidence. No meaningful conversation can be had with anyone who specifically rejects the concept of evidence and who believes anecdotal information supersedes knowledge obtained from large, controlled clinical trials. If someone explicitly rejects science and evidence, how can someone use science and evidence to change their minds? While this book is about the flaws and limitations of human cognition, the goal is to recognize these imperfections and do what we can to minimize them, not to throw up our arms and decided the truth is whatever we want it to be (Fig. 13.8).

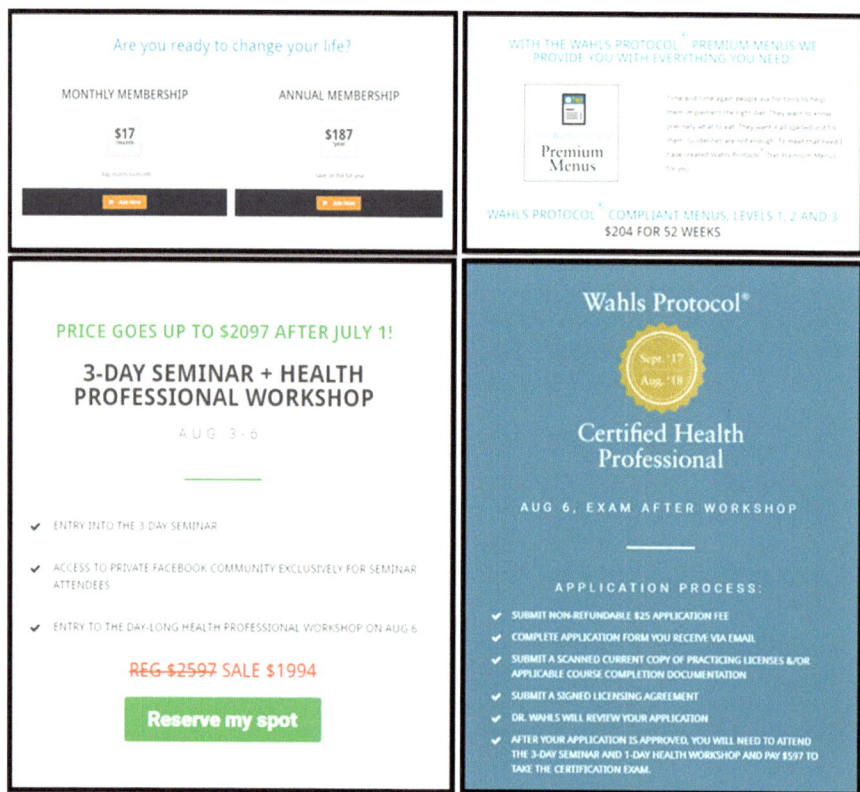

Fig. 13.7 Some of the many products for sale on Dr. Wahl's website. (Wahls T. Various screenshots of website [HTML files]. Terry Wahls MD. (n.d.). Retrieved from https://terrywahls.com/.)

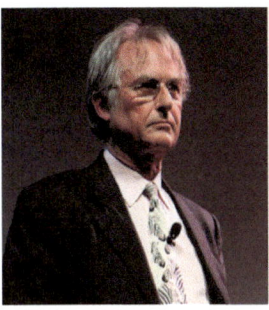
If any remedy is tested under controlled scientific conditions and proved to be effective, it will cease to be alternative and will simply become medicine. So-called alternative medicine either hasn't been tested or it has failed its tests.
Richard Dawkins

Fig. 13.8 Richard Dawkins gets it right. (Chiswick Chap. Bust-length cropped portrait photograph of Richard Dawkins in 2008 [Image file]. In: Wikimedia commons. 2008. Retrieved from https://commons.wikimedia.org/wiki/File:Dawkins_at_UT_Austin_detail.jpg.)

Are alternative treatments based on anecdotes harmless, as many people believe? In the case of Dr. Thomas, the harm done by believing his anecdotes over legitimate science would be the return of a serious vaccine-preventable disease. According to the CDC, prior to the introduction of the rotavirus vaccine, each year "among US children younger than five years of age, rotavirus led to more than 400,000 doctor visits, more than 200,000 emergency room visits, 55,000 to 70,000 hospitalizations, and 20 to 60 deaths."

But what about Dr. Wahls? After all, if she convinces people to exercise and pay more attention to what they eat, what could be wrong with that? A lot, potentially. Although Dr. Wahls does not actively encourage patients to stop medications, much of her philosophy is designed to instill fear and doubt around proven treatments for MS. In one of her papers, she says the medications used to treat MS have "limited benefit and serious side effects." Certainly these medications are not a cure and significant, even fatal side effects are possible. However, most of them are very safe and significantly benefit patients by preventing relapses and disability. Additionally, I have read multiple statements on her Facebook page where people with MS report stopping their medications and instead use diet alone to treat their disease. Consider the following Facebook exchange.

Louise   I have stopped taking Tecfidera for my ms but I have had ms for 18 years and the only time I have been sick are the 3 years on a drug for ms! But I have never eaten bread, pasta or anything like that but found out I have always been intolerant to dairy! I can trace that back to being 4 years old with symptoms, so I am a firm believer in sorting intolerances out and getting the right vitamins etc from your diet like I do now. But it has to be your decision to stop any medication, I have personally come off 14 prescription drugs in the past 10 months 😄 and feel much better for it

Like · Reply · 👍 9 · 23 January at 18:10

 Terry Wahls MD That is great to hear! Stick with it and health will stick with you.

Like · Reply · 👍 1 · 25 January at 11:23

Fig. 13.9 Fearmongering and advertising. (Wahls T. (Terry Wahls MD). If your doctor has told you there is no way to ever get off your immune suppressing, disease modifying drugs, hear what the research says [Facebook advertisement]. 2017. Retrieved from https://www.facebook.com/TerryWahls/posts/1568343559890356.)

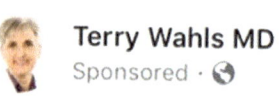

Terry Wahls MD
Sponsored · 🌐   •••

If your doctor has told you there is no way to ever get off of your immune suppressing, disease modifying drugs, hear what the research says about how someone CAN meet the scientific criteria to stop drugs without increasing the risk of disease flare, and how the Wahls Protocol® can help get there. This will be one of many informative lectures at The Wahls Protocol Seminar & Retreat. Don't miss out in 2018!

Learn more at https://terrywahls.com/wahls-protocol-seminar-retreat/

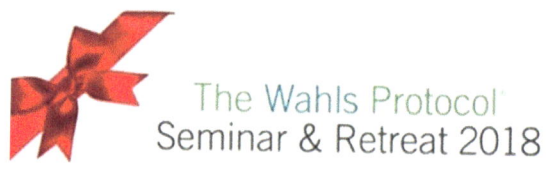

The Wahls Protocol
Seminar & Retreat 2018

Early Bird Pricing Ends 12/31/17
Reserve your spot today!

Perhaps Louise has been over-medicated and doesn't need her medication for MS (Tecfidera). On the other hand, perhaps she is setting herself up for a significant relapse by stopping it. I don't know anything about Louise's history, and I highly doubt Dr. Wahls does either. Yet, she doesn't let her lack of knowledge of Louise's case dissuade her from cheerleading on social media as Louise and other strangers stop their medications. She does not even advise them to consult with their neurologist before doing so. In her defense, at times I have seen her strongly advise people not to stop medications without first consulting their doctor. However, it is clear that she does not feel her protocol can stand on its own, but must constantly be contrasted against mainstream clinicians (Fig. 13.9).

The appeal of these CAM practitioners like Dr. Wahls becomes clear with the realization that she is not just promoting a specific treatment for MS, but rather an entire identity. Patients are led to believe their health is completely under their control, if only they have the discipline and willpower to make drastic changes to nearly every aspect of their life. As a part of this identity, "natural" foods are imbued with remarkable regenerative properties. Yet, as their treatments cannot stand on their own, it is rare to find a CAM practitioner who promotes their treatment without simultaneously demonizing mainstream medicine. As part of their marketing, evil pharmaceutical companies are said to be actively stifling effective treatments for profit, and mainstream clinicians are hiding "natural" cures, because they apparently just don't care if their patients deteriorate in front of their eyes. In 2017, a typical fearmongering article appeared article on Dr. Wahl's website titled *The High Cost of Today's Drug Therapy – What Your Physician May Not Be Telling You* [11]. It said:

> *What your physicians are not telling you is that the symptom reduction from the potent biologic drugs is often temporary. They are also not telling you that diet and lifestyle changes are often much more powerful than drugs at stopping disease progression and can even lead to regression of symptoms.*

As someone who counsels patients with MS on exercise and a healthy diet every day, this is a bizarre claim to read. Clinicians such as myself encourage patients to take appropriate medications and make appropriate lifestyle changes. Patients do not have to choose one or the other. Unfortunately, I often see the harm this false dichotomy causes. While writing this chapter, a patient of mine with neuromyelitis optica, a severe inflammatory disease that can rapidly and permanently disable people, became wheelchair bound due to her embrace of "natural" medicine. Her daughter sent me the following message:

> *We are all devastated but I guess we are hoping for a miracle.... I know this might not have happened if she would have followed your instructions but she tried to do it the natural way and now she is facing the consequences, so we would really want to be on top of this making sure she does follow your instructions this time. And her natural approach was changing her eating habits to more fruits and vegetables and I believe she met also a 'doctor' who was giving her every week a herbal syrup like of 20+ herbs which she drank every night with some drinks such as celery juice after breakfast, water and oatmeal after lunch or tea after dinner. She said she felt energized and strong so she stopped taking the meds she was supposed to take. She thought I guess she was healing.*

I have no evidence this patient was directly influenced by Dr. Wahls, nor is there any guarantee this horrible outcome would have been avoided had she taken a standard treatment for her disease. This case, after all, is an anecdote itself. But by rejecting science-based medicine in favor of magical thinking, she didn't put the odds in her favor.

The other harms of using "food as medicine" are less obvious. Some of my patients spend large amounts of money they don't have to make sure they eat "just right." For many patients, formerly pleasurable activities, such as going out to dinner with friends, have become dangerous landmines to be avoided at all costs. Many patients inappropriately blame themselves if their disease takes a turn for the worse, suffering undeserved guilt on top of their physical symptoms.

Finally, as a result of fetishizing the notion that food can cure their disease, several of my patients have developed an eating disorder known as orthorexia, which is excessive preoccupation with eating "healthy" or "righteous" food. In an article titled *Clean Eating Websites Like Gwyneth Paltrow's Goop 'Indistinguishable From Pro Anorexia Sites,* Christian Jessen, an internist, said:

> *I've had many, many patients, so many of them teenagers, convinced that their healthy lifestyle and their clean-eating regime was really helping them when actually all it was doing was helping them hide their increasingly disordered eating and to cover up an under-lying eating disorder* [12].

Eating disorder specialist Max Pemberton also reports that "clean eating" is behind a large number of severe eating disorders he treats, calling it "ugly, malevo-lent and damaging" [13]. He excoriates so-called wellness gurus, saying, "While not directly responsible for encouraging eating disorders, they epitomized the mod-ern trend for charismatic gurus to play on their looks and life stories to influence their audience and make them buy into their food philosophy." He further notes that advocating a reasonable diet based on eating everything in moderation "doesn't sell books or gain you thousands of followers on social media."

Importantly, anecdotes may be useful in communicating with patients. Every day, when discussing potential treatments, patients invariably ask me how my other patients are doing on them. People want to learn about the risks and benefits of medications in story form, which is almost always more reassuring than the raw statistics in controlled clinical trials. They don't want to hear about the relative risk reduction. They want to hear me say, "I have many patients on this medicine and they're all doing great." I can't remember a single patient, including several doctors and nurses, who requested the actual studies upon which my recommendations were based. While clinicians certainly have the obligation to inform patients of the facts behind the risks and benefits of a proposed treatment, many patients (and clini-cians) have trouble grappling with complicated medical statistics. As such, the risks and benefits of a treatment may be better conveyed by telling the story of a patient who selected or rejected a certain treatment. Similarly, mainstream medical organi-zations often use anecdotes to advertise their services. However this is ethical only to the extent that these anecdotes are supported by science.

Conclusion

The minimization of cognitive bias is the reason the scientific method is needed to obtain accurate answers about how reality operates. The entire idea of a double-blind controlled trial is to minimize the impact of bias on research subjects and researchers alike. We need an outside process which attempts to avoid and account for the biases that human intellect cannot. One of the key functions of science is quality control, and this is a primary reason why anecdotal information and personal experience can never be used to trump scientific answers. If someone disagrees with something science says because their personal experience was different, then the proper channel for that dis-agreement is more science. Simply put, if you're not disagreeing with science by using more science, then there is no way to know if your disagreement is due to bias. This may seem unfair, but it is a rule enforced by nature, not by science. It's no coincidence that many effects and phenomena disappear when we view them through the lens of science. It's because they never existed in the first place, and were merely an artifact of bias.

When faced with anecdotes, clinicians should remember that even though anecdotes may be emotionally compelling, the plural of anecdote is not data. What better way to show the potential harm of anecdotes than a powerful anecdote. Jim Gass suffered a stroke and underwent multiple stem cell therapies in several countries, costing him about $300,000, according to *The New York Times*. Unfortunately, the stem cells overgrew, causing a spinal cord tumor and further disability. Mr. Gass had sage advice to others who might be tempted follow his path, "Don't trust anecdotes." His sister-in-law also added, "If something sounds too good to be true, it is." These are wise words that clinicians and patients alike would be wise to remember.

> "Here are the facts.
> We checked them a lot!"
> -Science
>
> "But... but... My anecdotes!"
> -Comments section
>
> FB/A SCIENCE ENTHUSIAST

Survival Bias, Special Pleading, and Burden of Proof

One of the most fundamental flaws of anecdotal medicine is that it is prone to the survival bias. This is the fallacy of only paying attention to the winners and survivors of an event while ignoring the losers and dropouts. Let's do a thought experiment to understand how the survival bias works. Suppose a group people flipped a coin, the goal being to get seven heads in a row. At the end of seven coin tosses, eight people managed this feat. A plucky investigator studied those eight individuals and discovered they all used a magic chant that guaranteed they would flip heads. Would you then accept this chant worked? Probably not. You'd probably want to find out how people many were in the original group. After all, if it contained 1,000 people, eight people would be expected to flip seven heads in a row by chance alone. You'd also probably want to find out how many of the people who failed to flip seven heads in a row also used this chant. If many of these failures also tried this chant, you probably wouldn't find it too impressive. No matter what you found, you probably realize the best way to determine the truth would be to do another experiment, where certain people were instructed to perform this chant while others were not allowed to do so.

It's easy to see how with a large enough starting group, chance alone would predict that some people would flip many heads in a row. However, we often fail to apply this logic in other spheres. Imagine you got an e-mail that correctly predicted the winner of a football game. You might ignore it until the same thing happened the next week and the week after that. After several correct predictions in a row, you might think you've stumbled on something quite amazing. If your psychic messenger asked you for $100 to find out the winner of next week's game, you might be tempted to pay. Only when the prediction fails the next week do you realize you've been scammed. An episode of *Alfred Hitchcock Presents* from 1957 called "Mail Order Prophet" shows how the survival bias can be used to trick people this way. The episode is described as follows on IMDB:

> *One day, Ronald Grimes receives a letter from a Mr. Christianai who says he can predict the future. The letter correctly predicts the outcome of an upcoming election. More letters follow and through gambling, Grimes acquires a large amount of money. A final letter from Christianai asks for a contribution. Grimes gives it quite willingly. Later Grimes finds out that Christiani was a fraud. He was really a con man who sent out thousands of letters, half of them predicting one kind of outcome, and the other half predicting another. Grimes was lucky; he got the right predictions time after time* [14].

Inspirational stories of college dropouts who pursued their dreams and ended up founding billion dollar-companies or becoming movie stars are ubiquitous. However, because of the survival bias, we need to be careful in drawing life lessons from their experiences. After all, we don't hear much from college dropouts who failed in similar quests and are now unemployed, and there are likely many more of them. Several business books extol the virtues of CEOs who manage to outperform their competitors many years in a row. "What can we learn from their wisdom?" they ask. An investor who beat the stock market 10 years in a row *might* have some important investment advice. However, he also might be the financial equivalent a lucky coin flipper. Indeed, after several CEOs were lauded as financial wizards in these books, many subsequently underperformed the market. This represents a regression to the mean, implying a large degree of randomness in their performance.

At times, studying the survivors while ignoring victims can lead people to make the most erroneous decision possible. A famous example of this occurred during World War II when researchers from the Center for Naval Analyses studied planes to assess where they were most likely to be struck by enemy fire. They identified those placed where planes were prone to being hit and suggested adding extra armor to protect these areas. Statistician Abraham Wald realized this reasoning was completely backwards. After all, they were only examining planes that had returned from their missions. The damage they incurred showed where planes could be hit and still fly. In contrast, they couldn't examine the planes that had crashed. Wald realized that extra armor needed to be added to the areas where the surviving planes were relatively unscathed (Fig. 13.10).

Anti-vaccine commentators frequently fall victim to the survival bias, claiming that vaccine-preventable diseases are benign because they survived them without

Fig. 13.10 An illustration showing where airplanes could be hit and return home safely. (McGeddon. Illustration of hypothetical damage pattern on a WW2 bomber [Image file]. In: Wikimedia commons. 2016. Retrieved from https://commons.wikimedia.org/wiki/Category:Cognitive_biases#/media/File:Survivorship-bias.png.)

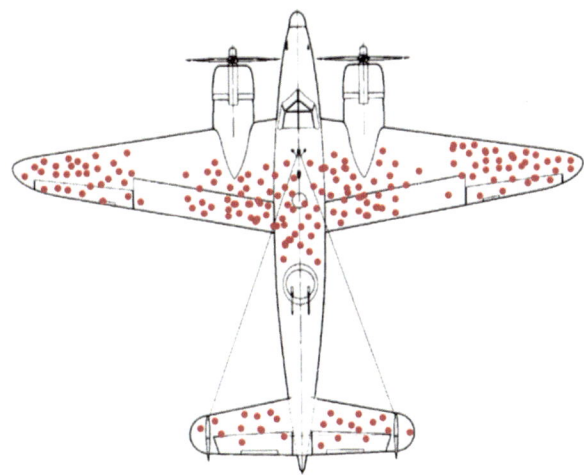

Fig. 13.11 An anti-vaccine commentator falls victim to the survival bias. (Adriana. Facebook comment (n.d.). (redacted for privacy).)

Adriana

I caught measles, mumps and chicken pox when I was a kid and I survived. Potentially deadly? What a bunch of snowflakes. To build immunity to anything you really have to have a good case of it. If a serious strain of any of these diseases were to arrive none of these "vaccinated small dose of" wimps would survive. Also after anyone gets a vaccine in order to not spread it they should be quarantined - think long on that one.

consequence. Of course, children who died of these diseases aren't here to tell us about their experience (Fig. 13.11).

Let's do another thought experiment to see how the survival bias might affect a clinicians' judgment. Suppose that the life expectancy of patients with lung cancer is five years. As with the coin flippers, we can expect some outliers based on natural variation. The unluckiest 5% may survive only two years, while the luckiest 5% may survive 10 years. Let's say a researcher was to study those fortunate survivors to try to figure out what accounted for their survival. Perhaps all of them read about a kale detox and credit their health to this program. Does this mean that kale detoxes slow the progression of lung cancer? Maybe. However, any responsible researcher would also want to also study the people who didn't survive a long time. After all, perhaps many of them had also tried kale detoxes, but because they're dead, they can't be interviewed. Of course, in order to properly determine the effects of kale detoxes on cancer, it would be necessary to perform a clinical trial, enrolling newly diagnosed patients and studying them in a prospective manner.

According to the National Cancer Institute, nearly 1.7 million Americans will be diagnosed with cancer each year. Given this, it is certain that many thousands of them will significantly outlive their prognosis by chance alone. A handful might even have spontaneous remission of their cancer, a rare, but well-documented occurrence. Not surprisingly, these spectacular cancer survivors have attracted a great deal of interest. And also not surprisingly, by studying them retroactively, reasons for their survival have been found. Kelly Turner reviewed 1,000 such cases for her book *Radical Remission: Surviving Cancer Against All Odds*. She claims to have uncovered "nine factors that can lead to a spontaneous remission from cancer— even after conventional medicine has failed." She found that cancer survivors made significant dietary interventions, embraced social support, and used herbs and other supplements.

Studying cases of long-term cancer survivors seems like an eminently reasonable idea to me, and if a researcher noticed that everyone who survived a particular cancer had used a certain treatment, this could potentially be very valuable information. However, because of the survivor bias no firm conclusions can be drawn from studying these patients. Like Dr. Wahls, if Dr. Turner can demonstrate her nine factors lead to cancer remission, she will have made one of the most momentous discoveries in the history of medicine, saving millions of lives per year, earning a certain Nobel Prize and fame for centuries to come. So, is she proposing a prospective trial to prove the curative properties of her nine factors? Not to my knowledge. Instead, she is working on a TV docuseries and, like Dr. Wahls, is selling an online course for $245 [15].

While Dr. Turner may have identified nine healing factors that can dramatically improve cancer survival rates, a more likely explanation is that she has fallen victim to the survival bias. The survivors are studied in detail, while the dead victims are completely ignored. I don't think it strains credulity to imagine that many of the people who died of cancer also changed their diet, joined support groups, and experimented with herbs and supplements. As oncologist Rebecca Johnson said:

> For every person we hear about who refuses cancer therapy and lives, there are additional people who refuse standard medical therapy and die. There's no way to count the latter number. Without formal scientific studies, it's impossible to generate statistics on the efficacy of alternative treatments [16]. Exactly.

Additionally, what researchers discover reflects what they are looking for, and what they are looking for reflects their preconceived biases. Researchers who suspect that cancer can be cured by eating organic food and taking herbs are likely to query cancer survivors about these factors. They may very well find that many cancer survivors indeed eat only organic foods and take supplements and herbs. In the mind of an uncritical thinker, prone to confirmation bias, this initial hypothesis becomes transmogrified into absolute certainty. However, this does not mean that organic food and herbs cure cancer. Perhaps a lucky genetic mutation is the true reason for their survival. But researchers won't find this gene if they don't look for it.

Let's further examine how the survival bias can lead to faulty conclusions. Nicholas Gonzalez was an oncologist who believed that "tumors are a sign that the body is too filled with toxins." He further claimed cancer could be treated by a combination of dietary modification, twice daily coffee enemas, and the use of pancreatic enzymes and other supplements, which required patients to take up to 175 pills per day. Many of his recommendations were based on dubious tests, such as hair analysis. The hair samples were sent to a self-trained technician who analyzed them using techniques Dr. Gonzalez admitted he did not understand. However, he claimed that the results provided invaluable insights on a patient's cancer and overall organ function. Like Drs. Wahls and Turner, if he could demonstrate his protocol worked, this would be one of the most important discoveries in the history of medicine.

In 1999, he and his partner, Linda Isaacs, published a paper of 11 cases of patients with pancreatic cancer [17]. Patients treated with his protocol survived an average 17 months, while most patients with advanced pancreatic cancer die in under a year. In 2007, they published a paper titled *The Gonzalez Therapy and Cancer: A Collection of Case Reports* in which they reported 31 cases of patients with various cancers, all of whom survived much longer than expected using their protocol [18]. Some of the cases are extremely impressive, describing patients with metastatic cancers surviving for 16 years after their diagnosis. Like Dr. Wahls, he also used his personal experience as evidence, telling an interviewer that he used his protocol himself and saying, "I've never had cancer" [19]. So does this mean that the Gonzalez protocol is a miraculous treatment for cancer surpassing all others in existence? Again, maybe.

However, before we accept this, let's consider whether the survival bias and other biases might be playing a role in his findings. His publication of patients with pancreatic cancer was a "nonconsecutive case series," meaning that he cherry-picked the best cases for publication. According to the National Cancer Institute:

> The investigators report that 25 additional patients with pancreatic cancer were seen during the study period but were excluded from study participation. Eleven of these patients were excluded on the basis of comorbidities, previous treatment, or delay between diagnosis and beginning the program; 14 otherwise eligible patients were excluded on the grounds that they chose not to start the program, complied only briefly, or predicted noncompliance.

How might the inclusion of these 25 patients have affected his results? It's impossible to say. While his 11 cases are certainly impressive, perhaps they are merely the medical equivalent of the planes who returned safely or the lucky people who flipped seven heads in a row (Fig. 13.12).

His results also show how difficult it is to fairly measure central tendency. While it seems intuitive that the average is a fair statistical measure, this is true only if there are no extreme outliers. This becomes obvious when one realizes that if Bill Gates were to visit a homeless shelter, the average net worth of every person there would be hundreds

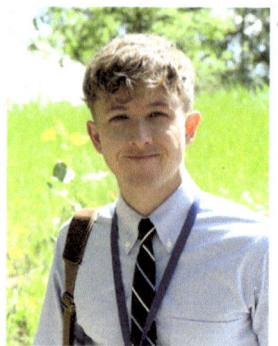

The law of good science is that you can't say "I've got an idea and I'm going to fall in love with it and selectively cite evidence to support it."

James Hamblin

Fig. 13.12 James Hamblin gets it right. (Bluerasberry. James Hamblin at spotlight health Aspen ideas festival 2015 [Image file]. In: Wikimedia commons. 2015. Retrieved from https://commons.wikimedia.org/wiki/File:James_Hamblin_at_Spotlight_Health_Aspen_Ideas_Festival_2015.JPG.)

of millions of dollars. In Dr. Gonzalez's series of 11 cases, four patients survived three years. Perhaps these four outliers increased the average survival time of the group to an impressive 17 months. Perhaps the 25 patients with pancreatic cancer he excluded contained some people who died in a few months and would have made the overall average much less impressive had they been included in his report. Even if this were known, further questions remain. How might the selection bias have impacted his results? Did he turn away patients whom he suspected were too ill to follow his demanding protocol? Did the most ill patients even bother to call his office at all, or did they go directly to the hospital and into the care of mainstream clinicians?

These possibilities show why even the most incredible cancer survival cases have to be recognized for what they are –anecdotes with little scientific merit. As oncologist Murray Brennan commented:

> *I have never seen anybody's tumor respond to pancreatic enzymes.* Not one time… *If he has something we have overlooked, it would be thrilling. But when people talk about his 'success' I wonder what they mean, because as far as I can tell it is based on ten or eleven people. I don't mean to be unkind or unfair, but ten people is not enough to change the way a nation does business* [20].

Stephen Barrett, a psychiatrist and science advocate, provided five reasons that might explain such miraculous results from cancer testimonials [21]:

- The patient never had cancer.
- The cancer was cured or put into remission by proven therapy, but questionable therapy was also used and erroneously credited for the beneficial result.
- The cancer is progressing but is erroneously represented as slowed or cured.
- The patient represented as cured may have died as a result of the cancer or been lost to follow-up.
- The patient had a spontaneous remission (very rare) or slow-growing cancer that was publicized as a cure.

Dr. Gonzalez's largest collection of cases was published in a book devoted to his mentor titled *One Man Alone: An Investigation of Nutrition, Cancer, and William Donald Kelley*. An investigation of these cases by Peter Moran and Louise Lubetkin found that "At least 41 of the patients had been treated with surgery, radiation, and/or chemotherapy that could have been responsible for the length of their survival. The rest lacked biopsy evidence and/or had cancers that typically have long survival times" [22].

As previously stated, anecdotes can be used to generate a hypothesis for a formal clinical trial. Dr. Gonzalez's case reports were impressive enough to justify a trial, and in contrast to many CAM practitioners, he was eager to test his protocol. As he said in an interview, "I am not in hiding, not in Mexico. If my results work, they work. If not, I'll walk away" [20]. So what happened when his protocol was formally tested in patients with pancreatic cancer? It failed miserably. A prospective trial found that patients treated with Dr. Gonzalez's protocol survived an average of 4.3 months, while those using standard chemotherapy survived an average for 14 months and reported a better quality of life [23]. The difference between the groups was so stark that the Data Safety and Monitoring Committee halted enrollment in the study, bringing it to a premature close before more people could be hurt.

Despite his promise before the trial to "walk away" if his treatment failed, Dr. Gonzalez was not at all dissuaded by this study. Instead of accepting the results, he engaged in special pleading, which is the logical fallacy of applying standards and rules to others, while exempting oneself from the same rigorous criteria without reasonable justification. After the study he claimed that mismanagement of the trial led to its poor results, even writing a book, titled *What Went Wrong: The Truth Behind the Clinical Trial of the Enzyme Treatment of Cancer*. Indeed, it was an imperfect study, with many patients refusing to be randomized, a key component in most clinical trials. He also complained that patients "assigned to the nutrition arm actually failed to meet the entry criteria, and were far too sick physically, or not sufficiently committed, to comply with the prescribed regimen" [24].

Dr. Gonzalez's objection reveals two important points. Firstly, whether he realized it or not, he was essentially admitting at least some of the success of his protocol might be due reverse causation; instead of 175 pills and twice daily coffee enemas causing patients to survive longer, it is possible that only the healthiest patients could adhere to his rigorous regimen. He himself stated that his protocol was a "hard program and you have to accept that getting well is a full-time job" [19]. Extremely ill patients can't do this. As oncologist David Gorski put it, "Robbed of his ability to pick the best patients, Gonzalez's results were no better than no treatment at all, and certainly not the equal of chemotherapy" [25].

Secondly, it shows the importance one of the most standard procedures in most clinical trials, a practice known as the intention-to-treat analysis. In such an analysis, the final study results are based on the patient's initially assigned treatment, regardless of whether the study subject actually received that treatment. In other words, if 100 people are assigned to receive treatment X at the start of a study, they will be all included in the analysis of treatment X at the end of the study even if they all did not receive treatment X.

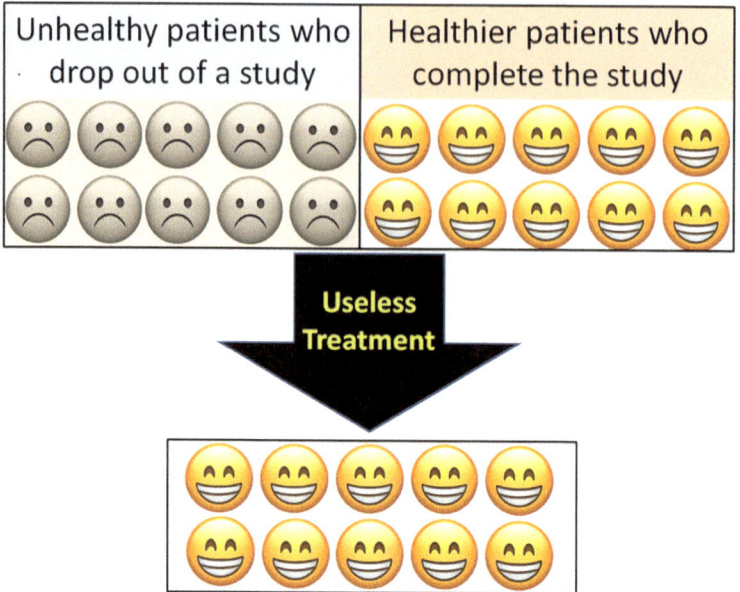

Fig. 13.13 The attrition bias occurs when only the heathiest subjects at the start of the trial are analyzed at the end of the trial. This can make a useless treatment appear effective

While it may be counterintuitive, the intention-to-treat protocol allows researchers to avoid something called the attrition bias, which is a systematic error that occurs when there is unequal loss of subjects in a clinical trial. It is essentially a form of the survival bias that affects medical studies. If the most ill patients drop out of a study, a useless treatment will appear effective if only those subjects who finish the trial are compared with those who began it (Fig. 13.13).

As Dr. Gorski wrote:

> *Excluding patients who couldn't make it through Gonzalez's protocol, which is, as has been pointed out before, quite onerous, would introduce bias in that the more debilitated patients, who couldn't swallow 150 pills a day, along with the raw juices and various other dietary woo, and undergo coffee enemas twice a day, would be excluded, leaving patients in better shape for analysis* [25].

Not surprisingly, Dr. Gonzalez felt that the intention-to-treat protocol shouldn't apply to his treatment. He engaged in more special pleading, arguing that:

> *Such a design can be disastrous for a lifestyle intervention trial such as ours, since patients who might initially be enthusiastic but who can't or choose not to proceed with the self-administered dietary/nutritional regimen will be counted as having been fully treated.*

He's right, but counting patients as "fully treated," even if they haven't been, is the whole point. He does not provide any reason why his "lifestyle intervention" should be exempt from this standard practice.

Simply put, Dr. Gonzalez rejected the idea that his protocol should be held to the same standards as other cancer treatments. He said in one interview, "Natural treatments like mine are not just chemotherapy, and you can't design clinical studies to test them as if they were" [26]. When an epidemiologist expressed interest studying his patients, Dr. Gonzalez replied that it would be impossible to tell whether his treatments actually worked using standard metrics such as 5-year survival rate. He claimed that this is because he treated a variety of different cancers, many patients had prior conventional treatments that would taint any evaluation of his therapy, and it would be impossible to tell if patients actually complied with his therapy. As he put it in an article titled *Statistics: Why Meaningful Statistics Cannot Be Generated From a Private Practice*:

> The epidemiologist finally realized it would be a cumbersome and fairly meaningless exercise to try and prove my overall "success" rate with breast cancer by reviewing my files. Determining compliance alone could take months, if not years, of work because we had treated so many women with "breast cancer" during the time of our practice. He also began to understand my point that the so-called gold standard 5-year survival rate would be essentially meaningless to assess treatment effect [27].

This is special pleading on steroids. It is also interesting that Dr. Gonzalez believed his inability to document patient compliance with his regimen meant no one could argue against it, without also realizing this makes it impossible to defend. If he was not sure his patients actually followed his therapy, how could he be so sure it worked?

There is little doubt that Dr. Gonzalez was a sincere believer in his protocol. Similarly, I am sure Dr. Wahls honestly believes she is "living proof" of the efficacy of her protocol for MS. However, because of the survival bias, the testimonies of the "Wahls Warriors" are close to useless from a scientific standpoint, though they are certainly emotionally compelling. As with Dr. Gonzalez, before we can assess the value of her treatment, we must have some idea how of many people have tried her protocol and either deteriorated or did not improve.

Like Dr. Gonzalez, Dr. Wahls also engages in special pleading, arguing that her protocol should be exempt from standard measures of scientific proof. In her largest study, she too felt the intention-to-treat protocol shouldn't apply, writing, "Including subjects who did not adhere to the study diet would not provide a clear answer to whether the diet can be efficacious" [5]. I disagree. After all, it's possible that the success of her protocol, slight as it is, is due to reverse causation. Instead of her protocol improving mood and fatigue in patients with MS, perhaps only patients with whose mood and energy improved over the course of the study could adhere to the dramatic lifestyle changes it required. This explanation becomes more plausible when one considers that only eight out of 17 people randomized to her "paleo" diet finished the study and were included in the final analysis (Fig. 13.14).

Let's further examine the Facebook post below, which was given in response to someone who quite reasonably asked, "Any peer reviewed papers out on this yet?" (Fig. 13.15).

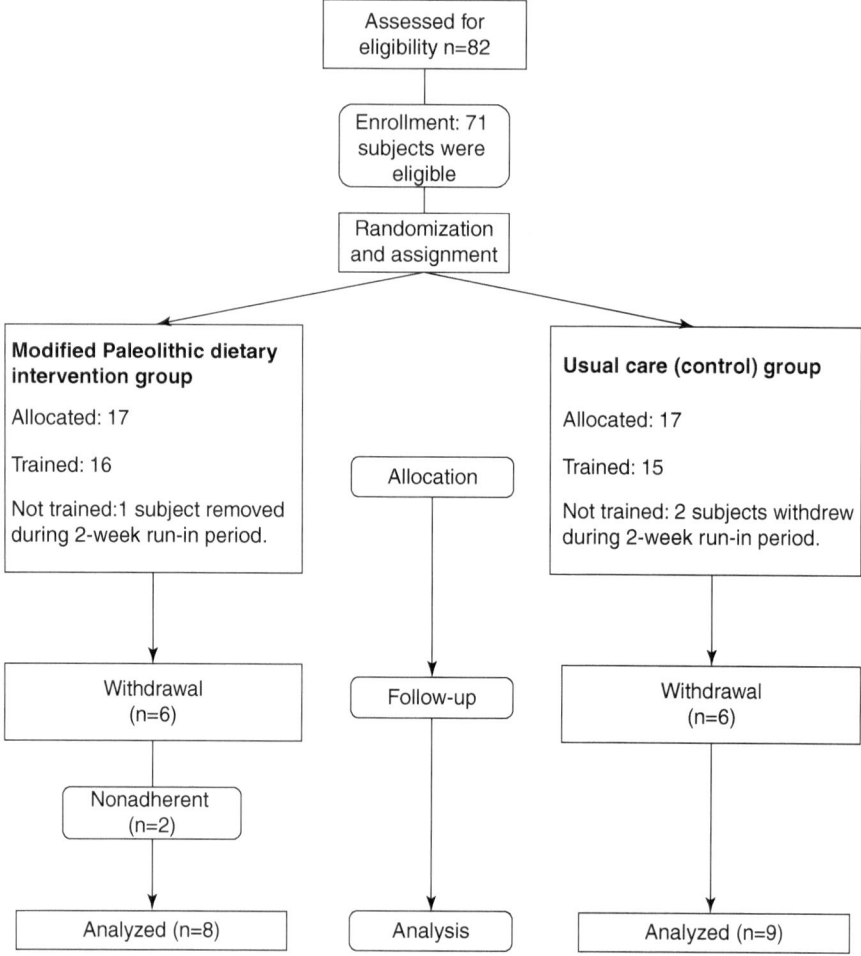

Fig. 13.14 Half of the patients in Dr. Wahls' study dropped out. Those that dropped out were not included in the final analysis

As we have seen, Dr. Wahls' evidence that she can reverse MS is nonexistent. Her excuse is that her research is "made difficult by pharmaceutical interest and a scientific methodology designed for drugs over food." This is nonsense. The "scientific methodology" was designed to find out answers to questions as accurately as possible. It was not "designed for drugs over food." In addition to this, she protests on her website that no one wants to fund her research, writing that "Dr. Wahls has sent multiple grant proposals for $450,000 to the National MS Society and the National Institutes of Health (NIH), but has thus far has not been funded." She does say that she is trying to raise funds to conduct larger studies "to prove that the intervention is effective," and she solicits donations for this purpose on her website. Notice that she says she is going to prove that the intervention *is* effective, not that she is going to determine *if* it is effective, as a fair researcher would do.

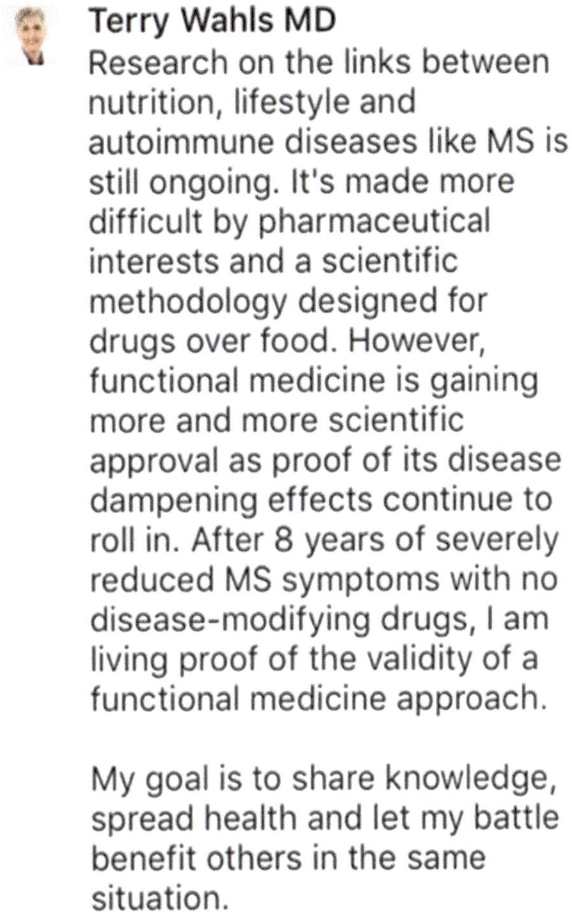

Fig. 13.15 Special pleading by Dr. Terry Wahls. (Wahls T. (Terry Wahls MD). [Facebook status update]. (n.d.). Retrieved from https://www.facebook.com/pg/TerryWahls/posts/?ref=page_internal.)

Terry Wahls MD

Research on the links between nutrition, lifestyle and autoimmune diseases like MS is still ongoing. It's made more difficult by pharmaceutical interests and a scientific methodology designed for drugs over food. However, functional medicine is gaining more and more scientific approval as proof of its disease dampening effects continue to roll in. After 8 years of severely reduced MS symptoms with no disease-modifying drugs, I am living proof of the validity of a functional medicine approach.

My goal is to share knowledge, spread health and let my battle benefit others in the same situation.

Finally, despite her protestations, the MS Society has decided to fund a study of her treatment, announcing in August 2016 that they would give one million dollars to her university for this purpose [28]. The results will be available in several years. If it produces compelling evidence that her protocol can meaningfully alter the course of MS, I and other clinicians will embrace it with open arms. If it fails to show that diet positively affects MS, will Dr. Wahls do the same, closing her online shop? I think we know the answer to that.

It is clear that neither Dr. Wahls nor Dr. Gonzalez feel the lack of scientific evidence to support their claims in any way indicates flaws in their protocol. Rather the flaws lie with the scientific method. When an alternative treatment cannot pass scientific muster, a key step of marketing that treatment is to delegitimize science. A common front-line defense used by promoters of alternative treatments is the assertion that "the science just hasn't caught up to the treatment." As psychologist Ray Hyman wrote, "Many pseudo- and fringe-scientists often react to the failure of science to confirm their prized beliefs, not by gracefully accepting the possibility that they were wrong, but by arguing that science is defective" [29].

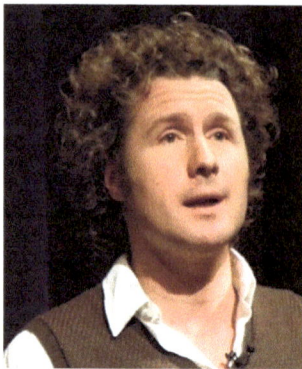

Quacks citing problems in pharma make me laugh. Flaws in aircraft design do not prove the existence of magic carpets.
Ben Goldacre

Fig. 13.16 Ben Goldacre gets it right. (Cornelius G. (Gaius). Ben Goldacre speaking at TAM London Oct 2009 [Image file]. In: Wikimedia commons. 2009. Retrieved from https://commons.wikimedia.org/wiki/Category:Ben_Goldacre#/media/File:Ben_Goldacre_TAM_London_2009.JPG.)

While marketing, even of legitimate products, often contains an alarming amount of manipulation, when it comes to marketing of CAM, belittling science and mainstream medicine is merely business as usual. If alternative treatments worked as well as claimed, that would be all the marketing they would need. There would be no reason to vilify doctors, pharmaceutical companies, and the scientific method itself. As Ben Goldacre memorably said, "Quacks citing problems in pharma make me laugh. Flaws in aircraft design do not prove the existence of magic carpets" [30]. Moreover, malfeasance of the part of pharmaceutical companies and mainstream clinicians does not prove the efficacy of alternative treatments (Fig. 13.16).

Yet when it comes to medicine, if a clinician doesn't have evidence, they just have marketing. In the marketing of CAM, a simple truth like "there is no evidence this treatment works" generates stock replies such as "science doesn't know everything," "the scientific method isn't appropriate for this treatment," and "this treatment has been around long before science." The fact that mainstream clinicians reject treatments that lack evidence generates stock replies such as "doctors just want your money," "doctors only treat the symptoms," and "doctors want you to be sick." This is designed to sidestep accountability and act as a substitute for evidence, when, according to their own claims, evidence for alternative treatments should be in abundant supply. If they were vastly superior, as they are said to be, then displaying that evidence would not only be the most effective way to gain customers, it would also be the easiest. If the treatments of Drs. Gonzalez and Wahls are as miraculous as claimed, proving it in a clinic trial should be relatively easy (Fig. 13.17).

Vilifying the scientific process creates a double standard, where mainstream medical treatments must have valid evidence, while CAM practitioners do not. No clinician would be satisfied if a pharmaceutical company released a product that failed to pass clinical trials on the justification that "it worked for our patients." And if the company had no testing at all, they would be properly accused of using the public as guinea pigs. Pharmaceutical companies would be rightly vilified if, instead of showing data their drug worked, they pointed out the limitations of alternative treatments.

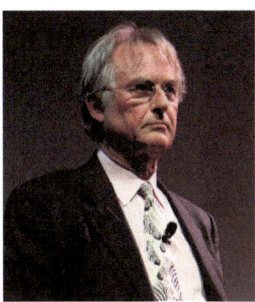

[Alternative medicine is defined as] that set of practices that cannot be tested, refuse to be tested or consistently fail tests.

Richard Dawkins

Fig. 13.17 Richard Dawkins gets it right. (Chiswick Chap. Bust-length cropped portrait photograph of Richard Dawkins in 2008 [Image file]. In: Wikimedia commons. 2008. Retrieved from https://commons.wikimedia.org/wiki/File:Dawkins_at_UT_Austin_detail.jpg.)

If CAM practitioners believe that it's necessary for mainstream clinicians and the pharmaceutical industry to meet a certain level of quality control before they market their products to the public, then they should hold themselves to the same standards. This means recognizing that when they endorse or recommend an alternative treatment because it "worked for my patients," they are failing to live up to their own standards. It's understandable that personal experience is very compelling to the human mind, but if a particular treatment is scientifically implausible, has not been studied in clinical trials, or has failed clinical trials, then a clinician's personal experience cannot be used as a trump card.

Drs. Wahls and Gonzalez are both certainly right that dietary and lifestyle interventions are difficult to study for most diseases. There is rarely significant funding to support large trials, and it is difficult, if not impossible, to blind patients to what they eat or to give placebo coffee enemas. However, the fact that something is difficult to study doesn't mean it is true. Not does it exempt people from being required to provide evidence for their statements. This is especially true if their claims represent extraordinary breakthroughs that would revolutionize medicine. As Carl Sagan was fond of saying, "extraordinary claims require extraordinary evidence" (Fig. 13.18).

This brings us to the philosophical concept of burden of proof (formally known as *onus probandi*). It refers to the obligation of somebody who makes a claim to provide evidence of its accuracy. A statement presented without evidence might be correct, but the burden of proof is on the person making the claim to provide evidence for it. It is not the responsibility of a skeptic who doubts the claim to prove it wrong. Dr. Gonzalez is the one claiming that diet, supplements, and coffee enemas cure cancer. It is up to him to prove it. Even though he was right that studying his protocol is difficult, one cannot conclude from this that it therefore works. The best and only trial of his protocol, however flawed it was, showed it failed so miserably the trial had to be prematurely halted. Similarly, Dr. Wahls is the one claiming that a "paleo" diet reverses progressive MS. It is up to her to prove it. The fact that formal trials of many alternative treatments are difficult to conduct does not shift the burden of proof onto those who are skeptical of these treatments (Fig. 13.19).

To demonstrate this point, let me join the ranks of Drs. Wahls and Gonzalez by proposing the Howard Protocol™ as a means to prevent cancer, MS, and almost

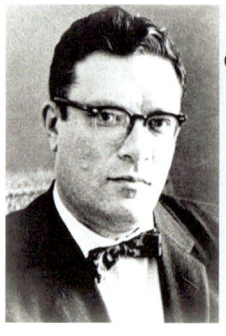

I believe in evidence. I believe in observation, measurement, and reasoning, confirmed by independent observers. I'll believe anything, no matter how wild and ridiculous, if there is evidence for it. The wilder and more ridiculous something is, however, the firmer and more solid the evidence will have to be.

Isaac Asimov

Fig. 13.18 The greater the claim, the greater the need for evidence. (Leonian P. Isaac Asimov [Image file]. In: Wikimedia commons. (n.d.). Retrieved from https://commons.wikimedia.org/wiki/Isaac_Asimov#/media/File:Isaac.Asimov01.jpg.)

Fig. 13.19 I agree. (The Logic of Science. From a recent post [Facebook status update]. 2015. Retrieved from https://www.facebook.com/thelogicofscience/photos/a.1618699508361446/1629169717314425/?type=3.)

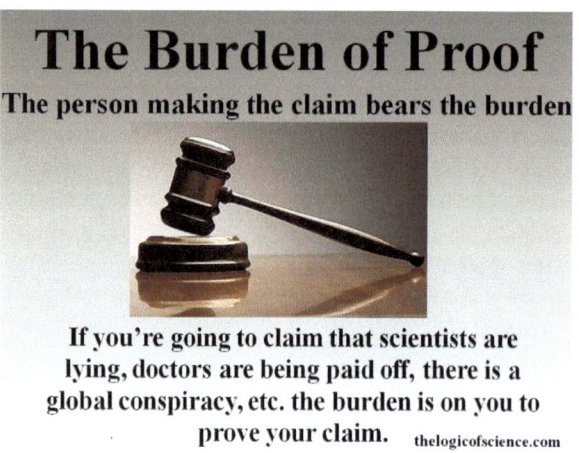

every disease but the common cold. Like them, I will use myself as an example. I have never had cancer or MS. Even more impressively, since I started medical school in 1999, I have never even taken a sick day. I have had one doctor's visit in this time. I can count on one hand the number of times I have taken any medication. To what do I attribute my remarkable health? Firstly, I have a strict diet where I eat GMOs and gluten as often as possible, while completely avoiding organic food. Secondly, I am obsessively up-to-date on my vaccines. As a bonus, I also think negative thoughts as often as I can. As evidence of the Howard Protocol™, I have my own set of before and after pictures. On those extremely rare days when I get a minor sniffle, a vaccine and a donut laden with sugar and gluten fixes things almost immediately (Fig. 13.20). I have also collected multiple testimonials from people just like me. I call them Howard's Heroes (Fig. 13.21).

Yet, while the mainstream medical community certainly recognizes the value of vaccines, they reject my protocol as a panacea for preventing cancer and MS. They claim my "anecdotes" are not scientific proof. Unfortunately, science is just not equipped to test the Howard Protocol™. This is because it is simply not possible to investigate my treatment in a randomized, double-blind, placebo-controlled study.

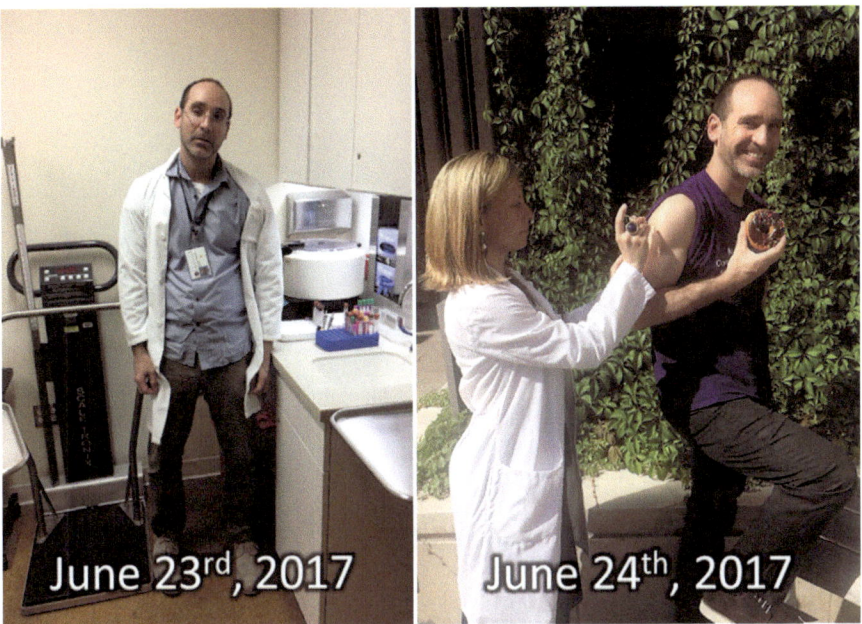

Fig. 13.20 Before and after pictures of the author proving that donuts and vaccines restore him to health

> **Kavin**   I eat GMOs every day, I was formula fed, and I like sugar. My fertility is excellent, took two months to conceive each child.
> Like · Reply · 3 hrs

> **Tati I**   I eat like a college kid. Never stopped. Ramen noodles, cereal and pizza 24/7.
> 40, healthy, cholesterol is even below the lower limit, BP is low consistently, and somehow I managed to get my MD and be a neurologist. My kid is gifted, and I ate basically a diet of Haagen Dazs during pregnancy. She is super healthy, and not only vaccinated, but vaccinated on the US *and* Brazilian schedule.
>
> Oh, and I was formula fed in the 70s 😊
> Like · Reply · 👍 7 · 17 hrs

> **Mandy**   I ate a steady diet of ramen noodles, pizza, and chocolate as a teen and in my 20's. I have had all my vaccines and had many of them at least three times because the Army lost my shot records twice. I get my yearly flu shots. I avoid organic and non-GMO foods. Thanks to all that, I was able to earn a doctorate in pharmacy. Because I work in a pharmacy, I am exposed to Big Pharma products all day long and it helps keep me healthy. My vaccinated kids are also doing great. My daughter started college at 16 and my son is taking algebra at 11. My husband lived grew up on a farm and was exposed to pesticides and herbacides on a regular basis. He is smart and very strong.
> Like · Reply · 👍 4 · 11 hrs

Fig. 13.21 Testimony from Howard's Heroes

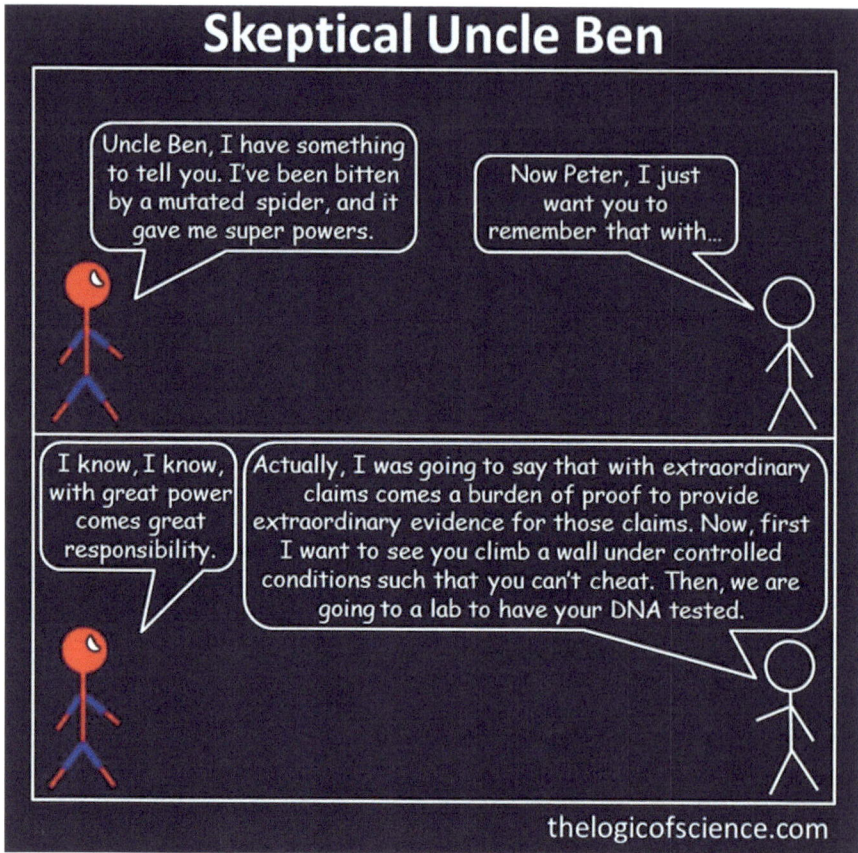

Fig. 13.22 Extraordinary claims require extraordinary proof. (The Logic of Science. [Image file, Facebook status update]. 2016. Retrieved from https://www.facebook.com/thelogicofscience/posts/1806423949589000:0.)

Furthermore, no one wants to fund a study of my protocol. Powerful forces are aligned against me. Think how many people would be out of a job if my protocol became a mainstream treatment! Pharmaceutical companies would also lose billions of dollars and mainstream clinicians would lose their jobs. Finally, no one can prove my protocol *doesn't* prevent cancer and MS.

So, would CAM practitioners accept that a diet rich in GMOs and gluten combined with vaccines prevents cancer and MS? Since my evidence is as strong as any in CAM, they should (Fig. 13.22).

When all else fails, the final common pathway of CAM practitioners is to claim a conspiracy. There is a near universal tendency to paint themselves as victims of nefarious plots, led by mainstream clinicians and pharmaceutical companies, who collaborate to prevent them from carrying out research and spreading their cure. As Neil deGrasse Tyson tweeted, "Conspiracy theorists are those who claim coverups whenever insufficient data exists to support what they're sure is true" [31]. Perhaps "pharmaceutical interests" are preventing Dr. Wahls from doing large, rigorous trials, as she claimed in her Facebook post. To my knowledge, she has not provided any evidence this is the case. And if indeed the pharmaceutical industry is trying to suppress Dr. Wahls, her multiple speeches, online store, and prominent social media profile indicate they are extremely incompetent in doing so. Dr. Gonzalez also claimed a conspiracy led to his protocol failing in a clinical trial. He wrote that the trial showed "deceit, collusion, and disregard for patient safety that reaches right into the highest levels of the academic medical community." He specifically accused the lead investigator on the study, John Chabot, of gross scientific fraud, purposely selecting the most ill patients to receive his treatment. He wrote, "We suspect Dr. Chabot believed it was in his best interest to discredit our alternative therapy and instead prove the value of a treatment he helped develop" (Figs. 13.23, 13.24, and 13.25) [32].

As is common with CAM practitioners, it is not surprising that Drs. Wahls and Gonzalez have embraced much more sinister medical conspiracies. Dr. Wahls wrote on her Facebook page:

Vaccines have a variety of compounds to create a more vigorous immune response. In turn, the body must either metabolize and eliminate these compounds from your body, or store in fat cells. If these compounds are stored in the body, they will continue to act as low grade toxins.

She also appeared in the anti-vaccine movie *Bought*, extoling the benefits of several vaccine-preventable diseases and repeating standard fearmongering arguments

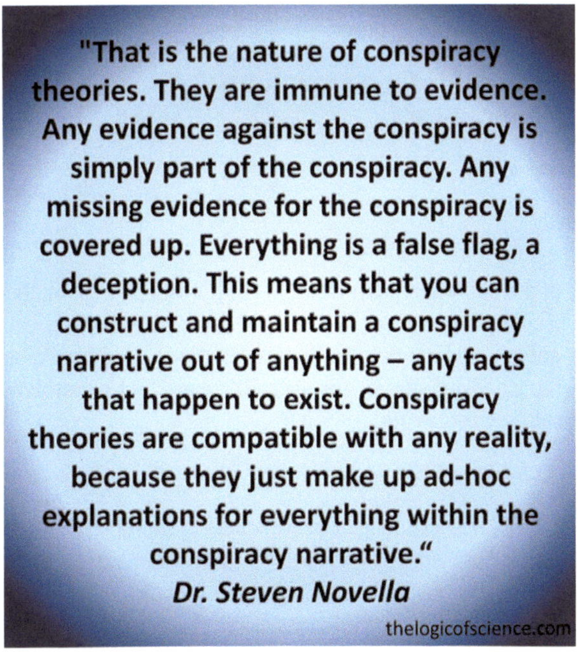

Fig. 13.23 Steven Novella gets it right. (The Logic of Science. [Image file, Facebook status update]. 2017. Retrieved from https://www.facebook.com/thelogicofscience/posts/1967658323465561:0.)

"That is the nature of conspiracy theories. They are immune to evidence. Any evidence against the conspiracy is simply part of the conspiracy. Any missing evidence for the conspiracy is covered up. Everything is a false flag, a deception. This means that you can construct and maintain a conspiracy narrative out of anything – any facts that happen to exist. Conspiracy theories are compatible with any reality, because they just make up ad-hoc explanations for everything within the conspiracy narrative."

Dr. Steven Novella

thelogicofscience.com

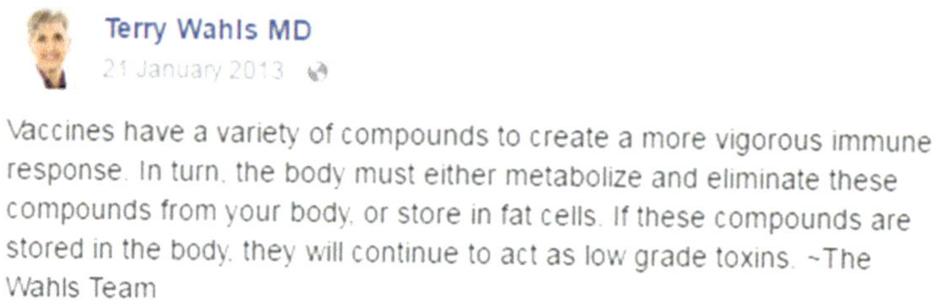

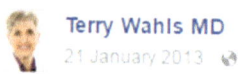

Terry Wahls MD
21 January 2013

Vaccines have a variety of compounds to create a more vigorous immune response. In turn, the body must either metabolize and eliminate these compounds from your body, or store in fat cells. If these compounds are stored in the body, they will continue to act as low grade toxins. ~The Wahls Team

Fig. 13.24 Anti-vaccine fearmongering from Dr. Terry Wahls. (Wahls T. (Terry Wahls MD). [Facebook status update]. 2013. Retrieved from https://www.facebook.com/TerryWahls/posts/469099296481460.)

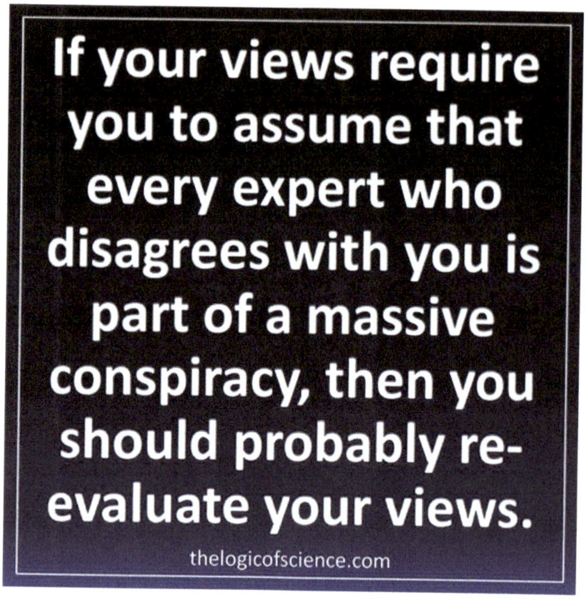

Fig. 13.25 I agree. (The Logic of Science. [Image file, Facebook status update]. 2015. Retrieved from https://www.facebook.com/thelogicofscience/posts/1884483368449724:0.)

> **If your views require you to assume that every expert who disagrees with you is part of a massive conspiracy, then you should probably re-evaluate your views.**
>
> thelogicofscience.com

of the anti-vaccine movement [33]. Ironically, given the complete absence of research backing her claims, one of Dr. Wahls' main objections to vaccines is that they have not been adequately studied, even though they have been the subject of hundreds of thousands of studies for over 200 years. For example, in the Reditt AMA forum, she said the following:

Toxins in vaccines, the adjuvant, is typically a metal such as mercury or aluminum used to increase the immune reaction, so that humans will respond to the dead virus. The adjuvants are compounds that are toxic to brain cells. We don't understand yet what a "safe" dose of an adjuvant is. This is why some people are concerned with the practice of stacking so many

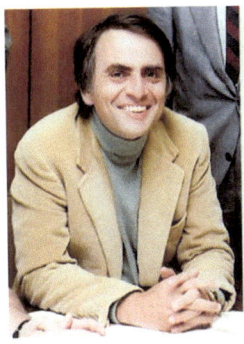

One of the saddest lessons of history is this: If we've been bamboozled long enough, we tend to reject any evidence of the bamboozle. We're no longer interested in finding out the truth. The bamboozle has captured us. It's simply too painful to acknowledge, even to ourselves, that we've been taken. Once you give a charlatan power over you, you almost never get it back.

Carl Sagan

Fig. 13.26 Carl Sagan gets it right. (NASA/JPL. Carl Sagan [Image file]. In: Wikimedia commons. 1979. Retrieved from https://commons.wikimedia.org/wiki/Carl_Sagan#/media/File:Carl_Sagan_Planetary_Society.JPG.)

vaccines together on the same day. More research definitely has to be done to answer this question one way or the other. We do not know the health consequence of not acquiring the infections that were are currently being immunized against long term, but I think people should get the appropriate vaccines [34].

Dr. Gonzalez similarly regurgitated anti-vaccine talking points, arguing against "force-feeding vaccination" in an essay on the medical conspiracy theory site Greenmedinfo. He both minimized the severity of diseases like polio and blamed vaccines for destroying the immune systems of young people, saying he saw "many patients in their 20s and 30s, the first of the highly-vaccinated generation, coming to my office unable to function, having been exposed to some viral illness." (Fig. 13.26).

Conclusion
A comedian once joked, "I hope I live to be 100. When people ask me about my secret, I'll make up something ridiculous. I'll tell them that I ate a pine cone every day. Then I'll see how many people start eating pine cones" [35]. While the flaw in his logic is readily apparent, because of the survival bias, clinicians and patients may make similar errors. While anecdotal data can suggest that a treatment is worth investigation, only prospective clinical trials can determine whether a treatment is truly effective or not. If a trial does not give the expected or desired conclusion, an honest scientist will admit this and adjust her view accordingly. Pseudoscientists will retain their beliefs and engage in special pleading, finding reasons why standard measures of scientific proof should not apply to their treatment. The burden of proof always lies with the person making a claim, not with someone skeptical of it. As Christopher Hitchens said, "What can be asserted without evidence, can be dismissed without evidence." Finally, when someone seems more interested in marketing their treatment than proving it scientifically, this raises serious questions about their motivations (Fig. 13.27).

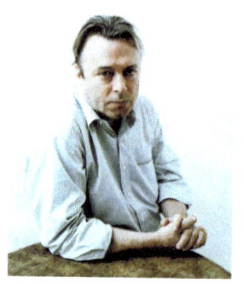

What can be asserted without evidence can be dismissed without evidence.

Christopher Hitchens

Fig. 13.27 Christopher Hitchens gets it right. (Tanke F. (Fri). British author and journalist Christopher Hitchens [Image file]. In: Wikimedia commons. 2008. Retrieved from https://commons.wikimedia.org/wiki/Category:Christopher_Hitchens#/media/File:Christopher_Hitchens_2008-04-24_001.jpg.)

References

1. Centers for Disease Control and Prevention. Pneumocystis pneumonia DOUBLEHYPHEN-Los Angeles. MMWR Morb Mortal Wkly Rep. 1981;30(21):1–3. Retrieved from https://www.cdc.gov/mmwr/preview/mmwrhtml/june_5.htm.
2. Smith GC, Pell JP. Parachute use to prevent death and major trauma related to gravitational challenge: systematic review of randomised controlled trials. BMJ. 2003;327(20–27):1459–61. https://doi.org/10.1136/bmj.327.7429.1459.
3. Janssen WF. (1977). Cancer quackery: past and present. FDA Consumer, 1977(July–August). Retrieved from https://www.cancertreatmentwatch.org/q/janssen.shtml.
4. Borreli L. (2013, Aug 9). Multiple sclerosis diet: Doctor Terry Wahls reverses MS with diet alone. Medical Daily. Retrieved from https://www.medicaldaily.com/multiple-sclerosis-diet-doctor-terry-wahls-ms-diet-alone-249419.
5. Irish AK, Erickson CM, Wahls TL, Snetselaar LG, Darling WG. Randomized control trial evaluation of a modified Paleolithic dietary intervention in the treatment of relapsing-remitting multiple sclerosis: a pilot study. Degener Neurol Neuromuscul Dis. 2017;7:1–18. https://doi.org/10.2147/DNND.S116949.
6. Lee JE, Bisht B, Hall MJ, Rubenstein LM, Louison R, Klein DT, Wahls TL. A multimodal, nonpharmacologic intervention improves mood and cognitive function in people with multiple sclerosis. J Am Coll Nutr. 2017;36(3):150–68. https://doi.org/10.1080/07315724.2016.1255160.
7. Bisht B, Darling WG, Grossmann RE, Shivapour ET, Lutgendorf SK, Snetselaar LG, Hall MJ, Zimmerman MB, Wahls TL. A multimodal intervention for patients with secondary progressive multiple sclerosis: feasibility and effect on fatigue. J Altern Complement Med. 2014;20(5):347–55. https://doi.org/10.1089/acm.2013.0188.
8. Bisht B, Darling WG, White EC, White KA, Shivapour ET, Zimmerman MB, Wahls TL. Effects of a multimodal intervention on gait and balance of subjects with progressive multiple sclerosis: a prospective longitudinal pilot study. Degener Neurol Neuromuscul Dis. 2017;7:79–93. https://doi.org/10.2147/DNND.S128872.
9. FuzzyCub20. (ca. 2014). Response to Dr. Terry Wahls [Reddit post]. Retrieved 15 Sept 2018 from https://www.reddit.com/r/IAmA/comments/20f6eg/i_am_dr_terry_wahlsa_physician_who_was_diagnosed/.
10. Thomas P, Margulis J. The vaccine-friendly plan: Dr. Paul's safe and effective approach to immunity and health – from pregnancy through your child's teen years. New York: Ballantine Books; 2016. p. 118.

11. Reger C. (2017, Apr 5). The high cost of today's drug therapy – what your physician may not be telling you – Part 1 [Blog post]. Terry Wahls M.D. Retrieved 25 Sept 2018 from https://terrywahls.com/the-high-cost-of-todays-drug-therapy-what-your-physician-may-not-be-telling-you-part-1/.

12. Pells R. (2017, June 7). Dr Christian Jessen: clean eating websites like Gwyneth Paltrow's Goop 'indistinguishable from pro anorexia sites'. The Independent. Retrieved from https://www.independent.co.uk/news/education/education-news/dr-christian-jessen-gqyneth-paltrow-goop-pro-anorexia-websites-clean-eating-embarrassing-bodies-a776641.html.

13. Pemberton M. (2017, July 18). Horrifying toll the clean eating fad is taking on young women: It's the ultra-selective diet made popular by bloggers, but Dr MAX PEMBERTON sees the unsettling results every week in his clinic. The Daily Mail. Retrieved from https://www.dailymail.co/health/article-4709100/Horrifying-toll-clean-eating-fad-taking-young-women.html.

14. Anonymous. (n.d.). Mail order prophet [Plot summary]. Retrieved 15 Sept 2018 from https://www.imdb.com/title/tt0508320/plotsummary?ref_=tt_ov_pl.

15. courses_wp (2016, Mar 14). Radical remission online course: applying the 9 healing factors into your own life. The Radical Remission Project. Retrieved from https://courses.kelly-turner.com/product/radical-remission-online-course/.

16. Deardorff J. (2014, Sept 29). Spontaneous cancer remission rare, but worth study. Chicago Tribune. Retrieved from http://www.chicagotribune.com/lifestyles/health/breastcancer/ct-cancer-remission-met-20140914-story.html.

17. Gonzalez NJ, Isaacs LL. Evaluation of pancreatic proteolytic enzyme treatment of adenocarcinoma of the pancreas, with nutrition and detoxification support. Nutr Cancer. 1999;33(2):117–24. https://doi.org/10.1207/S15327914NC330201.

18. Gonzalez NJ, Isaacs LL. The Gonzalez therapy and cancer: a collection of case reports. Altern Ther Health Med. 2007;13(1):1–33.

19. The Moneychanger. (1995). Dr. Nicholas Gonzales on nutritional cancer therapy [Interview]. OAWHealth. Retrieved from https://oawhealth.com/article/dr-nicholas-gonzalez-on-nutritional-cancer-therapy/.

20. Specter M. (2001, Feb 5). The outlaw doctor. The New Yorker. Retrieved from http://www.michaelspecter.com/2001/02/the-outlaw-doctor/.

21. Barrett S. (2000). "Miraculous recoveries". Quackwatch. Retrieved from https://www.quackwatch.org/01QuackeryRelatedTopics/Cancer/miracles.html.

22. Moran PJ, Lubetkin L. (2015, July 24). Book review [Review of the book One man alone: an investigation of nutrition, cancer, and William Donald Kelley]. Cancer Treatment Watch. Retrieved from https://www.cancertreatmentwatch.org/reports/gonzalez/book.shtml.

23. Chabot JA, Tsai WY, Fine RL, Chen C, Kumah CK, Antman KA, Grann VR. Pancreatic proteolytic enzyme therapy compared with gemcitabine-based chemotherapy for the treatment of pancreatic cancer. J Clin Oncol. 2010;28(12):2058–63. https://doi.org/10.1200/JCO.2009.22.8429.

24. Gonzalez NJ. (2017, Jan 2). The truth about the NCI-NCCAM clinical study. The Nicholas Gonzalez Foundation. Retrieved 15 Sept 2018 from http://www.dr-gonzalez.com/jco_rebuttal.htm.

25. Gorski DH. (2009, Sept 17). Nicholas Gonzalez' response to the failed trial of the Gonzalez protocol: disingenuous nonsense [Blog post]. ScienceBlogs. Retrieved from http://scienceblogs.com/insolence/2009/09/17/nicholas-gonzalez-response-to-the-failed/.

26. Lampe F, Snyder S. Nicholas J. Gonzalez, MD: seeking the truth in the fight against cancer [PDF file]. Altern Ther. 2007;13(1):66–73. Retrieved from http://www.alternative-therapies.com/at/web_pdfs/gonzalez.pdf.

27. Gonzalez NJ, Isaacs LL. Statistics: why meaningful statistics cannot be generated from a private practice [PDF file]. Altern Ther. 2015;21(2):11–5. Retrieved from http://www.alternative-therapies.com/openaccess/ATHM_21_2_Gonzalez.pdf.

28. National Multiple Sclerosis Society. (2016, Aug 24). National MS Society and University of Iowa launch $1 million clinical trial to test dietary approaches to treating fatigue in MS. Retrieved from https://www.nationalmssociety.org/About-the-Society/News/National-MS-Society-and-University-of-Iowa-Launch.

29. Hyman R. (n.d.). How people are fooled by ideomotor action. Quackwatch. Retrieved from http://www.quackwatch.org/01QuackeryRelatedTopics/ideomotor.html.
30. Goldacre B. [ben goldacre]. (2013, Jan 31). Quacks citing problems in pharma make me laugh. FLAWS IN AIRCRAFT DESIGN DO NOT PROVE THE EXISTENCE OF MAGIC CARPETS [Twitter moment]. Retrieved from https://twitter.com/bengoldacre/status/2970526 62564802561?lang=en.
31. neiltyson. [Neil deGrassee Tyson]. (2011, Apr 7). Conspiracy theorists are those who claim coverups whenever insufficient data exists to support what they're sure is true. [Twitter moment]. Retrieved from https://twitter.com/neiltyson/status/56010861382336513?lang=en.
32. Gonzalez N. (n.d.). Cancer pioneers and researchers. EnCognitive.com. Retrieved 15 Sept 2018 from http://www.encognitive.com/node/17963.
33. Jeff Hays Films. (2015, Jan 22). Bought Movie Bonus Short- Terry Wahls, M.D. [Video file]. Retrieved from https://www.youtube.com/watch?v=4kwgkI1RkF0.
34. DrTerryWahls. (ca. 2014). Response to blarghusmaximus [Reddit post]. Retrieved September 15, 2018 from https://www.reddit.com/r/IAmA/comments/20f6eg/i_am_dr_terry_wahlsa_physician_who_was_diagnosed/.
35. Survivorship bias. (n.d.). Skeptical Medicine. Retrieved 15 Sept 2018 from https://sites.google.com/site/skepticalmedicine//cognitive-biases/survivorship-bias.

Case

Hudson was a 45-year-old man who awoke with a slight headache, right-sided weakness, and trouble finding the "right words." An MRI, revealed a lesion in the basal ganglia on the left (Fig. 14.1).

He was otherwise healthy, and an HIV test and a spinal tap were normal, making an infectious cause unlikely. A biopsy was performed out of concern for a brain tumor. It revealed a stroke, a condition for which a biopsy is not needed. As a result of the biopsy, Hudson suffered a hemorrhage that left him with more severe language deficits.

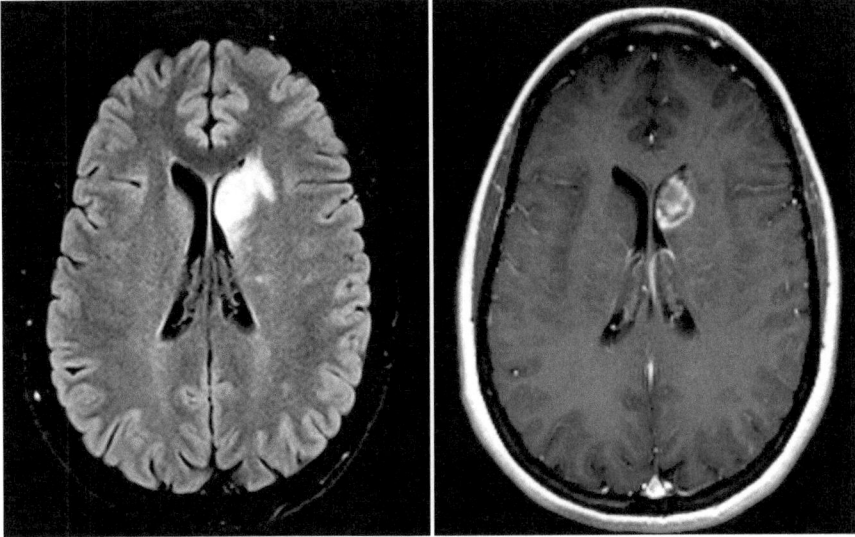

Fig. 14.1 A FLAIR MRI and post-contrast T1-weighted image demonstrate an enhancing lesion in the left caudate nucleus

© Springer International Publishing AG, part of Springer Nature 2019
J. Howard, *Cognitive Errors and Diagnostic Mistakes*,
https://doi.org/10.1007/978-3-319-93224-8_14

Given the final diagnosis, the hospital convened a review to discuss what went wrong. When the case was reviewed by several radiologists and neurologists who were not involved in the case, they all felt a stroke was the most likely diagnosis from the start and that the radiologist and neurologist had had erred in their decision-making. The treating doctors asked for a separate review of the case where the reviewers would be blind to the ultimate diagnosis. In this subsequent review, none of the blind reviewers felt a biopsy was inappropriate.

What Dr. Diallo Was Thinking

I was one of the neurologists who initially reviewed the case and recommended disciplinary action. I went into the case knowing that Hudson had a stroke, an unnecessary biopsy was performed, and the patient suffered as a result. As such, it seemed pretty obvious that his original treatment team had handled his case poorly. However, when my esteemed colleagues reviewed his case without this knowledge, all of them agreed with the decision to perform a biopsy. It was not possible to unlearn this information during my initial review and see things from the perspective on the doctors who had originally treated Hudson.

Discussion

The hindsight bias occurs as knowing the outcome of an event profoundly influences people's perception of the events that preceded it. There is a tendency after an event has occurred to perceive it as having been eminently predictable, even if this was not the case. Baruch Fischhoff, an expert in risk perception, described two aspects to the hindsight bias: (a) reporting an outcome's occurrence increases its perceived probability of occurrence; and (b) people who have received outcome knowledge are largely unaware of its having changed their perceptions in the manner described in the first hypothesis [1].

Pay attention after an unexpected news event, such as a major sports upset or natural disaster. Invariably, some people will say *afterward* that it was eminently foreseeable and warning signs were in plain sight all along. Perhaps some lone prognosticator will have predicted the event in some fashion and afterwards will be heralded as an ignored genius. As an example, consider an article on the website truththeory.com titled *How Was 9/11 Predicted So Many Times Before It Happened?* [2]. It's admittedly creepy to see how artists had drawn scenes similar to 9/11 before it occurred. However, such articles ignore the multitude of failed predictions that don't come to pass and are therefore forgotten (Fig. 14.2).

Closely related to the hindsight bias is the outcome bias. The outcome bias occurs when the quality of a decision or action is evaluated after the result of that decision is known. Francesca Gino and colleagues said that as a result of the outcome bias, "the same behaviors produce more ethical condemnation when they happen to produce bad rather than good outcomes, even if the outcomes are determined by chance" [3]. A drunk driver who hits a mailbox will get a much lighter sentence than a driver who hits a person, even though chance alone may

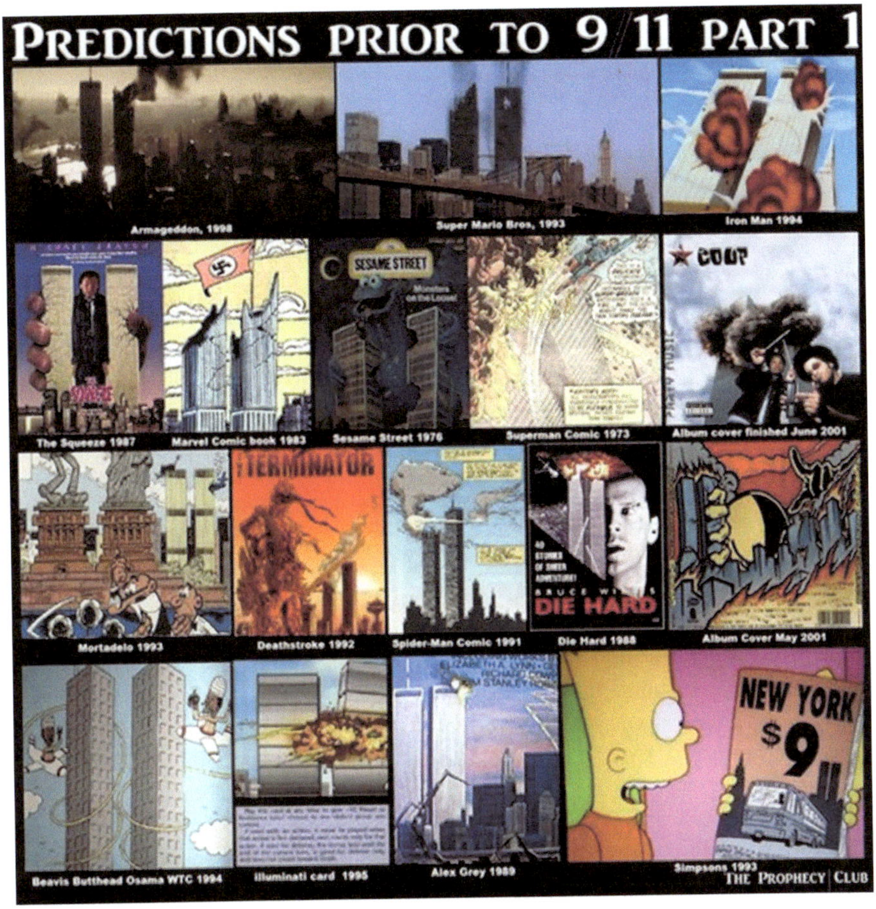

Fig. 14.2 9/11 was "predicted" many times. (911 predictions. [Image file]. (n.d.). Retrieved from https://i.pinimg.com/564x/da/54/04/da540466f45f9a9c2c1f29fdb9ee169d.jpg.)

be the only differentiating factor. The raid to kill Osama Bin Laden was rightfully seen as one of the greatest triumphs of Barack Obama's presidency. Praise came from people who had never done so before. Yet there is no doubt that had the raid failed, perhaps if one of the helicopters had crashed due to mechanical failure, this would have been seen as a huge blunder on his part. President Obama was judged largely on the outcome of his decision, not on the wisdom of the decision itself.

Consider the following case:

Claire was a 25-year-old woman who presented to the emergency room intoxicated, having made multiple superficial cuts to her wrist, claiming she wanted to die. She told the emergency room doctor that her boyfriend had broken up with her that evening and she couldn't imagine life without him. She had been to the ER three times previously that year

under similar circumstances. Claire was observed for several hours and discharged when
sober, with a referral to the outpatient clinic. Though she still reported feeling suicidal at
the time of discharge, she had said this every time she had been discharged previously.
The doctor felt that keeping her in the hospital would not lower her risk for dangerous
behavior and, in fact, would only encourage her to injure herself in response to future
frustrations.

Did the clinician make a mistake? Does it depend on what happens to Claire? Let's assume that she returned home, fell alseep, and went to work the next day with some recognition that cutting herself was a suboptimal response to life's stressors. It sure seems like the clinician acted reasonably. But what if instead, she jumped in front of a train and died. It then seems like the clinician acted irresponsibly, discharging a suicidal patient. However, what should determine whether the clinician acted properly; the decisions that were made during her case or its final outcome? I admit I didn't give you enough information to make a judgment of this case. But if you feel that you must know what happened to Claire before you judge the competence of this clinician, then you are feeling the tug of the outcome bias.

The hindsight and outcome biases can affect clinicians in several ways. Firstly, when reviewing a case, its outcome may seem obvious in retrospect, as the reviewer may be unable to appreciate ambiguities that may have plagued the clinician at the time. People may erroneously feel "I knew it the whole time" or "it's actually pretty obvious" after a challenging diagnosis is made. Several years ago, I reviewed a case where a neurologist missed an important finding on an MRI, and a patient suffered a severe injury. After reading the patient's records and reviewing the MRI, I was asked whether the finding was something the neurologist should have noticed. Though I did not appreciate it at the time, it was as if someone had given me a "Where's Waldo" picture, showed me where Waldo was, and asked me if I would have spotted him. Of course, as I knew the location of the missed MRI finding, the error seemed glaringly obvious. I was strongly convinced the neurologist had not just misread the MRI, but also that he had erred in nearly every aspect of the case. However, when I showed the MRI to several of my colleagues who knew nothing about the case, they too failed to see the abnormality, showing that I was a victim of hindsight bias.

In addition to affecting objective evaluation of cases when there is a poor outcome, the outcome bias may also allow for serious errors to go unnoticed as long as no one is harmed. In one of the most terrifying incidents during my medical internship, I was handed a syringe with a large dose of a sedative to be used during a minor procedure. I was supposed to give small doses until the patient was sleepy, but not knowing this I carelessly gave the entire syringe. The patient fell into a deep sleep and nearly stopped breathing. After a few tense minutes, an antidote was given, and the only consequence was that the patient slept for longer than was intended. My medical team teased me about this in a good-natured way for the next few days. Yet, this fortunate outcome was a combination of my colleagues' skill in ordering the antidote and sheer luck. Had the patient suffered a serious injury, the incident would have been reported to the senior faculty, I would have been castigated as reckless, and I would have potentially suffered serious disciplinary action. The fact that the patient suffered no injury made my serious mistake *appear* inconsequential. In this sense, I benefitted from the outcome bias. Yet, an important opportunity to improve patient safety was lost, as no investigation occurred into what went wrong and how it could have been prevented.

Susan Labine and Gary Labine demonstrated how the outcome bias influences the public's perception of clinicians' judgments [4]. They presented 297 community subjects with a scenario where a therapist evaluated a potentially violent patient. The subjects were given the following possible outcomes:

1. The patient became violent.
2. The patient did not become violent.
3. No outcome was given.

Subjects who received the scenario where the patient became violent believed the attack was more predictable, and the therapist was negligent for not having prevented the violence. In contrast, when the patient did not behave violently, the therapist's actions were seen as reasonable. Robert Caplan and colleagues studied the effect of the outcome bias in 112 anesthesiologists [5]. Subjects were given 21 cases and asked to rate the appropriateness of the care in a patient who suffered an injury. They found that changing the duration of the patient's injury from temporary to permanent had a significant effect on the response. The proportion of ratings for appropriate care fell by 31% when the outcome was changed from temporary to permanent and increased by 28% when the outcome was changed from permanent to temporary. This demonstrates how many of the anesthesiologists fell victim to the outcome bias, judging the appropriateness of the care on how the patient fared, not on the wisdom or skill of the clinician.

The hindsight bias has particular implications for reviews of poor outcomes and medical malpractice lawsuits. Obviously, in all such cases a patient has suffered harm, which is likely to hinder any objective evaluation of the case. Writing about hindsight bias in radiology, Leonard Berlin, a radiologist, quoted an expert who said, "I've never had an attorney bring me a normal radiograph. Whenever an attorney shows or sends me radiographs, the first and only question that comes to my mind is, what was missed on these films?" [6].

Consider a medical malpractice case where I was asked to be an expert witness. I was initially given only the following brief summary:

> This case involves a 52 year-old man with a left-sided parietal lesion, which was biopsied. The surgery was complicated by intraoperative hemorrhage, and he has been left weak on the right with speech deficits. Pathology demonstrated that the tissue was a demyelinating lesion.

For some background, demyelinating lesions are seen in diseases like multiple sclerosis (MS) and can almost always be diagnosed without a biopsy. However, occasionally demyelinating lesions can mimic tumors, and a biopsy is necessary to distinguish between these two conditions. Now, consider how this case summary has the potential to bias anyone who reads it. They will know a patient suffered a severe injury. They will know the biopsy may have been unnecessary. Yet, the ambiguities the clinicians faced prior to the biopsy are entirely absent and are unlikely to be grasped by anyone reviewing this case. Thomas Hugh and G. Douglas Tracy recognized the impact of the hindsight bias on medicolegal cases, writing:

> The degree of bias is linked to the severity of the outcome — with severely injured patients, judgements by reviewers tend to be harsher. When reviewers know of an adverse outcome, they tend to trivialize the management dilemmas facing the doctor at the time, overlooking the uncertainties inherent in diagnosis and treatment. Expert opinions frequently include the phrase "it should have been obvious." It has been suggested that hindsight bias is almost always present when that expression is used [7].

They suggested that in the same way the previous record of a defendant is withheld from juries in criminal cases, withholding the outcomes of medical malpractice cases might help reviewers judge cases in a more objective light.

Finally, the hindsight bias can affect research into medical errors and even how the term error is defined. There are many times when a clinician may be perceived to have made an error no matter what they did. Consider Max, a 45-year-old man who complained of severe, disabling back pain after a car accident. He had been unable to work as a result. He was in danger of becoming homeless and was very depressed. He had borrowed opioids from a friend and said they were the only medication that relieved his pain. His doctor, fearing Max was drug-seeking, refused to prescribe such medications. Max then continued to use his friend's medication, and soon thereafter died of an overdose. The doctor may then be blamed for not believing Max and inappropriately assuming that people with legitimate pain simply want to abuse medications. His family may feel that Max's life could have been spared had he been taking these medications under a doctor's supervision. Alternatively, suppose the doctor had acceded to Max's request for opioids and shortly thereafter, he was found dead of an overdose. The doctor may then be blamed for inappropriately prescribing an addictive, dangerous medication.

Recall the article from the *British Medical Journal* (BMJ) about medical errors at the start of the book. It was titled *Medical Error—the Third Leading Cause of Death in the US* [8]. While this seems like an utterly devastating indictment of health care in the US, the severity of the problem depends entirely on how the term "error" is defined. Most people consider an error to be when a patient is accidentally given a fatal dose of a medication or a horribly botched surgery. Yet, the definition of medical error used in the BMJ article was as follows:

> An unintended act (either of omission or commission) or one that does not achieve its intended outcome, the failure of a planned action to be completed as intended (an error of execution), the use of a wrong plan to achieve an aim (an error of planning), or a deviation from the process of care that may or may not cause harm to the patient.

This struck many clinicians as an extremely broad definition of medical error, one defined by the hindsight and outcome biases. Essentially whenever a person dies in a hospital, their death will be attributed to a medical "error" as long as *something* is discovered that should have been done differently. Given that thousands of decisions can be made during the treatment of a hospitalized patient, it is always easy to look back and find *some* way their care was suboptimal.

However, retrospectively identifying these imperfections does mean that an error was made at the time. If the BMJ article is correct, this means that about one in five people who die in a hospital are killed by a medical error, something that seems implausible on its face.

The number of deaths due to medical error are a subject of great debate, precisely because the term "error" is so hard define. A surgeon who operates on the wrong patient has clearly made an error. A neurologist who gives thrombolytic medications to a patient with symptoms that mimic a stroke who then suffers a fatal hemorrhage *may* have made an error, or they may have made a reasonable decision based on the information they had at the time. A patient who acquires an infection in the hospital has certainly been harmed, but this does not necessarily mean that some clinician made an error. However, often these bad patient outcomes are considered in the statistics as a medication error. As Vinay Prasad, an oncologist, wrote about the BMJ article:

> *When it comes to suspected errors, those who think they can always pinpoint which actions led to potentially preventable harm are either kidding themselves or are incredibly arrogant. One of the most difficult things about medicine is that much of the time we don't know for sure if an outcome would have been different had we acted another way. Good doctors agonize about this* [9].

Dr. Prasad wisely suggested this alternate definition of medical error:

> *A medical error is something a provider did or did not do that caused a bad outcome (death in this case) and — this is a big "and" — the action should have been done differently given what was known, or should have been known, at the time.*

Conclusion

Knowing the outcome of a case may prevent a realistic appraisal of what actually occurred, usually leading to the decision maker being seen as more or less culpable than they really were. Most people intuitively feel the final outcome determines the rectitude of a clinical decision. If a patient does well, the clinician is felt to have acted wisely, and conversely if a patient does poorly, the clinician may be felt to have acted foolishly. In medicine, as in all of life, a good decision might lead to a bad outcome, and a bad decision might lead to a good outcome. Because of the hindsight and outcome biases, we tend to focus on the outcome rather than the decision-making process and execution. These biases have been recognized in medicine, as clinicians joke that with the use of a "retrospectoscope," the solution to even the most complicated problem is obvious.

While some errors, such as amputating the wrong limb, are glaringly obvious, in many cases it is less clear that an error was made. It is often easy to look back at a case with a bad outcome and determine that out of thousands of decisions, something could have been done differently. This does not mean that an error was made, however. Similarly, not every complication is evidence that an error was made. For example, about 6% of stroke patients who receive thrombolytic medications will have a symptomatic hemorrhage from it. This does not mean an error was made in a patient who received the medication and bled.

As I am writing this chapter, I am treating one of the worst cases of MS I have ever seen. A 40-year-old man presented to another hospital with confusion over several days. By the time he arrived at our hospital, he was comatose. His brain MRI showed multiple large, actively inflamed lesions. I treated him with high-dose steroids for several days, the standard treatment for active MS, with no improvement. Then, against the advice of some more senior doctors, I treated him with high dose chemotherapy. Was I bold and fearless in the face of a seriously ill man? Or was I a reckless cowboy, needlessly exposing a patient to a serious risk? Do you feel you need to know how the patient fared to answer these questions?

False Memories

Case
Karen was a 34-year-old woman who arrived unconscious after being shot several times in the torso. The trauma team was unable to revive her and she died shortly after arriving to the hospital. On autopsy, a gunshot wound was also found on her thigh, and blood loss from this wound was felt to have contributed to her death. When the trauma team reviewed the case to see if their care could have been improved, multiple team members reported that the intern, Dr. Green, in charge of examining her legs for wounds had not done so. Dr. Green initially defended herself, but faced with the statements from several other team members conceded that she probably had neglected this part of the exam. When video from the security cameras in the trauma bay were reviewed, however, it was clear the intern not only examined Karen's legs, but was in the process of trying to staunch the bleeding when Karen died.

What Dr. Green Was Thinking
During a trauma code, we all have very clear roles, and mine was to examine the patient's extremities for wounds. I remember there was a lot of chaos when Karen arrived. There was blood everywhere, and we could hear people screaming and crying outside the room. The whole thing was kind of a blur. I certainly thought I remembered checking Karen's legs for wounds. But when multiple team members later said that I stood around and was "frozen," then this became my memory too. I even had a long discussion about this with the head of the trauma team where I described how I stood around like a deer-in-headlights. So I was surprised, but relieved, when the security tape showed I did what I was supposed to.

Discussion

An important component of the hindsight bias is recognizing that hindsight is definitely not 20/20. Our memories are vulnerable to multiple, predictable errors. In his book, *The Seven Sins of Memory: How the Mind Forgets and Remembers*, psychologist Daniel Schacter listed the following seven "sins" [10]:

1. **Transience**: Transience refers to the familiar experience of memories fading over time.
2. **Absent-Mindedness:** Absent-mindedness occurs when memories fail due to inadequate attention. People cannot learn new facts while simultaneously engaged in another activity and may forget import items when distracted. Anyone who has lost their glasses or wallet is familiar with this sin.
3. **Blocking**: Blocking occurs when another thought prevents the retrieval of information. This explains the "tip-of-the-tongue" syndrome.
4. **Misattribution**: Misattribution involves failing to accurately the source of information. As a result, real events can be conflated with fictional ones.
5. **Suggestibility**: Suggestibility occurs as memories can be influenced over the course of time by outside influences. A person who witnesses a crime may have their memory altered by hearing the accounts of other witnesses.
6. **Bias:** Bias occurs as a person's feelings and beliefs influence what is recalled about an event. Fans of rival football teams, for example, are likely to have very different recollections of the same game.
7. **Persistence:** Persistence occurs when unpleasant memories cannot be forgotten and intrude our minds without our control. This is the basis of posttraumatic stress disorder (PTSD).

While several of these are likely familiar to us all on a daily basis, others are rather counterintuitive. Though we recognize we forget many things, we generally think that the memories we do have are accurate, immutable, and protected from outside influences. We like to think of our memories as a video camera, faithfully recording events and facts, which we can then accurately retrieve. People often say, "I know what I saw."

The evidence, however, says otherwise. Our memories are likely to be both highly inaccurate and easily manipulated. In the same way that our minds automatically fill in the blind spot in our vision, our minds fill in gaps in our memory based on what we expect to remember. Our minds work hard to create a coherent narrative, often distorting the reality in the process, a phenomenon known as confabulation.

How an event is discussed and perceived afterwards will affect how it is remembered going forward. Once an incident becomes a part of a person's memory, its subsequent recollections will be recalled, not the original event. Our memories are highly prone to what is known as the misinformation effect, which occurs when post-event information distorts a person's recall of events. We are also more likely to remember aspects of event that have personal salience, a phenomenon known as subjective validation. For example, if a psychic makes five accurate statements and 20 false ones when "reading" a client, that client is more likely to remember the correct statements than the incorrect ones. Memories also have a strong social component. If an event is being discussed in a group and one person "remembers" something happening, their memory may be incorporated into the memory of other group members.

Importantly, there is no correlation between people's confidence in a memory and its accuracy. It is common for people to be quite certain about memories that turns out to be false. Contrary to expectations, memories of dramatic incidents and "flashbulb" events are some of the most vulnerable to error. The day after the Challenger shuttle explosion, psychologist Ulric Neisser asked his students to fill out a questionnaire about their experience learning about the disaster [11]. Three years later he repeated these questions. Only 10% completely matched their answers to the originals, and 25% were wrong about every major aspect. There was no correlation between how accurate someone's memory was and how confident they were in its accuracy. In a similar experiment, Deryn Strange and Melanie Takarangi showed subjects a footage of graphic, fatal car crash that was divided into separate scenes separated by blank spots [12]. The next day, subjects were again shown the scene, as well as some of the deleted footage, and asked to remember which scenes they had been shown. While most people did well on recalling the scenes they had been shown, they incorrectly remembered seeing 26% of scenes they had not been shown. They were more likely to misremember traumatic scenes, such as a crying child, than they were to misremember relatively mundane ones, such as the presence of a rescue helicopter.

In fact, there is evidence that more traumatic memories are the most likely to be distorted, and over time people tend to recall events as being more traumatic than they actually were. Steven Southwick and colleagues asked Operation Desert Storm veterans at one month and two years after returning from the Gulf War if they experienced certain traumatic events during that time, such as being shot at by a sniper or watching a fellow solider die [13]. They found 88% of veterans altered their answer at least once and 61% did so more than this. Most of the time, veterans "remembered" events that did not happen rather than forgot events that did happen, and this was associated with an increase in PTSD symptoms.

Perhaps even more disconcerting than mere fallibility of human memory is the relative ease with which people can be made to confidently remember events that did not occur, a phenomenon known as false memories. Take a look at the following list of words: butter, food, eat, sandwich, rye, jam, milk, flour, jelly, dough, crust slice, wine, loaf, toast. About 40% of people can be falsely made to recall a false lure, "bread," from this list [14]. In some situations, researchers have been able to make 72% of false lures being judged as "remembered."

The pioneer of the study of false memories is Elizabeth Loftus, a professor of law and cognitive science. She has shown the fallibility of "recovered" memories of repressed childhood sexual abuse and ritual satanic abuse, work which earned her scorn and even death threats from those whose memories she was questioning. Dr. Loftus says about her work:

> My students and I have now conducted more than 200 experiments involving over 20,000 individuals that document how exposure to misinformation induces memory distortion. In these studies, people "recalled" a conspicuous barn in a bucolic scene that contained no buildings at all, broken glass and tape recorders that were not in the scenes they viewed, a

white instead of a blue vehicle in a crime scene, and Minnie Mouse when they actually saw Mickey Mouse. Taken together, these studies show that misinformation can change an individual's recollection in predictable and sometimes very powerful ways [15].

Dr. Loftus' work has explored the means by which our minds create false memories. In a classic experiment, she showed students slides of car accidents. One showed a car turning at a stop sign and bumping into a pedestrian. Weeks later, subjects were asked about what they saw. When given misleading questions, such as "Did the car stop at the yield sign?" over half of subjects "remembered" seeing a yield sign instead of a stop sign. In another study, she showed subjects footage of a car crash and asked questions such as *"How fast were the cars going?"* Subjects' responses differed based on whether or not they were told the cars had "hit" each other compared to "smashed" into each other. Subjects were also asked if they remembered seeing broken glass, even though there was no glass. Most subjects correctly did not remember glass, but those who were told the cars had smashed into each other were more likely to report its presence. It is not difficult to imagine that memories of a medical case might similarly be distorted based on subtle word twists. Did a surgeon accidently "nick" an artery or "sever" it? Was an important radiographic finding "overlooked" or was it "neglected?" How these questions are phrased will prime and likely significantly impact how people remember an event.

It is even possible to implant vivid, yet completely false, memories (called rich false memories) into people's minds. In another experiment by Dr. Loftus, six of out 24 adult subjects were made to "remember" getting lost as a child, even providing rich details of their experience, despite this never happening [16]. Other researchers convinced people that, as a child, they were the victim of an animal attack, they had an accident at a family wedding, or they fell in water and needed to be rescued by a lifeguard. In another study, subjects were convinced they met Bugs Bunny at a Disney theme park after being showed phony advertisements [17]. Since the Bugs Bunny character is not owned by Disney, this would not happen. The probability of creating a false memory is increased if subjects are asked to vividly imagine an event, a phenomenon known as imagination inflation [15].

The power of false memory is such that people can be convinced they did things they did not actually do. In one study by Saul Kassin and Katherine Kiechel, subjects were falsely accused of crashing a computer by pressing a wrong key (the "ALT" key) [18]. When this action was "witnessed" by a confederate in the experiment:

94% of the innocent participants signed what was in fact a false confession. Perhaps more remarkably, 54% of those people believed they had pressed the "ALT" key when they hadn't, and 20% confabulated facts explaining their non-existent pressing of the "ALT" key.

Julia Shaw and Stephen Porter took this a step further and successfully convinced 70% of university students that when they were young teenagers, they committed a serious felony [19]. Specifically, subjects were told that they had committed assault, assault with a weapon, or theft. Real details from their teenage lives, obtained from the subjects' caregivers, were carefully interspersed with the false memory. With these prompts, some students were able to confabulate extremely rich "memories" of a crime they had never committed. As Dr. Shaw said:

> Our findings show that false memories of committing crime with police contact can be surprisingly easy to generate, and can have all the same kinds of complex details as real memories. All participants need to generate a richly detailed false memory is three hours in a friendly interview environment, where the interviewer introduces a few wrong details and uses poor memory-retrieval techniques [20].

Life examples of false memories are not hard to find. For example, my wife has an interesting false memory. When our daughter was about 3-years-old, she fell at the playground, as children often do. She walked up to me and in her little voice, told me what happened. I needed her to repeat herself several times before I understood her. Only after I grasped and acknowledged that she fell did she burst into tears. Strangely, my wife insists this happened to her, not me, and that I am the one with the false memory. However, since I am writing this book and she is not, I am the one who gets to decide whose memory is false.

Occasionally, false memories can have much more serious consequences. Lyn Balfour told a heartbreaking story of when she accidently left her son in a car, where he died of hyperthermia. She was not a careless mother. Rather, she said that, "I remembered dropping Bryce off, talking to the babysitter. It's what they call false memories" [21]. Tom Kessinger, a mechanic who worked in a rental truck store, gave a detailed description of two men who rented the Ryder truck used in the Oklahoma City terrorist attack. One was the bomber, Timothy McVeigh. The other, Pvt. Todd Bunting of the Army, had large biceps, wore a baseball cap and a black T-shirt, and had a tattoo on his left arm [22]. Mr. Bunting rented a truck the day prior to McVeigh. However, Kessinger combined the two memories and triggered a large manhunt for Mr. Bunting.

A fascinating example of false memories occurred in 2015 when New York City police officers shot and killed a man suspected of attacking several women with a hammer. When interviewed later about the shooting, several witnesses claimed the police acted inappropriately [23]. "He looked like he was trying to get away from the officers," said one witness. "I saw a man who was handcuffed being shot. And I am sorry, maybe I am crazy, but that is what I saw," said another. However, video clearly showed that the suspect was in fact chasing a woman, trying to bash her head in with a hammer when he was shot. When shown the video of the actual event, one surprised witness said:

> With all of the accounts in the news of police officers in shootings, I assumed that police were taking advantage of someone who was easily discriminated against. Based on what I saw, I assumed the worst. Even though I had looked away.

One wonders what the implications of these false memories might have been had video footage not been available, showing the shooting was justified.

At times, a false memory may spread throughout a culture, affecting many people at the same time. This phenomenon, termed the Mandela Effect, was coined by Fiona Broome, who describes herself as a "paranormal researcher." She had a particular false memory that Nelson Mandela died in prison in the 1980s, when in fact he died in 2013. She noticed that she was not alone in this false memory, writing that she "discovered a large community of people who remember the same Mandela history that I recall" [24]. There are several webpages devoted to the Mandela effect. Many people "remember" the comedian Sinbad playing a genie in a 1990s movie Shazaam, though no such movie exists. In researching this, I was shocked to learn that I have some false memories. For example, Darth Vader never actually said, "Luke, I am your father," Hannibal Lecter never said "Hello, Clarice," in the movie *The Silence of the Lambs*, and The Queen in *Snow White* never said, "Mirror, mirror on the wall" [25].

The notion of false memories is alien to most people. Since we can't fathom our own memories being so fallible, we assume others are lying when they are shown to have misremembered something. This is why we are often indignant or disbelieving when other people's memories are shown to be false. Consider the case of Hillary Clinton, who recalled a trip to Bosnia 12 years prior by saying, "I remember landing under sniper fire. There was supposed to be some kind of a greeting ceremony at the airport, but instead we just ran with our heads down to get into the vehicles to get to our base." As later video of the landing proved, this was not the case. However, she was excoriated as a liar in right-wing media outlets for this false memory. Similar examples are not hard to find. News anchor Brian Williams became infamous for claiming a military helicopter in which he was riding was forced down after being hit by a rocket-propelled grenade. However, the pilots in Iraq disputed this, saying said no rocket-propelled grenades had been fired at the helicopter. Mr. Williams was suspended from his job for six months for his false memory [26]. Ronald Reagan was known for repeatedly telling the following story [27]:

> It goes back to a war when a B-17 bomber was flying back across the channel badly shot up by anti-aircraft fire. The ball turret that hung beneath the belly of the plane had taken a hit, was jammed. They couldn't get the ball turret gunner out while they were flying, and he was wounded. And out over the channel the plane started to lose altitude. The skipper ordered bail-out, and as the men started to leave the plane, the boy in the ball turret knew he was being left to go down with the plane. The last man to leave the plane saw the captain sit down on the floor and take his hand, and he said, "Never mind son, we'll ride it down together."

Though he claims to have posthumously awarded the Congressional Medal of Honor to the captain, it turns out this event was from a movie released in 1944 and President Reagan conflated this movie with reality. This conflation of real life with fiction is known as source confusion.

Our memory for factual information, not just events in our lives, is similarly prone to distortion. Once a false belief has been lodged into our minds, it festers there, distorting our ability to learn accurate information. This phenomenon, termed the continued influence effect, posits that "facts" that are later discredited continue to influence our thoughts even after they have been corrected. For example, associating vaccines with autism, if only to debunk the myth that vaccines cause autism, may paradoxically cause some people to link them together. In one demonstration of this, psychologist Norbert Schwarz and colleagues studied peoples' memory of a document produced by the CDC to distinguish myths from facts about the flu [28]. They showed that after 30 minutes, older people believed 28% of the false statements were true and this rose to 40% after three days. Younger people did better initially, but within three days, they also believed nearly a quarter of the false statements were true. Other researchers have failed to replicate these findings, however, indicating that more research needs to be done [29].

A related phenomenon, known as belief perseverance, posits that beliefs often persist even when the initial evidence for them is contradicted. In an experimental model known as the "debriefing paradigm," study subjects are given false information. Their attitude change is measured initially and once the false information is revealed. Even after being told that the initial information was false, many people cling to their belief. In a demonstration of this by Lee Ross and colleagues, subjects were given 25 pairs of suicide notes and asked to determine which were real and which were phony [30]. After reading each note, they were told if they were correct or not. Subjects were told they did poorly (10 correct), average (17 correct), or very well (24 correct). They were then told that they had been deceived about their number of correct answers, and they had performed at an average level. They were then asked to predict how they actually did and how they would do if the task were done again. Despite being told that their initial reports of success or failure were fabricated, the subjects who believed they initially did well had higher estimations for their initial and future performance.

Belief perseverance and the continued influence effect pose significant challenges for anyone who attempts to counter pseudoscience and conspiracy theories. Repeating a myth in order to contradict it may lead some people to believe the myth is true. Moreover, when people already believe a myth, refuting it may inadvertently reinforce that belief. In the short term at least, science advocates may do more harm than good by simply correcting erroneous beliefs. Stephan Lewandowsky and colleagues suggest that when countering myths, the goal should be to replace:

> Misinformation by presenting simple and brief messages that focus on the new, correct information rather than on the incorrect information. When correcting misinformation, provide an alternative — but accurate — narrative of events to fill in the gap left when information once thought true is found to be false [31].

Other strategies have been suggested to combat the fallability of human memory. In response to the seven errors of memory, Colonel Scott S. Haraburda developed seven techniques to improve accurate recall of events [32].

1. Obtain information quickly after an event, when it's fresh in people's minds.
2. Use a prioritized task list.
3. Take notes from important events, including meeting minutes.
4. Record important events and milestones daily.
5. Use neutrally worded questions when soliciting information.
6. Understand the basis or perspective of the person providing the information.
7. Understand and recognize the symptoms of PTSD.

The medical field has used several approaches to account for memory errors. Surgeons have taken steps to minimize the potentially fatal error of surgical

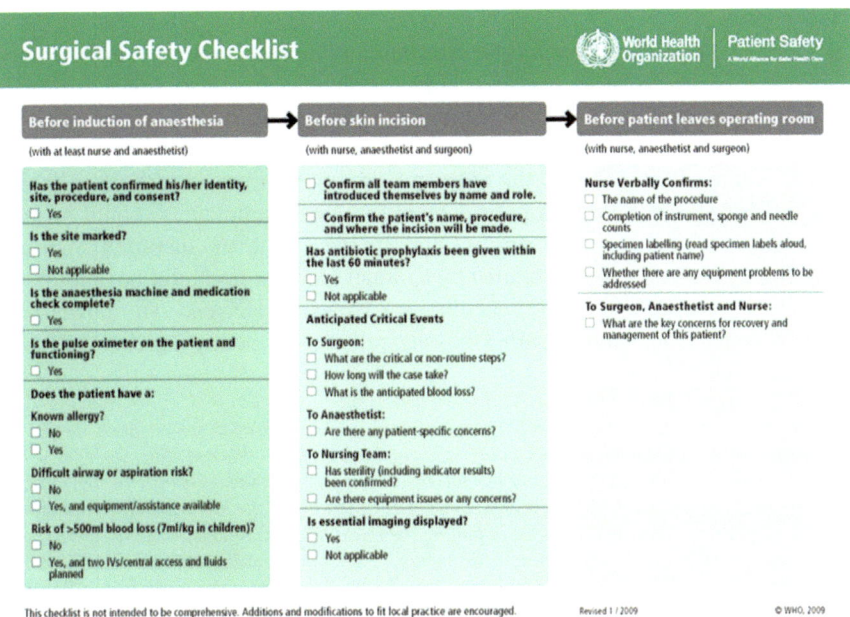

Fig. 14.3 The World Health Organization surgical safety checklist. (The Joint Commission. Universal protocol poster [PDF file]. (n.d.). Retrieved Sept 15, 2018 from https://www.jointcommission.org/assets/1/18/UP_Poster1.PDF.)

material being accidently left inside a patient. Researchers at the Mayo Clinic found that this error was not common, but not rare either, occurring in one in 5,500 operations [33]. As a result, surgical teams routinely count sponges and sharp objects during an operation to make sure all surgical material is accounted for [34]. "Time-outs" are also a necessary part of every operation and medical procedure. They are done prior to the procedure and help ensure that the right procedure is being done on the right patient on the right part of their body [35]. Though they are rare, there are definitely instances of the wrong patient or wrong side of the body being operated on [36]. (Such shocking errors have been termed "never events," reflecting the notion that they should never happen.) Similarly, various checklists are now common in medicine. Rather than relying on memory alone to ensure proper protocol is done during procedures, these checklists ensure that avoidable complications are minimized. The World Health Organization created a checklist in 2008 to minimize errors partially caused by faulty memories (Fig. 14.3) [37].

The use of these checklists has improved patient care. A study by Alex Haynes and colleagues investigated the use of these checklists in 3,955 non-cardiac surgeries at eight hospitals around the world. They found that the use of these checklists decreased the death rate from 1.5% to 0.8% and decreased the complication rate from 11% to 7% [38].

Conclusion

Though we perceive our memories to accurately represent the past, our memories are biased and prone to post-event distortion. Psychologists have shown that memories are not just flawed, but quite malleable. These findings have wide-ranging implications, including the reliability of eyewitness testimony, how police obtain confessions, and how the aftermath of a poor medical outcome is likely to be recalled. When there is a poor outcome in a case, clinicians should be aware that the memories of team members may be inaccurate and distorted. Whenever possible, the techniques developed by Colonel Haraburda should be employed to minimize inaccurate, false memories. Howard Herrell, an obstetrician-gynecologist, also warned against the over-reliance on memory, giving the following sage advice:

> In the pre-computer days, a highly valued quality in a physician was a good memory. Unfortunately, medical schools today still emphasizes this skill, selecting students who might excel in rote memorization but lag behind in critical thinking skills. In the 1950s, memory was everything: there was no quick way of searching the literature, of comprehensively checking drug interactions, of finding the latest treatment guidelines, etc. But today, memory is our greatest weakness. Our memories are poor and biased, and there is more data that we need to have mastery of than ever before in order to be a good doctor. So stop relying on your memory. We need to encourage the habitual use of cognitive aids, whether that's mnemonics, practice guidelines, algorithms, or computers [39].

References

1. Fischhoff B. Hindsight ≠ foresight: the effect of outcome knowledge on judgment under uncertainty. BMJ Qual Saf. 2003;12(4):304–11. https://doi.org/10.1136/qhc.12.4.304.
2. Walker K. (2016, Feb 23). How was 9/11 predicted so many times before it happened? Truth Theory. Retrieved from https://truththeory.com/2016/02/23/how-was-911-predicted-so-many-times-before-it-happened/.
3. Gino F, Moore DA, Bazerman MH. (2009, April 8). No harm, no foul: the outcome bias in ethical judgments. Harvard Business School NON Working Paper No. 08–080. https://doi.org/10.2139/ssrn.1099464.
4. LaBine SJ, LaBine G. Determinations of negligence and the hindsight bias. Law Hum Behav. 1996;20(5):501–16. https://doi.org/10.1007/BF01499038.
5. Caplan RA, Posner KL, Cheney FW. Effect of outcome on physician judgments of appropriateness of care. JAMA. 1991;265(15):1957–60. https://doi.org/10.1001/jama.1991.03460150061024.
6. Berlin L. Malpractice issues in radiology: hindsight bias. Am J Roentgenol. 2000;175(3):597–601. https://doi.org/10.2214/ajr.175.3.1750597.
7. Hugh TB, Tracy GD. Hindsight bias in medicolegal expert reports. Med J Aust. 2002;176(6):277–8.
8. Malary MA, Daniel M. Medical error-the third leading cause of death in the US. BMJ. 2016;353:i2139. https://doi.org/10.1136/bmj.i2139.
9. Prasad V. (2016, May 9). Don't believe what you read on new report of medical error deaths. STAT. Retrieved from https://www.statnews.com/2016/05/09/medical-errors-deaths-bmj/.
10. Murray B. The seven sins of memory. Monit Psychol. 2003;34(9):28. Retrieved from http://www.apa.org/monitor/oct03/sins.aspx.

11. Memories of the Challenger space-shuttle disaster. (2007, Jan 4). Retrieved from http://as-psychology.pbworks.com/w/page/9174277/KeyStudyNeisser.
12. Strange D, Takarangi MK. False memories for missing aspects of traumatic events. Acta Psychol. 2012;141(3):322–6. https://doi.org/10.1016/j.actpsy.2012.08.005.
13. Southwick SM, Morgan CA, Nicolaou AL, Charney DS. Consistency of memory for combat-related traumatic events in veterans of Operation Desert Storm. Am J Psychiatr. 1997;154(2):173–7. https://doi.org/10.1176/ajp.154.2.173.
14. Roediger HL, McDermott KB. Creating false memories: remembering words not presented in lists. J Exp Psychol Learn Mem Cogn. 1995;21(4):803–14. https://doi.org/10.1037/0278-7393.21.4.803.
15. Loftus EF. Creating false memories. Sci Am. 1997;277(3):70–5. Retrieved from http://www.jstor.org/stable/24995913.
16. Loftus EF. Planting misinformation in the human mind: a 30-year investigation of the malleability of memory. Learn Mem. 2005;12(4):361–6. https://doi.org/10.1101/lm.94705.
17. Braun KA, Ellis R, Loftus EF. Make my memory: how advertising can change our memories of the past. Psychol Mark. 2002;19(1):1–23. https://doi.org/10.1002/mar.1000.
18. Kassin SM, Kiechel KL. The social psychology of false confessions: compliance, internalization, and confabulation. Psychol Sci. 1996;7(3):125–8. https://doi.org/10.1111/j.1467-9280.1996.tb00344.x.
19. Shaw J, Porter S. Constructing rich false memories of committing crime. Psychol Sci. 2015;26(3):291–301. https://doi.org/10.1177/0956797614562862.
20. Shaw J. (2015, Jan 15). People can be convinced they committed a crime that never happened. APS: Association for Psychological Science. Retrieved from https://www.psychologicalscience.org/news/releases/people-can-be-convinced-they-committed-a-crime-they-dont-remember.html.
21. Balfour L. (2012, Jan 20). Experience: my baby died in a hot car. The Guardian. Retrieved from https://www.theguardian.com/lifeandstyle/2012/jan/20/my-baby-died-in-hot-car.
22. Thomas J. (1997, Jan 30). Suspect's sketch in Oklahoma case called an error. The New York Times. Retrieved from https://www.nytimes.com/1997/01/30/us/suspect-s-sketch-in-oklahoma-case-called-an-error.html.
23. Dwyer J. (2015, May 14). Witness accounts in midtown hammer attack how the power of false memory. The New York Times. Retrieved from https://www.nytimes.com/2015/05/15/nyregion/witness-accounts-in-midtown-hammer-attack-show-the-power-of-false-memory.html.
24. Broome, F. (2010, Sept 9). Nelson Mandela died in prison? The Mandela Effect. Retrieved from https://mandelaeffect.com/nelson-mandela-died-in-prison/.
25. Hudspeth C. (2016, Oct 13). 20 examples of the Mandela Effect that'll make you believe you're in a parallel universe. BuzzFeed. Retrieved from https://www.buzzfeed.com/christopherhudspeth/crazy-examples-of-the-mandeal-effect-that-will-make-you-ques?.
26. Yu R, Eversley M. (2015, Feb 10). NBC: Brian Williams suspended for six months. USA Today. Retrieved from https://www.usatoday.com/story/money/2015/02/10/brian-williams-nbc-suspended/23200821/.
27. Peters G, Woolley JT. (n.d.). Ronald Reagan: "Remarks on arrival in Berlin" [Transcript]. The American Presidency Project. Retrieved from http://www.presidency.ucsb.edu/ws/?pid=42622.
28. Skurnik I, Yoon C, Schwarz N. (2007). Myths and facts about the flu: health education campaigns can reduce vaccination intentions [PDF file]. Manuscript in review. Retrieved from http://webuser.bus.umich.edu/yoonc/research/Papers/Skurnik_Yoon_Schwarz_2005_Myths_Facts_Flu_Health_Education_Campaigns_JAMA.pdf.
29. Cameron KA, Roloff ME, Friesema EM, Brown T, Jovanovic BD, Hauber S, Baker DW. Patient knowledge and recall of health information following exposure to "facts and myths" message format variations. Patient Educ Couns. 2013;92(3):381–7. https://doi.org/10.1016/j.pec.2013.06.017.
30. Ross L, Lepper MR, Hubbard M. Perseverance in self-perception and social perception: biased attributional processes in the debriefing paradigm. J Pers Soc Psychol. 1975;32(5):880–92. https://doi.org/10.1037/0022-3514.32.5.880.

31. Lewandowsky S, Ecker UK, Seifert CM, Schwarz N, Cook J. Misinformation and its correction: continued influence and successful debiasing. Psychol Sci Public Interest. 2012;13(3):106–31. https://doi.org/10.1177/1529100612451018.
32. Haraburda SS. (2007, Jan/Feb). The "seven sins of memory": how they affect your program [PDF file]. Defense AT&L. p. 30–32. Retrieved from http://www.haraburda.us/Publications/sins2006.pdf.
33. Cima RR, Kollengode A, Garnatz J, Storsveen A, Weisbrod C, Deschamps C. Incidence and characteristics of potential and actual retained foreign object events in surgical patients. J Am Coll Surg. 2008;207(1):80–7. https://doi.org/10.1016/j.jamcollsurg.2007.12.047.
34. Treadwell JR. (2013, Mar). Prevention of surgical items being left inside patient: brief update review. In: Making health care safer II: an updated critical analysis of the evidence for patient safety practices (Chapter 15). Rockville: Agency for Healthcare Research and Quality (US). Available from https://www.ncbi.nlm.nih.gov/books/NBK133403/.
35. The Joint Commission. (n.d.). Universal protocol poster [PDF file]. Retrieved 15 Sept 2018 from https://www.jointcommission.org/assets/1/18/UP_Poster1.PDF.
36. U.S. Department of Health and Human Services, Agency for Healthcare Research and Quality. (2018). Wrong-site, wrong-procedure, and wrong-patient surgery. Retrieved from https://psnet.ahrq.gov/primers/primer/18/wrong-site-wrong-procedure-and-wrong-patient-surgery.
37. NHS Improvement. (2018, June 12). Learning from patient safety incidents. NHS Improvement. Retrieved from https://improvement.nhs.uk/resources/learning-from-patient-safety-incidents/.
38. Haynes AB, Weiser TG, Berry WR, Lipsitz SR, Breizat AHS, Dellinger EP, Herbosa T, Joseph S, Kibatala PL, Lapitan MC, Merry AF, Moorthy K, Reznick RK, Taylor B, Gawande AA. A surgical safety checklist to reduce morbidity and mortality in a global population. N Engl J Med. 2009;360(5):491–9. https://doi.org/10.1056/NEJMsa0810119.
39. Herrell H. (n.d.) Debiasing strategies. Howardisms.com. Retrieved 15 Sept 2018 from http://www.howardisms.com/cognitive-bias/debiasing-strategies/.

Illusionary Correlation, False Causation, and Clustering Illusion

Case

David was a 34-year-old man with temporal lobe epilepsy who presented to a neurologist's office for a routine consultation. He had been taking seizure medications for many years, but wished to stop them, saying he was "tired of taking medications." While his neurologist did not encourage him to do so, he suggested treatment with turmeric, saying that a number of his patients with epilepsy had remarkable reductions in seizure frequency with the use of this supplement. David eagerly embraced this approach and was seizure-free on daily turmeric supplements for six months.

What Dr. Benjamin Was Thinking

I was first introduced to turmeric from a patient who told me that it had cut his seizures in half. I reviewed some of the literature on it, and though there were no human studies of turmeric in epilepsy, there was promising animal data. Moreover, turmeric is a spice used around the world. So it is safe. As such, I started suggesting it to my patients, and almost all of them reported a reduction in the frequency of their seizures. Bharat Aggarwa, a highly respected oncologist, echoed my experience, saying in an interview, "I've been working with curcumin and turmeric for 25 years, I've seen and studied the effects, and I can't deny the benefits I see" [1].

However a large systematic review later found that "evidence that, contrary to numerous reports, the compound has limited—if any—therapeutic benefit" [2]. While turmeric itself is very unlikely to be harmful, I don't know if it is fair to say I didn't harm my patients. My job is to give them the best advice according to science, not what I have personally observed. And who knows, maybe patients were telling me what they thought I wanted to hear, minimizing the number of seizures they actually had after taking turmeric. Though I certainly didn't suggest that my patients stop their anti-epileptic medications, I am sure David was not the only patient who did so. Meanwhile, Dr. Aggarwa resigned in 2015 due to allegations of fraudulent research, and nearly 20 of his papers were retracted.

© Springer International Publishing AG, part of Springer Nature 2019
J. Howard, *Cognitive Errors and Diagnostic Mistakes*,
https://doi.org/10.1007/978-3-319-93224-8_15

Discussion

Illusionary correlation is the tendency to believe there is a relationship between two variables when they are both present when in fact, no such relationship exists. False causation is the mistake of assuming one variable caused another when a correlation is identified. It is formalized as the *post hoc ergo propter hoc* fallacy (Latin for "after this, therefore because of this."), which posits that because one event occurred after another, the first caused the second. In medical studies, illusionary correlation and false causation can lead to the incorrect rejection of the null hypothesis (a type I or "false positive" error).

When two variables appear to be correlated, there are several possibilities:

- **X causes Y (true causation):** Often, X causes Y. Often one thing coming after the other often means there is a causal relationship. Cigarettes can cause lung cancer, alcohol can cause cirrhosis, and vitamin C prevents scurvy (Fig. 15.1). As statistician Edward Tufte said, "Correlation is not causation, but it sure is a hint."

- **Y causes X (reverse causation):** Reverse causation occurs when Y causes X, but X is erroneously thought to cause Y. It would occur if someone was to conclude that because roosters crow when the sun rises, roosters cause the sun to rise. To point to a real-life example, anti-vaccine activists seized on a small subset of data

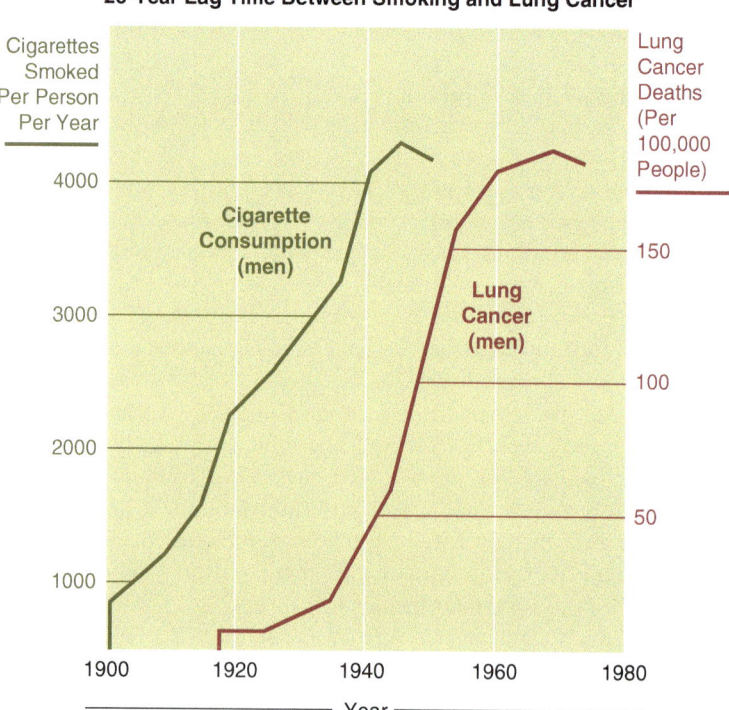

Fig. 15.1 True causation. (Sakurambo. Cancer smoking lung cancer correlation from NIH [Image file]. In: Wikimedia commons. 2007. Retrieved from https://commons.wikimedia.org/wiki/File:Cancer_smoking_lung_cancer_correlation_from_NIH.svg.)

Fig. 15.2 Reverse causation. (State Library of Queensland, Australia. Child driving a toy car [Image file]. In: Wikimedia commons. (n.d.). Retrieved from https://commons. wikimedia.org/wiki/ File:Child_driving_a_toy_ car_(6145780380).jpg.)

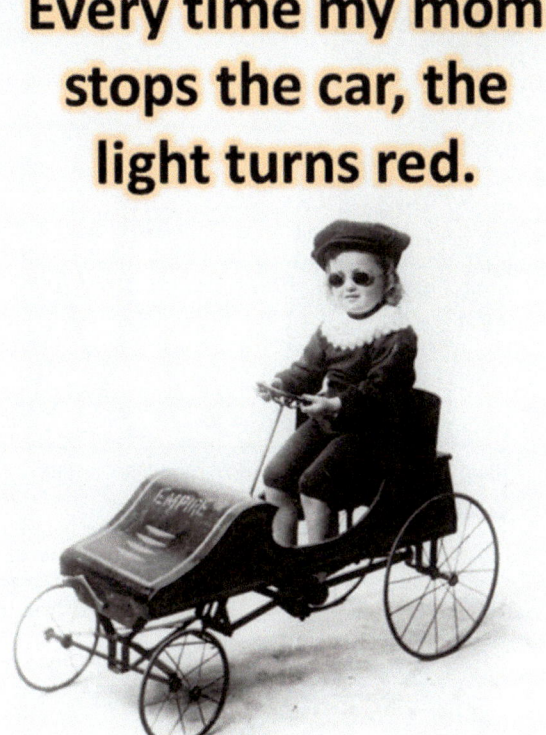

Every time my mom stops the car, the light turns red.

from a study that showed African-American boys with autism received the measles, mumps, and rubella (MMR) vaccine at a higher rate than non-autistic boys. However, this does not mean that vaccines caused autism (Fig. 15.2). As pediatrician Paul Offit explained:

In order to qualify for autism-support programs, this subset of under-vaccinated children with autism had to get vaccinated. In other words, it wasn't that MMR had caused autism; it was that the diagnosis of autism had caused them to get MMR [3].

- **X causes Y AND Y causes X (bi-directional correlation):** In some circumstances, X causes Y and Y causes X. This bi-directional correlation can be seen with predator/prey populations, for example. As the population of rabbits goes up, so does the population of wolves, which then causes the population of rabbits to fall (Fig. 15.3).

- **Z causes both X and Y (third cause fallacy):** X and Y can appear correlated when they are both caused by a third factor, Z. For example, at the height of the polio epidemic, some scientists blamed the disease on ice cream, noting that as ice cream sales increased, so did polio rates. The common cause of both was summertime, which increased both ice cream sales and opportunities for the transmission of polio (Fig. 15.4).

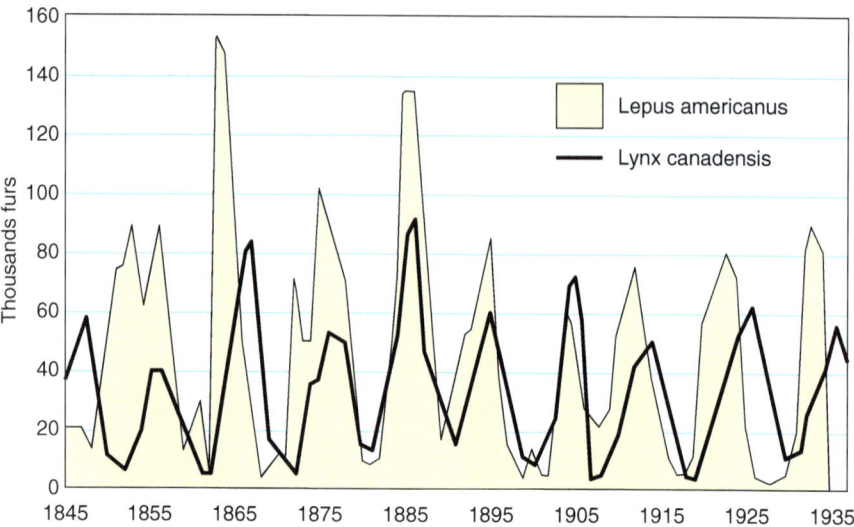

Fig. 15.3 Bi-directional correlation in a population of animals. (Lamiot. Canad lynx and American hare [Image file]. In: Wikimedia commons. 2015. Retrieved from https://commons.wikimedia. org/w/index.php?search=predator+prey+graph&title=Special:Search&go=Go#/media/ File:Milliers_fourrures_vendues_en_environ_90_ans_odum_1953_en.jpg.)

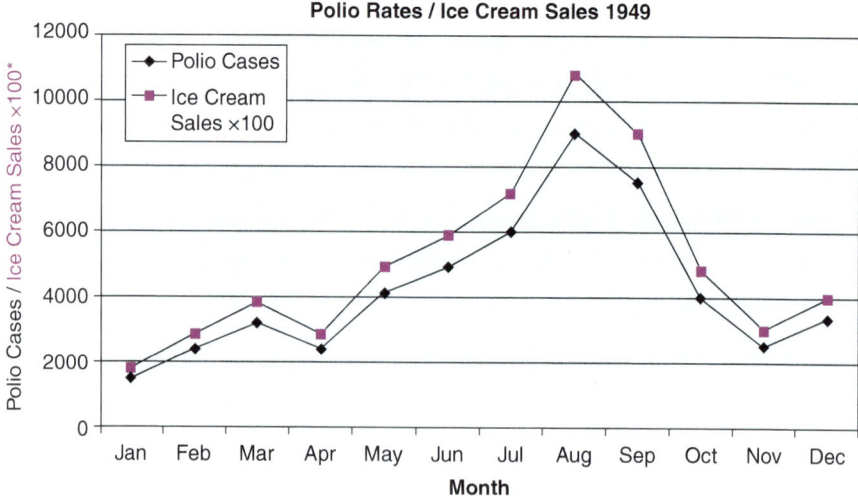

Fig. 15.4 Third cause fallacy; summertime led to an increase in both ice cream sales and polio. (Herrell H. How do I know if a study is valid? [Image file]. Howardisms.com. (n.d.). Retrieved Sept 15, 2018 from http://www.howardisms.com/evidence-based-medicine/how-do-i-know-if-a-study-is-valid/.)

Another example of the third cause fallacy can be seen with certain anti-psychiatry activists who are certain that psychotropic medications are responsible for mass shootings and other acts of violence. Though many of these killers never sought psychiatric care, several others had done so on their own or at the request of others and had been placed on medications at some point. While it may be true that

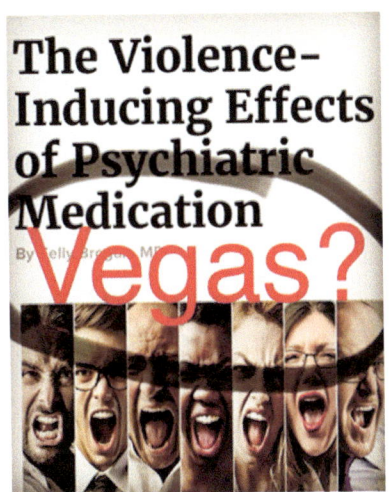

Kelly Brogan MD - Holistic Psychiatrist
Like This Page · 2 October ·

While Pharma-funded media points fingers at terrorists, guns, and mental illness, those of us who know of the evidence-based propensity for psychiatric medications (and associated withdrawal) to induce violence are waiting to learn what we already suspect to be true. To an incident, every mass shooting and murder (including the Germanwings crash) was committed by someone under the influence. This is how and why psychiatric prescribing has become an urgent matter of public health and basic safety. May this be the darkness before the dawn.

The Violence-Inducing Effects of Psychiatric Medication
By Kelly Brogan MD
Vegas?

Fig. 15.5 Psychiatrist Kelly Brogan commits the third cause fallacy, blaming psychiatric medications for violence. (Brogan K. [Kelly Brogan MD]. While Pharma-funded media points fingers at terrorists, guns, and mental illness, those of us who know of the evidence-based propensity [Facebook status update]. 2017. Retrieved from https://www.facebook.com/KellyBroganMD/photos/a.245158725690983/755097854697065/?type=3.)

psychotropic medications cause individuals to commit mass shootings, a more plausible explanation is that severe mental illness can rarely lead individuals to commit such shootings and severely mentally ill people are likely to have been prescribed medications in the past. After all, it is not difficult to imagine that the same symptoms that led them to eventually commit acts of terror also led a psychiatrist to suggest medications to them. Anti-psychiatry advocates insist that correlation equals causation, however, often to push an agenda (Fig. 15.5). For example, The Citizens Commission on Human Rights, an anti-psychiatry organization funded by Scientology, wrote a typically provocative article titled, *36 School Shooters/School Related Violence Committed by Those Under the Influence of Psychiatric Drugs* [4]. Psychiatrist Joseph Pierre correctly debunked such claims by writing:

> *If psychiatric medications were being taken, it might be more accurate to say that they weren't working very well rather than assuming causality in terms of violence…And then, of course, there's the issue of correlation vs. causality. After all, I'm fairly certain all known mass murderers were drinkers of tap water, which has also been linked to violent outbursts* [5].

Perhaps the most damaging example of the third cause fallacy has been the myth that vaccines cause autism. Many parents first notice autism symptoms in children at the same age when they receive many vaccines. This is because a third factor, namely being a certain age, exposes children to many vaccines and allows autism to be detected.

- **X and Y are coincidently related:** Sometimes X and Y are related by pure coincidence. The most famous example of illusionary correlation is a graph showing the decline of pirates correlates with the global average temperature (Fig. 15.6) [6].

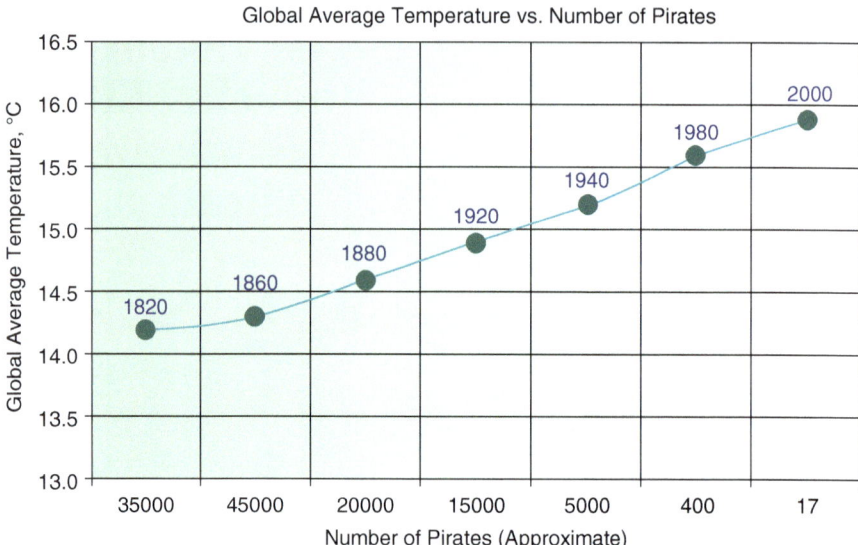

Fig. 15.6 Coincidental correlation, unless you think pirates cause global warming. (Kaiserscience. Correlation and causation [Image file]. (n.d.). Retrieved from https://kaiserscience.wordpress.com/ physics/the-scientific-method/correlation-and-causation/.)

When presented with variables that are appear to be highly correlated, it can be difficult to distinguish which of these relationships exist. Consider the following graph, popularized by Stephanie Seneff, a senior research scientist at the Massachusetts Institute of Technology Computer Science and Artificial Intelligence Laboratory. She claimed that glyphosate (sold by Monsanto as RoundUp), an herbicide commonly-used on genetically modified crops, is responsible for a rise in autism (Fig. 15.7). She also claimed that "At today's rate, by 2025, one in two children will be autistic" [7].

Dr. Seneff's graph garnered a significant amount of attention, particular among groups opposed to genetically modified foods. The website vaccine-injury.info, for example, published several videos of Dr. Seneff and wrote:

> *Numerous health problems increased after GMOs were introduced in 1996. The percentage of Americans with three or more chronic illnesses jumped from 7% to 13% in just 9 years; food allergies skyrocketed, and disorders such as autism, diabetes, reproductive disorders, digestive problems, and others are on the rise. Dr. Stephanie Seneff explains how glyphosate (Round Up) causes nutritional deficiencies leading to diseases such as autism, alzheimer's, crone's, parkinson's, multiple sclerosis, muscle wasting, irritable bowel disease and leaky gut syndrome* [8].

Certainly, the correlation between glyphosate and autism is quite strong, and the graph is visually compelling. But does this mean that glyphosate *causes* autism? Others have jokingly suggested that the real culprit is organic food. After all, the prevalence of autism correlates nearly perfectly with increased sales of organic food (Fig. 15.8) [9].

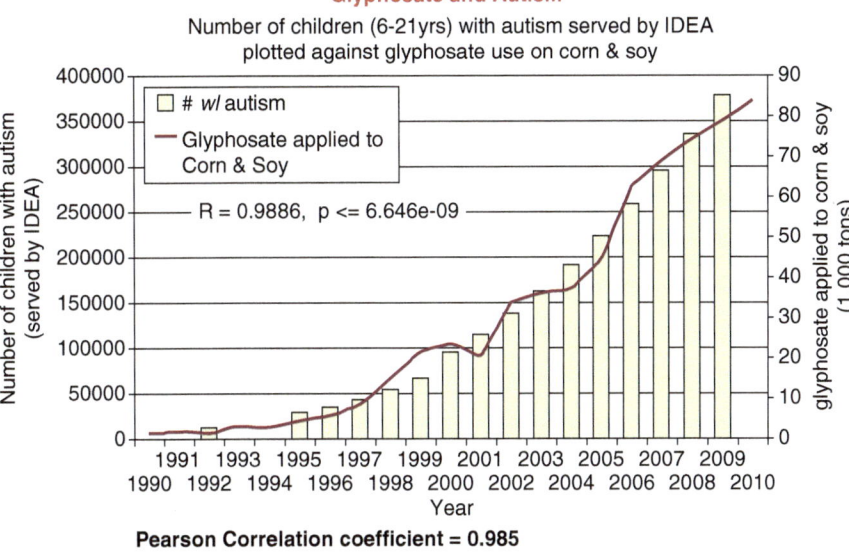

Fig. 15.7 The rates of autism have risen in lockstep with the use of glyphosate. (Honeycutt Z. Swanson charts: Glyphosate and GMOs linked to neurological disorders and more [Image file, Blog post]. Moms across America. 2014. Retrieved from https://www.momsacrossamerica.com/glyphosate_linked_to_neurological_disorders.)

Obviously, the idea that organic food causes autism is ridiculous, and the best available evidence suggests that the autism rate is not increasing at all, rather the condition is more widely recognized now than in the past. However, Dr. Seneff and many others are adamantly convinced that her graph proves that glyphosate causes autism.

Tyler Vigen created a fantastic website, appropriately called Spurious Correlations, full of purposefully ridiculous correlations [10]. He found, for example, that the number people who drowned by falling into swimming pools correlates with the number of films starring Nicolas Cage. Other findings include that the age of Miss America correlates with murders by steam, hot vapors and hot objects, and that the per capita consumption of mozzarella cheese correlates with the number of civil engineering doctorates awarded (Fig. 15.9).

Clinicians, like everyone else, can be easily fooled by illusionary correlation and false causation. Consider the statement from anti-vaccine doctor, Paul Thomas, which he felt important enough to make into a meme to help sell his book (Fig. 15.10).

Does "data" from his own practice trump controlled trials of tens of thousands of children? Or does his data (which I could not find published in a peer-reviewed article) merely show that Dr. Thomas has been duped by false causation? This speaks to a key aspect of illusionary correlation and false causation; because of confirmation bias, people are likely to find and believe patterns that confirm their pre-existing biases. People who are suspicious of vaccines will look for evidence

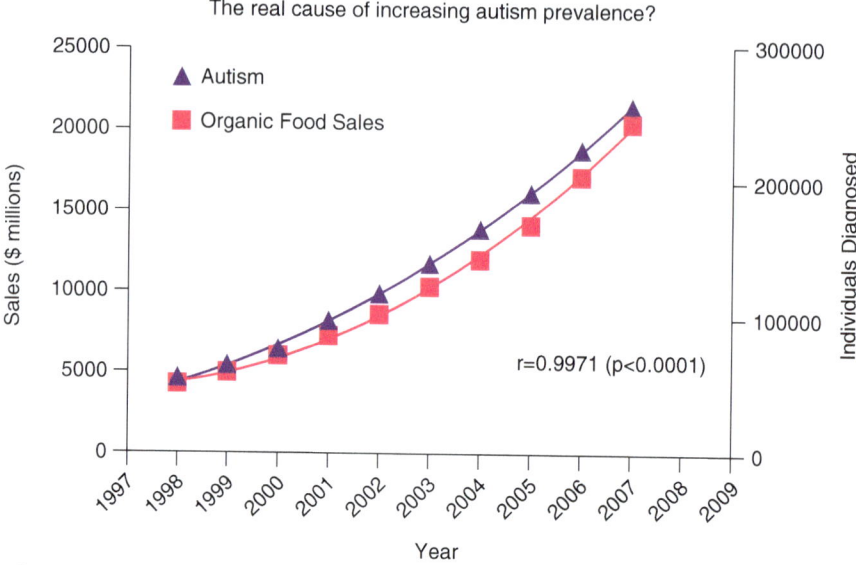

Fig. 15.8 The rates of autism have also risen in lockstep with the sales of organic food. (Suresh A. Autism increase mystery solved? No, it's not vaccines, GMOs, glyphosate – or organic foods [Image file]. Genetic Literacy Project. 2016. Retrieved from https://geneticliteracyproject.org/2016/09/22/autism-increase-mystery-solved-no-its-not-vaccines-gmos-glyphosate-or-organic-foods/.)

they cause harm and will be less critical of data that fits their narrative. People who believe chemical or electric companies are producing dangerous products will be primed to find disease clusters that support this this (Fig. 15.11).

In contrast, people will immediately recognize spurious correlations that do not fit their narratives. No anti-vaccine advocate will believe that vaccines lower the crime rate. However, the crime rate has drastically fallen over the past 30 years, while the number of routine childhood vaccinations has increased over this period. Honest investigators will always acknowledge the possibility of illusionary correlation or false causation, while someone pushing an agenda will almost never do so.

In contrast to Dr. Thomas, I hope that when my personal experience does not mesh with large clinical trials, I'm humble enough to assume that my necessarily limited experience is the outlier, not the scientific evidence. However, I know how easy it is to be fooled by false causation, especially when it makes one of my treatments seem helpful and effective. Like all clinicians, I want my patients to feel better, and I feel good when I feel I played a role in their recovery. Yet, many diseases improve spontaneously, and a clinician may easily confuse this natural history with the effects of their treatment. Often, I have seen patients with multiple sclerosis recover from a relapse after I have given them steroids.

Number of people who drowned by falling into a pool
correlates with
Films Nicolas Cage appeared in
Correlation: 66.6% (r=0.666004)

Data sources: Centers for Disease Control & Prevention and Internet Database

Age of Miss America
correlates with
Murders by steam, hot vapors, and hot objects
Correlation: 87.01% (r=0.870127)

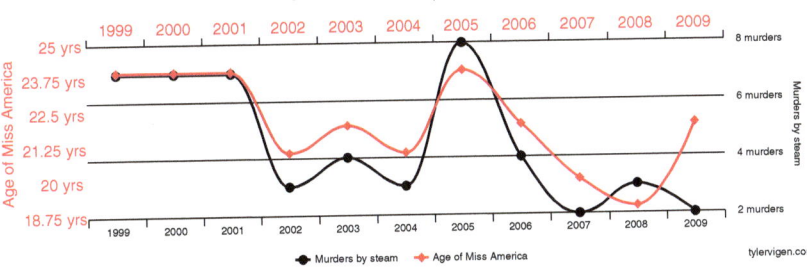

Data sources: Wikipedia and Centers for Disease Control & Prevention

Per capita consumption of mozzarella cheese
correlates with
Civil engineering doctorates awarded
Correlation: 95.86% (r=0.958648)

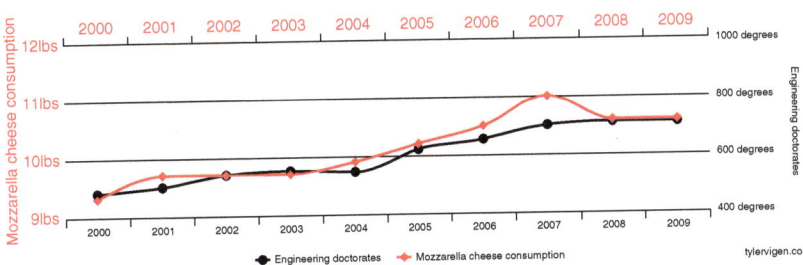

Data sources: US Department of Agriculture and National Secience Foundation

Fig. 15.9 Spurious correlations

Fig. 15.10 Dr. Paul Thomas and false correlation. (Thomas P, Margulis J. The vaccine-friendly plan: Dr. Paul's safe and effective approach to immunity and health – from pregnancy through your child's teen years. New York: Ballantine Books; 2016. p. 118–119.)

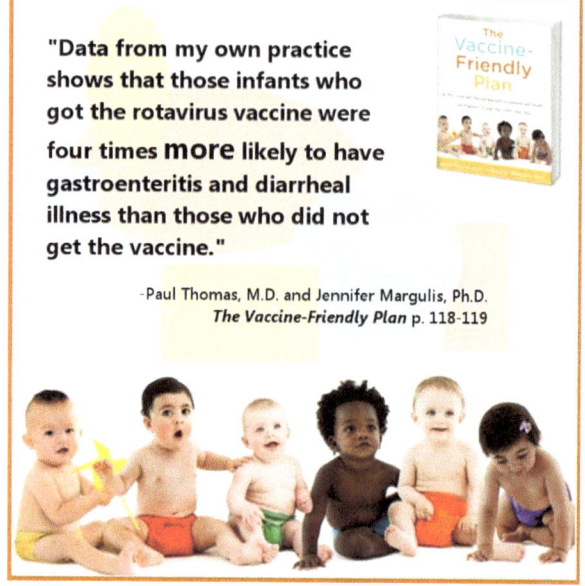

Fig. 15.11 I agree. (Contrived Platitudes. [Image file, Facebook status update]. 2016. Retrieved from https://www.facebook.com/contrivedplatitudes/posts/1721897721462036:0.)

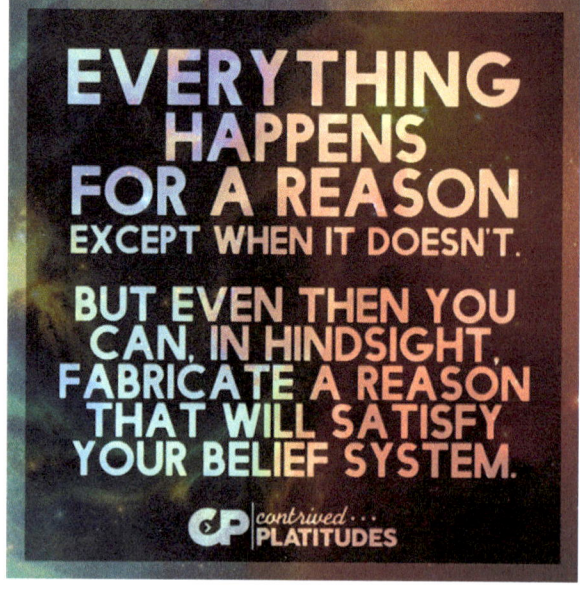

Other times, however, I have seen patients recover spontaneously without any treatment. Had I given them steroids, however, I have no doubt that I would have attributed their recovery to this treatment. Similarly, I have seen many stroke patients significantly recover shortly after receiving thrombolytic medications. Invariably, their recovery is attributed to this treatment, though the studies show its benefits are not apparent until three months later.

Such false causation is the reason that many treatments that really seem to work based on enthusiastic patient reports often fail when subject to rigorous clinical trials. Some very common procedures, such as arthroscopic surgery for degenerative knee arthritis and meniscal tears, failed when subject to blinded trials where patients were randomized to receive either genuine or sham surgery [11]. Almost no alternative treatment, such as acupuncture or reiki, passes muster when properly studied. The apparent success of these treatments shows the power of the placebo effect and the natural history of many diseases; patients will often improve no matter what is done and any intervention will receive credit.

In medicine, this phenomenon is known as the therapeutic illusion and was defined as "the unjustified enthusiasm for treatment on the part of both patients and doctors" [12]. It comes from a paper by Dr. KB Thomas who studied 200 patients in whom no definitive diagnosis could be made. Half of the patients were given a symptomatic diagnosis and treated, while others were told no there was no evidence of disease and no treatment was given. No difference was noticed between these two groups based on whether the patient returned in a month and their report that they did or did not improve.

At times, false causation can effect large swaths of the population. A famous example occurred with the use of hormone replacement therapy (HRT) in post-menopausal women. Several epidemiological studies showed that women taking HRT had a lower incidence of cardiovascular disease, and millions of women took HRT for this reason. However, when it was studied in a randomized, controlled trial, HRT was shown to cause a small but real increase in the risk of heart attacks, strokes, and blood clots [13]. More recent data suggests that HRT has no effect at all on mortality [14]. Regardless, women who took HRT hoping to prolong their lives (as opposed to treating the symptoms of menopause) were wasting their time. It turned out that women in the original epidemiological studies were wealthier than average and likely engaged in other activities, such as eating a healthy diet and exercising, that prevented cardiovascular disease. Given that the users of HRT had a better-than-average diet and exercise regimens, a third cause led to both the use of HRT and a lower incidence of heart disease.

Another example of erroneous false causation occurred when a highly effective vaccine against pertussis was discontinued due to its supposed propensity to cause seizures. It is true that a number of children developed severe epilepsy shortly after the vaccine. However, it is now known that these seizures were due to a rare genetic condition called Dravet syndrome [15]. While the vaccine might have triggered the earlier onset of seizures, these children would have developed epilepsy regardless, and the vaccine did not affect the overall prognosis of the disease. Despite this, this vaccine is no longer used, and its replacement is much less effective. There has been a resurgence of the disease, with tens of thousands of cases and dozens of deaths in the US alone (Fig. 15.12).

A particular form of illusionary correlation is known as the clustering illusion. It shows how people are prone to finding patterns even in completely random data. Our brains are pattern-seeking machines. We see faces in clouds and religious figures in everyday objects. Pareidolia refers to the psychological phenomenon where the brain involuntarily perceives a pattern when none exists. The term is most often

Fig. 15.12 It is easy to find patterns when they confirm our beliefs. (Contrived Platitudes. [Image file, Facebook status update]. 2015. Retrieved from https://www.facebook.com/contrivedplatitudes/posts/1480321362286341:0.)

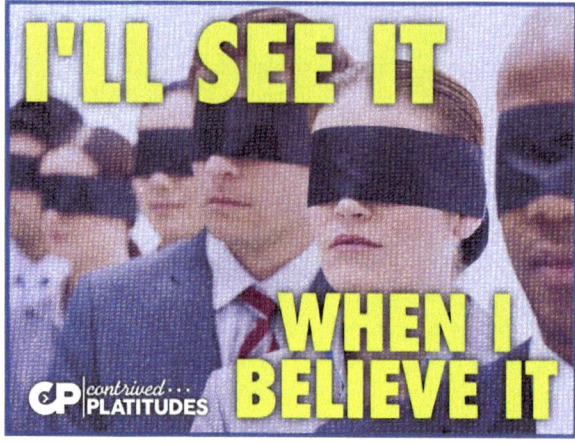

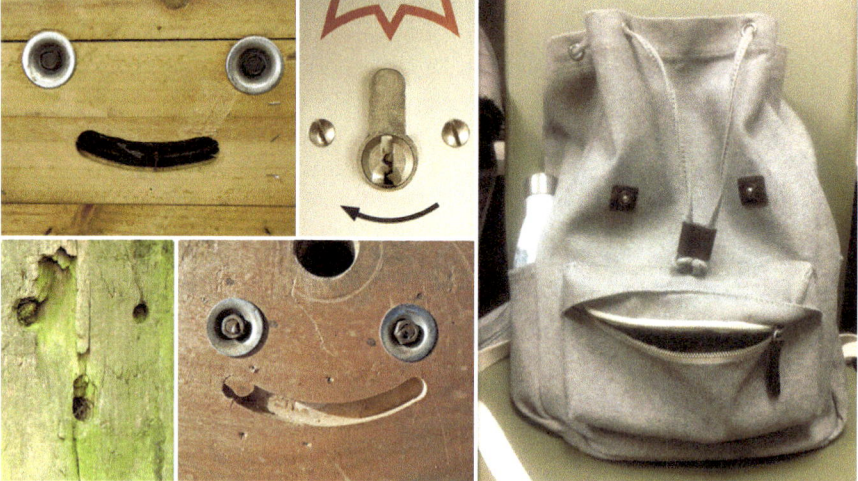

Fig. 15.13 Pareidolia. (**Left**: Pixeltoo. Collage de plusieurs photos montrant des paréidolies [Image file]. In Wikimedia commons. 2016. Retrieved from https://commons.wikimedia.org/wiki/Category:Anthropomorphic_pareidolias#/media/File:Collage_par%C3%A9idolies.jpg.)

applied to the fact that we involuntary see faces in mundane objects such as clouds or geological formations (Fig. 15.13).

Shown above is the *Face on M*ars taken by Viking 1 in 1976 (Fig. 15.14). This image led some people to believe that there had been previous civilization on Mars, spawning books such as *The Monuments of Mars: A City on the Edge of Forever* by Richard Hoagland.

Artists can take advantage of our brain's tendency to see certain patterns to create clever works of art. *Vertumnus* and *The Jurist* by Giuseppe Arcimboldo appear to be portraits. Upon closer inspection, the "person" in one picture is made entirely of fruit, while the "face" in the other is a collection of fish and poultry (Fig. 15.15).

Fig. 15.14 The Face on Mars. (Cydonia (region of Mars). (n.d.). [Image file]. In Wikipedia. Retrieved from https://en.wikipedia.org/wiki/Cydonia_(region_of_Mars)#/media/File:Martian_face_viking_cropped.jpg.)

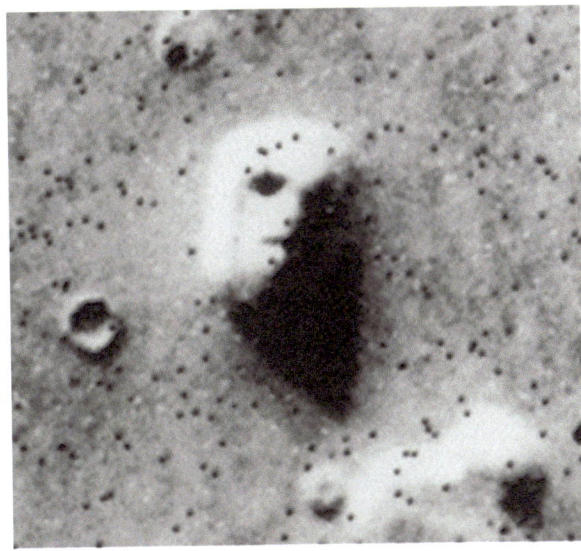

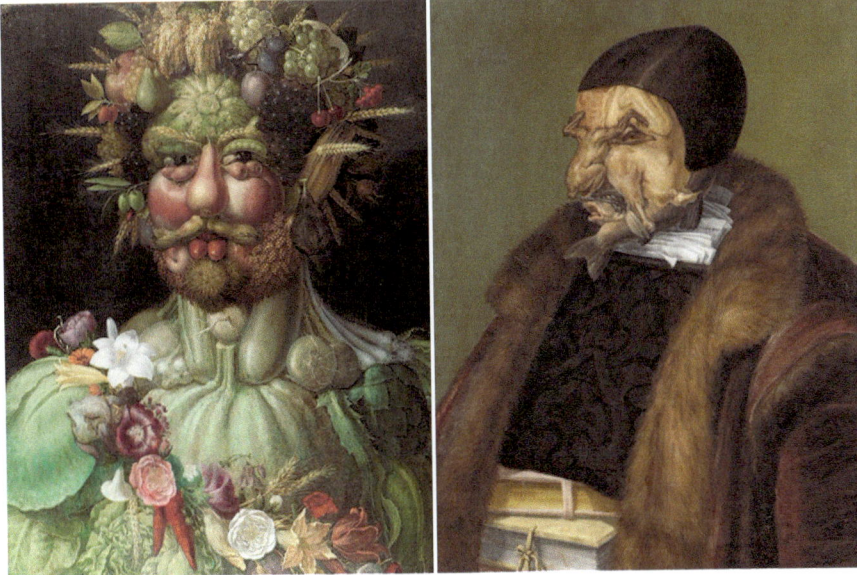

Fig. 15.15 *Vertumnus* and *The Jurist* by Giuseppe Arcimboldo. (Arcimboldo G. [Image files]. In: Giuseppe Arcimboldo: The complete works [Image files]. (n.d.). Retrieved from https://www.giuseppe-arcimboldo.org/?ps=96.)

Apophenia is a broader term that refers to the tendency to perceive meaningful patterns with random information. It is commonly seen in conspiracy-prone and mentally ill people who can "connect the dots," even when there are no dots to connect (Fig. 15.16).

To see how the clustering illusion might affect those searching for the cause of a disease, look these 1,000 points (Fig. 15.17).

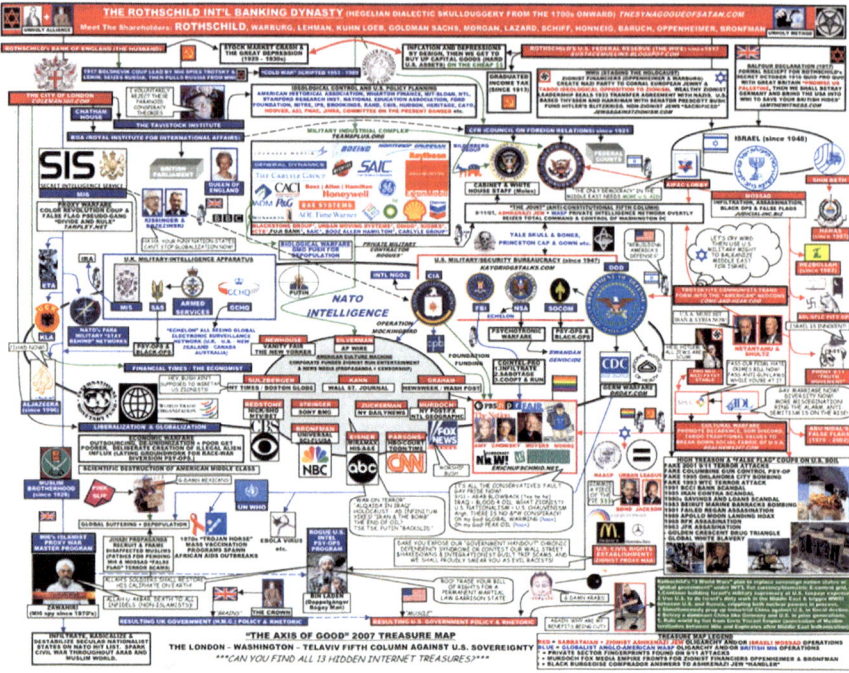

Fig. 15.16 Apophenia. (TruthMove. The axis of good 2007 treasure map [Image file]. In: Truthmove: international truth movement. (n.d.). Retrieved from http://www.truthmove.org/tmp/chart1.png.)

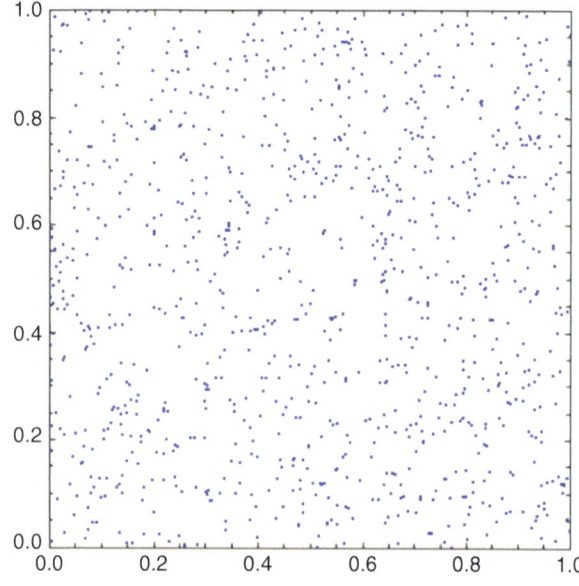

Fig. 15.17 1,000 random points. (CaitlinJo. RandomPoints [Animated image file]. In: Wikipedia. 2013. Retrieved Sept 15, 2018 from https://en.wikipedia.org/wiki/Clustering_illusion#/media/File:RandomPoints.gif.)

If we imagine that each of these dots represented a case of cancer in a city, it would be easy to assume that there was something in the environment that caused certain areas to have many cases the disease, while other areas seem relatively immune. This image was created with a program that adds 100 random dots at a time up to 10,000 dots [16]. No matter how many times the program is run, "clusters" invariably appear.

People generally do a very poor job at estimating the natural frequency of clusters. The most famous demonstration of this is the birthday problem. Pretend you were in a room of people. If there were 366 people, it is 100% certain that at least two people would share a birthday. How many people would there have to in the room be before the likelihood of at least two people having the same birthday was over 50%? Most people estimate that the answer is close to 100 people. However, with only 23 people, the odds are 50% that at least two people will share the same birthday. With 70 people, the odds are 99.9% that at least two people will share the same birthday [17]. Yet, most people would find it a remarkable coincidence if two people in a group of 20 had the same birthday.

Moreover, events that appear non-random attract our attention. For example, someone who picks four aces from a well-shuffled deck of cards will notice this fortunate pattern. They might assume something extremely unlikely happened, and they would be right. The first ace is a 4/52 chance, the second ace is 3/51, the third ace is 2/50, and the fourth is 1/49. Multiply these all together and one finds the probability of drawing four aces is only 1/270,725. In contrast, someone who drew the two of clubs, four of hearts, eight of spades, and ace of diamonds wouldn't blink an eye, even though the probability of drawing these four cards is exactly the same as drawing four aces.

The clustering illusion leads us to see patterns in random data and the birthday problem shows how our intuitive grasp of probability can sometimes be quite misguided. These phenomenon help explain the occurrence of "cancer clusters," which happen when many people in a small area contract a cancer at a rate seemingly greater than chance. This often triggers a search for an environmental cause, such as a power plant or chemical factory. Other than clear occupational exposures, upon further investigation, these clusters almost always turn out to be an illusion.

According to Michael Thun and Thomas Sinks:

> In approximately 5% to 15% of the reported situations, formal statistical testing confirms that the number of observed cases exceeds the number expected in a specific area, given the age, sex, and size of the affected population. Even in these instances, however, chance remains a plausible explanation for many clusters, and further epidemiologic investigation almost never identifies the underlying cause of disease with confidence. The few exceptions have involved clusters of extremely rare cancers occurring in well-defined occupational or medical settings, generally involving intense and sustained exposure to an unusual chemical, occupation, infection, or drug [18].

Of course, the ability to find such patterns is not necessarily a negative, as observant people can find important new connections between seemingly unrelated events. Occasionally, disease clusters provide invaluable information, and they should not be dismissed out of hand. A map of London created by in 1854 by the doctor John Snow shows how important it is to notice real clusters (Fig. 15.18).

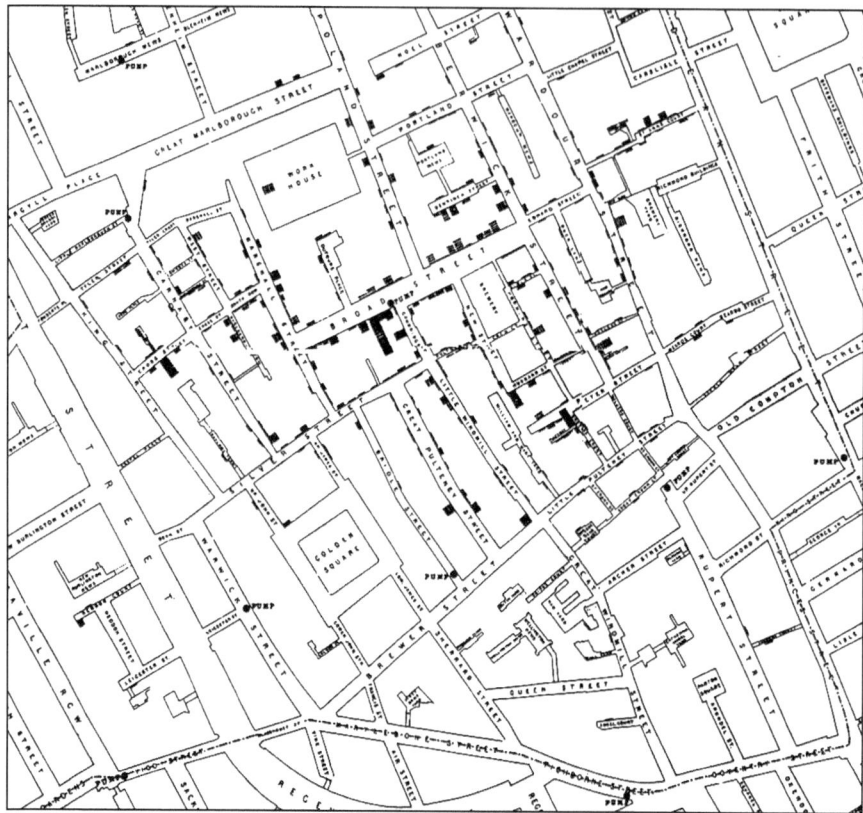

Fig. 15.18 You know something John Snow. (Snow cholera map [Image file]. In: Wikipedia. (n.d.). Retrieved Sept 15, 2018 from https://en.wikipedia.org/wiki/File:Snow-cholera-map-1.jpg.)

In Snow's map, cholera cases are highlighted in black, showing a cluster of cholera cases around a pump on Broad Street [19]. This was enough to convince people to disable the well and is considered the seminal event in the founding of epidemiology. In more modern times, the AIDS epidemic was first recognized when the CDC published a cluster of five young men in Los Angeles with a rare lung infection, *Pneumocystis carinii pneumonia.* All of these patients also had cytomegalovirus and candidal mucosal infections. Two of them were already dead. In the following days, numerous similar cases among gay men were reported to the CDC, including a cluster of cases of Kaposi's sarcoma, a rare and aggressive cancer caused by a herpesvirus infection.

Similarly, true clusters of vaccine-preventable diseases have occurred in areas of low vaccine uptake. The maps from a large measles outbreak in the Netherlands in 2013, show measles cases clustered together in areas where members of a church had refused to vaccinate their children (Fig. 15.19).

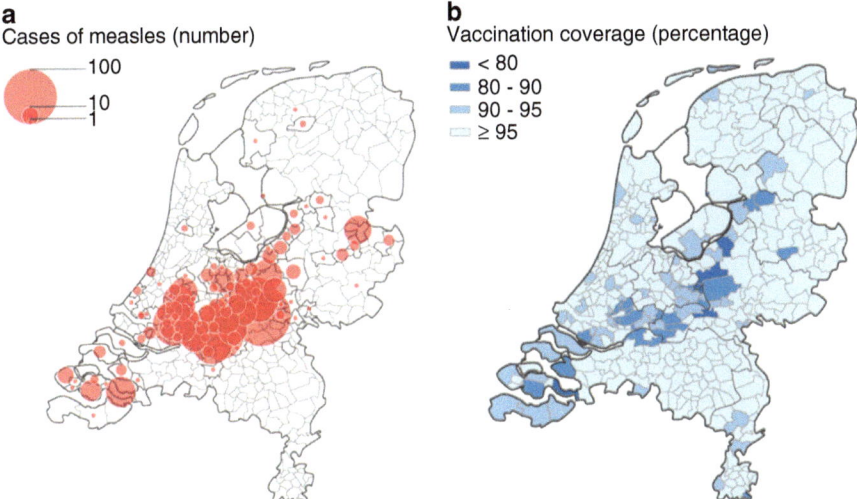

a
Cases of measles (number)

100
10
1

b
Vaccination coverage (percentage)

■ < 80
■ 80 - 90
▦ 90 - 95
▢ ≥ 95

MMR: measles-mumps-rubella.
aThere are 30 municipalities with MMR-1 vaccination coverage below 90%, of which 29 are within the 'Bible belt'. The other municipality is Vaals, in the far south-east of the Netherlands. A considerable number of the infants living in Vaals receive their vaccinations in Germany and are therefore not registered in the Dutch vaccination registration, which explains the low vaccination coverage (84.3%).

Fig. 15.19 Measles cases clustered together in areas where parents refused vaccines. (Knol MJ, Urbanus AT, Swart EM, Mollema L, Ruijs WL, van Binnedijk RS, et al. Large ongoing measles outbreak in a religious community in the Netherlands since May 2013 [Figure 3]. Eurosurveillance 2013;18(36):20580. https://doi.org/10.2807/1560-7917.ES2013.18.36.20580.)

Given that causation can be real or false and that clusters can be illusions or real, what is to be done? The answer is logic and science. Perhaps the best known criteria for determining causality are known as known as the Hill criteria after English epidemiologist Sir Austin Bradford Hill (1897–1991) [20].

1. **Strength**: The larger the effect size, the more likely that it is causal.
2. **Consistency**: Reproducible findings by different people with different samples in different locations strengthens (or diminishes) the likelihood of an effect.
3. **Specificity**: Causation is most likely when there is a very specific population at a specific site and disease with no other likely explanation. The more specific an association between a factor and an effect is, the bigger the probability of a causal relationship.
4. **Temporality**: The effect has to occur after the cause.
5. **Dose-Response**: A larger exposure should generally lead to larger incidence of the effect.
6. **Biological Plausibility**: A plausible mechanism between cause and effect is useful, but not required. A claim of implausible causation, such as that vaccines

cause sudden infant death syndrome or that black cats are bad luck *may* be true, but they are unlikely.

7. **Coherence**: Coherence between epidemiological and other scientific disciplines increases the likelihood of an effect.

8. **Experiment**: As Dr. Hill said, "Occasionally it is possible to appeal to experimental, or semi-experimental evidence." Experimental evidence lends the strongest support for causation, but obviously, many experiments, such as purposefully exposing people to potential dangers, cannot be done for ethical reasons.

9. **Analogy**: The effect of similar factors may be considered.

Conclusion

Our minds are cause-and-effect machines that involuntary search for patterns and meanings in images and data. Often we are right and there is a relationship between two variables. Similarly some disease clusters are real. The pioneer of epidemiology, John Snow, was able to trace a cholera epidemic to a specific pump by creating a cluster map. It would be wrong to say all disease clusters are products of our imagination.

However, we are highly prone to see a relationship between two variables when none exists, and are very capable of finding patterns in random data. Controlled scientific studies are the only means of determining whether correlation and causation are real or a figment of our imaginations. Although such studies may be difficult to perform and the answer might not emerge until many studies are done, only by striving to eliminate biases and illusions through the scientific method, can we determine the truth.

References

1. Heid M. (2015, Aug 5). You asked: should i take turmeric supplements? TIME. Retrieved from http://time.com/3984504/turmeric-supplements-curcumin/.

2. Nelson KM, Dahlin JL, Bisson J, Graham J, Pauli GF, Walters MA. The essential medicinal chemistry of curcumin: miniperspective. J Med Chem. 2017;60(5):1620–37. https://doi.org/10.1021/acs.jmedchem.6b00975.

3. Offit P. (2016, April 11). Anti-vaccine doc 'Vaxxed': a doctor's film review. The Hollywood Reporter. Retrieved from https://www.hollywoodreporter.com/news/anti-vaccine-doc-vaxxed-a-882651.

4. 36 School shooters/school related violence committed by those under the influence of psychiatric drugs (n.d.). CCHR International: The Mental Health Watchdog. Retrieved from https://www.cchrint.org/school-shooters/.

5. Pierre J. (2015, June 20). Mass shootings, psychiatric medications, and Rick Perry [Blog post]. Psychology Today. Retrieved from https://www.psychologytoday.com/blog/psych-unseen/201506/mass-shootings-psychiatric-medications-and-rick-perry.

6. PiratesVsTemp(en) [Image file]. (n.d.). In: Wikipedia. Retrieved 15 Sept 2018 from https://en.wikipedia.org/wiki/File%3aPiratesVsTemp%28en%29.svg.

7. Bloom J. (2017, June 7). MIT researcher: glyphosate will cause half of all children to be autistic by 2025. Yeah, sure. American Council on Science and Health. Retrieved from https://www.acsh.org/news/2017/06/07/mit-researcher-glyphosate-will-cause-half-all-children-be-autistic-2025-yeah-sure-11337.

8. Seneff S. (n.d.). Dr Tony Bark, MD interviews Dr Stepnanie Seneff, PhD and Vaccines CONFIRMED to be tainted with glyphosate [Video files]. Vaccine-Injury.info. Retrieved from http://vaccine-injury.info/gmo-autism-link.cfm.

9. Gonzalez R. (2014, Jan 5). On correlation, causation, and the "real" cause of autism. Gizmodo. Retrieved from https://io9.gizmodo.com/on-correlation-causation-and-the-real-cause-of-auti-1494972271.

10. Vigen T. (n.d.). Spurious correlations. Retrieved 15 Sept 2018 from http://www.tylervigen.com/spurious-correlations.

11. Siemieniuk RA, Harris IA, Agoritsas T, Poolman RW, Brignardello-Petersen R, Van de Velde S, Buchbinder R, Englund M, Lytvyn L, Quinlan C, Helsingen L, Knutsen G, Olsen NR, Macdonald H, Hailey L, Wilson HM, Lydiatt A, Kristiansen A. Arthroscopic surgery for degenerative knee arthritis and meniscal tears: a clinical practice guideline. BMJ. 2017;357:j1982. https://doi.org/10.1136/bmj.j1982.

12. Thomas KB. The consultation and the therapeutic illusion. Br Med J. 1978;1(6123):1327–8. https://doi.org/10.1136/bmj.1.6123.1327.

13. U.S. Department of Health & Humans Services, National Institutes of Health, National, Heart, Lung, and Blood Institute. (2012, Feb 29). Lower heart disease risk: menopausal hormone therapy and heart disease. Retrieved from https://www.nhlbi.nih.gov/health/educational/heart-truth/lower-risk/hormone-therapy.htm.

14. Wise J. No overall increase in all cause mortality with HRT, study finds. BMJ. 2017;358:j4230. https://doi.org/10.1136/bmj.j4230.

15. Ben-Menachem E. Vaccination and the onset of Dravet syndrome. Epilepsy Curr. 2011;11(4):120–2. https://doi.org/10.5698/1535-7511-11.4.120.

16. CaitlinJo. (2013, July 13). RandomPoints [Animated image file]. In: Wikipedia. Retrieved 15 Sept 2018 from https://en.wikipedia.org/wiki/Clustering_illusion#/media/File:RandomPoints.gif.

17. Birthday problem. (2018, Sept 17). In: Wikipedia. Retrieved 17 Sept 2018 from https://en.wikipedia.org/wiki/Birthday_problem.

18. Thun MJ, Sinks T. Understanding cancer clusters. CA Cancer J Clin. 2004;54(5):273–80. https://doi.org/10.3322/canjclin.54.5.273.

19. Snow cholera map [Image file]. (n.d.). In: Wikipedia. Retrieved 15 Sept 2018 from https://en.wikipedia.org/wiki/File:Snow-cholera-map-1.jpg.

20. Hill AB. The environment and disease: association or causation? Proc R Soc Med. 1965;58:295–300. Retrieved from https://www.edwardtufte.com/tufte/hill.

Case

Lucia, pictured below, was a 34-year-old woman who presented with numbness in her fingertips for the past week. She was told she likely had carpal tunnel syndrome and told that her symptoms would improve with weight-loss and the use of splints at night. Lucia's symptoms gradually abated over the next few weeks. She returned one year later with visual loss in her right eye. She was diagnosed with optic neuritis and multiple sclerosis (MS) at that time. Lucia was able to contrast her experience with that of her friend Clara, also pictured below, who presented with similar numbness the next year and was rapidly diagnosed with MS based on MRIs (Fig. 16.1).

What Dr. Simpson Was Thinking

I am someone who likes to be judicious in my use of medical tests. Obesity increases the risk of carpal tunnel syndrome, and that's what I thought Lucia had. In retrospect, I really had little reason to consider this diagnosis, other than that Lucia was overweight. Unfortunately, I was not able to see past this. In contrast, when Clara came into my office I knew right away that something was seriously wrong. I ordered MRIs, made the right diagnosis, and started her on treatment. Of course, I am not consciously biased against obese patients, but it was clear that I treated these two patients differently based on only their weight.

Case

Jeffrey, pictured below, was a 34-year-old man who presented from prison with the sudden onset of leg weakness and urinary retention. On exam, he was utterly unable to move his legs and said that he could not feel anything below his waist. A CT scan was normal and the patient was discharged back to prison, insisting that he was unable to walk. He returned three days later with acute renal failure due to urinary retention. A MRI during this visit revealed a demyelinating lesion in the lower part of his spinal cord known as the conus medullaris. He was treated with steroids with only partial recovery from his symptoms (Fig. 16.2).

© Springer International Publishing AG, part of Springer Nature 2019
J. Howard, *Cognitive Errors and Diagnostic Mistakes*,
https://doi.org/10.1007/978-3-319-93224-8_16

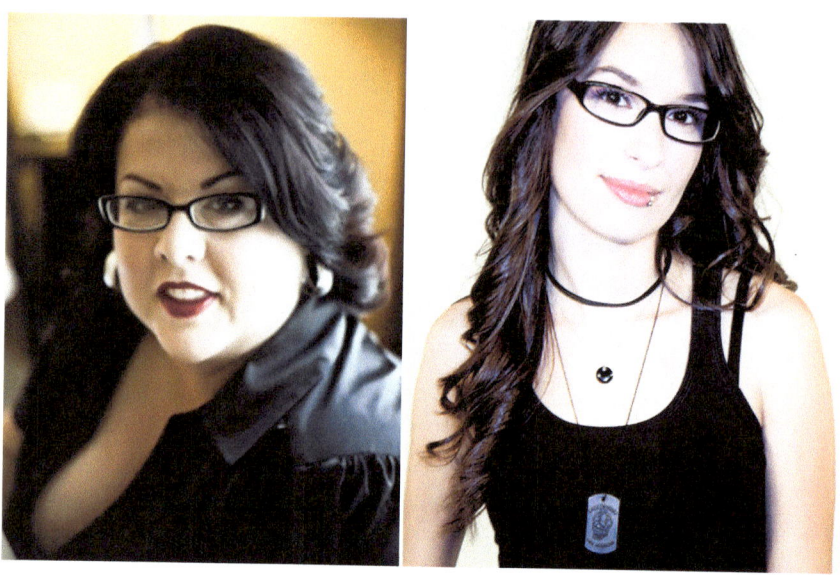

Fig. 16.1 Lucia and Clara. (**Left:** Bougon C. Chrystal Bougon, owner of Curvy Girl Lingerie at her boutique [Image file]. In: Wikimedia commons. 2017. https://commons.wikimedia.org/wiki/ Category:Chrystal_Bougon#/media/File:Chrystal_Bougon_(cropped).jpg.); **Right:** Nybe B. (Bob). Cara Santa Maria [Image file]. In: Wikimedia commons. 2011. Retrieved from https://commons. wikimedia.org/wiki/File:Cara_Santa_Maria.jpg)

Fig. 16.2 Jeffrey. (US Marshals Service. Mugshot of former Detroit mayor Kwame Kilpatrick [Image file]. In: Wikimedia commons. 2010. Retrieved from https://commons. wikimedia.org/wiki/ Category:Convicts#/media/ File:2010-kilpatrick-usmarshals-mugshot.JPG)

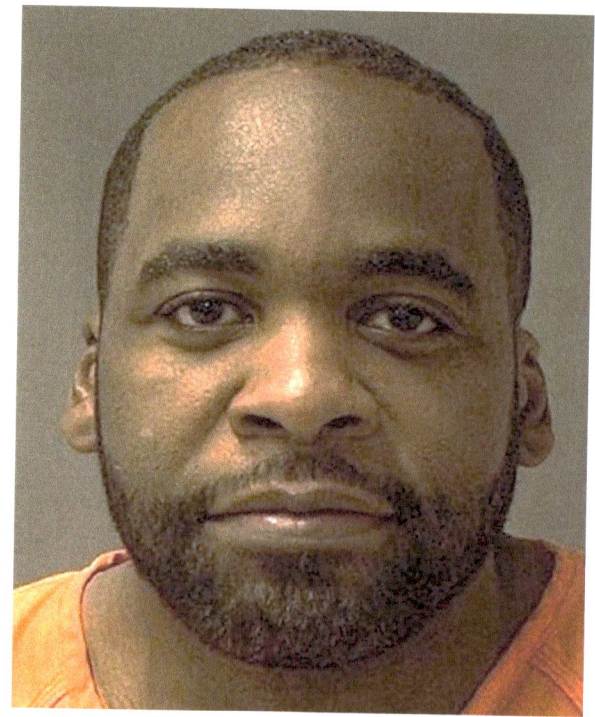

What Dr. Johnson Was Thinking

Everyone knows that it is common for prisoners to exaggerate symptoms or make them up altogether. Some of them would rather be in the hospital than in jail, and frankly I can't blame them. I'll be honest with you that whenever I hear a prisoner has been admitted to the neurology service with a supposed seizure or low back pain, I automatically assume they are faking it. I am not saying this is right, but having seen it so many times, it's an automatic reflex I have. At this point, I can't help it any more than I can change how I feel about a food I don't like. So, I dismissed Jeffrey's complaint more rapidly than I would have had he been a civilian. To be perfectly honest, the fact that he was black may have contributed to why I did not take him seriously either.

However, just because some prisoners fake their symptoms, this does not mean they all are faking. Or just because a prisoner is exaggerating some of his symptoms, this does not mean he is faking all of his symptoms. Now, whenever a prisoner is admitted to our service, I essentially take a "time-out" and consciously spend more time and effort than I might do with a civilian.

Case

Bruce, pictured below, was a 65-year-old man with schizophrenia who was brought in by ambulance for agitation on the street. He was shouting at and pushing people as they tried to get on the bus. On arrival to the ER, he was paranoid and disorganized. He was given medications to sedate him to prevent him from hurting himself and others. His vital signs were unremarkable other than a heart rate of 140 bpm. His tachycardia (rapid heart rate) was attributed to his agitation and he was admitted to the inpatient psychiatric unit. Admission blood work showed mild anemia, but was otherwise unremarkable. A urine toxicology screen was negative. His EKG showed only sinus tachycardia, and a chest radiograph was unremarkable.

Bruce was calmer the next day, though he was convinced the hospital staff was trying to poison him. He remained tachycardic with a heart rate ranging from 130–150 bpm. On hospital day three, he complained of shortness of breath and was found to be tachypneic (rapid breathing). He was transferred to the medical service at that time, where he was found to have a large pulmonary embolus (Fig. 16.3).

What Dr. Miles Was Thinking

I saw Bruce soon after his arrival to the psychiatric floor. He was calm, but floridly delusional and paranoid. In addition to being seen by the psychiatrist, he had been seen by an internist and he had been "medically cleared for psych." I always quickly review the medical work-up in the ER, and other than his tachycardia, there was nothing concerning. Though the patient remained tachycardic while on the unit, and I continued to attribute this finding to his "agitation." All too often, once patients with psychiatric conditions are deemed "medically cleared," then all their physical symptoms are attributed to their psychiatric condition. Once I heard Bruce had schizophrenia, my brain turned off. There are certain diagnoses that do this, and schizophrenia is one of them. Of course, having schizophrenia doesn't protect you from other diseases. Had he not had schizophrenia, I would have

Fig. 16.3 Bruce.
(Skalstad LA. (Leroy
Allen). Color portraiture of
homeless man [Image file].
In: Wikimedia commons.
2009. Retrieved from
https://commons.
wikimedia.org/wiki/
Category:Homeless_
people#/media/
File:HOMELESS.tif.)

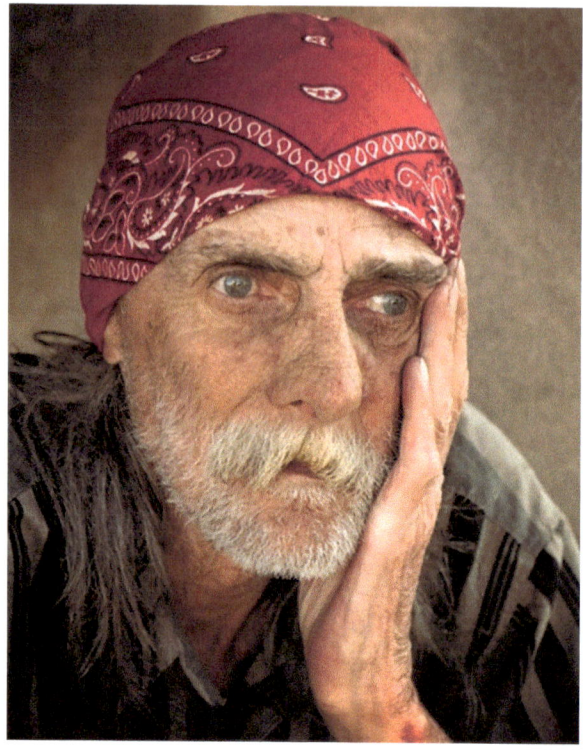

recognized there was a serious problem. Luckily, his pulmonary embolism was
detected before it killed him.

Discussion

We all have a natural tendency to prefer people in the same group to which we
belong, a phenomenon known as the in-group favoritism. Whether it's a city, profession, religion, race, or political partly, our self-image largely depends on the groups
to which we belong. If you consider someone to be part of your group, you are more
likely to have a favorable view of them. In contrast, if you believe someone to be
part of another group, you are more prone to view them negatively.

This phenomenon of in-group favoritism was studied by psychologist Henri
Taifel who investigated the minimal conditions required for discrimination to occur
between groups. Such minimal groups occur when "complete strangers are formed
into groups using the most trivial criteria imaginable [1]." In his studies, boys ages
14 and 15 years old were randomly divided into groups based on arbitrary criteria,
such as being told they had overestimated or underestimated the number of dots in
a display or which painting they preferred. Once the two groups had been formed,
the boys had to divide points to other participants who were identified by their group
membership. He found that random, meaningless group assignments led to an in-
group bias in the allocation of these points. In similar studies, he found that even
though the groups were assigned randomly, study subjects almost always "liked the

members of their own group better and they rated the members of their in-group as more likely to have pleasant personalities [2]."

While in-group favoritism can be harmless or even potentially beneficial with rival sports teams, competing businesses, and political parties, it is easy to see how excessive loyalty to a group can lead to horrors such as terrorism, racism, and genocide. Indeed, understanding how such atrocities occur is what inspired Taifel's research [3].

Stigmatized individuals may have three related, yet distinct experiences with regards to their social identity.

- **Identity threat:** *An identity threat* occurs when patients have devaluing experiences due to their social identity.
- **Stereotype threat:** *A stereotype threat* occurs when a patient knows they belong to a stigmatized group. As such, they may alter their behavior to ensure it does not conform to expected stereotypes, and they may be highly attuned to detecting bias within others.
- **Felt stigma:** *Felt stigma* refers the expectation of substandard treatment due to previous poor care or societal prejudice.

The in-group bias can be amplified by the expectancy effect, which occurs when a prejudice causes someone to behave in a manner that elicits the expected behavior from the target. It is a type of self-fulfilling prophecy that often occurs in interpersonal relationships. For example, if a clinician believes that a large, heavily-tattooed patient on the prison ward is likely to display antisocial behavior, the clinician may behave antagonistically towards the patient, eliciting the behavior they expected.

While anyone can be victimized by the in-group bias, there is no question that certain persons are more likely than others to suffer bias as a result of their social identity. Specific types of in-group biases in medicine are discussed below.

Race

Though there has been significant progress in recent years, by almost every measure, black Americans have significantly worse health care outcomes than whites [4]. Compared to whites, they have higher infant mortality rates and die younger of common diseases, such as cancer and heart disease [5]. While the reasons behind this are multifactorial and beyond the ability of any individual clinician to remedy, there is evidence of a racial bias in medicine.

A bias against black patients has been convincingly demonstrated with differing rates of prescriptions for opioid pain medications. In 2012, Saliman Meghani and colleagues analyzed 20 years of data on racial and ethnic disparities in pain relief in the US. They found that compared to whites, blacks were 34% less likely to receive opioids for backaches, abdominal pain, and migraines, and 14% less likely to receive opioids for pain caused by traumatic injuries or surgery [6]. When blacks are given pain medications, they are given them at lower doses compared to whites. In 2016, Astha Singhal and colleagues found similar disparities for patients with back and abdominal pain [7]. Monika Goyal and colleagues found that this disparity existed even in children of different races suffering from appendicitis [8]. Black children in severe pain were less likely to receive opioids than whites. While a case could be made that this is a blessing in disguise for blacks, as dangerous and addictive opioids are overprescribed for whites, it nonetheless demonstrates a significant difference in how clinicians treat patients of different races.

A similar pattern of bias has been found is psychiatric diagnoses. A study by Frederic Blow and colleagues of 134,523 US veterans found that, compared to whites, blacks were more than four times as likely to be diagnosed with schizophrenia, while Hispanics were more than three times as likely to receive this diagnosis [9]. A similar study by Karen Coleman and colleagues of 1.2 million patients with a psychiatric diagnosis found that non-Hispanic blacks were diagnosed with schizophrenia at nearly double the rate of non-Hispanic whites. There is no evidence that schizophrenia is actually more common in blacks, though they more readily receive this devastating and stigmatizing diagnosis. They were also significantly less likely to receive medication treatment [10]. Interestingly, they were more likely to receive psychotherapy, however.

Of course, races other than African-Americans may be subject to bias. For example, it is well known that clinicians often view Hispanic women as being highly prone to somatization. Behind closed doors, clinicians may say such patients have "status Hispanicus" or "Hispanic hysterical syndrome." Their complaints may be minimized if they are perceived to suffer from TBD, which stands for total body dolor.

Black and Hispanic women may also face discrimination when giving birth. According to Karen Scott, an obstetrician:

> African Americans in the highest socioeconomic group experience the same or higher rates of infant mortality, low birthweight, and high blood pressure and excess weight during pregnancy in comparison with white women in the lowest socioeconomic statuses [11].

Indeed, studies have found that neonatal mortality rates of black women are double those of whites, and maternal mortality rates of black mothers three to four times higher than white mothers [12]. While the reasons behind this are multifactorial, it is clear that clinician bias plays a role. In one survey, 21% of black mothers and 19% of Hispanic mothers experienced "poor treatment from hospital staff due to race, ethnicity, cultural background, or language" while delivering in the hospital [13]. In contrast, only 8% of white mothers reported such poor treatment. Hispanic women were tested for chronic or gestational diabetes at half the rate as black and white women. They were significantly less likely to rate their clinician as "completely trustworthy" and their prenatal and their babies' pediatric visits as "very good." Another study by Jennifer Hsu and colleagues found that black women who experienced an ectopic pregnancy were less likely to have surgery that preserved their fallopian tubes compared to white women [14]. They were also less likely to receive a laparoscopic operation for an ectopic pregnancy, though this surgery is much less invasive and is the standard of care [15].

Importantly, not all of this bias is unconscious. White clinicians have been shown to have some very erroneous beliefs regarding basic biological differences between the races. In 2015, Kelly Hoffman and colleagues surveyed 222 white medical students and residents about basic differences between the races [16]. Some differences in the study were true; blacks do have a higher bone density than whites and are less likely to have spinal cord disorders. However, some also endorsed false, even bizarre, beliefs. For example, 29% of first year medical students felt black people's blood coagulates more quickly than whites, and 21% felt they had stronger immune systems. Twenty-five percent of residents felt blacks have thicker skin than whites, and 11% felt blacks were better at detecting movement.

There is some evidence that patients have better outcomes when they are treated by clinicians of their same race. Philip Okafor and colleagues examined outcomes in patients with five common gastrointestinal diagnoses treated at 3,392 hospitals [17]. They found that patients were 20% less likely to have major complications or die when they were treated at hospitals with diverse patient populations. Similarly, Lisa Cooper and colleagues found that when patients were treated by same-race clinicians, the visits were several minutes longer and there were higher average ratings of "positive patient affect" as rated by voice tone qualities [18]. Patients treated by a same-race clinician were more satisfied and felt the clinician was more participatory in their care. There is some evidence that patients may be more adherent to treatment when treated by a same-race clinician. Ana Traylor and colleagues found that black patients were slightly more likely to take medications to prevent cardiovascular disease when they were prescribed by a black clinician [19]. Similarly, Spanish-speaking patients were more likely to take medications when prescribed by a clinician who spoke Spanish. No effect was seen for Asian patients or English-speaking Hispanic patients. Other studies have found that having a same-race clinician does not improve cardiovascular outcomes [20, 21].

Gender

The gender bias is the tendency to believe that gender is a determining factor in the probability of diagnosis of a particular disease when no such pathophysiological basis exists. Generally, it results in an overdiagnosis of the favored gender and underdiagnosis of the neglected gender [22]. Perhaps the most glaring example of this is the misdiagnosis of coronary heart disease (CHD) in women, which may present differently in men and women. In women, myocardial infarctions (MI) may present without the classic symptoms of crushing chest pain radiating to the left arm and jaw, a phenomenon termed Yentl Syndrome (named after a movie where Barbara Streisand impersonates a man to receive religious training). As Jennifer Mieres, a cardiologist, said:

> For decades, doctors used the male model of coronary heart disease testing to identify the disease in women, automatically focusing on the detection of obstructive coronary artery disease. As a result, symptomatic women who did not have classic obstructive coronary disease were not diagnosed with ischemic heart disease, and did not receive appropriate treatment, thereby increasing their risk for heart attack [23].

As a result, clinicians may be very too quick to label women with chest pain and shortness of breath as having a panic attack. As cardiologist Adam Splaver said, "In training, we were taught to be on the lookout for hysterical females who come to the emergency room [24]."

Studies by psychologist Gabrielle Chiaramonte showed clinicians are more likely to be inappropriately distracted by extra-symptom characteristics in women [25]. In one study, 230 family medicine doctors and internists were given case presentations of two patients with identical medical histories and the classic symptoms of an MI: a 47-year-old man and a 56-year-old woman. For each patient, they were correctly able to identify the symptoms of an MI. However, when told that they patient had experienced a recent, significant stressor, their diagnostic accuracy fell, though by unequal amounts for the male and female patients. With the female patient, only 15% of doctors made the correct diagnosis, only 13% suggested appropriate medications, and only 30% would refer the patient to a cardiologist. In the male patient, 56% of doctors made the correct diagnosis, 47% suggested appropriate medications, and 62% would refer the patient to a cardiologist. As Dr. Chiaramonte wrote:

> For women, the presence of stress or anxiety drives the interpretation of accompanying symptoms so that symptoms such as chest pain or shortness of breath undergo a "meaning shift" when presented in the context of stress or anxiety and they are perceived as a manifestation of the stress or anxiety and not as CHD symptoms. For men, cardiac symptoms drive the interpretation of accompanying symptoms so that anxiety or stress is perceived (rightly so) as a risk factor for CHD and may in fact augment the CHD assessment. The presence of anxiety or stress in men does not deter from the CHD assessment; for women, it appears to preclude a CHD assessment [26].

Not only might clinicians be less willing to consider cardiac disease in women, women themselves may be unaware that their symptoms could be an MI. In interviews with 30 women under the age 55 who suffered an MI, Judith Lichtman found that many of them delayed seeking appropriate care [27]. The problem is not necessarily that these women were ignorant of the textbooks, but rather that the textbooks neglected women like them. Other women were aware they might be having an MI, but nonetheless delayed seeking care, not wanting be perceived as being histrionic. Partly as a result of this, younger women with MIs have a higher rate of death than same-aged men [28].

Other examples of gender discrimination abound in medicine. As with heart disease, there are gender-specific patterns of misdiagnosis in multiple sclerosis (MS.) In one study, misdiagnosed women with MS were most likely to be told they had a psychiatric condition, while misdiagnosed men were most likely to be told they had an orthopedic problem [29]. Stories of clinicians ignoring or minimizing women's pain are not hard to find, and formal studies support these anecdotes. Women receive pain medications less than men and have to wait longer to receive them [30]. A study by Cornelia M. Borkhoff and colleagues presented 71 doctors a standardized patient with the exact same physical symptom of knee pain, differing only by sex. Forty-two percent of doctors recommended surgery to the male but not the female patient, while only 8% suggested surgery to the female but not the male [31].

A gender bias similarly exists in scientific studies, as women are much less likely to be enrolled in clinical trials of cardiovascular disease [32]. Chiara Melloni and colleagues examined 156 such trials and found that women are significantly under-enrolled in clinical trials compared to men. In fact, 20 of the trials enrolled only men while just one study enrolled only women.

As with race, there is some evidence that patients fare better when they are treated by clinicians of the same gender. Julie Schmittdiel and colleagues examined 157,458 adult diabetes patients and found that patient and clinician gender concordance were modestly associated with improvement in their diabetes and other cardiovascular risk-factors [33].

Obesity

Obesity affects nearly 33% of Americans, and obese people are a stigmatized group, often perceived as lazy, mentally deficient, and indifferent to their own health. One orthopedist, discussing the challenges obese patients may pose, placed the blame for their condition almost exclusively on their shoulders, saying that obesity was due to "several contributing factors, including poor nutrition (a high-fat diet, poor nutritional knowledge, overeating, and eating out), physical inactivity, psychological problems, lack of willpower, and metabolic or endocrine disorders [34]." Similarly, one psychiatrist blamed their mental state and claimed to help "women find and overcome the unconscious emotions, beliefs, traumas and more that keep women from releasing weight [35]." Privately and informally, clinicians have been known to deride obese patients as "beached whales [36]." Studies show these attitudes are common. According to *Physician Bias: Trends from the 2016 Medscape Lifestyle Report*, a patient's weight was the second-most common patient characteristic that triggered bias in doctors (56% of male doctors and 48% of female doctors [37].)

There is also evidence that obese patients receive worse care. Some of the problems that obese patients face while getting medical care are systemic. Many hospitals do not have scanners that can fit very obese patients, and medication doses may not be calibrated with obese patients in mind. Additionally, there is evidence individual clinicians are often biased against obese patients. Mary Huizinga and colleagues examined visits from 40 doctors and 238 patients. They found that patients with a higher body mass index were less likely to be respected by the clinician [38]. A survey of 122 primary care doctors found that:

> Physicians reported that seeing patients was a greater waste of their time the heavier that they were, that physicians would like their jobs less as their patients increased in size, that heavier patients were viewed to be more annoying, and that physicians felt less patience the heavier the patient was [39].

There is also evidence that many orthopedic surgeons will not perform hip and knee surgeries on obese patients unless they are able to lose weight [40]. According to Adolph Yates Jr., an orthopedics professor, "There are offices that will screen by phone. They will ask for weight and height and tell patients before they see them that they can't help them [41]." In England, it is the official policy to delay such elective surgeries for obese patients and smokers [42].

Another potential problem faced by obese patients is that their health concerns will not be taken seriously. As a result of their obesity, they are vulnerable to a form of premature closure, where other conditions are erroneously excluded due to their obesity. As author Sarai Walker said, "No matter what the problem is, the doctor will blame it on fat and will tell you to lose weight [41]." Anecdotes of treatable conditions being missed in obese patients are common. Author Kelly Coffey, for example, reported going to her gynecologist's office with severe menstrual cramps. The doctor spent only a few minutes with her, did not examine her, and told her to lose 100 pounds [43]. Years went by before she was diagnosed with endometriosis, a treatable condition. Not surprisingly, many obese people avoid going to the doctor as they are fearful that their symptoms will automatically be attributed to their weight.

Sara Bleich and colleagues surveyed 600 overweight and obese patients to determine whether their relationship was affected by the clinician's weight [44]. They found that overweight and obese patients generally trusted their clinician, though about 20% felt judged due to their weight. Importantly, they were more likely to trust dietary advice if the clinician was also overweight. Interestingly, overweight and obese patients were more likely to feel judged due to their weight when their clinician was also obese.

Prisoners

Ill prisoners are assumed often to be feigning illness, a phenomenon known as malingering. To qualify as malingering, a patient must purposefully fake an injury or illness with goal of gaining a specific desired outcome, such as shelter, drugs, or an absence from work. Malingering is a "diagnosis of exclusion," meaning that it can only be made when all other conditions have been definitively ruled out. Conditions such as seizures, chest pain, paralysis, and psychosis are commonly feigned as they take time to evaluate and dangerous diseases cannot be easily excluded. Depending on the feigned condition, malingering can be very dangerous to patients. I commonly see patients who feign symptoms and then receive multiple unnecessary tests and procedures as a result. Occasionally, I have seen them receive medications with potentially devastating side effects, such as thrombolytic medications for acute strokes.

While malingering is by no means restricted to inmates, it is not uncommon for them to feign symptoms to avoid incarceration in a correctional facility. For example, in one study of psychiatric patients in the correctional setting, 66% were found to be malingering [45]. Despite this, a common error that occurs, with prisoners is that they are prematurely viewed as malingering in ways that civilians are not. Patients with a history of substance abuse or mental illness may face a similar bias. Jeffrey Keller, a doctor who works with inmates, recognized that the term must be used with care. He wrote:

> The most important consideration of the term "malingering" is not its actual definition. The most important part is its _emotional_ meaning. This is a word that causes others to instantaneously have a strong emotional reaction. When you say that a patient is malingering, whether you are using the term correctly or not, what that patient (and others) understand is that you are calling them a liar [46].

While I agree with Dr. Keller, it is also true that if a clinician is confident that a patient is feigning symptoms, they should not shy away from saying so. Giving malingering patients a diagnosis other than malingering would require clinicians to be dishonest as well. However, given that it is such an emotionally laden term, clinicians should recognize that by labeling a patient a malingerer, they will certainly affect encounters with future health care providers. Patients with a documented history of malingering are almost never trusted when they present with new symptoms.

Similarly, clinicians must be cautious when treating a patient who has been perceived as malingering in the past. Anyone who had worked extensively with inmates will eventually have the experience of disbelieving a patient who turns out to have a genuine illness. A prisoner who reports back pain and leg weakness may actually have a spinal disorder. A prisoner who said he "fell out," may actually have had a seizure. Additionally, challenging a patient who malingers almost always backfires. Many malingerers have a relatively rapid recovery from their symptoms when they get tired of being in the hospital. Confronting them is usually counterproductive, as they may feel required to "prove" the clinician wrong and maintain the sick role.

Unfortunately, despite it being a relatively common presentation, malingering is almost never formally discussed as part of the medical curriculum. There are lectures and case conferences on all manners of disease, including those that occur in literally one-in-a-million people. Yet, the only lecture I can remember attending on the topic was one I gave. The effect malingering has on clinicians is similarly ignored. Malingering can have a corrosive effect on clinicians, leading them to believe everyone is lying to them. Some informal rules in medicine assume patients will lie. For example, clinicians are taught to automatically double the amount of alcohol a patient says they consume. As obstetrician Amy Tuteur wrote:

> The patients who are deliberately deceptive seem to have an outsize influence on the practice of medicine. During internship and residency, young doctors are repeatedly fooled, and therefore embarrassed, by patients. Drug addicts are notorious for presenting themselves as model citizens with serious pain problems. After several episodes of unwittingly giving an addict a fix, or a prescription for drugs that will be sold, young doctors begin to listen to a patient's stories with increasing cynicism. The subtext for many physician's consciously or unconsciously, is that they must be convinced that the patient is telling the truth [47].

Finally, clinicians should be sensitive to the fact that many people have legitimate reasons to malinger. Faking a seizure to go to the hospital may be a rational response for a prisoner who is housed with rival gang members. A woman who feigns chest pain may be doing so to escape an abusive husband.

Lesbian, Gay, Bisexual, and Transgender

Lesbian, gay, bisexual, and transgender (LGBT) patients are another marginalized group who often face discrimination when receiving health care. In a study of over 2,000 first-year medical students by Sara Burke and colleagues, 46% expressed at least some explicit bias against gay and lesbian individuals [48]. This bias has real-world implications. A 2015 survey by the National Center for Transgender Equality had some disturbing results [49]. Thirty-three percent of respondents reported having at least one negative experience with a clinician related to being transgender. Six percent said they were verbally harassed in a health care setting, while 5% said a health care provider used harsh or abusive language when treating them. Two percent even reported that a health care provider was physically rough or abusive when treating them.

Psychiatric Patients and Diagnostic Overshadowing

According to *Physician Bias: Trends from the 2016 Medscape Lifestyle Report*, "emotional problems" were the single most likely patient characteristic that triggered bias in clinicians, with 62% of respondents reporting such a bias [37]. Patients with psychiatric illness and those with intellectual disability commonly have physical symptoms erroneously attributed to their mental condition, a phenomenon known as diagnostic overshadowing [50]. Additionally, medical problems, even when identified, may be ignored or undertreated in patients with severe mental illness. In one study by Greer Sullivan and colleagues, patients with mental illness and diabetes were less likely to be admitted to the hospital than patients with diabetes alone [51]. There is also some evidence that patients with mental illness do not receive proper cancer screenings, and that if diagnosed, they are perceived as problematic patients who are unlikely to be compliant with treatment or lack the capacity to make treatment decisions for themselves [52]. Additionally, mentally ill patients, especially those with devastating illnesses such as schizophrenia, are less likely to receive appropriate treatments for multiple different types of cancers [52].

Not surprisingly, patients with significant mental illnesses have much poorer health than the general population. They are more likely to smoke cigarettes, more likely to be obese, more likely to live sedentary lifestyles, and more likely to have metabolic syndrome [53–56]. A systematic review by Carsten Hjorthøj and colleagues found that schizophrenia was associated with an average of 14.5 years of potential life lost [57]. Another review found that 14.3% of deaths worldwide are due to mental illness, and only 67.3% of deaths in patients with mental illness were due to natural causes [58]. As Graham Thornicroft, a psychiatrist, wrote about these findings, "If such a disparity in mortality rates were to affect a large segment of the population with a less stigmatized characteristic, then we would witness an outcry against a socially unacceptable decimation of this group [59]."

Similarly, because of stigma and fear of professional sanction, clinicians may be reluctant to discuss and seek treatment for their own mental illness. Kay Redfield Jamison, a psychiatrist with bipolar disorder, expressed this sentiment by saying:

> It was difficult to make the decision to be public about having a severe psychiatric illness.... but privacy and reticence can kill. The problem with mental illness is that so many who have it—especially those in a position to change public attitudes, such as doctors, lawyers, politicians, and military officers—are reluctant to risk talking about mental illness, or seeking help for it. They are understandably frightened about professional and personal reprisals [60].

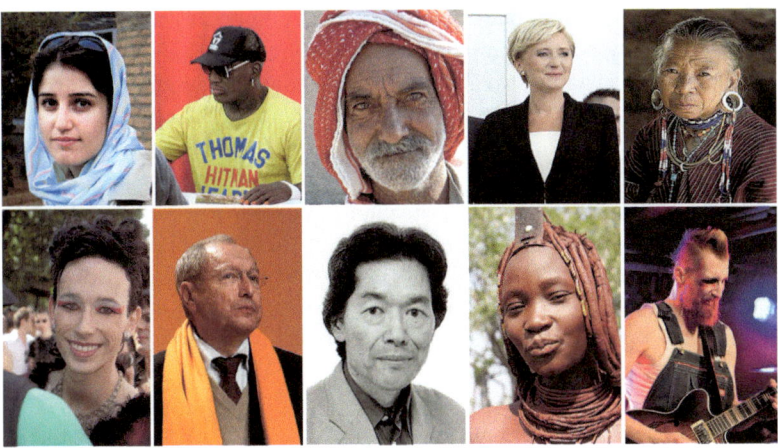

Fig. 16.4 **Top Row**: Saber H. (Hamed). Iranian woman [Image file]. In: Wikimedia commons. 2006. Retrieved from https://commons.wikimedia.org/wiki/Woman#/media/File:Portrait_of_a_Persian_lady_in_Iran,_10-08-2006.jpg; GabboT. Dennis Rodman 01 [Image file]. In: Wikimedia Commons. 2017. Retrieved from https://commons.wikimedia.org/w/index.php?title=Special:Search&limit=20&offset=0&profile=default&search=dennis+rodman#/media/File:Dennis_Rodman_01_(34679281591).jpg; Briggs C. (Christiaan). Iraqi militiaman at Sabaa Nissan [Image file]. In: Wikimedia commons. 2003. Retrieved from https://commons.wikimedia.org/wiki/Man#/media/File:Sabaa_Nissan_Militiaman.jpg; The Chancellery of the Senate of the Republic of Poland. Agata Kornhauser-Duda [Image file]. In: Wikimedia commons. 2015. Retrieved from https://commons.wikimedia.org/wiki/Woman#/media/File:Agata_Kornhauser-Duda_Sejm_2015.JPG; Evans S. (Steve). Kayaw woman [Image file]. In: Wikimedia commons. 2007. Retrieved from https://commons.wikimedia.org/wiki/Woman#/media/File:Tribes_woman_with_ear_piercing.jpg. **Bottom Row**: Krech T. (Till). At a glance [Image file]. In: Wikimedia commons. 2006. Retrieved from https://commons.wikimedia.org/wiki/Category:LGBT_Pride#/media/File:At_a_glance_(195838401).jpg; Nguyen M-L. (Marie-Lan). March 2008 – Jean Peyrelevade [Image file]. In: Wikimedia commons. 2008. Retrieved from https://commons.wikimedia.org/wiki/Jean_Peyrelevade#/media/File:Sarnez_Mutualite_2008_03_04_n8.jpg; Agnostizi. Professor Dr. Ichiro Yamaguchi [Image file]. In: Wikimedia commons. 2000. Retrieved from https://commons.wikimedia.org/wiki/Man#/media/File:Ichiro_Yamaguchi.jpg; Picq Y. (Yves). Himba woman [Image file]. In: Wikimedia commons. 2007. Retrieved from https://commons.wikimedia.org/wiki/Woman#/media/File:Namibie_Himba_0717a.jpg; Schwichtenberg F. (Frank). Johnny Flesh & the Redneck Zombies [Image file]. In: Wikimedia commons. 2014. Retrieved from https://commons.wikimedia.org/wiki/File:Johnny_Flesh_%26_the_Redneck_Zombies_%E2%80%93_Wilwarin_Festival_2014_03.jpg

Conclusion

Test yourself. What associations do you bring to these names: Tristan Higginbotham III, Xishan Pang, Mohammed Hussein, D'Shawn Jackson, Jesus Fernandez, Bubba Lou Jones, Abeeku Nkrumah? Look at the people below. How would you feel if you were called to evaluate each of them for a headache? [61]

Clinicians should not feel guilty for having involuntary associations with these names and faces. In-group favoritism does not mean that clinicians are prejudiced. Rather, in-group favoritism bias is an inevitable part of the human condition, and there are several studies showing that such biases begin in infants as young as six months old [62]. As such, clinicians should strive to be aware of their biases and how they might impact the care of their patients.

Organizational changes can also be made to minimize in-group favoritism. Few people would suggest that we should return to the days of segregated hospitals or that patients routinely be matched with clinicians of the same sex, race, and sexual orientation. However, there is evidence that in-group bias can be diminished by exposure to people of other groups, a phenomenon known as passive tolerance [63]. The psychological phenomenon known as the mere exposure effect, in which people develop a preference for things that are familiar, can be harnessed to diminish in-group favoritism. This makes a compelling case that, all things being equal, a diverse patient population will be best served by a diverse group of clinicians.

References

1. Pratkanis AR. Age of propaganda: the everyday use and abuse of persuasion. New York: W.H. Freeman; 1992. p. 216). [Google books version].
2. Tajel H, Billig MG, Bundy RP, Flament C. Social categorization and intergroup behavior. Eur J Soc Psychol. 1971;1(2):149–78. https://doi.org/10.1002/ejsp.2420010202.
3. Minimal Group Paradigm. (n.d.). Age-of-the-sage.org. Retrieved 15 Sept 2018 from https://www.age-of-the-sage.org/psychology/social/minimal_group_paradigm_study.html.
4. Tavernise S. (2016, May 8). Black Americans see gains in life expectancy. The New York Times. Retrieved from https://www.nytimes.com/2016/05/09/health/blacks-see-gains-in-life-expectancy.html.
5. Centers for Disease Control and Prevention. (2017, May 3). Health of Black or African American non-Hispanic population. Retrieved 15 Sept 2018 from https://www.cdc.gov/nchs/fastats/black-health.htm.
6. Meghani SH, Byun E, Gallagher RM. Time to take stock: a meta-analysis and systematic review of analgesic treatment disparities for pain in the United States. Pain Med. 2012;13(2):150–74. https://doi.org/10.1111/j.1526-4637.2011.01310.x.
7. Singhal A, Tien Y-Y, Hsia RY. Racial-ethnic disparities in opioid prescriptions at emergency department visits for conditions commonly associated with prescription drug abuse. PLoS One. 2016;11(8):e0159224. https://doi.org/10.1371/journal.pone.0159224.
8. Goyal MK, Kuppermann N, Cleary SD, Teach SJ, Chamberlain J, M. Racial disparities in pain management of children with appendicitis in emergency departments. JAMA Pediatr. 2015;169(11):996–1002. https://doi.org/10.1001/jamapediatrics.2015.1915.
9. Blow FC, Zeber JE, McCarthy JF, Valenstein M, Gillon L, Bingham CR. Ethnicity and diagnostic patterns in veterans with psychoses. Soc Psychiatry Psychiatr Epidemiol. 2004;39(10):841–51. https://doi.org/10.1007/s00127-004-0824-7.
10. Coleman KJ, Stewart C, Waitzfelder BE, Zeber JE, Morales LS, Ahmed AT, Ahmedani BK, Beck A, Copeland LA, Cummings JR, Hunkeler EM, Lindberg NM, Lynch F, Lu CY, Owen-Smith AA, Trinacty CM, Whitebird RR, Simon GE. Racial-ethnic differences in psychiatric diagnoses and treatment across 11 health care systems in the Mental Health Research Network. Psychiatr Serv. 2016;67(7):749–57. https://doi.org/10.1176/appi.ps.201500217.
11. Choo E. (2017, Dec 26). The elephant in the delivery room: how doctor bias hurts black and brown mothers. NBC News: THINK. Retrieved from https://www.nbcnews.com/think/opinion/elephant-delivery-room-how-doctor-bias-hurts-black-brown-mothers-ncna832616.
12. Howell EA, Zeitlin J, Hebert P, Balbierz A, Egorova N. Paradoxical trends and racial differences in obstetric quality and neonatal and maternal mortality. Obstet Gynecol. 2013;121(6):1201–8. https://doi.org/10.1097/AOG.0b013e3182932238.

13. Childbirth Connection. (n.d.). How do childbearing experiences differ across racial and ethnic groups in the United States? A Listening to Mothers III data brief. [Blog post]. Transforming Maternity Care. Retrieved 15 Sept 2018 from http://transform.childbirthconnection.org/reports/listeningtomothers/race-ethnicity/.

14. Hsu JY, Chin L, Gumer AR, Tergas AI, Hou JY, Burke WM, Ananth CV, Hershman DL, Wright JD. Disparities in the management of ectopic pregnancy. Am J Obstet Gynecol. 2017;217(1):49.e1–49.e10. https://doi.org/10.1016/j.ajog.2017.03.001.

15. Ranjit A, Chaudhary MA, Jiang W, Zhan T, Schneider EB, Cohen SL, Little SE, Haider AH, Robinson JN, Witkop CT. Disparities in receipt of a laparoscopic operation for ectopic pregnancy among TRICARE beneficiaries. Surgery. 2017;161(5):1341–7. https://doi.org/10.1016/j.surg.2016.09.029.

16. Hoffman KM, Trawalter S, Axt JR, Oliver MN. Racial bias in pain assessment and treatment recommendations, and false beliefs about biological differences between blacks and whites. Proc Natl Acad Sci. 2016;113(16):4296–301. https://doi.org/10.1073/pnas.1516047113.

17. Okafor PN, Stobaugh DJ, Van Ryn M, Talwalkar JA. African Americans have better outcomes for five common gastrointestinal diagnoses in hospitals with more racially diverse patients. Am J Gastroenterol. 2016;111:649–57. https://doi.org/10.1038/ajg.2016.64.

18. Cooper LA, Roter DL, Johnson RL, Ford DE, Steinwachs DM, Powe NR. Patient-centered communication, ratings of care, and concordance of patient and physician race. Ann Intern Med. 2003;139(11):907–15. https://doi.org/10.7326/0003-4819-139-11-200312020-00009.

19. Traylor AH, Schmittdiel JA, Uratsu CS, Mangione CM, Subramanian U. Adherence to cardiovascular disease medications: does patient-provider race/ethnicity and language concordance matter? J Gen Intern Med. 2010;25(11):1172–7. https://doi.org/10.1007/s11606-010-1424-8.

20. Schoenthaler A, Montague E, Baier Manwell L, Brown R, Schwartz MD, Linzer M. Patient–physician racial/ethnic concordance and blood pressure control: the role of trust and medication adherence. Ethn Health. 2014;19(5):565–78. https://doi.org/10.1080/13557858.2013.857764.

21. Traylor AH, Subramanian U, Uratsu CS, Mangione CM, Selby JV, Schmittdiel JA. Patient race/ethnicity and patient-physician race/ethnicity concordance in the management of cardiovascular disease risk factors for patients with diabetes. Diabetes Care. 2010;33(3):520–5. https://doi.org/10.2337/dc09-0760.

22. Nickson C. (2016, May 2017). Cognitive dispositions to respond [Blog post]. Life in the Fast Lane. Retrieved 15 Sept 2018 from https://lifeinthefastlane.com/ccc/cognitive-dispositions-to-respond/.

23. American Heart Association. (2014, June 16). Gender-specific research improves accuracy of heart disease diagnosis in women. ScienceDaily. Retrieved 15 Sept 2018 from www.sciencedaily.com/releases/2014/06/140616204359.htm.

24. Dador D. (2011, Nov 2). 'Medical sexism': Women's heart disease symptoms often dismissed. ABC: Eyewitness News. Retrieved from https://abc7.com/archive/8416664/.

25. Chiaramonte GR. (2007). Physicians' gender bias in the diagnosis, treatment, and interpretation of coronary heart disease symptoms (Doctoral dissertation) [PDF file]. Retrieved from https://dspace.sunyconnect.suny.edu/bitstream/handle/1951/44285/000000052.sbu.pdf?sequence=2.

26. Romero J. (2008, Oct 12). Study reveals that signs of heart disease are attributed to stress more frequently in women than men. AAAS: EurekAlert! Retrieved 15 Sept 2018 from https://www.eurekalert.org/pub_releases/2008-10/crf-srt101008.php.

27. Lichtman JH, Leifteit-Limson EC, Watanabe E, Allen NB, Garavalia B, Garavalia LS, Spertus JA, Krumholz HM, Curry LA. Symptom recognition and healthcare experiences of young women with acute myocardial infarction. Circ Cardiovasc Qual Outcomes. 2015;8(2, Suppl. 1):S31–8. https://doi.org/10.1161/CIRCOUTCOMES.114.001612.

28. Vaccarino V, Parsons L, Every NR, Barron HV, Krumholz HM. Sex-based differences in early mortality after myocardial infarction. N Engl J Med. 1999;341(4):217–25. https://doi.org/10.1056/NEJM199907223410401.

29. Levine N, Mor M, Ben-Hur R. Patterns of misdiagnosis of multiple sclerosis. Isr Med Assoc J. 2003;5(7):489–90.

30. Chen EH, Shofer FS, Dean AJ, Hollander JE, Baxt WG, Robey JL, Sease KL, Mills AM. Gender disparity in analgesic treatment of emergency department patients with acute abdominal pain. Acad Emerg Med. 2008;15(5):414–8. https://doi.org/10.1111/j.1553-2712.2008.00100.x.

31. Borkhoff CM, Hawker GA, Kreder HJ, Glazier RH, Mahomed NN, Wright JG. The effect of patients' sex on physicians' recommendations for total knee arthroplasty. Can Med Assoc J. 2008;178(6):681–7. https://doi.org/10.1503/cmaj.071168.

32. Melloni C, Berger JS, Wang TY, Gunes F, Stebbins A, Pieper KS, Dolor RJ, Douglas PS, Mark DB, Newby LK. Representation of women in randomized clinical trials of cardiovascular disease prevention. Circ Cardiovasc Qual Outcomes. 2010;3(2):135–42. https://doi.org/10.1161/CIRCOUTCOMES.110.868307.

33. Schmittdiel JA, Traylor A, Uratsu CS, Mangione CM, Ferrara A, Subramanian U. The association of patient-physician gender concordance with cardiovascular disease risk factor control and treatment in diabetes. J Women's Health. 2009;18(12):2065–70. https://doi.org/10.1089/jwh.2009.1406.

34. Porucznik MA. (n.d.). Obese patients present a weighty problem. American Academy of Orthopaedic Surgeons. Retrieved 15 Sept 2018 from https://www.aaos.org/CustomTemplates/AcadNewsArticle.aspx?id=8735&ssopc=1.

35. Brogan K. [Kelly Brogan MD]. (2017, Oct 22). My friend and New York Times Best Selling Author, Jessica Ortner is an expert in helping women to actually be able to make the changes they need to make to be able to lose weight. Jessica shares details on her approach to helping women find and overcome the unconscious emotions, beliefs, traumas and more that keep women from releasing weight in a COMPLIMENTARY webinar. [Facebook status update]. Retrieved from https://www.facebook.com/KellyBroganMD/posts/763643437175840.

36. O'Rourke M. (2014, Nov). Doctors tell all – and it's bad. The Atlantic. Retrieved 15 Sept 2018 from https://www.theatlantic.com/magazine/archive/2014/11/doctors-tell-all-and-its-bad/380785/.

37. Cornwall L. (2016, Jan 25). Physician bias: trends from the 2016 Medscape Lifestyle report. CompHealth. Retrieved from https://comphealth.com/resources/physician-bias-trends-from-the-2016-medscape-lifestyle-report/.

38. Huizinga MM, Cooper LA, Bleich SN, Clark JM, Beach MC. Physician respect for patients with obesity. J Gen Intern Med. 2009;24(11):1236–9. https://doi.org/10.1007/s11606-009-1104-8.

39. Hebl MR, Xu J. Weighing the care: physicians' reactions to the size of a patient. Int J Obes. 2001;25(8):1246–52. https://doi.org/10.1038/sj.ijo.0801681.

40. Adolph J, Yates C Jr. Value measurements: the impending barrier to orthopaedic surgery for obese patients. Curr Orthop Prac. 2016;27(2):125–8. https://doi.org/10.1097/BCO.0000000000000330.

41. Kolata G. (2016, Sept 25). Why do obese patients get worse care? Many Doctors don't see past the fat. The New York Times. Retrieved from https://www.nytimes.com/2016/09/26/health/obese-patients-health-care.html.

42. Campbell D. (2017, Apr 22). Smokers and obese patients face more curbs on NHS surgery. The Guardian. Retrieved 15 Sept 2018 from https://www.theguardian.com/society/2017/apr/22/nhs-letter-more-rations-on-operations-obese-smokers.

43. Coffey K. (2017, July 18). The shocking ways large women are mistreated by health-care providers [Blog post]. SELF. Retrieved from https://www.self.com/story/weight-bias-and-health-care.

44. Bleich SN, Gudzune KA, Bennett WL, Jarlenski MP, Cooper LA. How does physician BMI impact patient trust and perceived stigma? Prev Med. 2013;57(2):120–4. https://doi.org/10.1016/j.ypmed.2013.05.005.

45. McDermott BE, Sokolov G. Malingering in a correctional setting: the use of the structured interview of reported symptoms in a jail sample. Behav Sci Law. 2009;27(5):753–65. https://doi.org/10.1002/bsl.892.

46. Keller JE. (2016, May 22). The M-word–Malingering [Blog post]. Jail Medicine. Retrieved 15 Sept 2018 from http://www.jailmedicine.com/the-m-word-malingering/.

47. Tuteur A. (2009, June 4). Doctor, listen to your patient [Blog post]. The Skeptical OB. Retrieved from http://www.skepticalob.com/2009/06/doctor-listen-to-your-patient.html.

48. Burke SE, Dovidio JF, Przedworski JM, Hardeman RR, Perry SP, Phelan SM, Nelson DB, Burgess DJ, Yeazel MW, Van Ryn M. Do contact and empathy mitigate bias

against gay and lesbian people among heterosexual medical students? A report from Medical Student CHANGES. Acad Med. 2015;90(5):645–51. https://doi.org/10.1097/ACM.0000000000000661.

49. James SE, Herman JL, Rankin S, Keisling M, Mottet L, Anafi M. The report of the 2015 US transgender survey. Washington, DC: National Center for Transgender Equality; 2016.

50. Kanne S. Diagnostic overshadowing. In: Volkmar FR, editor. Encyclopedia of autism spectrum disorders. New York: Springer; 2013. https://doi.org/10.1007/978-1-4419-1698-3_398.

51. Sullivan G, Han X, Moore S, Kotrla K. Disparities in hospitalization for diabetes among persons with and without co-occurring mental disorders. Psychiatr Serv. 2006;57(8):1126–31. https://doi.org/10.1176/ps.2006.57.8.1126.

52. Weinstein LC, Stefancic A, Cunningham AT, Hurley KE, Cabassa LJ, Wender RC. Cancer screening, prevention, and treatment in people with mental illness. CA Cancer J Clin. 2016;66(2):133–51. https://doi.org/10.3322/caac.21334.

53. Pedersen T. (2015, Oct 6). Adults with mental illness smoke one-third of cigarettes in U.S. Psych Central. Retrieved 15 Sept 2018 from https://psychcentral.com/news/2013/02/09/adults-with-mental-illness-smoke-one-third-of-cigarettes-in-u-s/51411.html.

54. Dipasquale S, Pariante CM, Dazzan P, Aguglia E, McGuire P, Mondelli V. The dietary pattern of patients with schizophrenia: a systematic review. J Psychiatr Res. 2013;47(2):197–207. https://doi.org/10.1016/j.jpsychires.2012.10.005.

55. Stubbs B, Firth J, Berry A, Schuch FB, Rosenbaum S, Gaughran F, Veronesse N, Williams J, Craig T, Yung AR, Vancampfort D. How much physical activity do people with schizophrenia engage in? A systematic review, comparative meta-analysis and meta-regression. Schizophr Res. 2016;176(2–3):431–40. https://doi.org/10.1016/j.schres.2016.05.017.

56. Vancampfort D, Stubbs B, Mitchell AJ, De Hert M, Wampers M, Ward PB, Rosenbaum S, Correll CU. Risk of metabolic syndrome and its components in people with schizophrenia and related psychotic disorders, bipolar disorder and major depressive disorder: a systematic review and meta-analysis. World Psychiatry. 2015;14(3):339–47. https://doi.org/10.1002/wps.20252.

57. Hjorthøj C, Stürup AE, McGrath JJ, Nordentoft M. Years of potential life lost and life expectancy in schizophrenia: a systematic review and meta-analysis. Lancet Psychiatry. 2017;4(4):295–301. https://doi.org/10.1016/S2215-0366(17)30078-0.

58. Walker ER, McGee RE, Druss BG. Mortality in mental disorders and global disease burden implications: a systematic review and meta-analysis. JAMA Psychiat. 2015;72(4):334–41. https://doi.org/10.1001/jamapsychiatry.2014.2502.

59. Thornicroft G. Physical health disparities and mental illness: the scandal of premature mortality. Br J Psychiatry. 2011;199(6):441–2. https://doi.org/10.1192/bjp.bp.111.092718.

60. Gray AJ. Stigma in psychiatry. J R Soc Med. 2002;95(2):72–6. https://doi.org/10.1177/014107680209500205.

61. Saber H. (Hamed). Iranian woman [Image file]. In: Wikimedia commons. 2006. Retrieved from https://commons.wikimedia.org/wiki/Woman#/media/File:Portrait_of_a_Persian_lady_in_Iran,_10-08-2006.jpg; GabboT. Dennis Rodman 01 [Image file]. In: Wikimedia Commons. 2017. Retrieved from https://commons.wikimedia.org/w/index.php?title=Special:Search&limit=20&offset=0&profile=default&search=dennis+rodman#/media/File:Dennis_Rodman_01_(34679281591).jpg; Briggs C. (Christiaan). Iraqi militiaman at Sabaa Nissan [Image file]. In: Wikimedia commons. 2003. Retrieved from https://commons.wikimedia.org/wiki/Man#/media/File:Sabaa_Nissan_Militiaman.jpg; The Chancellery of the Senate of the Republic of Poland. Agata Kornhauser-Duda [Image file]. In: Wikimedia commons. 2015. Retrieved from https://commons.wikimedia.org/wiki/Woman#/media/File:Agata_Kornhauser-Duda_Sejm_2015.JPG; Evans S. (Steve). Kayaw woman [Image file]. In: Wikimedia commons. 2007. Retrieved from https://commons.wikimedia.org/wiki/Woman#/media/File:Tribes_woman_with_ear_piercing.jpg; Krech T. (Till). At a glance [Image file]. In: Wikimedia commons. 2006. Retrieved from https://commons.wikimedia.org/wiki/Category:LGBT_Pride#/media/File:At_a_glance_(195838401).jpg; Nguyen M-L. (Marie-Lan). March 2008 – Jean Peyrelevade [Image file]. In: Wikimedia commons. 2008. Retrieved from https://commons.wikimedia.org/wiki/Jean_Peyrelevade#/media/File:Sarnez_Mutualite_2008_03_04_n8.jpg; Agnostizi. Professor Dr. Ichiro Yamaguchi [Image file]. In: Wikimedia commons. 2000.

Retrieved from https://commons.wikimedia.org/wiki/Man#/media/File:Ichiro_Yamaguchi.jpg; Picq Y. (Yves). Himba woman [Image file]. In: Wikimedia commons. 2007. Retrieved from https://commons.wikimedia.org/wiki/Woman#/media/File:Namibie_Himba_0717a.jpg; Schwichtenberg F. (Frank). Johnny Flesh & the Redneck Zombies [Image file]. In: Wikimedia commons. 2014. Retrieved from https://commons.wikimedia.org/wiki/File:Johnny_Flesh_%26_the_Redneck_Zombies_%E2%80%93_Wilwarin_Festival_2014_03.jpg

62. Xiao NG, Quinn PC, Liu S, Ge L, Pascalis O, Lee K. Older but not younger infants associate own-race faces with happy music and other-race faces with sad music. Dev Sci. 2018;21(2):e12537. https://doi.org/10.1111/desc.12537.

63. University of Oxford. (2014, Mar 3). Race relations affected by where you live. ScienceDaily. Retrieved from www.sciencedaily.com/releases/2014/03/140303154100.htm.

Case

Cathy was a 25-year-old woman who presented with three days of double vision when she looked to the left. She was otherwise healthy, but said that she had a numbness in her right foot several months prior and had been diagnosed with a "pinched nerve." On examination, when she looked to the left, her right eye did not go fully to her nose and there was rhythmic beating of her left eye (nystagmus). This finding is called an internuclear ophthalmoplegia and is characteristic of multiple sclerosis (MS). She also had increased reflexes in her legs, indicative of damage to her motor pathway in the brain or spinal cord. An MRI revealed multiple demyelinating lesions (Fig. 17.1).

A spinal tap showed oligoclonal bands, a marker of inflammation found in 90% of patients with MS. Two days later, Cathy developed a severe headache whenever

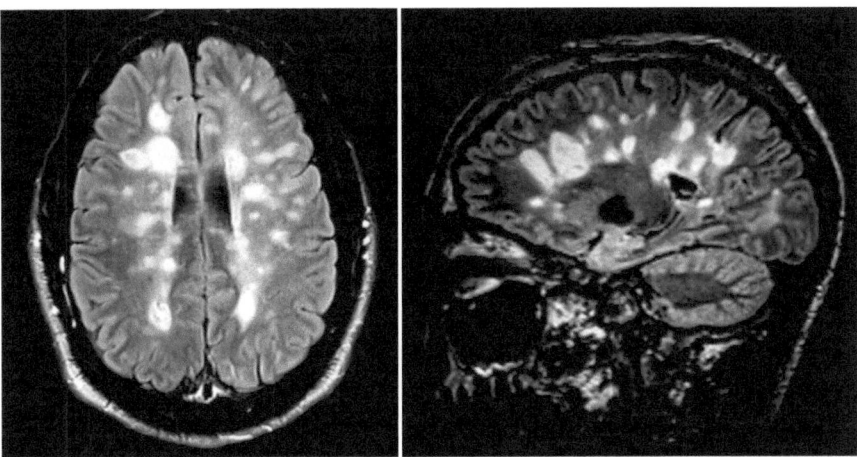

Fig. 17.1 FLAIR MRIs showing multiple demyelinating lesions as seen in MS

© Springer International Publishing AG, part of Springer Nature 2019
J. Howard, *Cognitive Errors and Diagnostic Mistakes*,
https://doi.org/10.1007/978-3-319-93224-8_17

she stood upright, characteristic of a low-pressure headache due to the spinal tap. Her own blood was injected into the lumbar puncture site with relief of her headache.

What Dr. Taylor Was Thinking

Nothing went horribly wrong with this case. Cathy developed cerebral hypotension, which can cause a severe headache, but is fortunately treatable with a blood patch. Cathy missed nearly a week of work and was not happy about that. When she asked me why the spinal tap was done in the first place, I told her I was hoping it would help confirm the diagnosis of MS, which it did. However, to be honest with myself, even before the spinal tap was done, it was pretty obvious she had the disease. She had a classic clinical presentation and classic MRI. While a spinal tap is generally a benign procedure, it is uncomfortable, and is of virtually no clinical value in a patient like Cathy. In other words, Cathy needed to be treated for MS regardless of whether oligoclonal bands were present or not. However, seeing that oligoclonal bands are present was satisfying, as it further confirmed what I knew was true.

Discussion

The information bias is the tendency to believe that the more evidence one can accumulate to support a diagnosis the better, even if the extra information is irrelevant for the decision. Clinicians often have a natural desire to obtain as much information as possible, even if this information won't alter their management. However, when ordering diagnostic tests, it is important to anticipate the potential value of information and whether it will be useful or not in establishing a diagnosis or altering how a patient is treated. Information should not be obtained for its own sake or out of curiosity. As Jerome Kassirer, a kidney specialist, wrote:

> The more information we get, the more confidence in the validity of our diagnoses we feel, even when such confidence may not be justified on the basis of the information obtained. Of course, the more tests we perform, the higher the risk to the patient: we often find ourselves performing a cascade of risky tests when a set of results is abnormal or ambiguous. Despite the limitations of our diagnostic procedures, we continue to test excessively, partly because of our discomfort with uncertainty. We have assiduously woven the goal of minimizing uncertainty into the fabric of clinical practice and teaching [1].

Jonathan Baron and colleagues provided an example of how the information bias can cause people to order worthless tests [2]. Study subjects were given the following case:

> A patient's presenting symptoms and history suggest a diagnosis of globoma, with about .8 probability. If it isn't globoma, it's either popitis or flapemia. Each disease has its own treatment, which is ineffective against the other two diseases. A test called the ET scan would certainly yield a positive result if the patient had popitis, and a negative result if she has flapemia. If the patient has globoma, a positive and negative result are equally likely. If the ET scan were the only test you could do, should you do it? Why or why not?

Table 17.1 Regardless of the result of the ET scan, 80% of patients have a globama

Test result	Patient with globoma	Patient with popitis	Patient with flapemia
Positive ET scan	40	10	0
Negative ET scan	40	0	10
All patients	80	10	10

Some simple math shows that the ET test is worthless in this scenario. In a group of 100 people, 80 will have a globoma, 10 will have popitis, and 10 will have flapemia. The ET test will be positive in 50 of the 100 patients and negative in 50. Regardless of the results of the ET test, there is an 80% chance the patient has a globoma, and the patient should therefore be treated for this disease. Nevertheless, when presented with this scenario, a number of subjects continued to insist that the ET would be a worthwhile test (Table 17.1).

In another problem, they asked subjects the following:

> A [different] patient has a .8 probability of umphitis. A positive Z-ray result would confirm the diagnosis, but a negative result would be inconclusive; if the result is negative, the probability would drop to .6. The treatment for umphitis is unpleasant, and you feel it is just as bad to give the treatment to a patient without the disease as to let a patient with the disease go untreated. If the Z-ray were the only test you could do, should you do it? Why or why not?

As with the first case, the Z-ray is useless. Regardless of its result, the probability that the patient has umphitis is over 50%, and the patient should be treated. While most subjects were able to do the math and understood this test was of no value, several people defended its use.

Unfortunately, few cases in medicine come in clean packages like the fictional case above. Clinicians routinely deal with relatively unknown probabilities and probabilities that shift dramatically as test results come back. Not surprisingly, there is a strong tendency for many clinicians to order multiple tests of questionable benefit so as not to "miss something." A real-world example of this is the use of CT scans in stroke patients who have received the thrombolytic medication tissue plasminogen activator (tPA). The main complication of this medication is intracerebral bleeding. For some patients these bleeds cause symptoms, while for others, the bleeds are clinically silent. The American Heart Association guidelines advise that clinicians get a CT 24 hours after giving tPA to screen asymptomatic patients for bleeding. The problem is, no one knows what to do with this information. A study by Theresa Sevilis and colleagues found that these CTs did not change patient management in 95% of asymptomatic patients [3]. Even when their management was changed (by delay in the administration of an antiplatelet agent), it is not clear if this is the right thing to do. As Dr. Sevilis said about her findings:

> So all of those patients got radiation exposure for really no reason... We're getting this CT head, you're finding out information, and then it kind of depends on the clinician as to what

to do. Some people will delay the antiplatelet agent and others will just give it right away. And really we don't actually have any evidence for which is the right answer [4].

Conclusion

There is a strong tendency in medicine to believe more information is better information, even if that information is irrelevant to the care of the patient. Getting a result that confirms a course of action is reassuring, even if a negative result would not alter the patient's treatment course. However, few tests are without risks, and all tests cost time and money. As such, before ordering any test, a clinician should ask themselves, "How will this test will change my management?" If no answer can be given, the test should not be ordered.

References

1. Kassirer JP. Our stubborn quest for diagnostic certainty. N Engl J Med. 1989;320(22):1489–91. https://doi.org/10.1056/NEJM198906013202211.
2. Baron J, Beattie J, Hershey JC. Heuristics and biases in diagnostic reasoning: II. Congruence, information, and certainty. Organ Behav Hum Decis Process. 1988;42(1):88–110. https://doi.org/10.1016/0749-5978(88)90021-0.
3. Collins TR. News from the AAN annual meeting: routine CT scans after tPA do not effect clinical management, study finds. Neurol Today. 2016;16(8):35–6. https://doi.org/10.1097/01.NT.0000483058.68552.99.
4. Samson K. News from the AAN annual meeting: phase 3 trial of Valbenazine for tardive dyskinesia clears way for new drug application. Neurol Today. 2016;16(8):1–27. https://doi.org/10.1097/01.NT.0000483048.63608.4b.

Case

Sadie was a 45-year-old woman who presented with three days of right-sided weakness and numbness. She had a history of systemic lupus erythematosus and had a prior episode of visual loss due to inflammation of her optic nerve (optic neuritis) several years prior. An MRI on admission showed a large lesion in the left frontal lobe. A biopsy was performed showing that this was a demyelinating lesion, and it was felt to be either due to multiple sclerosis (MS) or systemic lupus erythematosus (Fig. 18.1).

She was treated with intravenous steroids, which reduced the inflammation, though she never fully recovered. Two years later, she presented with the acute onset of bilateral leg weakness such that she could not walk. An MRI at that time revealed

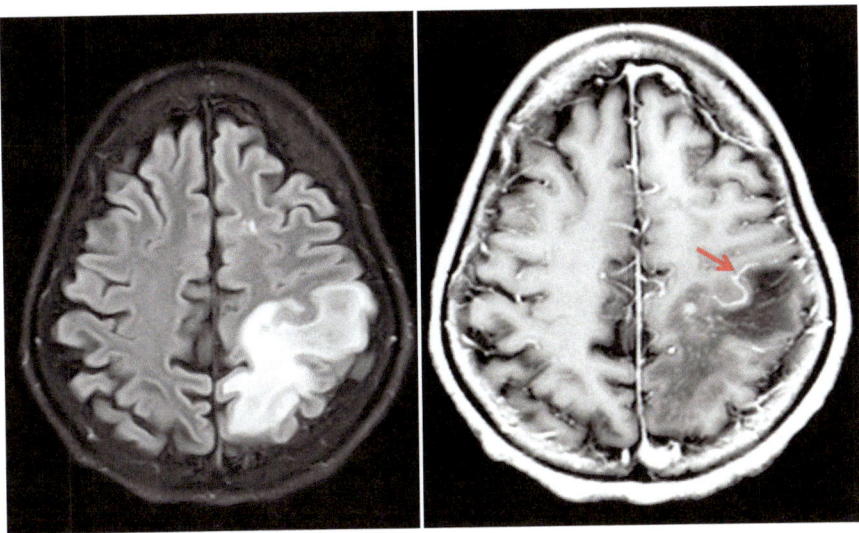

Fig. 18.1 FLAIR and post-contrast T1WI demonstrate a large white matter lesion in the left frontal lobe with peripheral enhancement (red arrow)

© Springer International Publishing AG, part of Springer Nature 2019
J. Howard, *Cognitive Errors and Diagnostic Mistakes*,
https://doi.org/10.1007/978-3-319-93224-8_18

inflammation throughout most of her cervical spinal cord. NMO antibodies, which had not been sent during her first admission, were positive. This confirmed the diagnosis of neuromyleitis optica (NMO), an inflammatory disease that presents with pathology of the optic nerves/chiasm, spinal cord, brainstem, or, less commonly, the brain.

What Dr. Yesky Was Thinking

In 2009, when I met Sadie, she did not have NMO, at least by the criteria at the time.
In 2006, the following formal diagnostic criteria were as follows:

- Optic neuritis.
- Acute myelitis.
- At least two of three supportive criteria:
  - Continuous spinal cord MRI lesion extending greater than three spinal cord segments in length.
  - Brain MRI not meeting the criteria for multiple sclerosis.
  - NMO-IgG antibody detected in the blood.

As new discoveries about NMO accumulated, these criteria were revised in 2015 to include brainstem syndromes, lesions of the thalamus that may present with narcolepsy, and symptomatic brain lesions. As such, many patients who might have been explicitly excluded from the 2006 diagnostic criteria for NMO, especially if their brain MRI met the diagnostic criteria for MS, are now known to have NMO.

At the time, it did not occur to me to send the blood test that would have made the diagnosis. By obeying the 2006 criteria, as if they had been delivered from stone tablets on Mount Sinai, I missed a chance to initiate immunosupressive treatment in Sadie. When the revised criteria were released the next year, it was obvious she had NMO all along. I suppose the mistake I could make now would be to assume that these 2015 criteria are set in stone and no further developments will occur.

Discussion

Nosology is a branch of medicine that deals with classification of diseases, disorders, syndromes, and injuries. The most widely used classification system is the International Statistical Classification of Diseases and Related Health Problems created by the World Health Organization. It contains 22 chapters and nearly 15,000 codes for diseases, abnormal signs, symptoms, social circumstances, and external causes of injury or diseases (Fig. 18.2).

Categorizing diseases this way is extremely important as it allows clinicians to communicate meaningfully to each other across time and space about the patients they treat. Additionally, little medical research would be possible without formal definitions of diseases. Certainly, many patients will have a disease that fits squarely within a well-established diagnostic category. However, the formal boundaries of many diseases can be rather arbitrary. It is often difficult to separate one disease from another, and sometimes there is great controversy as to whether a person even has a disease or not. Occasionally, a completely new disease emerges. Medicine is not a static field, and

Certain infectious and parasitic diseases
Neoplasms
Diseases of the blood and blood-forming organs and certain disorders involving the immune mechanism
Endocrine, nutritional and metabolic diseases
Mental and behavioral disorders
Diseases of the nervous system
Diseases of the eye and adnexa
Diseases of the ear and mastoid process
Diseases of the circulatory system
Diseases of the respiratory system
Diseases of the digestive system
Diseases of the skin and subcutaneous tissue
Diseases of the musculoskeletal system and connective tissue
Diseases of the genitourinary system
Pregnancy, childbirth and the puerperium
Certain conditions originating in the perinatal period
Congenital malformations, deformations and chromosomal abnormalities
Symptoms, signs and abnormal clinical and laboratory findings, not elsewhere classified
Injury, poisoning and certain other consequences of external causes
External causes of morbidity and mortality
Factors influencing health status and contact with health services
Codes for special purposes

Fig. 18. 2 Chapters in International Statistical Classification of Diseases and Related Health Problems. (World Health Organization. Classifications. ICD-11. 2018. Retrieved from http://www.who.int/classifications/icd/en/.)

clinicians who allow themselves to be hemmed in by formal diagnostic criteria may miss a new disease or a new manifestation of an old one. Additionally, diagnostic criteria may be overly broad, encompassing multiple different diseases. The nosology trap occurs when clinicians uncritically rely on formal diagnostic criteria to separate the sick from the healthy, to make a diagnosis, and to determine treatments.

Consider MS, the main disease I treat. At present, MS is classified primarily by the time course over which patients develop symptoms. The majority of patients present with relapsing-remitting disease. These patients develop the rather abrupt onset of neurological symptoms, which last for several days to weeks, and then gradually abate. In order to make a diagnosis of MS, a patient must have evidence, either based on their history or MRI, of central nervous system inflammation in at least two different places at different times. Patients with a single episode of inflammation cannot be said to have MS, but are instead said that have clinically isolated syndrome. Other patients have progressive disease, where symptoms slowly progress over the course of months to years without any abrupt changes (Fig. 18.3).

Yet, this disease classification system is clearly incomplete. It says nothing about which symptoms a given patient experiences. Some of my patients are in wheelchairs, but have no cognitive or visual impairment. Other patients can walk fairly

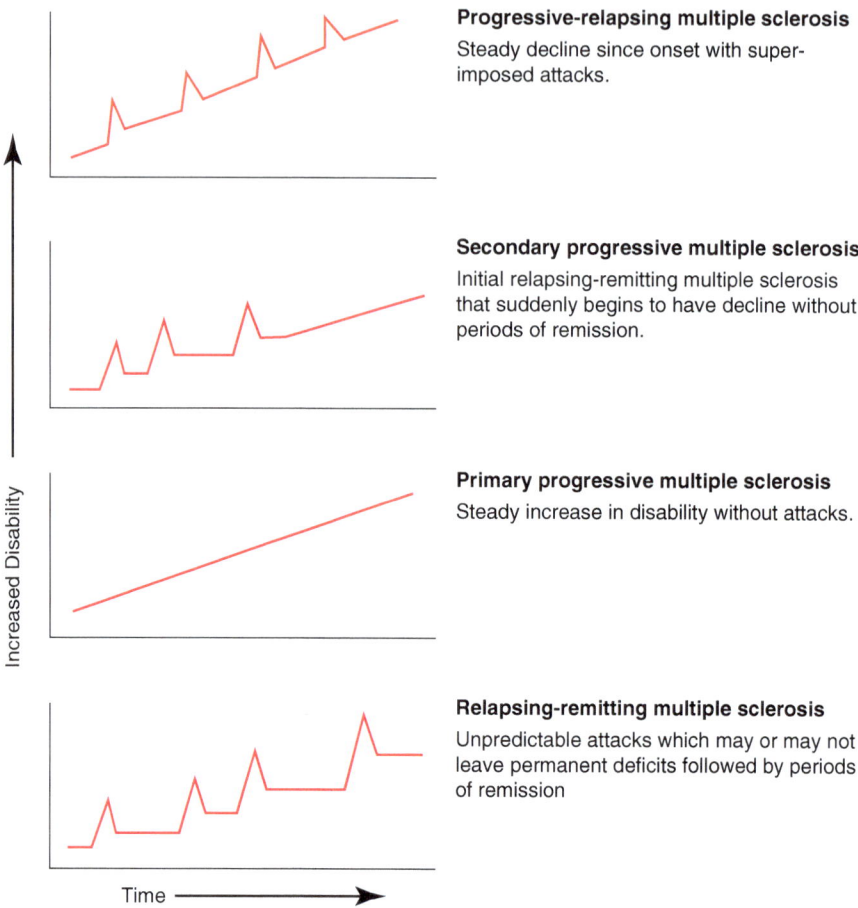

Fig. 18. 3 The main subtypes of multiple sclerosis. (Diagnosis of multiple sclerosis. [Image file]. In: Wikipedia. (n.d.). Retrieved from https://en.wikipedia.org/wiki/Diagnosis_of_multiple_sclerosis#/media/File:Ms_progression_types.svg.)

well, but have visual impairment or cognitive limitations. It also says nothing about the severity of impairment caused by the disease. I know several patients in their twenties who need full-time care due to their disability. At the other extreme, there are many patients in their sixties and seventies who have mild impairment that does not prevent them from leading a full and productive life. It's not entirely clear what is the best way to classify MS.

Even the diagnostic criteria for this seemingly well-established disease were modified in 2010, and further tweaked in 2017. Based on changes made that year, many patients who had clinically isolated syndrome prior to 2010 could now be diagnosed with MS. The existing categories of MS were further changed in 2014, and several new subcategories were added. I am sure that the current classification scheme will not be the final one. Similarly, the International League Against

Epilepsy revamped its basic seizure classification scheme in 2017. Terms that had been used for 35 years were eliminated and replaced with a new vocabulary [1]. These examples show that even the definition of diseases that have been described since antiquity are still subject to change today.

The implications of these changes are not just academic. All of the treatments for MS are approved based on the classification of the disease into relapsing and progressive forms. Additionally, because of changes in the definition of diseases, it is often impossible to compare studies conducted in different times. A study of patients with MS today can enroll a different patient population from a trial conducted only several years prior, making it problematic to compare results from one study to the next.

Many times, it is not clear where one disease stops and another begins. In the classification of medical conditions, there is a tension between the "lumpers" and "splitters," which are opposing camps that emerge when diseases have to be placed within rigorously specified categories. Lumpers combine things into broad categories, while splitters divide things into smaller categories.

There are many times when the "splitters" have won, and diseases that were once considered to be a single condition were recognized as different diseases. For example, NMO was once thought to be a variant of MS. Prior to discover of the antibody responsible for NMO, it was called opticospinal MS due to its propensity to attack the optic nerves and spinal cord. We now know that NMO is a completely separate disease from MS, and while the symptoms often overlap, some of the treatments for MS may actually worsen NMO. A clinician who treated NMO patients with medications for MS may have inadvertently done significant harm. Even today, it's still not clear whether MS is a single disease with a wide variety of manifestations or several different diseases that we currently lump together because we don't know any better. Time will tell.

At other times, a single disease has been split into multiple different types and subtypes based on advances in medical knowledge. For example, Charcot–Marie–Tooth disease is a relatively common peripheral nervous system disorder first described in 1886. It affects approximately one in 2,500 people in the US. It is characterized by the slow progression of weakness, gait disturbances, and numbness. It has evolved from its original designation as one disease and is now known to be caused by several different genetic mutations that lead to a broadly similar clinical presentation. Though they are still all called Charcot–Marie–Tooth disease, they have different symptoms, inheritance patterns, and prognoses. So, is Charcot–Marie–Tooth really one disease? Or it is multiple different genetic diseases that are artificially lumped together as one condition for the sake of convenience?

At other times, the lumpers have won, and multiple different diseases have been consolidated into a single entity. For example, several neurodegenerative diseases that existed when I was in medical school, such as Shy-Drager syndrome, striatonigral degeneration, and olivopontocerebellar atrophy, have now been merged into an entity called multiple system atrophy. Medical students today won't learn about these diseases, as they have effectively "disappeared" into a single category. Currently, multiple system atrophy is itself divided into two types depending if the patient has cerebellar dysfunction or symptoms that resemble Parkinson's disease.

Perhaps the splitters will again tackle multiple system atrophy, and future generations of medical students will learn about diseases that have yet to be named.

The classification of many cancers is also being radically altered by examining
their underlying molecular aberrations. The most common type of primary brain
tumor, known as a glioma, was divided into four categories for decades, based primarily on its appearance under a microscope. Today, gliomas are defined largely by the
presence or absence of certain genetic markers, which have enormous prognostic
value. In fact, it is often not clear which conditions should even earn the terrifying
designation "cancer [2]." Several conditions, previously classified as cancer and often
treated as such, have recently been changed, so that the word "cancer" was eliminated
from their description. In 2013, experts suggested renaming a breast condition called
ductal carcinoma in situ, eliminating the word "carcinoma" so that potentially harmful
treatments were avoided and patients were not needlessly frightened. Similarly, in
2016, an international team of doctors decided that a thyroid tumor (encapsulated follicular variant of papillary thyroid carcinoma), had been classified and treated as cancer, is not actually a cancer as it has a benign prognosis even without treatment [3].

Not only are old diseases reclassified, but new diseases are occasionally still
identified. Most obviously, this includes new infectious diseases. For example,
severe acute respiratory syndrome (SARS) is a viral infection that emerged in China
in 2002 and spread to nearly 40 countries, causing 8,098 cases of the disease and
774 deaths. Additionally, new antibody-mediated and genetic diseases are being
discovered as well. These diseases have likely existed for decades or centuries, but
are just being recognized now as a distinct disease entity. Anti-NMDA receptor
encephalitis, a disease that is gaining increasing recognition today, was only formally characterized in 2007 [4]. It presents with psychosis, cognitive disturbances,
and seizures, often in young women with benign ovarian tumors. Undoubtedly,
many patients were treated for years as having a primary psychotic disorder, such as
schizophrenia, without the neurological nature of their disease being recognized.

Along these lines, many diseases that were once thought to be "psychiatric" are
now realized to have a physiological basis. As late as the 1970s, many dystonias,
which are characterized by abnormal movements and postures due to sustained,
involuntary muscle contractions, were thought to be psychiatric in nature, when in
fact they have a genetic basis [5]. Certain dystonias caused by muscle overuse in
writers, musicians, and athletes were referred to as "occupational neurosis [6]."
Today, almost 30 different genetic mutations have been identified that lead to a wide
spectrum of dystonias. As the classification for this disease changed from psychiatric to neurologic, the treatment changed from psychotherapy to medications.

Large sums of money can be at stake if something is labeled a disease or not, and
where the boundaries of a certain disease are set. Widening the diagnostic boundaries of diseases is known as disease-mongering.

Science writer Lynn Payer defined disease-mongering as having the following
characteristics [7]:

• Stating that normal human experiences are abnormal and in need of treatment.
• Advertising a common symptom as a serious disease.

- Claiming to recognize suffering, which is not present.
- Defining a disease such that a large number of people have it.
- Defining a disease's cause as an ambiguous hormonal imbalance or deficiency.
- Associating a disease with a public relations spin campaign.
- Directing the framing of public discussion of a disease.
- Intentionally misusing statistics to exaggerate treatment benefits and setting a dubious clinical endpoint in research.
- Advertising a treatment as without side effect.

A 2002 editorial in the *British Medical Journal* (BMJ) titled *Selling Sickness: The Pharmaceutical Industry and Disease Mongering* warned of disease-mongering, saying:

> *Inappropriate medicalisation carries the dangers of the unnecessary labelling, poor treatment decisions, iatrogenic illness, and economic waste, as well as the opportunity costs that result when resources are diverted away from treating or preventing more serious disease. At a deeper level it may help to feed unhealthy obsessions with health, obscure or mystify sociological or political explanations for health problems, and focus undue attention on pharmacological, individualised, or privatised solution* [8].

Disease-mongering is a common tactic of both pharmaceutical companies and practitioners of complementary and alternative medicine (CAM) who profit when previously healthy people are considered ill. Conditions such as adrenal fatigue, chronic Lyme disease, electromagnetic hypersensitivity, leaky gut syndrome, multiple chemical sensitivity, and non-celiac gluten sensitivity are unrecognized conditions that CAM practitioners promote right before they try to sell you the cure. Once a condition is labeled a disease, the genie is out of the bottle, and it can be hard to put back in.

Similarly, the cut-off for bona fide diseases can be lowered, creating conditions such as "pre-dementia" and "pre-diabetes." With MS, the criteria have been relaxed to make it possible to diagnosis the disease in people who have had a single neurological event combined with MRI data. It is not clear that this is an improvement for patients, but it forces insurance companies to pay for medications in people who might have previously been ineligible for them. In the 1990s, the definition of osteoporosis was redefined such that nearly 25% of post-menopausal women were considered to have the "disease." Soon after this, Merck launched the osteoporosis drug Fosamax, which became a blockbuster, selling billions of dollars. In 2008, the US National Osteoporosis Foundation again altered their guidelines such that 72% of white women older than 65% and 93% of those older than 75 were suggested to take drugs for osteoporosis [9]. Similarly, in 2017 guidelines from the American Heart Association and the American College of Cardiology redefined hypertension as a blood pressure greater than 130/80 mmHg, down from the previous value of 140/90 mmHg [10]. Almost half of adults in the US will meet criteria for hypertension based on this revision, up from about one-third. While the guidelines stressed that vast majority of the new cases could be managed by lifestyle interventions, invariably this will lead to the use of more medications (though by some estimates the numbers will be rather low) [11].

When expert panels meet to define diseases, they almost never advocate for making the criteria for the disease more stringent. Raymond Moynihan and colleagues reviewed 16 publications representing 14 diseases where expert panels suggested changing diagnostic criteria. The disease definition widened for 10 diseases, narrowed for only one, and had an unclear impact in five diseases [12]. Additionally, expert panels rarely consider the potential harms of over-diagnosis. Even more concerning is that many panels have been found to have members with undeclared conflicts of interest with pharmaceutical companies [12].

In response to disease-mongering, an international group of multidisciplinary experts created a checklist of eight questions to consider when modifying the definition of a disease [13].

1. **Definition**: What are the differences between the previous and new definition?
2. **Number of people affected**: How will the new disease definition change the incidence and prevalence of the disease?
3. **Trigger**: What is the trigger for considering the modification of the disease definition?
4. **Prognostic ability**: How well does the new definition of disease predict clinically important outcomes compared with the previous definition?
5. **Disease definition precision and accuracy**: What is the repeatability, reproducibility, and accuracy of the new disease definition?
6. **Benefit**: What is the incremental benefit for patients classified by the new disease definition versus the previous definition?
7. **Harm**: What is the incremental harm for patients classified by the new definition versus the previous definition?
8. **New benefit and harms**: What is the net benefit and harm for patients classified by the new definition versus the previous definition? (Fig. 18.4)

It is often difficult to determine if a patient has a disease at all. Family medicine doctor Ian McWhinney wrote, defining the word "disease" can be as difficult as defining "beauty, truth, and love [14]." A survey of 3,280 doctors, nurses, and laypeople in Finland by Kari Tikkinen and colleagues showed it is difficult to determine what does and does not constitute disease and that professional clinicians can have a different opinion from the general public [15]. There was broad agreement amongst responders that conditions such as malaria and lung cancer are diseases. There was also broad agreement that conditions such as aging, wrinkles, and homosexuality are not diseases. However, there was disagreement about whether conditions such as gambling addiction, infertility, and drug addiction are diseases.

In an attempt to demonstrate the "slipperiness of the notion of disease," The BMJ conducted a survey in 2002 asking their readers to identify "non-diseases," which they defined as "a human process or problem that some have defined as a medical condition but where people may have better outcomes if the problem or process was not defined in that way [16]." The suggestions, compiled in an international classification of non-disease, included several conditions that most clinicians would today consider diseases, such as alcohol dependency, anorexia,

Checklist Item	Rationale
1. Definition: What are the differences between the previous and the new definition?	It is important to delineate the proposed change precisely.
2. Number of people affected: How will the new disease definition change the incidence and prevalence of the disease?	The number of people affected is important in understanding benefits, harms, and resources needed.
3. Trigger: What is the trigger for considering the modification of the disease definition?	Stating the trigger for considering modification helps understand the necessity for modifying the disease definition.
4. Prognostic ability: How well does the new definition of disease predict clinically important outcomes compared with the previous definition?	The most important feature of a disease definition is its ability to accurately predict clinically meaningful outcomes.
5. Disease definition precision and accuracy: What is the repeatability, reproducibility, and accuracy (when estimations are possible) of the new disease definition?	Disease definitions that are repeatable and reproducible improve the consistency of clinical decision-making. Accuracy is often not able to be estimated owing to the lack of a reference standard.
6. Benefit: What is the incremental benefit for patients classified by the new definition vs the previous definition?	Benefits of the disease definition can be outlined, using methods such as GRADE. It is particularly important to estimate benefits in conditions where the new definition will be used to determine treatment thresholds.
7. Harm: What is the incremental harm for patients classified by the new definition vs the previous definition?	Harms may also be outlined using methods such as GRADE. It is often more difficult to quantify harms, and particularly the psychosocial harms and harms on the societal level, including resource related harms.
8. Net benefit and harms: What is the net benefit and harm for patients classified by the new definition vs the previous definition?	A panel should consider all of the above, and the balance of net benefits and harms prior to modifying a disease definition.

Fig. 18. 4 Checklist of items to consider when modifying a disease definition

attention deficit disorder, and tics. It also included many conditions that few would consider diseases today, including loneliness, boredom, flat feet, colic, aging, and false memory syndrome. While these conditions can cause undoubtedly immense suffering, it is not clear that people suffering from them are necessarily ill. Perhaps future generations will disagree.

Clinicians struggle to know what to do with people who are suffering but not necessarily ill. People with conditions that are generally not regarded as diseases often chafe at the idea that they are healthy. Strong communities form, often on social media and under the influence of passionate, charismatic leaders. They often rail against a seemingly callous and dogmatically rigid medical system that fails to legitimatize their suffering. People with Morgellons disease, for example, believe their skin has been infested with yet to be identified parasites. According to The Morgellons Research Foundation, "The symptoms include itching, biting and crawling sensations, 'filaments' or fibers which emerge from the skin, skin lesions which range from minor to disfiguring, joint pain, debilitating fatigue, changes in cognition, memory loss, mood disturbance and serious neurological manifestations [17]." Under close analysis, the fibers are often found to be cotton and other clothing items. A $600,000 study conducted by the CDC failed to elucidate the etiology, and most clinicians view the disorder as a delusional parasitosis. Not surprisingly, Morgellons sufferers did not accept this conclusion. Jan Smith, a leading patient advocate, said in an interview, "I'm pretty sure they'll say we're all delusional. There's so much more to this than a medical condition. There's something being hidden [18]."

Clifton K. Meador, a professor of medicine, argued in 1965 that patients with such conditions should be labeled as having a specific non-disease [19]. He wrote:

> Patients are frequently seen on referral with a specific disease diagnosis, and yet investigation fails to substantiate the referral diagnosis; in fact it may not reveal any disease. What, then, does the patient have? He must have something. The argument will be presented that he or she has a particular nondisease. This is certainly more reasonable than the common error of continuing to label such patients with nonexistent diseases.

However, a small study by KB Thomas in 1987 showed that this might be a mistake, at least in communicating with patients. He studied 200 patients for whom no definitive diagnosis could be made. Some of the patients had a positive consult, where they received a diagnosis and told they would improve. Others had a negative consult, where no diagnosis was made and no prognosis for improvement was rendered. Two weeks later, 64% of the patients who received a "positive" consultation improved, while only 39% who received a "negative" consultation improved [20].

Even if no disease diagnosis can be made, clinicians should remember that patients are still suffering. As Mark L. Eberhard, director of the division of parasitic diseases and malaria at the CDC, said about patients with Morgellons, "These people are definitely suffering from something. It has impacted their lives greatly [18]."

Political and cultural norms can further complicate determinations of what is and is not considered a disease. Culture-bound syndrome is a well-recognized set of psychiatric and somatic symptoms that are recognized as a disease within a specific society or culture. Dozens such syndromes exist. Koro, for example, is seen in parts of Africa and Asia. It is a delusional disorder in which people believe their genitals are retracting and will disappear. Running amok occurs in Indonesia and Malaysia, and is defined as "an episode of sudden mass assault against people or objects usually by a single individual following a period of brooding."

Western cultures have their own culture-bound syndromes. A condition known as neurasthenia was described by a New York neurologist George Beard in 1869. It was characterized by headaches, palpitations, hypertension, neuralgia, fatigue, anxiety, and depression. He believed it was caused by busy society women, overworked businessmen, and the general challenges of living in an increasingly industrial world. It was also called Americanitis, as it was common in the US. It was thought to be a condition that could only afflict people with active, intelligent minds and racist explanations were given as to why only white people could get the "disease." National parks were established in part to let people with neurasthenia rest [21]. While neurasthenia essentially died as a diagnosis 100 years ago, its echoes are seen with conditions such as chronic fatigue syndrome and chronic Lyme disease.

More recently, homosexuality was classified as a disease by the American Psychiatric Association (APA) in its official *Diagnostic and Statistical Manual of Mental Disorders* until 1973. Even today, some fundamentalist Christian groups continue to advocate for conversion therapy as a means to "cure" homosexuality. While the notion of homosexuality as a disease likely seems abhorrent to most people, it is possible that there currently stigmatized behaviors that future generations might view as a sign of mental illness. For example, psychiatrist Alvin Poussaint argued that extreme racism should be considered a delusional disorder and that it is amenable to treatment. He wrote, "It is time for the American Psychiatric Association to designate extreme racism as a mental health problem by recognizing it as a delusional psychotic symptom [22]."

Other critics argue that psychiatric illnesses in particular have a significant cultural component and that medicalizing them using Western values carries potentially grave consequences for non-Western cultures. Ethan Waters wrote in *The New York Times* that:

> For more than a generation now, we in the West have aggressively spread our modern knowledge of mental illness around the world. We have done this in the name of science, believing that our approaches reveal the biological basis of psychic suffering and dispel prescientific myths and harmful stigma. There is now good evidence to suggest that in the process of teaching the rest of the world to think like us, we've been exporting our Western "symptom repertoire" as well. That is, we've been changing not only the treatments but also the expression of mental illness in other cultures. Indeed, a handful of mental-health disorders — depression, post-traumatic stress disorder and anorexia among them — now appear to be spreading across cultures with the speed of contagious diseases. These symptom clusters are becoming the lingua franca of human suffering, replacing indigenous forms of mental illness.

Finally, defining someone as "diseased" has important implications for how patients view themselves, how they are viewed by their loved ones, and by society at large. Receiving a medical diagnosis may have significant practical implications for a person's life, determining whether someone is exempt from work or entitled to benefits. For the most part, sick people are thought of as needing care, sympathy, and treatment.

However, this is not always the case, and at times defining someone as "diseased" can be used as a weapon to stigmatize and discriminate against them. As the example of homosexuality shows, psychiatric diagnoses in particular have all too often been used as weapons to denigrate certain classes of people and stigmatize individuals. The most famous example of this occurred in a 1964 magazine article titled, *1189 Psychiatrists Say Goldwater is Psychologically Unfit to Be President!* In it, psychiatrists said that the Republican candidate for president, Barry Goldwater, was mentally unfit for the job. He was called "unpredictable," "emotionally unstable," and "a dangerous lunatic! [23]" Barry Goldwater successfully sued for libel, and the APA established an ethical principle, known informally as the "Goldwater rule," that prohibited psychiatrists from giving their medical opinion about someone unless they have personally evaluated them and consent has been obtained. (There have been calls to end this rule with the election of Donald Trump.)

Even more dramatically, psychiatric diagnoses have been used at times to subject people to unethical medical procedures such as forced sterilization. Most famously, Carrie Buck was forcibly sterilized in 1927 at the age of 19 for being "feeble-minded" and "promiscuous." Her case made it to the Supreme Court, where famed jurist Oliver Wendell Holmes defended her sterilization by famously arguing that "Three generations of imbeciles are enough." The ruling legitimized Virginia's sterilization procedures, which were only repealed in 1974. Her sister Doris was also sterilized without her knowledge when she was hospitalized for appendicitis. Carrie Buck's one child, conceived at the age of 17 as the result of a rape, was considered to be above-average intelligence, and there is no evidence Ms. Buck herself was particularly impaired. She was described as an avid reader until her death in 1983.

Conclusion

The principle of linguistic relativity (the Sapir–Whorf hypothesis) posits that the structure of a language affects the cognition and thoughts of those who speak it. While this is a controversial notion, it is clear that, to some degree in medicine, the classification schemes used to categorize diseases affect how clinicians think about them. Given that medical diagnoses are often in flux, clinicians must be careful not to be hemmed in by formal diagnostic criteria for diseases. Obviously, this is not to say that formal diagnostic criteria are meaningless or without use. Clinicians need a framework to conceptualize diseases and to communicate with each other. These criteria are also necessary for medical research. In a clinical study of any disease, it is important that only persons who meet the criteria for that disease be enrolled in the study.

However, by rigidly assuming that medical diagnostic categories are fixed entities without room for change, clinicians may fail to recognize heretofore undescribed variations of a disease or even an entirely new disease. Alternatively, they may respond to the name of the disease- certainly encapsulated follicular variant of papillary thyroid carcinoma and ductal carcinoma in situ sound scary- rather than to the actual threat the "disease" poses. Additionally, some diseases are culturally bound. A condition that is considered a disease today might be considered a variant of normal in the future, and vice versa. Finally, clinicians who sit on expert panels should be very cautious before expanding the boundary of disease, carefully considering the risks and benefits of the proposed change.

References

1. Fisher RS, Shafer PO, D'Souza C. (2016). 2017 revised classification of seizures, J. I. Sirven (Reviewer). Epilepsy Foundation. Retrieved from https://www.epilepsy.com/article/2016/12/2017-revised-classification-seizures.
2. Esserman LJ, Thompson IM, Reid B. Overdiagnosis and overtreatment in cancer: an opportunity for improvement. JAMA. 2013;310(8):797–8. https://doi.org/10.1001/jama.2013.108415.

3. Nikiforov YE, Seethala RR, Tallini G, Baloch ZW, Basolo F, Thompson LDR, Barletta JA, Wenig BM, Al Ghuzlan A, Kakudo K, Giordano TJ, Alves VA, Khanafshar E, Asa SL, El-Naggar AK, Gooding WE, Hodak SP, Lloyd RV, Maytal G, Mete O, Nikiforova MN, Nosé V, Papotti M, Poller DN, Sadow PM, Tischler AS, Tuttle RM, Wall KB, VA LV, Randolph GW, Ghossein RA. Nomenclature revision for encapsulated follicular variant of papillary thyroid carcinoma: a paradigm shift to reduce overtreatment of indolent tumors. JAMA Oncol. 2016;2(8):1023–9. https://doi.org/10.1001/jamaoncol.2016.0386.

4. Dalmau J, Tüzün E, Wu H, Masjuan J, Rossi JE, Voloschin A, Baehring JM, Shimazaki H, Koide R, King D, Mason W, Sansing LH, Dichter MA, Rosenfeld MR, Lynch DR. Paraneoplastic anti-N-methyl-D-aspartate receptor encephalitis associated with ovarian teratoma. Ann Neurol. 2007;61(1):25–36. https://doi.org/10.1002/ana.21050.

5. Munts AG, Koehler PJ. How psychogenic is dystonia? Views from past to present. Brain. 2010;133(5):1552–64. https://doi.org/10.1093/brain/awq050.

6. Pritchard MH. Writer's cramp: Is focal dystonia the best explanation? JRSM Short Rep. 2013;4(7):1–7. https://doi.org/10.1177/2042533313480071.

7. Martin T. Disease-mongers: how doctors, drug companies, and insurers are making you feel sick. N Engl J Med. 1993;328(3):218. https://doi.org/10.1056/NEJM199301213280322.

8. Moynihan R, Heath I, Henry D. Selling sickness: the pharmaceutical industry and disease mongering. BMJ. 2002;324(7342):886–91. https://doi.org/10.1136/bmj.324.7342.886.

9. Donaldson MG, Cawthon PM, Lui LY, Schousboe JT, Ensrud KE, Taylor BC, Cauley JA, Hillier TA, Black DM, Bauer DC, Cummings SR. Estimates of the proportion of older white women who would be recommended for pharmacological treatment by the new U.S. National Osteoporosis Foundation guidelines. J Bone Miner Res. 2009;24(4):675–80. https://doi.org/10.1359/jbmr.081203.

10. Bernstein L, Cha AE. (2017, Nov 13). Blood pressure of 130 is the new 'high,' according to first update of guidelines in 14 years. The Washington Post. Retrieved from https://www.washingtonpost.com/news/to-your-health/wp/2017/11/13/blood-pressure-of-130-is-the-new-high-according-to-first-update-of-guidelines-in-14-years/.

11. American Heart Association News. (2017, Nov 13). Nearly half of U.S. adults could now be classified with high blood pressure, under new definitions. American Heart Association. Retrieved from https://www.heart.org/en/news/2018/07/18/nearly-half-of-us-adults-could-now-be-classified-with-high-blood-pressure-under-new-definitions.

12. Moynihan RN, Cooke GPE, Doust JA, Bero L, Hill S, Glasziou PP. Expanding disease definitions in guidelines and expert panel ties to industry: a cross-sectional study of common conditions in the United States. PLoS Med. 2013;10(8):e1001500. https://doi.org/10.1371/journal.pmed.1001500.

13. Doust J, Vandvik PO, Qaseem A, Mustafa RA, Horvath AR, Frances A, Al-Ansary L, Bossuyt P, Ward RL, Kopp I, Gollogly L, Schunemann H, Glasziou P. Guidance for modifying the definition of diseases. JAMA Intern Med. 2017;177(7):1020–5. https://doi.org/10.1001/jamainternmed.2017.1302.

14. McWhinney IR. Health and disease: problems of definition. CMAJ. 1987;136(8):815.

15. Tikkinen KAO, Leinonen JS, Guyatt GH, Ebrahim S, Järvinen TLN. What is a disease? Perspectives of the public, health professionals and legislators. BMJ Open. 2012;2(6):e001632. https://doi.org/10.1136/bmjopen-2012-001632.

16. Smith R. In search of "non-disease". BMJ. 2002;324(7342):883–5. https://doi.org/10.1136/bmj.324.7342.883.

17. Admin. (2014, April 29). Frequently asked questions [Blog post]. Morgellons Disease? The Morgellons Research Foundation (MRF). Retrieved from https://www.morgellons.org/faq-home.htm.

18. Mystery skin disease Morgellons has no clear cause, CDC study says. (2012, Jan 25). NBC News. Retrieved from http://vitals.nbcnews.com/_news/2012/01/25/10236063-mystery-skin-disease-morgellons-has-no-clear-cause-cdc-study-says.

19. Meador CK. The art and science of nondisease. N Engl J Med. 1965;272(2):92–5. https://doi.org/10.1056/NEJM196501142720208.

20. Thomas KB. General practice consultations: is there any point in being positive? Br Med J (Clin Res Ed). 1987;294(6581):1200–2. https://doi.org/10.1136/bmj.294.6581.1200.
21. Beck J. (2016, Mar 11). 'Americanitis': the disease of living too fast. The Atlantic. Retrieved from https://www.theatlantic.com/health/archive/2016/03/the-history-of-neurasthenia-or-americanitis-health-happiness-and-culture/473253/.
22. Poussaint AF. Is extreme racism a mental illness?: yes: it can be a delusional symptom of psychotic disorders. West J Med. 2002;176(1):4.
23. Held A. (2017, July 25). 'Goldwater rule' still in place barring many psychiatrists from commenting on Trump. National Public Radio. Retrieved from https://www.npr.org/sections/thetwo-way/2017/07/25/539238529/goldwater-rule-still-in-place-barring-many-psychiatrists-from-commenting-on-trum.

Case

Herbert was a 34-year-old man who suffered from multiple sclerosis (MS) for eight years. His initial symptom was trouble walking, and he was found to have multiple demyelinating lesions in his spine and brain. He was placed on glatiramer acetate, a safe, but only partially effective treatment. He continued to have multiple relapses with resultant progression in his disability. Five years into his disease course, he was using a cane and had developed cognitive and visual impairment. The decision was made to place him on natalizumab, a monoclonal antibody given intravenously every month that is highly effective in preventing relapses in MS. However, it carries a significant risk for a potentially fatal viral infection known as progressive multiple focal leukoencephalopathy (PML). The causative virus is the JC virus, and Herbert had serum antibodies against the JC virus detected in his serum. In patients with significantly elevated antibody levels, the risk of PML is about one in 100. Based on Herbert's blood tests, he had an approximately 1:1,000 risk of contracting PML if continued on natalizumab.

Herbert did well for the next two years. For the first time several years, he suffered no relapses and had only minimal progression of his disability. However, as natalizumab treatment beyond two years is a risk factor for PML, the neurologist elected to discontinue this treatment and return to glatiramer acetate. Within one year, he suffered several significant relapses and became mostly wheelchair bound.

What Dr. Smith Was Thinking

I realized that Herbert had severe MS, and I was obviously pleased that he had done well on natalizumab. However, as he approached two years of being on the medication, I felt that the risks of remaining on natalizumab outweighed the benefits. Obviously, this is not a decision I would make independent of patient input. However, Herbert was quite cognitively impaired and unable to remember what happened to him last week. He was clearly not capable of appreciating the risks and benefits of changing medications and would have done whatever I suggested, effectively leaving the decision to me alone.

© Springer International Publishing AG, part of Springer Nature 2019   321
J. Howard, *Cognitive Errors and Diagnostic Mistakes*,
https://doi.org/10.1007/978-3-319-93224-8_19

I had seen my first case of natalizumab-induced PML several months prior, and although the patient lived, she was permanently disabled. A colleague of mine had a patient die of natalizumab-induced PML as well, and was being sued by the patient's family. Had Herbert continued on natalizumab and contracted PML, it would have been very easy to second-guess my decision. There is no doubt we would have had to discuss the case at the hospital where I work, the case would have been reported to the drug-company and the FDA, and I would have left myself vulnerable to a lawsuit. Finally, I would have felt like I injured or even killed this young man. That would have been a heavy burden for me to bear.

I knew he had a 1:1,000 risk of contracting PML. To me, this was too much, and stopping natalizumab was an easy decision. However, I admit I don't have a number in my head that would have been an acceptable risk, and could not objectively defend any particular number.

However, within one year, Herbert was permanently wheelchair bound due to a worsening of his MS. In contrast, even with this horrific outcome, there was no conference to discuss his case, no report was made to the drug company or any regulatory agency, and the patient's family didn't sue me. While I was certainly not happy with this bad outcome, I didn't feel *responsible* for it. After all, the patient's disease disabled him, not the medication I gave him.

Discussion

The principle of non-maleficence is one of the basic principles of medical ethics, and is summarized in the oft-quoted dictum *primum non nocere,* "first, do no harm" [1]. The omission bias occurs when clinicians inappropriately fear a harm they might cause more than a harm they fail to prevent. When a treatment harms a patient, there is a natural tendency for clinicians to feel responsible and that an error was made, even if the treatment was appropriate. Conversely, when a disease harms a patient, clinicians certainly feel sympathy, but they are less likely to feel responsible. This serves as a powerful motivation to avoid harming the patient through action, even if inaction is more likely to result in substantial harm. Of course, a patient who is harmed by their illness may be suffering more than a patient who is injured by a treatment. This suffering is not less because it is "natural."

The omission bias can be understood by recognizing that people feel differently about the same outcome depending on whether or not they feel responsible for it. Perhaps no scenario illustrates this better than the trolley problem, which was created by the philosopher Philippa Foot. In this famous thought experiment, there is a trolley traveling along railway tracks. Up ahead, there are five people tied up on the tracks. You are standing next to a lever, and if you pull this lever, the trolley will move to a different set of tracks. However, on this set of tracks, there is one person tied up. Would you allow the trolley to continue on its current path, killing five people? Or would you pull the lever, diverting the trolley so that it will kill one person? [2]

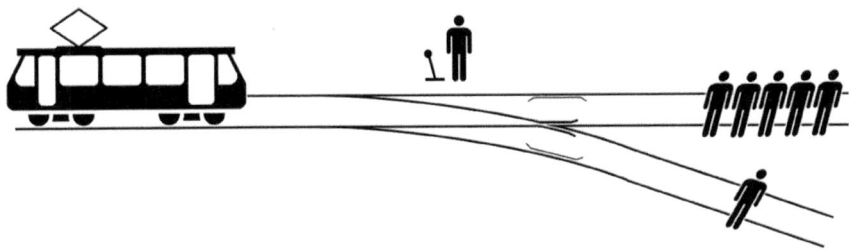

Recognizing that a simple tug on a lever can save four lives, most people say they would pull it. However, consider this variation created by the philosopher Judith Thomson:

> As before, a trolley is hurtling down a track towards five people. You are on a bridge under which it will pass, and you can stop it by putting something very heavy in front of it. As it happens, there is a very fat man next to you – your only way to stop the trolley is to push him over the bridge and onto the track, killing him to save five. Should you proceed?

In contrast to the original scenario, where most people will pull the lever to save four lives, many people will reject pushing the heavy man to save four lives. Yet, other than feeling they are doing more and are therefore more responsible, nothing has really changed. Consider another scenario:

> Five ill people are waiting for an organ transplant and will soon die. By killing a healthy man and harvesting his organs, the lives of these five people will be saved. Would you kill this one man to save the lives of five other people?

No one in their right mind would kill this healthy man. Yet, it's hard to parse out exactly what the difference is. In each of these scenarios, one person is sacrificed so that five others may live. Multiple variations of the trolley problem exist. They demonstrate that people feel differently about bad outcomes depending on whether they feel they directly caused the calamity or whether they failed to prevent it.

Psychologist Joshua Greene has proposed that in the same way our cognitive systems have a "fast" and slow" mode, so do our moral reasoning systems (this is called the dual process account) [3]. The first is emotional, instinctual, and mostly unconscious. The second is a slower, conscious, controlled process of moral reasoning. Each of these systems corresponds to a different brain area on functional MRI investigations. Conflicts arise when people must choose between violating moral rules and maximizing the overall good.

The practice of medicine can be analogous to the trolley problem in that clinicians must often choose between harms they directly cause and harms they fail to prevent. Studies of the omission bias have confirmed its presence in health care workers. In one study, pulmonary and critical care doctors were given scenarios involving the evaluation of pulmonary embolism and treatment of septic shock, two potentially fatal conditions. When an omission option was present, a majority of respondents chose a suboptimal treatment strategy [4]. Similarly, in another study university faculty and staff were queried regarding their willingness to accept a free influenza vaccine or a medication. While both the vaccine and the medication prevented a negative health outcome, they could also cause the negative health outcome, though at a lower rate [5]. Many respondents demonstrated the omission bias by refusing the vaccine or medication even when it lowered the overall risk of a poor outcome. In contrast, many respondents were willing to accept a treatment as long as it was called a "natural herb," even when the risks and benefits were identical to a treatment synthesized in a laboratory (the naturalness bias.) The omission and naturalness biases are likely the driving factors behind the anti-vaccine movement [6]. For many anti-vaccine advocates, the fear of a vaccine causing harm is greater than their fear of natural diseases (Fig. 19.1).

Clinicians and patients alike may fall victim to a form of the omission bias called the zero-risk bias. It is a tendency chose a course of action that completely eliminates a particular risk even when the alternative causes a greater overall reduction in risk. Completely eliminating a risk, even a small one, has larger psychological rewards than reducing a risk from a high level to a medium level. In other words, reducing the risk of a serious side effect from 1% to 2% may seem more significant than reducing a risk from 70% to 65%. In the case presented at the start of this chapter, stopping natalizumab reduced Herbert's risk of PML to zero, though the risk was relatively low to begin with. However, it left him exposed to a much higher risk of his MS becoming active.

Many clinicians today practice the zero-risk bias when they refuse to prescribe opioid pain medications for patients with chronic pain. In the understandable desire to prevent addiction and life-threatening overdoses, many clinicians now refuse to prescribe these medications for long-term conditions. This can leave chronic pain patients in enormous suffering when a clinician, who formerly prescribed these medications, is no longer able to do so. Several patients have committed suicide as a result. A doctor, William Weeks, wrote about the death of his 49-year-old sister, who injured her back after being thrown from a horse [7]. Over 14 years she received high doses of both opioids and sedatives from a qualified pain clinician. While she was still in pain, she was able to function. When the clinician became ill himself and retired, she was left with a one-month supply of medications and a list of doctors. As Dr. Weeks wrote:

> My sister made appointments with several of the physicians [but at] every appointment, she was told that the physician would be unwilling to prescribe her current medication regimen. At every appointment, she was told that she would need to dramatically reduce her use of opioids and benzodiazepines. At every appointment, she felt that the medical establishment, which had prescribed these medications for a decade and a half, had abandoned her. Having not found a physician to manage her medications, she tried to wean herself, if only to extend her medication supply.

Unable to find anyone to give her medications, she increased her alcohol use, wound up in an ER, and several weeks later, in a jail cell. She died four days after her incarceration, possibly due to drug withdrawal. It is not clear what clinicians should do in situations like these. However, this tragic anecdote and others like it demonstrate that doing nothing can sometimes be very dangerous (Fig. 19.2).

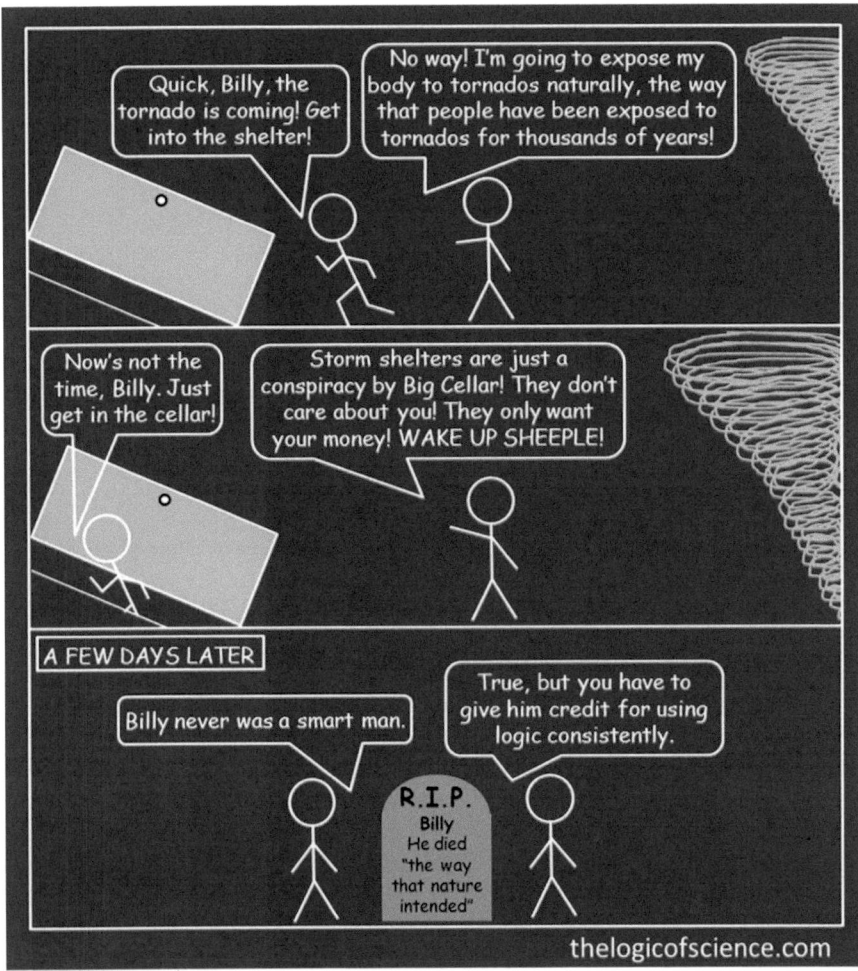

Fig. 19.1 Natural is not always better. (The Logic of Science. [Image file, Facebook status update]. 2016. Retrieved from https://www.facebook.com/thelogicofscience/posts/1758034211094641:0)

Additionally, as a result of the omission bias, many clinicians focus on smaller risks from their treatments than on greater risks from seemingly mundane matters that they do not cause. For example, I have had innumerable discussions about the risks of various MS medications that are very serious, but as infrequent as one in 10,000 people. This is because we would feel responsible for any harm our patients suffered as a result. In contrast, I am not sure if I have had more than a few discussions about fall prevention, even though this represents a much greater threat to most of my patients. After all, falls are the cause of death in one out of 127 Americans according to the National Safety Counsel [8]. Perhaps few interventions would protect my patients more than home safety visits and physical therapy to minimize their

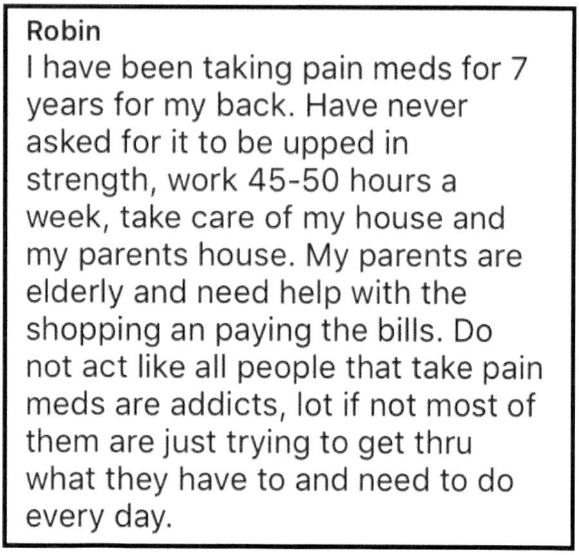

Fig. 19.2 A commentator
on social media lamenting
the stigmatization of
people with chronic pain.
(Robin. I have been taking
pain meds for 7 years for
my back. Have never asked
for it to be upped. (n.d.).
[Facebook comment,
redacted for privacy])

> **Robin**
> I have been taking pain meds for 7 years for my back. Have never asked for it to be upped in strength, work 45-50 hours a week, take care of my house and my parents house. My parents are elderly and need help with the shopping an paying the bills. Do not act like all people that take pain meds are addicts, lot if not most of them are just trying to get thru what they have to and need to do every day.

fall risk. Yet because clinicians do not cause falls, they receive less attention than rare medication side effects.

Additionally, the omission bias may occur not only when clinicians fail to initiate a necessary treatment, but also when they fail to stop unnecessary medications. All too often, once a treatment is started, it may be exceedingly difficult to stop, as clinicians fear potential harms from stopping an effective treatment. Often the idea of stopping medications does not occur to them at all. Many patients come to me with large list of medications, and they are often unsure what each medication is for. Clinicians who do nothing in these situations and fail to stop unnecessary medications may be missing an opportunity to help their patients. A study by Doron Garfinkel and Derelie Mangin, found that 58% of medications could be stopped in elderly patients and only 2% were restarted because of a return of the original indication [9]. Most importantly, quality of life improved with medication discontinuation.

Finally, it is important to recognize whether someone perceives themselves as taking an action greatly depends on what they perceive the status quo to be. With organ donation, for example, organ donation rates are nearly 100% in several countries where people need to opt out of donating [10]. In contrast, donation rates fell to 4–27% in places where people must opt in to donate. Similarly, more people are willing to save money for retirement when they have to opt out of doing so [11]. The practice of medicine can be improved by changing clinicians' default options. For example, when generic drugs are the default option of the electronic medical record, clinicians are much more likely to prescribe them than the brand-name medications, and patients are more likely to adhere to generic medications [12].

Conclusion
Problems caused by clinicians are likely to garner significant attention and concern compared to problems they fail to prevent. Balancing the risks of treatment versus

the risks of the disease is a core part of every clinicians' responsibility. Reasonable people can come to different conclusions on what constitutes an acceptable risk in a particular case. However, there is no rational reason to think harm incurred by a treatment is somehow categorically worse than harm incurred by a disease; either way, a patient is hurt. Clinicians must take care not to let their fears of harming a patient interfere with what is actually in the patient's best interest.

Whether or someone perceives themselves to be acting or not depends on the status quo. However, a clinician who fails to stop an unnecessary medication is no different than a clinician who starts an unnecessary medication. Even if the two actions feel quite different, the patient is taking an unnecessary medication.

Commission Bias

Case

Peter was 38-year-old man who presented to the ER with depression on the advice of his mother. He had been found earlier in the day holding a handgun he had owned for several years, prompting his mother to suggest he get treatment. He had been struggling in his marriage and recently had to take a pay cut at work. He had no history of substance use. In the ER, Peter consistently denied suicidal ideation, saying that he took the gun out "just to look at it." He said that he came to the hospital "just to have someone to talk to" and to get referrals for outpatient therapy. He said that the gun had been turned in to the police, something that his mother confirmed. On mental status examination, he was downcast, but not overtly depressed and not psychotic. Peter said that he wanted to go home after a few hours, and his mother was willing to pick him up. The psychiatrist evaluating him in the ER did not feel that he was safe to leave and admitted him against his will to the hospital. He spent five days on the inpatient psychiatric unit, where he consistently denied suicidal ideation. At the time of discharge, he said that he didn't trust psychiatrists and no longer wanted to associate with his mother, whom he blamed for his hospitalization.

What Dr. Wilson Was Thinking

This was a difficult case. Peter had several risk factors for suicide, namely that he was a middle-aged white male going through marital and financial difficulties. Obviously, what scared me the most was that he had been holding a gun earlier in the day. I know there are some places where gun ownership is relatively common, but this really worried me, even though the gun had been turned into the police. However, I was mostly treating myself by admitting him. He came to the hospital looking to establish outpatient psychiatric care, and instead, he ended up distrusting psychiatrists completely and severing ties with his mother, who had been a significant source of support. Certainly the job of a psychiatrist in the ER is difficult. We are asked to predict the future when we cannot do so. And who knows, had I discharged him maybe he would have killed himself. However, the most likely outcome of this case is that I felt better, but Peter was poorly served.

Case

Jane was a 46-year-old woman who presented with a headache two weeks after being involved in a minor car accident. She said that she did not lose consciousness and that while her headache was improved, she just wanted to get herself "checked out." She had a normal neurological examination. The doctor ordered an MRI which revealed a benign tumor called a meningioma in the right frontal lobe. She was referred to a neurosurgeon who removed the tumor. She had a subdural hemorrhage after the operation, requiring a second operation (Fig. 19.3).

What Dr. Brody Was Thinking

Jane seemed fine to me, but she didn't go to the ER after her car accident. However, you never know, and I wanted to be safe than sorry. The MRI showed an incidental meningioma, which wasn't causing her any problems. Still, she was afraid, and the neurosurgeon was happy to remove the tumor. I could have tried harder to reassure her that she did not need a CT and that she did not need an operation. Almost certainly, Jane would have been better off had she never come to see me.

Discussion

The commission bias is the tendency toward action rather than inaction. It results from the obligation toward beneficence in that harm to the patient can best be prevented by active intervention. Clinicians often feel obligated to do *something* for a patient. Yet, essentially all tests and treatments have the potential to harm patients. Searching the internet for "Band-Aid reaction" shows that even the most seemingly

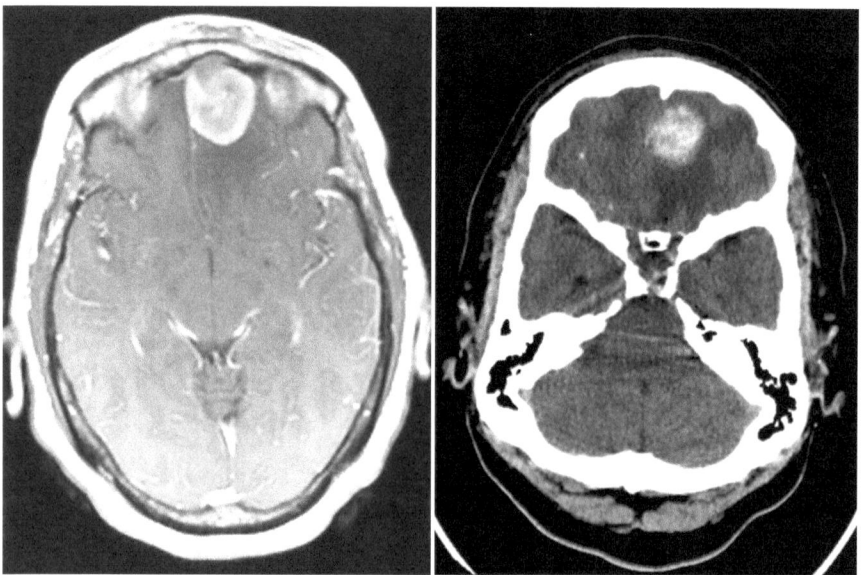

Fig. 19.3 Axial post-contrast T1WI MRI and CT scan demonstrate a meningioma abutting the right frontal lobe

benign treatments are not always so. Clinician induced harm is called iatrogenesis, which is Greek for "brought forth by the healer."

Many clinicians find it difficult to concede that, in some cases, another diagnostic test or treatment may do more harm than good. Doing "nothing" is formally known as clinical inertia and is used mostly as a pejorative term to describe clinicians who fail to adequately treat diseases such as hypertension, diabetes, and dyslipidemia, which are often clinically silent until they cause a devastating condition such as a stroke or heart attack. When doing too little hurts a patient, it is much more impactful on a clinician's psyche than an unnecessary test or unhelpful medication. As surgeon Atul Gawande wrote [13]:

> *Well, as a doctor, I am far more concerned about doing too little than doing too much. It's the scan, the test, the operation that I should have done that sticks with me—sometimes for years. More than a decade ago, I saw a young woman in the emergency room who had severe pelvic pain. A standard X-ray showed nothing. I examined her and found signs of pelvic inflammatory disease, which is most often caused by sexually transmitted diseases. She insisted that she hadn't been sexually active, but I didn't listen. If I had, I might have ordered a pelvic CT scan or even recommended exploratory surgery to investigate further. We didn't do that until later, by which time the real source of her symptoms, a twisted loop of bowel in her pelvis, had turned gangrenous, requiring surgery. By contrast, I can't remember anyone I sent for an unnecessary CT scan or operated on for questionable reasons a decade ago. There's nothing less memorable.*

The commission bias is most likely to occur in over-confident clinicians and in those who reap financial rewards from doing more (the financial bias). It also occurs as most clinicians are affected by the overconfidence bias and generally have an overly favorable view of the risks and benefits of their interventions. A review by Tammy Hoffmann and Chris Del Mar comprising 48 studies and 13,011 clinicians, found that they correctly estimated only 11% of the expected benefits and 13% of the expected harms of multiple common tests and treatments [14]. For the most part, they overestimated the benefit, while undervaluing the potential harms (see the overconfidence bias).

Patient factors may also increase the risk of the commission bias. It is more likely to occur in young patients with tragic conditions. Such patients naturally elicit a large degree of empathy from clinicians who may be tempted to "do everything." This sentiment was expressed by Langston Holly, who wrote about the use of steroids in patients with traumatic spinal cord injuries. He said that this practice, which is unsupported by the evidence, is fueled by a "desire to do everything humanly possible for these tragically injured patients" [15].

The drive to do more often comes from patients (and patient advocacy groups), many of whom undervalue the physical exam, overvalue imaging, and may not want to hear that further tests or treatments are not indicated. Clinicians and patients often agree that one more test is indicated and one more medicine can be tried. Too often, no one is willing to admit that the best treatment is "nothing." Once an abnormality is found, it can also be difficult for a clinician to convince patients that an abnormality is not necessarily pathological or dangerous. Many medical tests are overly sensitive, detecting lesions that are not "normal," but are also not dangerous and in need of treatment. It can be difficult for a clinician to tell patients with incidental finding that any "treatment" is more likely to do more harm than good. Additionally, this is something many anxious patients don't want to hear. In the same way that clinicians overvalue the benefits and undervalue the harms of many tests and treatments. Hoffmann and Del Mar found patients do this as well [14]. In an era of "shared decision-making" between patients and clinicians, both parties can drive each other to do more and more.

There are numerous examples in medicine when patients would have been better off had clinicians opted to do nothing, or at least a lot less. Daniel Morgan and colleagues published lists in 2015 and 2016 of *Medical Practices That Should Be Questioned* [16]. They selected the most influential articles each year and identified the following overuse of tests, overtreatment, and questionable use of services:

- Doubling of specialty referrals.
- Advanced imaging for simple headache.
- Unnecessary hospital admission for low-risk syncope, often leading to adverse events.
- Overly frequent colonoscopy screening.
- 25% of patients with atrial fibrillation at low risk for thromboembolism received anticoagulation.
- 94% of testosterone replacement therapy was administered off guideline recommendations.
- 91% of patients resumed taking opioids after overdose.
- 61% of patients with diabetes were treated to potentially harmfully low glucose levels.
- Questionable use of cyclobenzaprine and oxycodone/acetaminophen for acute low-back pain.
- Testing for Clostridium difficile with molecular assays.
- Lack of benefit for screening pelvic examinations.
- Inappropriate carotid artery screening.
- Thyroid ultrasonography and serial follow-up of benign thyroid nodules leading to unnecessary surgery and complications.
- Head computed tomography was an overused diagnostic test.
- Perioperative aspirin use.
- Medications to increase high-density lipoprotein cholesterol level.
- Inappropriate stenting for renal artery stenosis.
- Prolonged opioid use after surgery.

Specific examples of the commission bias are discussed below.

- **Overdiagnosis, misdiagnosis, and overtreatment from the overuse of diagnostic tests.**

Clinicians and patients alike often have a strong intuitive sense that more information equals better information. "It's better to know," they may think. Yet, knowing more information doesn't necessarily lead to better outcomes. Overtesting can lead to both overdiagnosis and misdiagnosis.

Overdiagnosis is the diagnosis of indolent "disease" that will never cause symptoms during a patient's lifetime. An example would be the detection of a slowly-progressive prostate cancer in an elderly man who is almost certainly going to die to of another cause. Clinicians often feel obligated to treat such cancers, fearful that they may one day blossom into full-blown disease.

Misdiagnosis is the incorrect diagnosis of a disease that the patient does not actually have. If enough tests are done on any person, something abnormal will be found. However, "abnormal" is not synonymous with "pathological." No one has perfect, blemish-free skin, for example, though the presence of a mole, scar, or birthmark does not indicate dermatological disease. Incidental findings detected on imaging tests are termed incidentalomas. James Andrews, a sports medicine orthopedist, did a small study that demonstrated this well. He performed MRI scans on the shoulders of 31 baseball pitchers, none of whom had any pain or trouble throwing. However, 90% of the pitchers had abnormal shoulder cartilage and 87% had abnormal rotator cuff tendons. As Dr. Andrews said, "If you want an excuse to operate on a pitcher's throwing shoulder, just get an MRI." Incidentalomas are particularly common on the kidneys, thyroid, adrenal glands, and lungs. In fact, it is extremely uncommon to see some radiology reports return with "normal findings." Clinicians often feel obligated to investigate such incidentalomas, fearful that they may represent more malignant diseases. As such, the detection of incidentalomas often results in a cascade of further tests and treatments, with minimal benefit to many patients.

The drive to order unnecessary tests often comes from anxious patients who may fail to see their potential harms. However, patients are not customers, and clinicians should be willing to resist requests for tests and treatments they feel are unnecessary, even when a patient demands them. This is especially the case for interventions that may harm the patient. Of course, there are times when ordering a safe test, such as an MRI, may be indicated to relieve a patient's severe anxiety, even if the clinician feels there is a very low probability the test will yield a significant result. However, clinicians must be prepared to deal with the possibility of incidental findings, ideally preparing patients in advance that scans often reveal abnormalities of little or uncertain significance.

- **Diagnostic tests may directly harm patients.**

In addition to overdiagnosis and misdiagnosis, many diagnostic tests have the potential to directly harm patients. Some of these dangers are obvious; no one thinks a brain biopsy is a trivial procedure. However, other harms are less obvious, either because the harms are generally rare or because the injury may occur many years after the test. For example, CT scans are an invaluable tool for rapidly and painlessly investigating multiple organs and other structures. Yet, they expose patients to radiation, and by some estimates a CT examination may be associated with an increased risk of fatal cancer in about one in 2,000 people. While a single CT does not carry great risk for any individual, given the number of CT scans performed annually, the overall population risk is quite large. Over 85 million CT scans were ordered in 2011 [17]. Moreover, many patients have multiple CT scans. A study by Aaron Sodickson and colleagues of 31,000 patients who had CT scans, found that 33% of patients had over five scans, 5% had more than 22 scans, and 1% had greater than 38 scans [18]. This is especially concerning given that by some estimates, 30–50% of CT scans fail to help the patient and are, therefore, medically unnecessary [19].

- **The over-prescription of medications such as antibiotics and opiates, which can lead to antibiotic resistance and addiction.**

It is probably not hyperbole to say that, at present, the greatest health care crisis in the US is the abuse and overuse of heroin and opioid medications. Partially in response to legitimate concerns that clinicians too often ignored pain, and partially in response to marketing by drug companies, clinicians were instructed to treat pain as the "5th vital sign." Clinicians were inundated with instructions to constantly ask patients about their pain and treat it aggressively. Hospital accrediting agencies required proof that patients' pain was not ignored, and "Patient's Bill of Rights" were plastered throughout hospitals, ensuring that patients knew they were entitled to pain relief. Asking patients "How would you rate your pain on a scale of 1 to 10?" became a standard question for every encounter. Moreover, clinicians were led to believe opioid medications were safe and that addiction was rare. In one commercial for the potent opioid OxyContin™, one doctor declared, "The rate of addiction amongst pain patients who are treated by doctors is much less than 1%" [20].

While this campaign was well-intended, the harms have been devastating. Nearly two million Americans abuse or are addicted to prescription opioids. In 2014, there were 1.27 million ER visits or inpatient hospitalizations for opioid-related issues [21]. Compared to 2005, there was 64% increase for inpatient care and a 99% increase in ER visits. Tens of thousands of people are dying. According to data compiled by *The New York Times*, drug overdoses are the single greatest cause of death in Americans under the age of 50 [22]. There are nearly 60,000 deaths due to drug overdoses annually. More Americans under age 50 die of drug overdoses than died from AIDS or motor vehicle accidents at their peaks. According to the CDC there were 15,000 deaths from prescription opioid overdoses in 2016, a number that quadrupled from 1999 [23]. The epidemic is only growing. In 2017, there were 17% more deaths than in 2015 [24].

Unfortunately, a number people began their addiction with a prescription. Seventy-five percent of heroin users reported that they started with prescription opioids [25]. Addiction afflicts as many as 25% of patients who receive prescription opioids for long-term, non-cancer pain in primary care settings. A CDC study found that prescriptions for eight days or longer increased the likelihood of using a drug a year later to 13%, a number that increased to 30% when the prescription was for thirty one days or longer [26]. Additionally, clinicians often over-prescribe pain medications after surgery. A study by Chad Brummett and colleagues found that 6% of post-surgical patients who were prescribed opioids after surgery were still taking them three to six months later. Given that there are nearly 50 million surgeries performed in the US annually, the potential to turn patients into addicts is large (Fig. 19.4) [27].

It is clearly unfair to lay all of the blame for the opioid epidemic at clinicians' feet. Clinicians are no better than anyone else at determining who is in pain and who isn't. There is no test to determine a patient's pain level other than to ask them. Patients are ultimately responsible for honestly reporting their pain and for what they put in their bodies. Certainly, a small number of clinicians run criminal "pill mills," where opioids are given to essentially all-comers. However, most clinicians simply want to relieve pain and suffering and were told that their failure to do so was an abrogation of their professional duties. Additionally, many opioids are not obtained directly from clinicians, but rather illegally manufactured or used by individuals for whom the medication was not prescribed.

Nonetheless, there is no doubt that clinicians' overprescribing of opioids is partly responsible for the opioid epidemic. Recognizing this, clinicians, pharmaceutical companies, and governmental agencies have taken steps to minimize the harm cause by prescription opioids. In 2010, OxyContin™ was converted to a form that is difficult to abuse, though this had the unintended consequence of causing many addicts to turn to street heroin. In 2016, the American Medical Association pushed to eliminate pain as the 5th vital sign [28]. In many states, abusable medications can be tracked via online databases and accessed by clinicians to prevent patients from "doctor-shopping" to obtain multiple prescriptions. Additionally, clinicians are writing fewer opioid prescriptions. A CDC report found that opioid prescriptions dropped 18% from 2010 to 2015, though the rate was still triple that seen in 1999 [29]. However, there is large regional variation, and the rates remain extremely high in many areas.

The over-prescription of antibiotics is another area where clinicians have created a potentially devastating health crisis. In many cases, clinicians simply get it wrong when prescribing antibiotics. In 30–50% of cases, the wrong antibiotic is used, it is given for an improper duration, or no antibiotic was needed at all [30]. In the US, antibiotics are the leading cause of adverse events from drugs. In a study of 32 states in 2011, they accounted for nearly 24% adverse drug reactions in patients admitted to the hospital and 28% of those reactions that occurred during a hospitalization [31]. Additionally, there is overwhelming evidence that the overuse of antibiotics (both with humans and animals) has led to the emergence and spread of resistant strain of bacteria. Currently, over two million people in the US become infected with resistant bacteria, and 23,000 are estimated to die annually due to these infections [32]. The World Health Organization (WHO) has found resistant bacteria throughout the world, leading them to speculate that we may soon be living in a post-antibiotic era [33].

As with opioids, clinicians are not blind to the problem of overprescribing antibiotics. The CDC and FDA have all warned against antibiotic overuse, and President Obama even set up a committee to study the issue. Despite this, the consumption of antibiotic drugs increased by 36% from 2000 to 2010 [34]. While most of this increase occurred outside of the US, in some states the number of prescribed antibiotics courses averaged to more than one treatment per person annually [30].

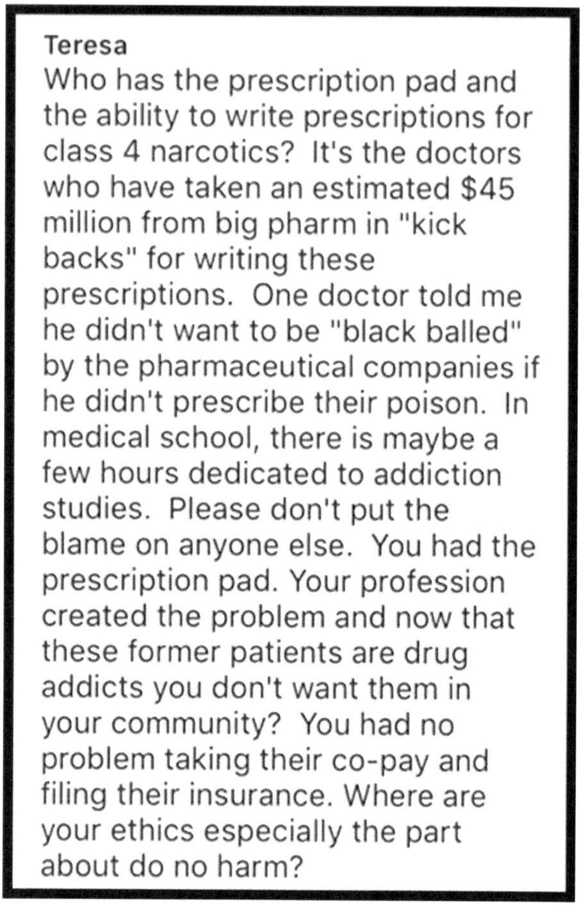

Fig. 19.4 A commentator
on social media blaming
doctors for the opioid
epidemic. (Teresa. Who
has the prescription pad
and the ability to write
prescriptions for class 4
narcotics? It's the doctors.
(n.d.). [Facebook
comment, redacted for
privacy].)

> **Teresa**
> Who has the prescription pad and the ability to write prescriptions for class 4 narcotics? It's the doctors who have taken an estimated $45 million from big pharm in "kick backs" for writing these prescriptions. One doctor told me he didn't want to be "black balled" by the pharmaceutical companies if he didn't prescribe their poison. In medical school, there is maybe a few hours dedicated to addiction studies. Please don't put the blame on anyone else. You had the prescription pad. Your profession created the problem and now that these former patients are drug addicts you don't want them in your community? You had no problem taking their co-pay and filing their insurance. Where are your ethics especially the part about do no harm?

- **The use of multiple medications leading to potentially dangerous polypharmacy.**

Obviously, the use of more medications does not always translate into better outcomes for patients. Yet, for some clinicians and patients, an appointment where a medication is not added or at least adjusted is perceived to be a wasted visited. Once a medication is started, it may be difficult to stop it. Polypharmacy is defined as the use of multiple drugs that are medically unnecessary, a problem that occurs in up to 50% of elderly patients [35]. There is an unquestionable relationship between polypharmacy and negative outcomes, including falls, cognitive impairment, incontinence, poor nutritional status, drug interactions, and adverse drug events [35]. By some estimates, up to 10% of ER visits are due to adverse drug events, accounting for millions of such visits per year.

- **The zealous use of new treatments that have not been properly tested.**

Too often, clinicians rush to embrace new treatments because they are fancy and make intuitive sense. Often clinicians' judgment is further affected by the potential for financial remuneration many of these treatments offer. Unfortunately, many treatments that intuitively "make sense" fail to benefit patients in large clinical trials, and occasionally can lead to significant harms. Medicine is full of procedures that were adopted rapidly and widely, which then failed to show benefit in rigorous clinical studies.

For many decades, oncologists believed that cancer spread locally and predictably from the site of the original tumor. As a result, potentially operable breast cancers were treated for many years with a procedure known as a radical mastectomy, which was developed in the nineteenth century by famed surgeon William Halstead [36]. It was felt removing the breast, along with as many of the adjacent structures as possible, led to the best chance for a cure. This involved horribly disfiguring and disabling surgery, where the entire breast, adjacent lymph nodes, and chest wall musculature were removed. Some aggressive surgeons performed a more aggressive procedure known as the extended radical mastectomy. This involved the extensive removal of additional lymph nodes and even the entire arm, in some cases. Some surgeons, feeling that the tumors grew in response to hormonal factors, also removed the patient's ovaries, pituitary gland, and adrenals.

However certain clinicians, namely Bernard Fisher, began to question the assumption that "more-is-better," noting that radical mastectomies did not seem to result in prolonged lifespans. Cancer biologists also began to realize that cancer growth was not always local and that cancer cells could spread via the bloodstream. Instead of relying on intuition, tradition, and authority, Dr. Fisher and his team decided to use science. Beginning in 1971, they began to collect data, which demonstrated that much more moderate surgeries, combined with adjunctive radiation and chemotherapy achieved comparable results to more radical surgeries. Formal randomized-controlled trials published in 1985 confirmed these earlier findings, sparing countless women painful, disfiguring, and useless surgery [37].

Unfortunately, this did not end the more-is-better mindset for women with breast cancer. In the 1980s and 1990s, a treatment involving large doses of chemotherapy followed by bone marrow transplantation was used to hopefully prevent the spread of the disease. As Imogen Evans and colleagues explain in their book *Testing Treatments*:

> In the USA especially, thousands of desperate women pressed for this very unpleasant treatment from doctors and hospitals, even though as many as five out of 100 patients died from the treatment. Many thousands of dollars were spent, including some from the patients' own pockets. Eventually, some patients were reimbursed by their health insurance companies, who caved in to pressure to do so, despite the lack of evidence that the treatment was useful. Many hospitals and clinics became rich on the proceeds. In 1998, one hospital corporation made $128 million, largely from its cancer centres providing bone marrow transplants. For US doctors it was a lucrative source of income and prestige and it provided a rich field for producing publications. Insistent patient demand fuelled the market. Competition from private US hospitals to provide the treatments was intense, with cut-price offers advertised. In the 1990s, even US academic medical centres trying to recruit patients for clinical trials were offering this treatment. These questionable programmes had become a "cash cow" for the cancer services [36].

Again, science provided enlightenment when personal experience could not. Rigorous studies failed to show any benefit to the procedure at all [38].

A more recent example is the use of coronary artery stents in patients with stable coronary artery disease (CAD), a procedure that was performed hundreds of thousands of times annually in the US and Europe. The procedure is not risk-free, with complications including strokes and heart attacks. The death rate is approximately one in 1,000, and it costs between $30,000–$50,000. In 2007, a randomized trial (COURAGE) of over 2,000 patients with stable CAD found stents did not prevent heart attacks or save lives compared to medical therapy alone [39]. A meta-analysis of eight trials and over 7,000 patients in 2012 concluded, "Initial stent implantation for stable CAD shows no evidence of benefit compared with initial medical therapy for prevention of death, nonfatal myocardial infarction, unplanned revascularization, or angina" [40].

Fortunately, clinicians largely responded to the data indicating the harms of placing coronary stents in patients with stable CAD. After a guideline titled *Appropriate Use Criteria for Coronary Revascularization* was published in 2009, the number of inappropriate procedures declined significantly, though nearly 60,000 inappropriate procedures were still performed in 2016 [41]. Still, many clinicians continued to believe that coronary stents helped people who had chest pain (stable angina) when performing vigorous activities. However, a study in 2017 (ORBITA) randomized such patients to receive stents or undergo a sham procedure [42]. The results were clear; patients who received the stents felt no better than those who had the sham procedure. It appears that, outside of patients suffering an acute heart attack, coronary artery stenting does nothing other than expose patients to risk and cost money. Many interventional cardiologists resisted this study's findings and did their best to spin the data to claim it supported the use of stents [43].

Unfortunately, other recent examples of clinicians overusing inadequately tested treatments and procedures are not hard to find. Another example of a technique adopted too soon is known as morcellation, a procedure to remove uterine fibroids or the entire uterus. While it led to smaller surgical incisions and faster recovery times, it also had the potential to spread undetectable cancer cells throughout a woman's abdomen. According the FDA, this is not a rare occurrence, with one in 350 women harboring such a tumor. In 2014, the FDA put out an advisory against the use of this procedure [44]. Numerous other procedures that "made sense" also failed when subjected to formal clinical trials. Examples include arthroscopy for degenerative knee disease and vertebroplasty for vertebral fractures. Prior to guidelines against it, arthroscopic knee surgery for degenerative knee disease was the most common orthopedic surgery in many countries, being performed over two million times annually. It was performed 500,000 times per year in the US alone. However, systematic reviews found that it was of no benefit in these patients [45].

As with procedures, medical treatments that seem obviously beneficial can sometimes be harmful. It seems to be beyond question that strict blood pressure and glucose control will lead to better outcomes in patients with diabetes. However, one study found that intensive blood pressure lowering in patients with type 2 diabetes did not prevent death or cardiovascular events compared to a somewhat higher blood pressure and was associated with more side effects [46]. Similarly, diabetics treated with intensive control of blood sugar had a 22% higher death rate, increased weight gain, and episodes of low blood sugar compared to patients treated with standard-therapy. Given these results, Dario Giugliano and Katherine Esposito argued that clinical inertia can serve as a safeguard against the "lower is better" mentality, which makes intuitive sense for many conditions, but does not always pan out in clinical trials [47].

- **End of life care.**

A compelling example of the commission bias occurs with end-of-life care, and how the choices clinicians would make for themselves differ from what they actually do to patients. Any young clinician will soon learn, dying is not the worst thing that can happen to a person. For many people, the thought of being alive, potentially for years, in a debilitated state where feeling pain is a real possibility, is worse than death. In 2013, Vyjeyanthi Periyakoil and colleagues surveyed 1,081 doctors and found that nearly 90% would refuse the treatments they routinely give to patients with terminal illness [48]. Dr. Periyakoil said about her findings, "Physicians know it's not the right thing to do, but we find ourselves participating in treatment that causes pain and suffering for our patient. Families are traumatized and there is a huge financial cost to the individual and the nation" [49]. Ken Murray, a family medicine doctor, expressed this sentiment by writing:

> *Of course, doctors don't want to die; they want to live. But they know enough about modern medicine to know its limits. And they know enough about death to know what all people fear most: dying in pain, and dying alone. They've talked about this with their families. They want to be sure, when the time comes, that no heroic measures will happen–that they will never experience, during their last moments on earth, someone breaking their ribs in an attempt to resuscitate them with CPR [50].*

There are several likely explanations for this disparity. The default position ethically is that clinicians must do everything they can for a dying patient. For obvious reasons, many terminally ill patients are not in a position to speak for themselves. Unless family members are present to prevent it, clinicians will never let a patient die, even if they are going to be neurologically devastated. Of course, in times of grief and shock, family members are unlikely to fully grasp the consequences of telling clinicians that "everything" should be done to save a loved one. Even when a dire outcome can be predicted in advance, such as a patient with metastatic cancer, clinicians rarely do a good job of discussing end-of-life care with their patients. This is true even when clinicians are patient themselves. In a 2003 survey of 765 older doctors by Joseph Gallo and colleagues, 46% said their own doctors were unaware of their treatment preferences or were not sure, and 59% of these respondents had no intention of discussing their wishes with their doctors within the next year [51]. Additionally, most doctors said that they would refuse major end-of-life medical interventions (Fig. 19.5).

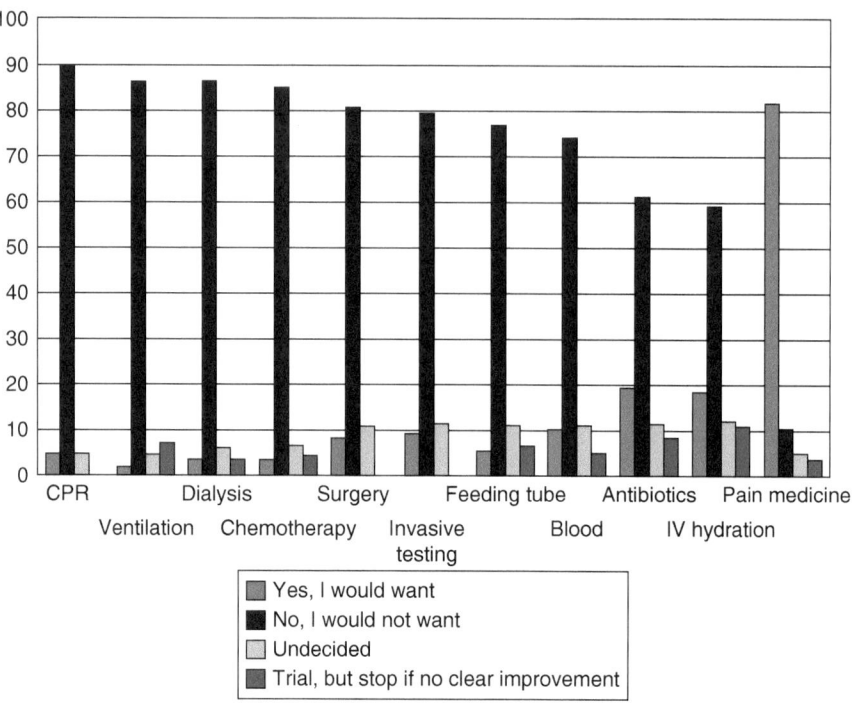

Fig. 19.5 Most doctors said that they would refuse major end-of-life medical interventions, though these are regularly given to patients

Cost

Finally, all of these treatments and tests cost a lot of money. In 2015, health spending in the US reached $3.2 trillion or $9,990 per person, accounting for nearly 18% of the nation's Gross Domestic Product [52]. This is more than double what was spent in 2000. This is expected to only increase so that by 2040, 30% of the money spent in the US will be for health care. By some estimates, overtreatment costs an extra $158–$226 billion annually [53]. Arthroscopic knee surgery for degenerative knee disease alone cost 3 billion dollars annually in the US. Many of the costs of overtreatment can't be measured. After all, how does one measure and account for the anxiety suffered by a person awaiting the biopsy results from an incidentally discovered lesion?

Do Patients Do Better with Fewer Doctors?

Given the potential for the commission bias, it is not surprising that there is some evidence that patient outcomes improve when clinicians are unavailable. Anupam Jena and colleagues examined Medicare beneficiaries hospitalized with heart attacks, heart failure, or cardiac arrest from 2002–2011 comparing patient outcomes when there were national cardiology meetings and the rest of the year [54]. They found that patients admitted during these meetings had a lower thirty day mortality compared to the rest of the year and were less likely to receive coronary artery stents. They wrote, "One explanation for these findings is that the intensity of care provided during meeting dates is lower and that for high-risk patients with cardiovascular disease, the harms of this care may unexpectedly outweigh the benefits." They specifically speculated that overtreatment could be responsible for their finding, writing that, "Interventions foregone during meeting dates are more likely to be those for which the risk-benefit trade-off is less clear and may involve harms that outweigh benefits in high risk patients."

Similarly, Solveig Cunningham and colleagues examined mortality rates from five physician strikes around the world [55]. In all cases, the mortality rate either stayed the same or decreased during the strikes. They suggested several possible explanations for this result: there were no elective surgeries performed during the strike, emergency care was still available, and the strikes were relatively short (nine days to seventeen weeks). Still, it is striking that the morality rate did not increase during any of these strikes.

Solutions

Medicine is hardly blind to overdiagnosis and overtreatment, problems that have garnered significant attention in recent years. The organization Preventing Overdiagnosis is devoted to calling attention to the harms of overtesting and overdiagnosis. Entire conferences have been devoted to the overuse of medical imaging, and multiple books have been written on the subject of overtreatment [56]. Perhaps the best-known campaign to limit unnecessary tests and treatments is known as The Choosing Wisely campaign, which is sponsored by the American Board of Internal Medicine Foundation. Its mission is to make sure that tests and treatments are supported by evidence, not duplicative of other tests or procedures, free from harm, and truly necessary. It asked each medical specialty to create and publish a list of five tests or treatments they commonly overuse.

Certain hospitals are using these guidelines to minimize overtesting. Cedars-Sinai Hospital in Los Angeles, for example, alerts clinicians when they ordered tests or drugs that run contrary to some of the Choosing Wisely recommendations [57]. They studied alerts from over 25,000 patient encounters from 2013 to 2016 and found that the guidelines were followed only 6% of the time. In cases when the guidelines were followed less than 50% of the time, patients had a 14% higher incidence of readmission and 29% higher risk of complications. They also increased costs by 7%. By implementing the Choosing Wisely guidelines, Cedars-Sinai Hospital saved $6 million in 2013 alone [58].

Importantly, whether a clinician is committing an error of omission or commission may only be clear with the benefit of hindsight. A clinician who is hesitant to try a new treatment may be showing judicious restraint or unwarranted caution. For example, there is good evidence that bariatric surgery is the most effective mechanism for obese people, including teenagers, to permanently lose significant amounts of weight and resolve many significant medical issues. Still, many clinicians are wary of the surgery, at least in certain populations. A survey of nearly 500 pediatricians and family medical doctors found that 48% of them would never refer an obese adolescent for the surgery [59]. Many expressed a reluctance to do so because of a fear of long-term consequences, which, if there are any, will take many decades to emerge. In response to this, David Arterburn, a weight-loss specialist said, "The contrarian view is that we don't know about the long-term health consequences of surgery. But my response to that is that we do know the long-term consequences of severe obesity" [60]. So who is committing what error? Are the clinicians who don't refer their patients for surgery committing the omission error? Or are the surgeons who operate on teenagers committing the commission error? Time will tell.

Conclusion

Clinicians are often advised to "just don't do something, stand there." As Danielle Ofri said in an essay titled *When Doing Nothing is the Best Medicine*, "Many make the argument that deciding not to act is as momentous as deciding to act. Except that it never feels that way" [61]. She's right. Doing nothing is one of the hardest things for many clinicians to do. I often find it difficult to tell patients that I am not going to order any tests or adjust any medications. Some patients are extremely displeased when they hear this "plan." However, doing more is not always doing better. The risk specialist Gerd Gigerenzer supposedly has a simple rule, "Never ask the doctor what you should do. Ask him what he would do if he were in your place" [62]. Within the bounds of medical ethics, clinicians should avoid tests and treatments in their patients that they would decline for themselves.

Note that it is easy in hindsight to find examples of the commission bias. Once the harms of certain tests and treatments are known, it is trivial to say that clinicians should not have used them. While clinicians may be too eager to embrace new treatments, mainstream medicine is committed to honestly studying those treatments and adjusting its practices when new evidence emerges.

References

1. Peel M. Human rights and medical ethics. J R Soc Med. 2005;98(4):171–3. https://doi.org/10.1258/jrsm.98.4.171.
2. Trolley problem [Image file]. (n.d.). In: Wikipedia. Retrieved from https://en.wikipedia.org/wiki/Trolley_problem#/media/File:Trolley_problem.png.
3. Greene JD, Sommerville RB, Nystrom LE, Darley JM, Cohen JD. An fMRI investigation of emotional engagement in moral judgment. Science. 2001;293(5537):2105–8. https://doi.org/10.1126/science.1062872.
4. Aberegg SK, Haponik EF, Terry PB. Omission bias and decision making in pulmonary and critical care medicine. Chest. 2005;128(3):1497–505. https://doi.org/10.1378/chest.128.3.1497.
5. DiBonaventura MD, Chapman GB. Do decision biases predict bad decisions? Omission bias, naturalness bias, and influenza vaccination. Med Decis Mak. 2008;28(4):532–9. https://doi.org/10.1177/0272989X07312723.
6. Ritov I, Baron J. Reluctance to vaccinate: omission bias and ambiguity. J Behav Decis Mak. 1990;3:263–77. https://doi.org/10.1002/bdm.3960030404.
7. Kertesz S, Satel S. (2017, Aug 17). Some people still need opioids. SLATE. Retrieved from http://www.slate.com/articles/health_and_science/medical_examiner/2017/08/cutting_down_on_opioids_has_made_life_miserable_for_chronic_pain_patients.html.

8. National Safety Council. (n.d.). What are the odds of dying from. Retrieved 15 Sept 2018 from https://www.nsc.org/work-safety/tools-resources/injury-facts/chart.

9. Garfinkel D, Mangin D. Feasibility study of a systematic approach for discontinuation of multiple medications in older adults: addressing polypharmacy. Arch Intern Med. 2010;170(18):1648–54. https://doi.org/10.1001/archinternmed.2010.355.

10. Johnson EJ, Goldstein DG. Defaults and donation decisions. Transplantation. 2004;78(12):1713–6. https://doi.org/10.1097/01.TP.0000149788.10382.B2.

11. Dholakia U. (2017, Nov 6). Why automating retirement savings may not be enough [Blog post]. Psychology Today. Retrieved from https://www.psychologytoday.com/us/blog/the-science-behind-behavior/201711/why-automating-retirement-savings-may-not-be-enough/.

12. Patel MS, Day S, Small DS, Howell JT, Lautenbach GL, Nierman EH, Volpp KG. Using default options within the electronic health record to increase the prescribing of generic-equivalent medications: a quasi-experimental study. Ann Intern Med. 2014;161(10_Supplement):S44–52. https://doi.org/10.7326/M13-3001.

13. Gawande A. (2015, May 11). Overkill. The New Yorker. Retrieved from https://www.newyorker.com/magazine/2015/05/11/overkill-atul-gawande.

14. Hoffmann TC, Del Mar C. Patients' expectations of the benefits and harms of treatments, screening, and tests: a systematic review. JAMA Intern Med. 2015;175(2):274–86. https://doi.org/10.1001/jamainternmed.2014.6016.

15. Holly L. Commentary. Neurosurgery. 2013;72(Supplement 3):2–3. https://doi.org/10.1227/NEU.0b013e3182772981.

16. Morgan DJ, Dhruva SS, Wright SM, Korenstein D. Update on medical practices that should be questioned in 2015. JAMA Intern Med. 2015;175(12):1960–4. https://doi.org/10.1001/jamainternmed.2015.5614; Morgan DJ, Dhruva SS, Wright SM, Korenstein D. 2016 update on medical overuse: a systematic review. JAMA Intern Med. 2016;176(11):1687–92. https://doi.org/10.1001/jamainternmed.2016.5381.

17. U.S. Department of Health and Human Services, Agency for Healthcare Research and Quality. (2018, Aug). Radiation safety. Retrieved 15 Sept 2018 from https://psnet.ahrq.gov/primers/primer/27/radiation-safety.

18. Sodickson A, Baeyens PF, Andriole KP, Prevedello LM, Nawfel RD, Hanson R, Khorasani R. Recurrent CT, cumulative radiation exposure, and associated radiation-induced cancer risks from CT of adults. Radiology. 2009;251(1):175–84. https://doi.org/10.1148/radiol.2511081296.

19. U.S. Department of Health and Human Services. Food and Drug Administration. (2018, Aug 15) Initiative to reduce unnecessary radiation exposure from medical imaging. Retrieved 15 Sept 2018 from https://www.fda.gov/Radiation-EmittingProducts/RadiationSafety/RadiationDoseReduction/.

20. Our Amazing World. (2016, Sept 22). Purdue Pharma OxyContin commercial [Video file]. Retrieved from https://www.youtube.com/watch?v=Er78Dj5hyeI.

21. Weiss AJ, Bailey MK, O'Malley L, Barrett ML, Elixhauser A, Steiner CA. (2017). Patient characteristics of opioid-related inpatient stays and emergency department visits nationally and by state, 2014 [PDF file]. Statistical Brief #224. Retrieved from https://www.hcup-us.ahrq.gov/reports/statbriefs/sb224-Patient-Characteristics-Opioid-Hospital-Stays-ED-Visits-by-State.pdf.

22. Katz J. (2017, June 5). Drug deaths in America are rising faster than ever. The New York Times. Retrieved from https://www.nytimes.com/interactive/2017/06/05/upshot/opioid-epidemic-drug-overdose-deaths-are-rising-faster-than-ever.html.

23. Centers for Disease Control and Prevention. (2017, Aug 30). Prescription opioid data. Retrieved 15 Sept 2018 from https://www.cdc.gov/drugoverdose/data/prescribing.html.

24. Kaplan S. (2017, Nov 3). C.D.C. reports a record jump in drug overdose deaths last year. The New York Times. Retrieved from https://www.nytimes.com/2017/11/03/health/deaths-drug-overdose-cdc.html.

25. National Institutes of Health, National Institute on Drug Abuse. (2018, Jan). Prescription opioids and heroin. Retrieved from https://www.drugabuse.gov/publications/research-reports/relationship-between-prescription-drug-heroin-abuse/prescription-opioid-use-risk-factor-heroin-use.

26. Shah A, Hayes CJ, Martin BC. Characteristics of initial prescription episodes and likelihood of long-term opioid use – United States, 2006-2015. MMWR Morb Mortal Wkly Rep. 2017;2017(66):265–9. https://doi.org/10.15585/mmwr.mm6610a1.

27. Brummett CM, Waljee JF, Goesling J, Moser S, Lin P, Englesbe MJ, ASB B, Kheterpal S, Nallamothu BK. New persistent opioid use after minor and major surgical procedures in US adults. JAMA Surg. 2017;152(6):e170504. https://doi.org/10.1001/jamasurg.2017.0504.

28. Frieden J. (2016, June 13). Remove pain as 5th vital, sign, AMA urged. Medpage Today. Retrieved from https://www.medpagetoday.com/meetingcoverage/ama/58486.

29. Guy GP, Zhang K, Bohm MK, Losby J, Lewis B, Young R, Murphy LB, Dowell D. Vital signs: changes in opioid prescribing in the United States, 2006-2015. MMWR Morb Mortal Wkly Rep. 2017;2017(66):697–704. https://doi.org/10.15585/mmwr.mm6626a4.

30. Ventola CL. The antibiotic resistance crisis: part 1: causes and threats. Pharm Ther. 2015;40(4):277.

31. Weiss AJ, Elixhauser A, Bae J, Encinosa W. (2006). Origin of adverse drug events in US hospitals, 2011: Statistical Brief# 158. Retrieved from https://www.hcup-us.ahrq.gov/reports/statbriefs/sb158.jsp.

32. Centers for Disease Control and Prevention. (2018, Sept 10). Antibiotic/Antimicrobial resistance: biggest threats and data. Retrieved 15 Sept 2018 from https://www.cdc.gov/drugresistance/biggest_threats.html.

33. Reardon S. WHO warns against 'post-antibiotic' era. Nature. 2014; https://doi.org/10.1038/nature.2014.15135.

34. Van Boeckel TP, Gandra S, Ashok A, Caudron Q, Grenfell BT, Levin SA, Laxminarayan R. Global antibiotic consumption 2000 to 2010: an analysis of national pharmaceutical sales data. Lancet Infect Dis. 2014;14(8):742–50. https://doi.org/10.1016/S1473-3099(14)70780-7.

35. Maher RL, Hanlon J, Hajjar ER. Clinical consequences of polypharmacy in elderly. Expert Opin Drug Saf. 2014;13(1):57–65. https://doi.org/10.1517/14740338.2013.827660.

36. Evans I, Thornton H, Chalmers I, Glasziou P. Testing treatments: better research for better healthcare. 2nd ed. London: Pinter & Martin Ltd; 2011.

37. Baum M, Houghton J. Contribution of randomised controlled trials to understanding and management of early breast cancer. BMJ. 1999;319:568. https://doi.org/10.1136/bmj.319.7209.568.

38. Farquhar CM, Basser R, Marjoribanks J, Lethaby AE. High dose chemotherapy and autologous bone marrow or stem cell transplantation versus conventional chemotherapy for women with early poor prognosis breast cancer. Cochrane Database of Systematic Reviews. 2016;2016(5):CD003139. https://doi.org/10.1002/14651858.CD003139.pub.3.

39. Boden WE, O'Rourke RA, Teo KK, Hartigan PM, Maron DJ, Kostuk WJ, Knudtson M, Dada M, Casperson P, Harris CL, Chaitman BR, Shaw L, Gosselin G, Nawaz S, Title LM, Gau G, Blaustein AS, Booth DC, Bates ER, Spertus JA, Berman DS, Mancini GB, Weintraub WS. Optimal medical therapy with or without PCI for stable coronary disease. N Engl J Med. 2007;356(15):1503–16. https://doi.org/10.1056/NEJMoa070829.

40. Stergiopoulos K, Brown DL. Initial coronary stent implantation with medical therapy vs medical therapy alone for stable coronary artery disease: meta-analysis of randomized controlled trials. Arch Intern Med. 2012;172(4):312–9. https://doi.org/10.1001/archinternmed.2011.1484.

41. Desai NR, Bradley SM, Parzynski CS, Nallamothu BK, Chan PS, Spertus JA, Patel MR, Ader J, Soufer A, Krumholz HM, Curtis JP. Appropriate use criteria for coronary revascularization and trends in utilization, patient selection, and appropriateness of percutaneous coronary intervention. JAMA. 2015;314(19):2045–53. https://doi.org/10.1001/jama.2015.13764.

42. Al-Lamee R, Thompson D, Dehbi H-M, Sen S, Tang K, Davies J, Keeble T, Mielewczik M, Kaprielian R, Malik IS, Nijjer SS, Petraco R, Cook C, Ahmad Y, Howard J, Baker C, Sharp

A, Gerber R, Talwar S, Assomull R, Mayet J, Wensel R, Collier D, Shun-Shin M, Thom SA, Davies JE, Francis DP. Percutaneous coronary intervention in stable angina (ORBITA): a double-blind, randomised controlled trial. Lancet. 2018;391(10115):31–40. https://doi.org/10.1016/S0140-6736(17)32714-9.

43. Gorski D. (2017, Nov 6). ORBITA: another clinical trial demonstrating the need for sham controls in surgical trials. Science-Based Medicine. Retrieved from https://sciencebasedmedicine.org/orbita-another-clinical-trial-demonstrating-the-need-for-sham-controls-in-surgical-trials/.

44. Flapan D. (2014, Apr 17). FDA warns against morcellation in hysterectomy, myomectomy. Medscape. Retrieved from https://www.medscape.com/viewarticle/823776.

45. Siemieniuk RA, Harris IA, Agoritsas T, Poolman RW, Brignardello-Petersen R, Van de Velde S, Buchbinder R, Englund M, Lytvyn L, Quinlan C, Helsingen L, Knutsen G, Olsen NR, Macdonald H, Hailey L, Wilson HM, Lydiatt A, Kristiansen A. Arthroscopic surgery for degenerative knee arthritis and meniscal tears: a clinical practice guideline. BMJ. 2017;357:j1982. https://doi.org/10.1136/bmj.j1982.

46. ACCORD Study Group. Effects of intensive blood-pressure control in type 2 diabetes mellitus. N Engl J Med. 2010;362(17):1575–85. https://doi.org/10.1056/NEJMoa1001286.

47. Giugliano D, Esposito K. Clinical inertia as a clinical safeguard. JAMA. 2011;305(15):1591–2. https://doi.org/10.1001/jama.2011.490.

48. Periyakoil VS, Neri E, Fong A, Kraemer H. Do unto others: doctors' personal end-of-life resuscitation preferences and their attitudes toward advance directives. PLoS One. 2014;9(5):e98246. https://doi.org/10.1371/journal.pone.0098246.

49. Walsh D. (2014, May 29), Why your doctor probably has a "Do Not Resuscitate" order. Time. Retrieved from http://time.com/131443/why-your-doctor-probably-has-a-do-not-resuscitate-order/.

50. Murray K. (2011, Nov 30). How doctors die. Zocalo. Retrieved from http://www.zocalopublicsquare.org/2011/11/30/how-doctors-die/ideas/nexus/.

51. Gallo JJ, Straton JB, Klag MJ, Meoni LA, Sulmasy DP, Wang NY, Ford DE. Life-sustaining treatments: what do physicians want and do they express their wishes to others? J Am Geriatr Soc. 2003;51(7):961–9. https://doi.org/10.1046/j.1365-2389.2003.51309.x.

52. U. S. Department of Health and Human Services, Centers for Medicare & Medicaid Services. (2018, Jan 8). National health expenditure data: historical. Retrieved from https://www.cms.gov/Research-Statistics-Data-and-Systems/Statistics-Trends-and-Reports/NationalHealthExpendData/NationalHealthAccountsHistorical.html.

53. Berwick DM, Hackbarth AD. Eliminating waste in US health care. JAMA. 2012;307(14):1513–6. https://doi.org/10.1001/jama.2012.362.

54. Jena AB, Prasad V, Goldman DP, Romley J. Mortality and treatment patterns among patients hospitalized with acute cardiovascular conditions during dates of national cardiology meetings. JAMA Intern Med. 2015;175(2):237–44. https://doi.org/10.1001/jamainternmed.2014.6781.

55. Cunningham SA, Mitchell K, Narayan KV, Yusuf S. Doctors' strikes and mortality: a review. Soc Sci Med. 2008;67(11):1784–8. https://doi.org/10.1016/j.socscimed.2008.09.044.

56. Hendee WR, Becker GJ, Borgstede JP, Bosma J, Casarella WJ, Erickson BA, Maynard CD, Thrall JH, Wallner PE. Addressing overutilization in medical imaging. Radiology. 2010;257(1):240–5. https://doi.org/10.1148/radiol.10100063.

57. Terhune C. (2017, May 25). Americans waste $200 billion every year on medical tests they don't need, experts say. Los Angeles Times. Retrieved from http://www.latimes.com/business/la-fi-medical-tests-20170526-story.html.

58. Terhune C. (2017, May 20). Needless medical test not only cost $200 billion, they can do harm. CNN: Money. https://money.cnn.com/2017/05/20/news/economy/medical-tests/index.html.

59. Woolford SJ, Clark SJ, Gebremariam A, Davis MM, Freed GL. To cut or not to cut: physicians' perspectives on referring adolescents for bariatric surgery. Obes Surg. 2010;20(7):937–42. https://doi.org/10.1007/s11695-010-0152-9.

60. Belluz J. (2017, Dec 18). Jewel's story: how one teen battled obesity with medicine's best — and most underused — tool. Vox. https://www.vox.com/science-and-health/2017/12/18/16707428/ bariatric-surgery-teen-weight-loss-jewel.
61. Ofri D. (2011, Oct 20). When doing nothing is the best medicine [Blog post]. The New York Times. Retrieved from https://well.blogs.nytimes.com/2011/10/20/when-doing-nothing-is-the-best-medicine/.
62. Taleb NN. (n.d.). [Personal quote]. Retrieved 15 Sept 2018 from https://www.goodreads.com/ quotes/699367-the-psychologist-gerd-gigerenzer-has-a-simple-heuristic-never-ask.

Overchoice and Decision Avoidance

20

Case

Jenna was a 23-year-old woman who was diagnosed with multiple sclerosis (MS) after she presented with tingling in her hands and feet. Her neurologist provided her with a list of treatment options as follows:

Injectable Medications

- Avonex™ (interferon beta-1a).
- Betaseron™ (interferon beta-1b).
- Copaxone™ (glatiramer acetate).
- Extavia™ (interferon beta-1b).
- Glatopa™ (glatiramer acetate -- generic equivalent of Copaxone 20 mg dose).
- Plegridy™ (peginterferon beta-1a).
- Rebif™ (interferon beta-1a).
- Zinbryta™ (daclizumab).

Oral Medications

- Aubagio™ (teriflunomide).
- Gilenya™ (fingolimod).
- Tecfidera™ (dimethyl fumarate).

Infused Medications

- Lemtrada™ (alemtuzumab).
- Novantrone™ (mitoxantrone).
- Ocrevus™ (ocrelizumab).
- Tysabri™ (natalizumab).

© Springer International Publishing AG, part of Springer Nature 2019   345
J. Howard, *Cognitive Errors and Diagnostic Mistakes*,
https://doi.org/10.1007/978-3-319-93224-8_20

As she was having pain, the neurologist also discussed multiple medications to treat neuropathic pain. Jenna never came back for a follow-up appointment and presented the next year with visual loss in her left eye. When asked why she missed her follow-up visit, she said that she was too overwhelmed to make a decision and just hoped the problem would go away.

What Dr. Ready Was Thinking

I have been treating patients with MS for over 30 years. I remember how devastated patients were in the days when there were no treatments. The situation is quite different today. I spent about 45 minutes going over all of the medications with Jenna. I thought I would be failing in my job to not present her with all of the treatment options and allow her to make a decision. However, for her, it was too overwhelming, so much so that she chose nothing, the worst possible choice. I now tell my patients, "it is your job to make a decision, but my job to make a recommendation." I still give the same list, but always try to narrow it down to two or three medications they should choose from. Ultimately, I try to provide a single recommendation for every patient. I don't want patients to spend so much time trying to choose the perfect medication that they end up choosing no medication at all.

Discussion

The concept of overchoice (also called the multiple alternative bias) was coined by Alvin Toffler in his book *Future Shock*. Overchoice occurs when more choices leads to less satisfaction and indecisiveness or paralysis. As Toffler wrote, "Ironically, the people of the future may suffer not from an absence of choice, but from a paralyzing surfeit of it. They may turn out to be the victims of that peculiar super-industrial dilemma: 'Overchoice [1].'" Closely related to this is a phenomenon known as information overload, a term coined by Bertram Gross, a political scientist. He wrote that, "Information overload occurs when the amount of input to a system exceeds its processing capacity. Decision makers have fairly limited cognitive processing capacity. Consequently, when information overload occurs, it is likely that a reduction in decision quality will occur." When faced with excess choices, some people prefer not to choose at all, even if making a choice would lead to a better outcome. This is especially the case if there is a time constraint. Moreover, once a choice is made, people who chose from a smaller subset of choices report greater satisfaction and less regret compared to those who had multiple options.

Understandably, no one likes not having any choices. Telling patients they suffer from a disease for which there is no treatment is difficult for everyone involved. Not surprisingly, more choices lead to more satisfaction, at least initially. When a new treatment is approved for a formerly untreatable condition, it often seems like a miracle. Though it may seem that there can't be too many choices, this is not the case. There are diminishing returns to more choices such that, at some point, people feel pressure and uncertainty. When there are many similar choices, making a decision can become overwhelming. People may feel obligated to weigh multiple potential outcomes and fret about making the wrong choice. Many people feel obligated to make the "perfect" choice, leading to frustration and anger. At times, a surplus of choices may prevent people from deciding at all. Most of us have had the experience of going to a large store intending to buy a product, only to walk out empty-handed because we were overwhelmed by the number of choices, a phenomenon known as decision avoidance.

In a classic demonstration of how overchoice leads to decision avoidance, Sheena Iyengar and Mark Lepper showed that people were more likely to purchase foods or write optional class essays when offered six choices than when offered 24 or 30 choices. In their study, 30% of people who choose from six jams or chocolates made a purchase, while only 3% of people who chose from 24 options did so. Moreover, participants reported greater subsequent satisfaction with their selections and wrote better essays when their choices were limited [2]. As Kathleen Vohs and colleagues wrote, these "findings suggest that choice, to the extent that it requires greater decision-making among options, can become burdensome and ultimately counterproductive [3]."

Predictably, some businesses are aware of the effect overchoice has on its customers. Denise Lee Yohn wrote the following about some of the strategies Costco uses to entice customers:

> For one, it deliberately limits the number of product choices offered. A typical Costco store stocks 4,000 types of items, including, say, just four toothpaste brands, while a Wal-Mart typically stocks more than 100,000 types of items and may carry 60 sizes and brands of toothpaste. Instead of turning off customers, the limited selection actually works in Costco's favour. Studies have consistently shown that customers buy fewer products when faced with too many choices, a dynamic that's probably magnified when shopping in a no-frills warehouse environment [4].

In medicine, overchoice can occur when clinicians are forced to choose between multiple potential diagnoses. As Pat Croskerry wrote:

> A multiplicity of options on a differential diagnosis may lead to significant conflict and uncertainty. The process may be simplified by reverting to a smaller subset with which the physician is familiar but may result in inadequate consideration of other possibilities. One such strategy is the three-diagnosis differential: "It is probably A, but it might be B, or I don't know (C)." Although this approach has some heuristic value, if the disease falls in the C category and is not pursued adequately, it will minimize the chances that some serious diagnoses can be made [5].

Similarly, overchoice can occur when clinicians and patients must choose between multiple treatment options. Overchoice has been demonstrated to occur with clinicians. In one study by Donald A. Redelmeier and Eldar Shafir, family physicians were given a scenario of a patient with osteoarthritis. Those who had to decide between two treatment options were less likely to prescribe a medication than those who were given only one medication to choose from [6]. They also found similar discrepancies when neurologists and neurosurgeons had to make decisions regarding carotid artery surgery. A similar study by Todd Roswarski and Michael Murray found that some clinicians opted to defer treatment when multiple alternatives were provided [7].

Overchoice and information overload both commonly occur in my care of patients with MS. In the past eight years, the number of treatment options has more than doubled. Whereas patients previously had to choose from a small number of medications that were relatively similar, there are now over ten medications, each with a complicated and unique risk/benefit profile. Some treatments are older and safe, but less effective and with unpleasant side-effects. Other medications are newer, more effective, and mostly well-tolerated. But they come with serious, even potentially fatal, risks. Some are injections, some are infusions, and some are pills.

As the number of treatment options has grown, patients agonize more over their choices. I tell my patients that their predicament is like going to one of those diners with a 20-page menu; all of the options can make it much more difficult and unpleasant to choose a meal compared to a menu with a handful of options. Some patients end up so paralyzed by indecision, they decide not to start any medication at all. As such, it is extremely important, though not easy, for clinicians to review treatment options with patients both thoroughly and concisely.

Giving patients too little information is unethical and does not allow them to actively participate in decisions about their healthcare. However, giving them too much information is counterproductive and likely to overwhelm them. The package insert for just one of the medications (fingolimod) is 25 pages of dense text, for example [8]. Providing patients with such handouts for over ten different medications is unlikely to be helpful. Ultimately, it is a clinician's job to not just present patients with a totality of their treatment options, but also to provide them with firm recommendations.

Conclusion

In his book *The Paradox of Choice*, Barry Schwartz wrote, "The more options there are, the more likely one will make a non-optimal choice, and this prospect undermines whatever pleasure one may get from one's actual choice." While it may seem impossible to have too many choices or too much information, a surplus of either can be paralyzing such that the perfect becomes the enemy of the good. Clinicians should try to be aware when a surplus of choices limits either their own decision-making or that of their patients.

References

1. Muench F. (2010, Nov 1). The burden of choice [Blog post]. Psychology Today. Retrieved from https://www.psychologytoday.com/us/blog/more-tech-support/201011/the-burden-choice.
2. Iyengar SS, Lepper MR. When choice is demotivating: can one desire too much of a good thing. J Pers Soc Psychol. 2000;79(6):995–1006.
3. Vohs KD, Baumeister RF, Twenge JM, Schmeichel BJ, Tice DM, Crocker J. (2005). Decision fatigue exhausts self-regulatory resources—But so does accommodating to unchosen alternatives [PDF file]. (Manuscript submitted for publication). Retrieved from https://www.researchgate.net/profile/Jean_Twenge/publication/237738528_Decision_Fatigue_Exhausts_Self-Regulatory_Resources_-_But_So_Does_Accommodating_to_Unchosen_Alternatives/links/554b9ee40cf21ed21359ccbd/Decision-Fatigue-Exhausts-Self-Regulatory-Resources-But-So-Does-Accommodating-to-Unchosen-Alternatives.pdf.

4. Yoh DL. (2015, Oct 30). Great brands don't chase customers; Why Costco limits customer choices. MyCustomer. Retrieved from https://www.mycustomer.com/service/management/great-brands-dont-chase-customers-why-costco-limits-consumer-choices.

5. Croskerry P, Cosby KS, Graber ML, Singh H. Diagnosis: interpreting the shadows (Appendix 1). Boca Raton: CRC Press; 2017.

6. Redelmeier DA, Shafir E. Medical decision making in situations that offer multiple alternatives. JAMA. 1995;273(4):302–5. https://doi.org/10.1001/jama.1995.03520280048038.

7. Roswarski TE, Murray MD. Supervision of students may protect academic physicians from cognitive bias: a study of decision making and multiple treatment alternatives in medicine. Med Decis Mak. 2006;26(2):154–61. https://doi.org/10.1177/0272989X06286483.

8. Novaris AG. (2018, May). Gilenya product insert [PDF file]. Retrieved from https://www.pharma.us.novartis.com/sites/www.pharma.us.novartis.com/files/gilenya.pdf.

Case

George was a 56-year-old man who presented with the gradual onset of gait impairment and neck pain. An MRI revealed severe narrowing of his cervical spine due to several herniated discs. He was scheduled for surgery several weeks later. The doctor had been up most of the night previously operating on an emergency case. He refused to reschedule George's surgery, saying that it was a simple, quick operation that he had performed hundreds of times previously without any complication. During the operation, one of the patient's nerve roots was accidently cut, leading to a permanent wrist drop. The surgeon had not made this mistake previously and attributed the error to being fatigued.

What Dr. Whiteson Was Thinking

I was too tired to operate, but I didn't want to admit it. Of course I realize I am human. I need to eat and sleep just like anyone else. However, admitting this and changing my operating schedule because of it felt like confessing to a personal flaw of sorts. I remember very clearly being told on my surgery rotation in medical school that "surgeons don't get tired." At the time, I admired that toughness and wanted to embody it myself. I would say this to the medical students in a tone of voice that let them know I was joking and not joking at the same time.

I now recognize, in some ways, that refusing to acknowledge when I am tired is actually a sign of weakness and selfishness. Of course, we all have to work in the middle of the night at times. However, a doctor who refuses to admit that fatigue or hunger can significantly impair patient care is prioritizing their own need to feel "tough" over the well-being of their patient. And that is wrong. I should have cancelled George's surgery. He would have been unhappy, but his case was not an emergency, and postponing his surgery a week or two would have resulted in a better outcome.

© Springer International Publishing AG, part of Springer Nature 2019   351
J. Howard, *Cognitive Errors and Diagnostic Mistakes*,
https://doi.org/10.1007/978-3-319-93224-8_21

Case

Karen was a 36-year-old woman who presented to a "holistic" pediatrician's office prior to the delivery of her first child. The pediatrician strongly advised against getting both vaccines and the vitamin K shot, which is given to newborns to prevent intracranial hemorrhages. Though the pediatrician had no scientific publications on the vitamin K shot, he told her that his research had shown that as long as she breast-fed her baby, the shot was likely to do more harm than good. He said that the American Academy of Pediatrics and CDC were mistaken in its recommendations. Though Karen delivered a healthy baby who left the hospital without problems, she later read of a cluster of seven infants who suffered intracranial bleeding due to vitamin K deficiency, causing her to lose confidence in the pediatrician [1].

What Dr. Pelvesky Was Thinking

Let me be honest about the vitamin K shot. I have done hundreds of hours of research on this chemical and have come to the conclusion that conventional medicine is highly flawed in the use of this drug. Even though the American Academy of Pediatrics feels every newborn needs to get it, it is not a harmless drug. Like vaccines, it is a manufactured synthetic chemical, and it is given at a much higher dose than what a child would naturally receive. Synthetic vitamin K contains up to 9 mg of benzyl alcohol. So hospitals are injecting these babies, who are literally only several minutes old, with a drug that contains alcohol that targets their liver, the organ which is necessary for them to detoxify. There are a lot of babies developing jaundice several days after birth. The many known side effects of synthetic vitamin K shots include shock, cardiac or respiratory distress, and jaundice. My research has shown that this shot is completely unneeded. I have come to know the difference between injection and ingestion and how that affects people physiologically. If the "best scientists" do not understand that, then we have more problems than we could possibly imagine.

Discussion

The overconfidence bias, also called illusory superiority, reflects a common tendency to believe we know more than we do or that we are more skilled than others at various tasks. It reflects a tendency to act on incomplete information, intuitions, or hunches. Too much faith is placed in opinion instead of carefully gathered evidence. Overconfidence may be augmented by other biases, and catastrophic outcomes may result.

Overconfidence leads the vast majority of people to consider themselves better than average at a variety of skills and attributes, when for any given task, exactly half of us are better than average. In one survey 93% of drivers in the US considered themselves to be above average drivers [2]. In a survey at the University of Nebraska, 68% of faculty members rated themselves in the top 25% for teaching ability, and more than 90% rated themselves in the top 50% [3]. In a similar survey, 87% of business students at Stanford University rated their academic performance as above average. People tend to view themselves as more popular than they actually are [4]. Persons with below-average IQs tend to overestimate their IQ, while people with above-average IQs to underestimate their IQ (a finding known as the Downing Effect). Similar findings have been demonstrated for overall health, popularity, and overall level of bias (the blind spot

Fig. 21.1 The Dunning-Kruger Effect: People with low levels of knowledge or skill suffer the illusion their ability is higher than it actually is. (Dilmen N. (Nevit). Dunning Kruger effect [Image file]. In: Wikimedia commons. 2013. Retrieved from https://commons.wikimedia.org/wiki/Category:Dunning%E2%80%93Kruger_effect#/media/File:Mr_Pipo_Dunning_kruger.svg)

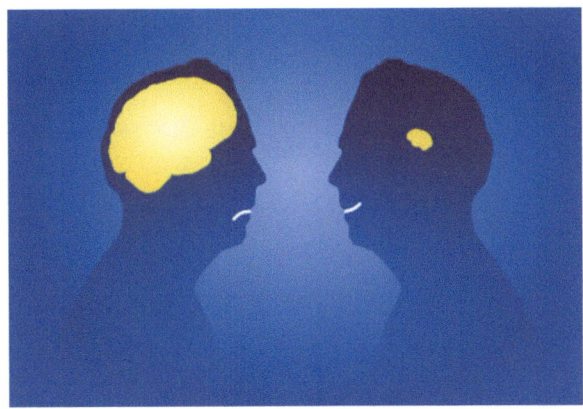

bias). The comedian George Carlin had a great line where he said, "Think of how stupid the average person is, and realize half of them are stupider than that." This is funny primarily because almost no one believes their intelligence is below average.

As a result of the overconfidence bias, the majority of people with less than average ability at a given task consider themselves to be high-achievers. This was formally described by psychologists David Dunning and Justin Kruger in a paper titled *Unskilled and Unaware of It: How Difficulties in Recognizing One's Own Incompetence Lead to Inflated Self-Assessments*. They were inspired by the case of McArthur Wheeler, a thief who rubbed lemon juice on his face, reasoning that since it can be used to create invisible ink, it would render his face invisible to security cameras. He robbed several banks in the middle of the day, was easily caught that evening, and sentenced to 24.5 years in jail.

Dunning and Kruger studied subjects in different domains and found "that participants scoring in the bottom quartile on tests of humor, grammar, and logic grossly overestimated their test performance and ability [5]." The Dunning–Kruger effect is now used to describe the phenomenon where people with low levels of knowledge or skill suffer the illusion their ability is higher than it actually is (Fig. 21.1). It posits that low-ability individuals:

- Do not recognize their lack of skill.
- Do not recognize the degree of their incompetence.
- Appreciate their own lack of knowledge only after they have been extensively taught about that topic.
- Fail to accurately evaluate skill in others.

President Donald Trump often demonstrates the Dunning–Kruger effect. For example, after a major tax bill was passed in December 2017, he made the following claim:

> *I know more about the big bills. … Than any president that's ever been in office. Whether it's health care and taxes. Especially taxes…I know the details of taxes better than anybody. Better than the greatest C.P.A. I know the details of health care better than most, better than most. And if I didn't, I couldn't have talked all these people into doing ultimately only to be rejected [6].*

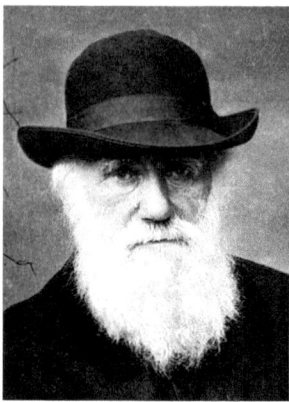

Ignorance more frequently begets confidence than does knowledge: it is those who know little, and not those who know much, who so positively assert that this or that problem will never be solved by science.

Charles Darwin

Fig. 21.2 Charles Darwin gets it right. (Elliot & Fry – Swarthmore.edu. Charles Darwin [Image file]. In: Wikimedia commons. (n.d.). Retrieved from https://commons.wikimedia.org/wiki/Charles_Darwin#/media/File:Charles_Darwin_1880.jpg.)

None of us wants to think of ourselves as "average." It implies mediocrity. However, depending on what company we keep, being average or even below average, might still reflect an extremely high level of skill. The "worst" neurosurgeon at a top medical center is likely to be an exceptional doctor, the same way the "worst" player in the NBA is an exceptional basketball player. However, what the Dunning–Kruger effect tells us, in essence, is that ignorant people, with a small amount of knowledge on a particular topic, are too ignorant to appreciate their own ignorance. As has been said, "The first rule of the Dunning–Kruger club is you don't know you're in the Dunning–Kruger club" (Fig. 21.2).

The overconfidence bias is pervasive in medicine. A review by Tammy Hoffmann and Chris Del Mar found that clinicians tend to overestimate the benefits of many of their treatments, while underestimating their risks [7].

The cold truth is that most patients don't benefit from most drugs, though it's likely that few clinicians are aware of this. Perhaps the most humbling statistic in medicine is the number needed to treat, which is defined as the number of people who need to receive a treatment for one person to benefit. The inverse of this is the number needed to harm. For many standard medical treatments, such as giving antiplatelet agents for acute ischemic stroke, only one patient in 79 avoided death or dependency. Another standard procedure, giving steroids for bacterial meningitis, helped prevent hearing loss in only one in 21 patients. These results are not outliers. The website thennt.com has a discussion of such many treatments, and the results are extremely humbling [8]. Only a few treatments, such as rapid defibrillation for cardiac arrest, seem to benefit close to half of patients. Since clinicians cannot know which patients will benefit, however, many patients are treated to help the few. Even more sobering is the fact that many standard tests and treatments do not benefit patients at all.

Related to the overconfidence bias and the Dunning-Kruger effect is a phenomenon known as the illusion of explanatory depth, a term coined by Leonid

Fig. 21.3 A bike drawn
by a medical student.
Do not try to ride this

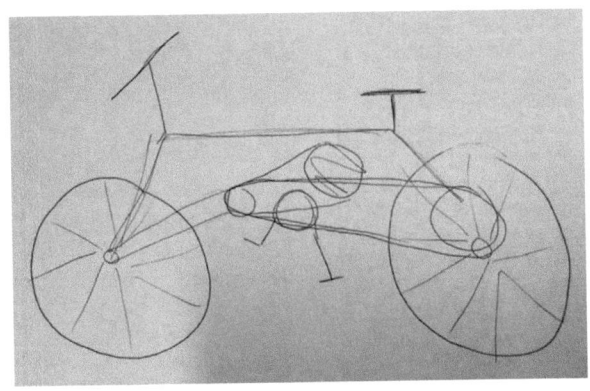

Rozenblit and Frank Keil [9]. It posits that people both fail to understand the world around them and also fail to recognize their lack of understanding. People believe they have a deeper understanding of the world than they really do and appreciate their lack of understanding only when they are explicitly asked to explain something. In a typical study, subjects are asked to evaluate their understanding of common objects such as cell phones, sewing machines, flush toilets, zippers, and locks. Most people feel they have a reasonable grasp how these objects work, until they are asked to demonstrate their knowledge in writing. When forced to confront their lack of knowledge, their self-ratings dropped. If you want to try this, ask yourself if you understand how a bicycle works. Now, prove your understanding by drawing a bicycle. The artist Gianluca Gimini gave this seemingly simple task to several hundred people and actually built the bicycles they drew [10]. Most were hopelessly non-functional and the results are quite amusing (Fig. 21.3).

In 2013, Philip Fernbach and colleagues extended this work to show that the illusion of explanatory depth affects political beliefs on issues such as single-payer health care, a national flat tax, and a cap-and-trade system to prevent pollution [11]. As with previous studies, subjects were first asked to rate their understanding of these issues. They were then asked to give a detailed explanation of how these policies actually worked and the implications of enacting them. After realizing how difficult this was, not only did subjects' self-reported understanding drop, but so did the extremity of their belief. People who felt strongly about an issue moderated their belief. Fernbach and his colleague Steven Sloman explained, "As a rule, strong feelings about issues do not emerge from deep understanding."

The Dunning–Kruger effect and the illusion of explanatory depth are very common if you look for them. A survey conducted in 2014 shortly after Russia annexed the Ukrainian territory of Crimea showed that there was an inverse correlation between how accurately people could identify Ukraine on a map and how likely they were to support military intervention [12]. The farther off they were about the location, the more they supported military intervention. A similar survey in 2017 found that Americans who could not identify North Korea on a map were also less likely to favor diplomacy (Fig. 21.4) [13].

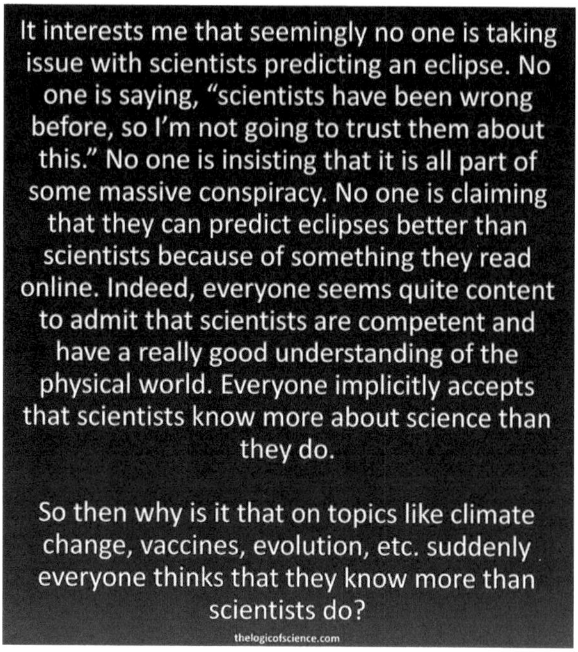

Fig. 21.4 Strangely, the
overconfidence bias applies
to some scientific fields, but
not others. (The Logic of
Science. [Image file,
Facebook status update].
2017. Retrieved from https://
www.facebook.com/
thelogicofscience/
posts/2027932000771526:0)

It interests me that seemingly no one is taking issue with scientists predicting an eclipse. No one is saying, "scientists have been wrong before, so I'm not going to trust them about this." No one is insisting that it is all part of some massive conspiracy. No one is claiming that they can predict eclipses better than scientists because of something they read online. Indeed, everyone seems quite content to admit that scientists are competent and have a really good understanding of the physical world. Everyone implicitly accepts that scientists know more about science than they do.

So then why is it that on topics like climate change, vaccines, evolution, etc. suddenly everyone thinks that they know more than scientists do?

thelogicofscience.com

The Dunning–Kruger effect seems to particularly afflict practitioners of complementary and alternative medicine (CAM) who regularly believe they know more than the entire scientific community about enormous swaths of medicine. Psychiatrist Kelly Brogan, for example, believes essentially every other doctor and scientist is wrong about the safety and efficacy of vaccines. In a Facebook post promoting an anti-vaccine movie, she wrote, "I remember when I believed that vaccines were the crowning achievement of Western Medicine. Almost a decade and more than 10,000 hours of personal research later, I've come to a very different conclusion" (Fig. 21.5) [14].

Despite her claim, implausible as it may be, that she has done "research" on vaccines for over 9 hours *every day* for three years and sixteen days (that's what it would take get to 10,000 hours), she has no peer-reviewed publications on vaccines, outside of a single opinion piece linking vaccines and depression that was published in the journal *Alternative Therapies, Health and Medicine.* She does not have a laboratory where she conducts basic experiments in immunology nor has she been involved in clinical trials of vaccines or done epidemiological research. She has not made any new discoveries, and therefore cannot be said to have done "research" on vaccines in any meaningful sense of the word. She makes errors in basic medical terminology, blaming vaccines for "the epidemic of sudden infant death (SIDS)," despite the fact that SIDS rates have declined significantly since 1990, the very opposite of an "epidemic [15]." In the same Facebook post where she boasted of 10,000 hours of research, she erroneously wrote that vaccines are "recommended for every human on the planet, cradle to grave, one-size-fits all." In fact, the inability of some people to safely receive vaccines is one of the reasons herd immunity is so important. The many contraindications to vaccines takes literally seconds to find by going to the

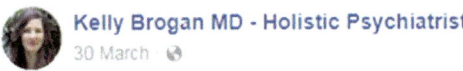

Kelly Brogan MD - Holistic Psychiatrist   ...
30 March

I remember when I believed that vaccines were the crowning achievement of Western Medicine. Almost a decade and more than 10,000 hours of personal research later, I've come to a very different conclusion.

You have to educate yourself on this issue. It's time to make a decision about how you will orient yourself around the only pharmaceutical product recommended for every human on the planet, cradle to grave, one-size-fits-all.

You could sit down, as I did, for years, but I invite you to start your journey in a more accessible way.

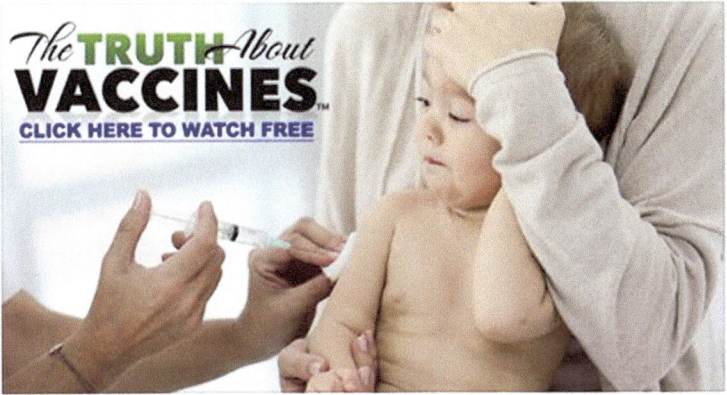

New Documentary Miniseries Event - The Truth About Vaccines

60 Top Vaccine Experts Unite To Inform Parents And Ensure Your Child's Health and Safety - Register to Watch it free online...

GO.THETRUTHABOUTVACCINES.COM

Fig. 21.5 Despite having done no research on vaccines, Kelly Brogan boasts of having done 10,000 hours of research. (Brogan K. [Kelly]. I remember when I believed that vaccines were the crowning achievement of Western Medicine [Facebook status update]. 2017. Retrieved from https://www.facebook.com/KellyBroganMD/posts/665999993606852.)

CDC webpage, and I would expect medical students to be aware of some of these before their first day of school (Fig. 21.6) [16].

Her most recent publication is a case report in a low-level journal, *Advances in Mind-Body Medicine*, of a patient with bipolar disorder who improved with dietary modifications, detox, meditation, supplementation, dry-skin brushing, and coffee enemas. This treatment is expensive and highly impractical, as many manic patients lack insight into their illness and won't even allow their blood to be drawn or vital signs to be taken. Though it was applied to a *single* patient, Dr. Brogan described it as "history-making" on social media. Most likely, medical historians will not be aware of this case report (Fig. 21.7).

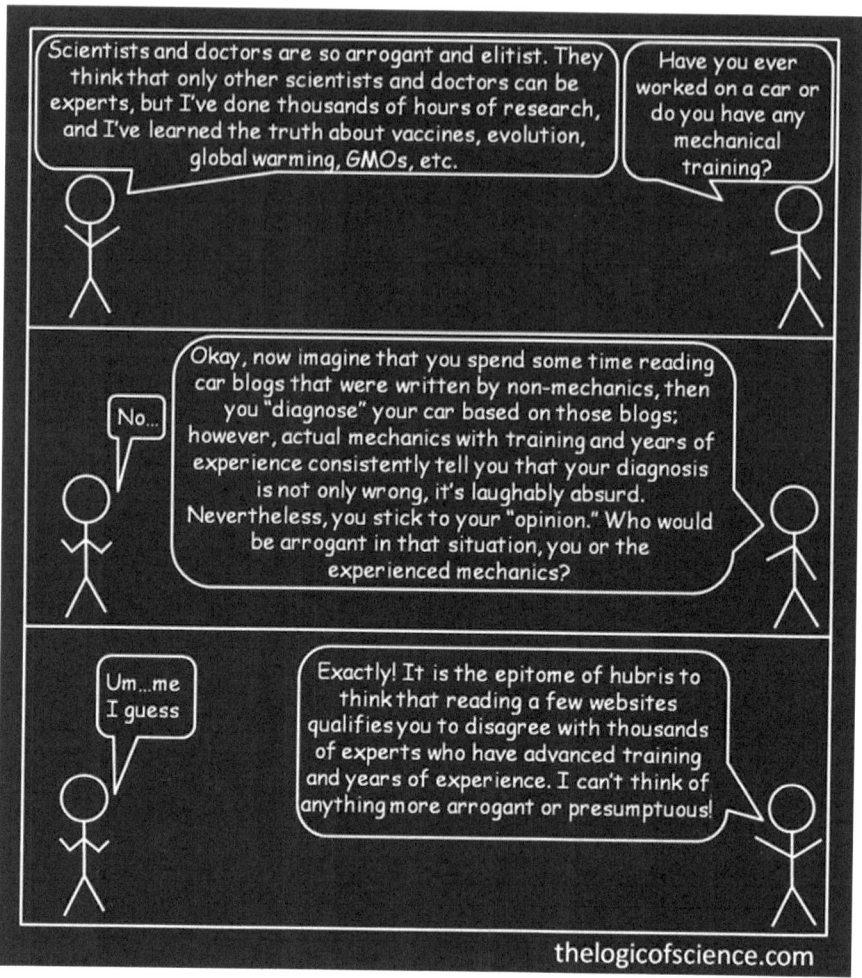

Fig. 21.6 I agree. (The Logic of Science. [Image file, Facebook status update]. 2015. Retrieved from https://www.facebook.com/thelogicofscience/posts/1727983517433044:0.)

Dr. Brogan is also a germ-theory denier, and somehow believes the fact that bacteria are everywhere bolsters this argument. She has even propagated the deadly myth that HIV does not cause AIDS. She wrote in a blog post that "drug toxicity associated with AIDS treatment may very well be what accounts for the majority of deaths [17]." This belief was propagated by the former South African president Thabo Mbeki, leading to over 300,000 deaths there [18]. She has even promoted the idea that insulin is lethal for diabetics, sharing an article called "Insulin Can Kill Diabetics; Natural Substances Heal Them" on her Facebook page [19]. For CAM practitioners like Dr. Brogan, casually overturning core tenets of medical science that have existed for decades across multiple disciplines is just another day at the office (Fig. 21.8).

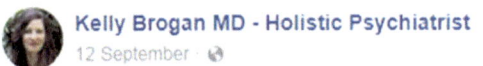

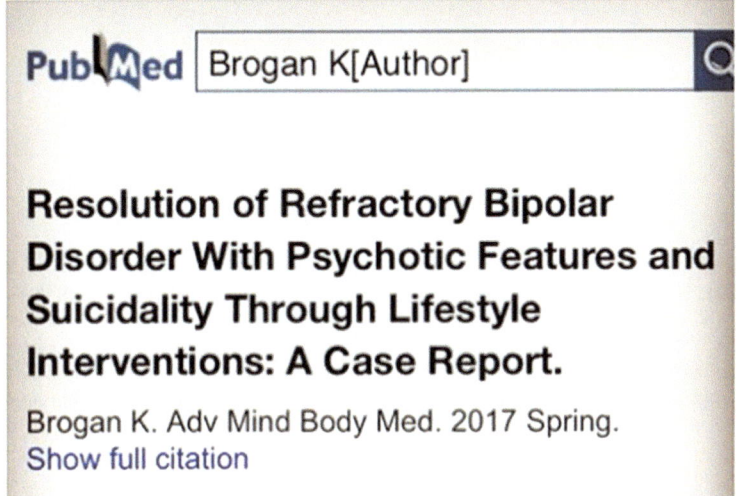

Fig. 21.7 CAM practitioner Dr. Kelly Brogan claims that publishing a case report in a low-ranking journal is "history-making." This is likely an overstatement. (Brogan K. [Kelly]. After being kicked off two hospital faculties and blacklisted by mainstream media, I promise I'm not looking for validation of holistic medicine from the mainstream. That's why it's just a cherry on top [Facebook status update]. 2017. Retrieved from https://www.facebook.com/KellyBroganMD/posts/746747322198785.)

While Dr. Brogan's credentials to overturn the global scientific consensus on the fundamental tenets of medicine can certainly be questioned, the confidence she displays when writing blogs and posting on social media, is beyond dispute. It certainly takes a great deal of confidence to use one's "personal research," whatever that means, to come a "very different conclusion" than the many thousands of immunologists who research vaccines in labs and the infectious-disease specialists who conduct clinical trials of vaccines and actually treat patients suffering from infectious diseases. However, writing blogs and posting on Facebook, is very different than actually working with sick patients (Fig. 21.9).

This speaks to an important point of the Dunning-Kruger effect with regards to almost all CAM practitioners: they never work in ERs, hospital wards, or intensive care units where they might encounter patients suffering from vaccine-preventable diseases, AIDS, and other conditions whose seriousness they deride. Lacking the responsibility for actually having to care for these patients, they are blind to their

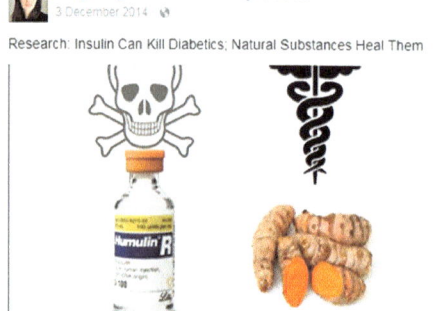

Kelly Brogan MD - Holistic Psychiatrist
3 December 2014

Research: Insulin Can Kill Diabetics; Natural Substances Heal Them

Research: Insulin Can Kill Diabetics; Natural Substances Heal Them

A paradigm-shifting study indicates that the standard of care for diabetics, including synthetic insulin and oral anti-diabetic drugs, increases morbidity and mortality...

WWW.GREENMEDINFO.COM

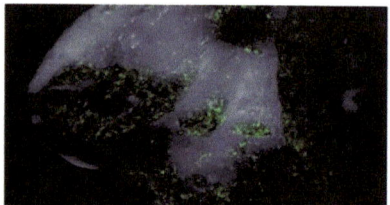

Kelly Brogan MD - Holistic Psychiatrist

Goodbye to germ theory! Can we really maintain the childish illusion that there are a handful of identified "bad germs" out there trying to kill us?

A single sand grain harbors up to 100,000 microorganisms from thousa...

sciencedaily.com

Fig. 21.8 Kelly Brogan warns diabetics of the dangers of insulin and denies germ theory. (**Left:** Brogan K. [Kelly]. Research: Insulin can kill diabetics; natural substances heal them. 2014. [Facebook status update, deleted from timeline]; **Right:** Brogan K. [Kelly]. Goodbye to germ theory! Can we really maintain the childish illusion that there are a handful of identified "bad germs" out there trying to kill us? [Facebook status update]. 2018. Retrieved from https://www. facebook.com/KellyBroganMD/posts/797098707163646.)

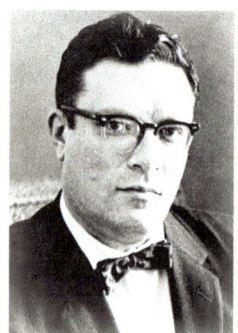

There is a cult of ignorance in the United States, and there always has been. The strain of anti-intellectualism has been a constant thread winding its way through our political and cultural life, nurtured by the false notion that democracy means that "my ignorance is just as good as your knowledge."

Isaac Asimov

Fig. 21.9 Isaac Asimov gets it right. (Leonian P. Isaac Asimov [Image file]. In: Wikimedia commons. (n.d.). Retrieved from https://commons.wikimedia.org/wiki/Isaac_Asimov#/media/ File:Isaac.Asimov01.jpg.)

existence, shielded from having to face an ill patient that might force them to correct their views. In the past year, two young men arrived to my hospital with a serious brain infection (toxoplasmosis) as the presenting symptom of AIDS. As neither of them had seen a doctor previously, blaming their illness on "drug toxicity associated with AIDS treatment" is obviously not a possibility. Dr. Brogan wasn't there to guide their treatment nor was any other CAM practitioner. Because they rarely work in environments where they are likely to encounter sick people, Dr. Brogan and similar CAM practitioners are blind to the consequences of their beliefs. As a result, their overconfidence

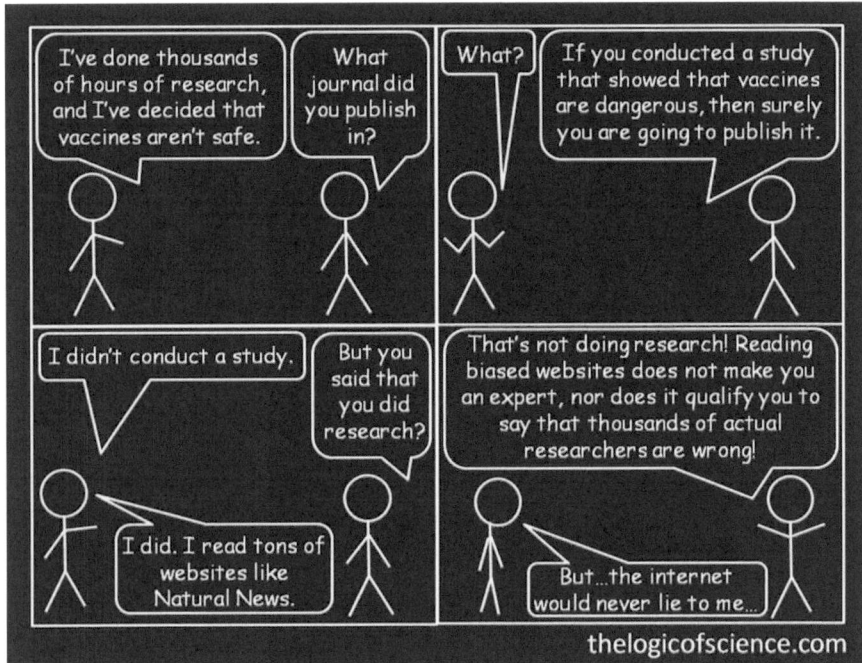

Fig. 21.10 "Research" as practiced by overconfident CAM practitioners. (The Logic of Science. [Image file, Facebook status update]. 2015. Retrieved from https://www.facebook.com/thelogicof-science/photos/a.1680841055480624/1642180706013326/?type=3.)

goes unchallenged. Their situation is analogous to someone who is certain they understand how a bicycle works, before they are asked to explain it (Fig. 21.10).

The case that opens this chapter, about the doctor who recommended against the vitamin K shot, was adapted from an article shared on the Facebook page of "holistic" pediatrician Lawrence Palevsky [20]. Though his medical training exposed him to critically ill children, from his current office at the Northport Wellness Center he is virtually guaranteed not to see any child who suffers an intracranial hemorrhage due to their parent's refusal of a vitamin K shot. This is in stark contrast to someone like Ivana Culic, a neonatologist at Boston Children's Hospital and medical director of a special care nursery, who said about such cases:

Personally, it is actually really hard to take care of any infant or baby that is sick. But when you realize that a severe illness was completely preventable, that is something that is really hard for everyone to comprehend and deal with in our field (Fig. 21.11) [21].

In contrast to clinicians like Drs. Brogan and Palevsky, high-knowledge people tend to underestimate their knowledge and skills. They may assume that since a skill is easy for them, this must be the case for others as well. Additionally, high-knowledge people will be aware of the enormous amount of knowledge in their field, and they will grasp the large amount of information they don't know. As Thomas Jefferson said, "He who knows most, knows best how little he knows" (Fig. 21.12).

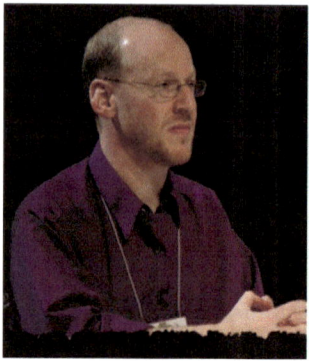

I'm tired of ignorance held up as inspiration, where vicious anti-intellectualism is considered a positive trait, and where uninformed opinion is displayed as fact.
Philip Plait

Fig. 21.11 Philip Plait gets it right. (Ensceptico. Philip Plait at The Amazing Meeting on Jan 20, 2007 [Image file]. In: Wikimedia commons. 2007. Retrieved from https://commons.wikimedia.org/w/index.php?search=Philip+Plait+&title=Special:Search&go=Go#/media/File:Philip_Plait_2007.jpg.)

Fig. 21.12 Jessica knows how much she doesn't know. [Facebook comment, redacted for privacy].)

Jessica
I love it when people say "I did my research." Did you? Did you really? Because I have two graduate degrees and spent many years with a pipette, Petri dishes and a powerful electron microscope and only then did I begin to scratch the surface of the field of microbiology and immunology. Apparently I should've just spent two hours on Google.

In contrast to low-knowledge people who are convinced they are experts, high-knowledge people are often fearful they will be revealed as fraudulent and undeserving of the success they have achieved, a phenomenon referred to as impostor syndrome. As such, the Dunning–Kruger effect applies to us all, though in different magnitudes and directions. The Dunning-Kruger effect can be diagramed with low-knowledge/high-confidence individuals said to reside on Mount Stupid (Fig. 21.13).

Closely related to the biases discussed so far are the illusion of control, the self-serving bias, and the optimism bias. The illusion of control, which was identified by Ellen Langer refers to the tendency for people believe they control or influence events that are, in fact, outside of their control [22]. Anyone who has ever watched

Fig. 21.13 Mount Stupid

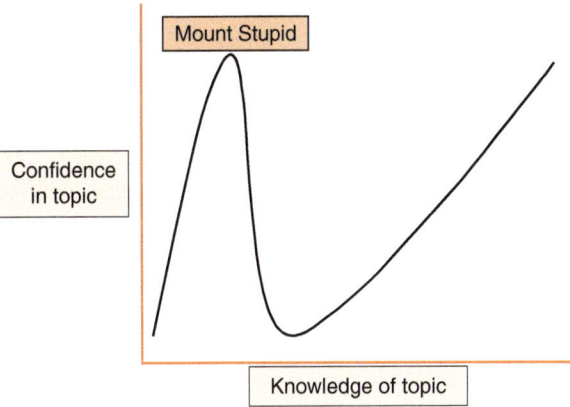

gamblers in a casino will see them blowing on the dice or performing other rituals, all in the hopes of influencing random events. In one study, subjects were instructed to press a button in order to turn on a light. Although it turned on and off randomly, many subjects were nonetheless convinced they had found a successful technique to manipulate the light [23]. With regards to medicine, a clinician may feel that a critically ill patient recovered due to her care. While this may be the case, often random chance and the natural history of many diseases plays larger roles than many clinicians recognize.

The self-serving bias refers to the tendency to claim more responsibility for successes than for failures. Clinicians may overestimate the number of times they have made a brilliant or insightful diagnosis and fail to remember their failures. Similarly, they may ascribe successes to their own skill, while blaming failures on circumstances beyond their control. A surgeon who successfully performs a risky operation on a critically ill patient may pat themselves on the back for the good outcome. Were the operation to go poorly, however, she may instead attribute its failure to the patient's poor condition, rather than second-guess her wisdom in performing the operation in the first place. Similarly, a clinician whose patient improves shortly after receiving a treatment will likely credit the patient's success to that treatment. Of course, this could just be illusionary correlation.

The optimism bias occurs when people believe they are less likely to experiencing a negative event than other people. People generally underestimate the likelihood that they will get divorced, contract a serious illness, or be the victim of crime. In medicine, clinicians may feel their patients are less likely to suffer a serious consequence as a result of a selected treatment. This is particularly the case if the adverse reaction is uncommon.

Together, these biases are termed positive illusions. They are a form of self-deception that promote favorable attitudes and allow people to maintain positive feelings. On many occasions, such illusions are highly advantageous. If it weren't for highly confident people, for example, it's hard to imagine humanity could have successfully put a man on the moon. The optimism bias allows us to be hopeful about the future and pursue our dreams, while the self-serving

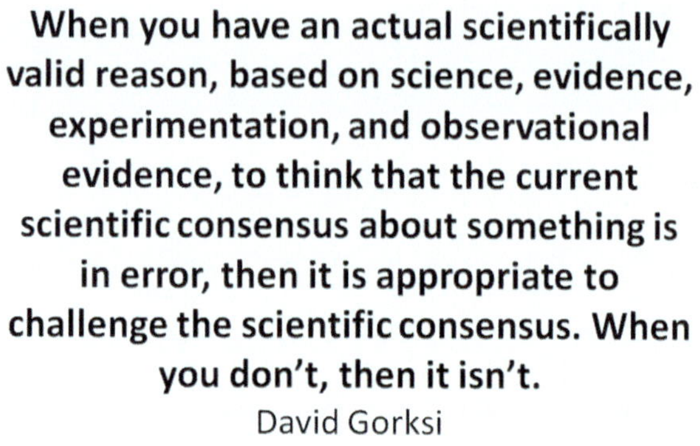

Fig. 21.14 David Gorski
gets it right

When you have an actual scientifically valid reason, based on science, evidence, experimentation, and observational evidence, to think that the current scientific consensus about something is in error, then it is appropriate to challenge the scientific consensus. When you don't, then it isn't.

David Gorksi

bias allows us to persevere in the face of a setback. However, clinicians should do their best to have a realistic sense of the probability of a treatment working for or harming a patient, not an opinion clouded by rose-colored glasses.

Interestingly, and perhaps predictably, depressed people are less prone to the overconfidence bias than euthymic people. Several studies suggest that depressed people have more accurate estimations of their abilities and are less likely to overestimate themselves or have unrealistic optimism. This hypothesis, known as depressive realism, was formulated by Lyn Yvonne Abramson and Lauren Alloy. Additionally, the Dunning-Kruger effect seems culture-specific. According to Dr. Dunning, "North Americans seem to be the kings and queens of overestimation. If you go to places like Japan, Korea, or China, this whole phenomenon evaporates."

A particular manifestation of the overconfidence bias that seems to affect many clinicians is the degree to which they view themselves immune from visceral impulses such as fatigue and hunger (see decision fatigue). Similarly, many clinicians to believe themselves to be superhuman, immune to hospital-acquired infections. This leads to imperfect handwashing on the part of clinicians and the spread of serious infections in the hospital. Adam Grant and David Hoffman found that posters reminding clinicians to wash their hands were effective only if the benefit to patients was emphasized [24]. In contrast, posters declaring that "Hand hygiene prevents you from catching diseases" were ineffective at getting clinicians to wash their hands (Fig. 21.14).

Conclusion

Author Charles Bukowski said, "The problem with the world is that the intelligent people are full of doubts, while the stupid ones are full of confidence" (Fig. 21.15).

Psychological research has supported this observation, a phenomenon known as the Dunning-Kruger effect. As such, clinicians should constantly strive to remain humble, especially in areas outside their expertise. They would be wise to heed the words of author David Brin who said, "If an outsider perceives 'something wrong'

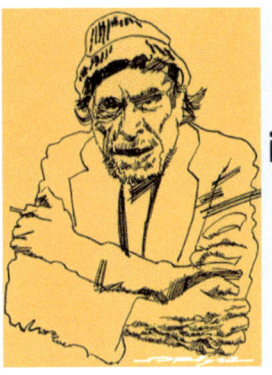

The problem with the world is that the intelligent people are full of doubts, while the stupid ones are full of confidence.

Charles Bukowski

Fig. 21.15 Charles Bukowski gets it right. (Origafoundation. Charles Bukowski, portrait by Italian artist Graziano Origa, pen&ink+pantone, 2008 [Image file]. In: Wikimedia commons. 2007. Retrieved from https://commons.wikimedia.org/wiki/Category:Charles_Bukowski#/media/File:Bukowski-by-origa.jpg.)

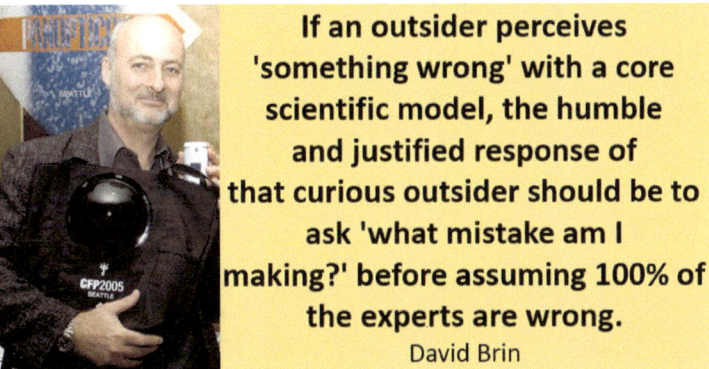

If an outsider perceives 'something wrong' with a core scientific model, the humble and justified response of that curious outsider should be to ask 'what mistake am I making?' before assuming 100% of the experts are wrong.

David Brin

Fig. 21.16 David Brin gets it right. (Rpetrov. David Brin at ACM CFP [Image file]. In: Wikimedia commons. 2005. Retrieved from https://commons.wikimedia.org/wiki/File:David_Brin_at_ACM_CFP_2005dsc278c.jpg.)

with a core scientific model, the humble and justified response of that curious outsider should be to ask 'what mistake am I making?' before assuming 100% of the experts are wrong" (Fig. 21.16) [25].

Given the great difficulty we all have in adequately assessing our own skills and knowledge, what is to be done? According to Dr. Dunning, "The road to self-insight runs through other people [26]." Since we are blind to our own short-comings, clinicians should not be afraid to ask for help with challenging cases and should be willing to accept criticism about their decisions and performance. Ideally, clinicians should be able to discuss difficult cases in regularly scheduled conferences with trusted colleagues who provide them with candid feedback.

References

1. Wilemon T. (2014, May 4). More babies hemorrhaging after parents refuse vitamin K shots. Tennessean. Retrieved from https://www.tennessean.com/story/news/health/2014/05/02/babies-hemorrhaging-parents-refuse-vitamin-k-shots/8610155/.
2. Svenson O. Are we all less risky and more skillful than our fellow drivers. Acta Psychol. 1981;47(2):143–8. https://doi.org/10.1016/0001-6918(81)90005-6.
3. Cross KP. Not can, but will college teaching be improved? N Dir High Educ. 1977;1977(17):1–15. https://doi.org/10.1002/he.36919771703.
4. Zuckerman EW, Jost JT. What makes you think you're so popular? Self-evaluation maintenance and the subjective side of the "friendship paradox". Soc Psychol Q. 2001;64:207–23.
5. Kruger J, Dunning D. Unskilled and unaware of it: how difficulties in recognizing one's own incompetence lead to inflated self-assessments. J Pers Soc Psychol. 1999;77(6):1121–34. https://doi.org/10.1037/0022-3514.77.6.1121.
6. Klein E. (2017, Dec 29). Incoherent, authoritarian, uninformed: Trump's New York Times interview is a scary read. Vox. Retrieved from https://www.vox.com/policy-and-politics/2017/12/29/16829806/trump-interview-new-york-times.
7. Hoffmann TC, Del Mar C. Clinicians' expectations of the benefits and harms of treatments, screening, and tests: a systematic review. JAMA Intern Med. 2017;177(3):407–19. https://doi.org/10.1001/jamainternmed.2016.8254.
8. The NNT Group. (2018). Quick summaries of evidence-based medicine. Retrieved from http://www.thennt.com.
9. Rozenblit L, Keil F. The misunderstood limits of folk science: an illusion of explanatory depth. Cogn Sci. 2002;26(5):521–62. https://doi.org/10.1207/s15516709cog2605_1.
10. Artist asks people to draw a bicycle from memory and renders the results. (2016, April 18). Retrieved from https://twistedsifter.com/2016/04/artist-asks-people-to-draw-a-bicycle-from-memory-and-renders-results/.
11. Fernbach PM, Rogers T, Fox CR, Sloman SA. Political extremism is supported by an illusion of understanding. Psychol Sci. 2013;24(6):939–46. https://doi.org/10.1177/0956797612464058.
12. Kolbert E. (2017, Feb 27). Why facts don't change our minds. The New Yorker. Retrieved from https://www.newyorker.com/magazine/2017/02/27/why-facts-dont-change-our-minds.
13. Quealy K. (2017, July 5). If Americans can find North Korea on a map, they're more likely to prefer diplomacy. The New York Times. Retrieved from https://www.nytimes.com/interactive/2017/05/14/upshot/if-americans-can-find-north-korea-on-a-map-theyre-more-likely-to-prefer-diplomacy.html.
14. Brogan K. [Kelly]. (2017, Mar 30). I remember when I believed that vaccines were the crowning achievement of Western Medicine [Facebook status update]. Retrieved from https://www.facebook.com/KellyBroganMD/posts/665999993606852.
15. Brogan K. (n.d.). Could this be driving the epidemic of sudden infant death (SIDS)?. Kelly Brogan MD. Retrieved 15 Sept 2018 from https://www.nytimes.com/interactive/2017/05/14/upshot/if-americans-can-find-north-korea-on-a-map-theyre-more-likely-to-prefer-diplomacy.html.
16. Centers for Disease Control and Prevention. (2018, Sept 14). Contraindications and precautions. Vaccine recommendations and guidelines of the ACIP. Retrieved from https://www.cdc.gov/vaccines/hcp/acip-recs/general-recs/contraindications.html.
17. Harris HP. (2014, Sept 23). Kelly Brogan denies germ theory and the value of HIV drugs [Blog post]. SciBlogs. Retrieved from https://sciblogs.co.nz/diplomaticimmunity/2014/09/23/kelly-brogan-denies-germ-theory-and-the-value-of-hiv-drugs/.
18. Boseley S. (2008, Nov 26). Mbeki Aids denial 'caused 300,000 deaths. The Guardian. Retrieved from https://www.theguardian.com/world/2008/nov/26/aids-south-africa.
19. Debunking the synthetic insulin myth. (2014, Dec 4). Bad Science Debunked. Retrieved from https://badsciencedebunked.com/2014/12/04/you-mad-bro-debunking-the-synthetic-insulin-myth-part-i/.

20. Palevsky LB. [Lawrence B.] (2014, Sept 3). Vitamin K shot at birth - - The controversy reignites [Facebook status update]. Retrieved from https://www.facebook.com/110703415650945/posts/vitamin-k-shot-at-birth-the-controversy-reigniteshttparticlesmercolacomsite-sarti/699495206771760/.
21. Goldberg C. (2016, Aug 12). When new parents refuse vitamin K shots and their babies get brain bleeds. WBUR.com. Retrieved from http://www.wbur.org/commonhealth/2016/08/12/vitamin-k-newborn.
22. Yarritu I, Matute H, Vadillo MA. Illusion of control: the role of personal involvement. Exp Psychol. 2014;61(1):38–47. https://doi.org/10.1027/1618-3169/a000225.
23. Jenkins HM, Ward WC. Judgment of contingency between responses and outcomes. Psychol Monogr Gen Appl. 1965;79(1):1–17.
24. Grant AM, Hofmann DA. It's not all about me: motivating hand hygiene among health care professionals by focusing on patients. Psychol Sci. 2011;22(12):1494–9. https://doi.org/10.1177/0956797611419172.
25. Brin D. (n.d.). Skeptics versus deniers: creating a climate of 'no!'. Davidbrin.com. Retrieved 15 Sept 2018 from http://www.davidbrin.com/nonfiction/climatechange2.html.
26. Ghose T. (2013, Feb 6). Why we're all above average. LiveScience. Retrieved from https://www.livescience.com/26914-why-we-are-all-above-average.html.

Case

David was an otherwise healthy 69-year-old man who presented with the sudden onset of left-sided numbness. He was a prominent local businessman who had donated millions of dollars to build a children's ward at the local hospital. An MRI revealed an ischemic stroke in his right thalamus. An evaluation for the cause of his stroke revealed 50% stenosis (narrowing) of his carotid artery on the right, as well as elevated blood pressure. The neurologist attributed his stroke to his hypertension and prescribed anti-hypertension medications and aspirin. David demanded that he be seen by a surgeon and called the head of vascular surgery service himself to arrange this. He then demanded that the surgeon perform an operation saying, "50% stenosis can't be good for someone who had a stroke. I'll make sure Lisa (the hospital's CEO) hears about this." When the surgeon tried to explain that the risks of the procedure outweighed the benefits, David contacted the hospital CEO. Though there was no evidence that surgery was beneficial in David's case, the surgeon relented and agreed to perform a carotid endarterectomy, an operation which removes plaque build-up on the inside of arteries. David suffered a second stroke during the operation that left him with weakness on his left side.

What Dr. Wolper Was Thinking

It's not every day the hospital CEO hospital calls me. Though she said that she wanted me to "use my best judgment," I could read between the lines. David was a major donor to the hospital, and the last thing I needed was to have some VIP complain about me to hospital administration. Ironically enough, there was an undocumented immigrant without insurance I cared for that week with a stroke very similar to David's. This patient didn't make demands for improper care, and I would have had no problem telling him "no," had such requests been made. This patient ended up getting much better care than David.

Doctors can really be in a bind at times. Our salaries depend, in part, on our "patient satisfaction" scores, and it is not uncommon to have a conflict between a

© Springer International Publishing AG, part of Springer Nature 2019
J. Howard, *Cognitive Errors and Diagnostic Mistakes*,
https://doi.org/10.1007/978-3-319-93224-8_22

"satisfied" patient, and a patient who actually receives proper care. I have since learned that doing the right thing for some patients requires thick skin. And I won't treat VIP patients worse than anyone else by refusing to tell them "no."

Discussion

The satisfied patient error occurs when a clinician provides inappropriate care to avoid unsatisfied patients. Many clinicians are "people-pleasers" and have a difficult time tolerating patients who are upset at them, even if that means ordering unnecessary tests and treatments. Additionally, clinicians may provide inappropriate care to avoid receiving bad reviews on the internet, negative marks on a patient satisfaction survey, or to appease a VIP patient. It is common for hospitals and clinicians to be rated, and sometimes compensated, based on "patient satisfaction" scores. In 2012, Press Ganey, the nation's largest provider of patient satisfaction surveys, processed 70 million patient surveys encompassing over 10,000 health care organizations and half of the hospitals in the US [1]. Medicare's patient survey is six pages long, and includes questions such as these [2]:

- During this hospital stay, how often did the doctors treat you with courtesy and respect?
- During this hospital stay, how often did doctors explain things in a way you could understand?
- During this hospital stay, how often did your doctors listen to you carefully?
- During this hospital stay, how often did the staff do everything they could to help you with your pain?
- During this hospital stay, did you get information in writing about what symptoms or health problems to look out for after you left the hospital?
- During this hospital stay, staff took my preferences and those of my family or caregiver into account in deciding what my health care needs would be when I left.

At first glance, asking patients questions like these seems entirely reasonable. If a clinician is a jerk or a poor diagnostician, low patient satisfaction scores would likely reflect this and allow corrective actions to be taken. If a hospital serves its patients poorly, it can also use information from patient satisfaction surveys to improve its performance.

Yet, what if a clinician is firm in denying inappropriate requests for medications, tests, or excuse notes from work? Should they be punished for using their clinical judgment? I certainly have had patients respond with disbelief and anger when I refused to order a test or medication they requested, as if I was a waiter who refused to bring them their preferred meal. Additionally, I have had patients in tears in my office when I refused to write a letter saying they were utterly incapable of any employment. Though I did my best to explain my reasoning, I am sure many of these patients left my office "unsatisfied."

So, does this mean I was a bad doctor? When you go to a restaurant, or get a haircut or massage, your satisfaction is all that matters. In these industries, the mantra "the customer is always right," seems reasonable. Is the same true for health-care? Wouldn't you rather go to a clinician whose main goal was your health, even if it meant they refused to accede to your every whim? Would you feel comfortable going to a clinician whose primary goal was to "satisfy" you, either because they were afraid to upset you or worried they would score poorly on your patient satisfaction survey? How would you feel, as a patient, knowing that your satisfaction rating might influence your clinician's salary or Medicare payments to their hospital? If you requested an inappropriate medication, such an antibiotic for a viral illness, would you want your clinician to give you this medication just to satisfy you? If you had an unhealthy lifestyle habit, would you want your clinician to avoid discussing this with you for fears of offending you?

Regardless of how you answer these questions, many clinicians face a conflict between satisfying their patients or providing appropriate care. As William Sonnenberg, a family physician, wrote, "doctors face the reality that uncomfortable discussions on behavioral topics — say, smoking or obesity — come with the risk of a pay cut" [3].

Because their salaries may depend in part on patient satisfaction scores, it is not surprising that clinicians commonly provide inappropriate care to appease patients. According to Forbes magazine:

> *In a recent online survey of 700-plus emergency room doctors by Emergency Physicians Monthly, 59% admitted they increased the number of tests they performed because of patient satisfaction surveys. The South Carolina Medical Association asked its members whether they'd ever ordered a test they felt was inappropriate because of such pressures, and 55% of 131 respondents said yes. Nearly half said they'd improperly prescribed antibiotics and narcotic pain medication in direct response to patient satisfaction surveys* [1].

Not surprisingly, patients who receive inappropriate care have worse outcomes. Simply put, a satisfied patient is not necessarily a well-treated patient. In the largest study of the impact of patient satisfaction, Joshua Fenton and colleagues studied nearly 52,000 adult patients from 2000-2007 through the national Medical Expenditure Panel Survey [4]. They found that the most satisfied patients were 12% more likely to be admitted to the hospital, their healthcare and prescription drug costs were 9% higher, and strikingly, they were 26% more likely to die.

Additionally, clinicians who avoid potentially uncomfortable conversations to avoid offending patients may miss an important piece of diagnostic information or may avoid offering an important treatment. The practice of medicine routinely necessitates both breaking bad news and uncomfortable discussions. Clinicians who deliver bad news often have negative emotions directed at them and can even be blamed for it.

The natural reluctance many people have to break bad news to others is known as the MUM effect after the expression "Mum's the word" [5]. Several studies have shown that people readily share positive information, but withhold negative information. In one such study, postcards were placed in the public transportation systems of five European cities [6]. They contained information that was either positive or negative and either high or low importance. More postcards were returned when the information was favorable than unfavorable, though only in the high importance conditions. In another study, subjects more readily communicated bad news to a third party than to the person impacted by the news. There is a reason medical schools have classes on how to break bad news, but no class is needed to tell patients their biopsy came back completely normal.

The MUM effect has been demonstrated in clinicians. A survey of 582 pediatricians and family physicians by Mandy Allison and colleagues found that about one-third of them don't discuss the HPV vaccine with pre-teen patients in part due to fears that their parents would object [7]. Given that the HPV vaccine can prevent cervical and several other cancers, failing to discuss it because of such fears is a significant mistake.

Moreover, clinicians who "satisfy" their anti-vaccine patients (or their parents) may be jeopardizing the health of other patients in their waiting room and the community at large. While children obviously cannot be vaccinated without the permission of their guardians, many pediatricians are firing families that refuse to vaccinate despite their best efforts to convince them otherwise. While this is a controversial topic, such pediatricians recognize that patient satisfaction is not their primary duty. As pediatrician Jesse Hackell asked, "If they won't accept my advice about vaccinations, how are they going to accept my advice on anything else?" [8] Pediatrician Chris Hickie explained his decision to stop seeing such families by saying [9]:

> I decided to stop seeing electively non-vaccinating families when an older unvaccinated child came into my waiting room with florid pertussis — coughing paroxysmally to the point of turning blue and retching. Thankfully my waiting room was not crowded and no infants were present, but the episode helped me to realize that spread of vaccine-preventable diseases via my waiting room is much more likely to happen if there are electively non-vaccinating families in my practice.

The harms that worry Dr. Hickie are not imaginary. Unvaccinated children have spread measles in medical facilities. In 2008, for example, several children caught measles in the waiting room of Bob Sears, a pediatrician who routinely spreads misinformation about vaccines [10]. Ultimately, 11 people were infected, including three infants under 12 months, one of whom was hospitalized for several days for dehydration. In Australia in 2011, seven people were infected in a waiting room [11]. Perhaps most tragically, an immunocompromised woman died of the measles in Washington State in 2015, most likely after being exposed to the disease in a medical facility [12].

Recognizing the risk unvaccinated children may pose, the American Academy of Pediatrics updated their position statement in 2016 to support the practice of discharging non-vaccinating families under very limited circumstances, namely when the pediatrician has exhaustively tried to educate the family and the child will not be left without treatment [8]. Although more research needs to be done, studies of the impact of pediatricians dismissing non-vaccinating families tend to show that this does not lead to clusters of unvaccinated children, as was feared, and may increase the overall rate of vaccine acceptance (Fig. 22.1) [13].

It's even possible that clinicians' fears of poor patient satisfaction scores might be contributing to the nation's opioid crisis and the overuse of antibiotics. A study

Fig. 22.1 A pro-vaccine meme illustrating the point that a clinician's job is not to satisfy patients

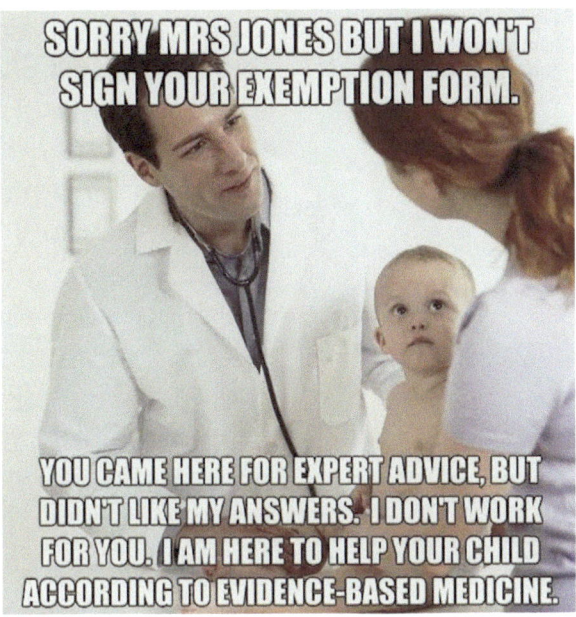

by Mark Ashworth and colleagues found that in primary care offices in England, antibiotic prescribing volume was the strongest predictor of overall patient satisfaction out of 13 prescribing variables [14]. Indiana health commissioner Jerome M. Adams said that many clinicians told him, "I'm scared to not give out those opioids because my patient satisfaction scores will come back poorly" [15]. One nurse, commenting on social media, wrote the following about the role patient-satisfaction scores and Press Ganey have played in the opioid epidemic:

> *Finally! I have been saying for years that the Joint Commission and Press Ganey need to be held accountable for their role in this epidemic! As an ER nurse, all I heard for years was that we are not meeting patient's pain needs. Pain as the fifth vital sign, are you kidding me!? I agree that the blame given to the doctors should be near the end of the article. Working closely with ER doctors for years, I heard many times that they felt like their hands were tied due to satisfaction surveys. The majority of them did not want to prescribe opioids but felt they had no choice! At my final job before retirement, I finally had a manager who did not live and die by the results of patient surveys. She left them in the break room for us to peruse but we were never called on the carpet because of a negative response from one of our drug seekers. Not so with other administrations and nurse managers! With them the blame fell squarely on the doctors and/or the nurses! I had been a nurse for over 30 years and the changes I saw over those years were not good. I miss the people I worked with over the years but I do not miss the job itself! I hardly recognize the profession anymore* [16].

It is important to point out that evidence linking patient satisfaction scores to the inappropriate prescribing of opioids is anecdotal and that formal studies have not shown a relationship between patient satisfaction scores and doctors' opioid prescribing habits. Nonetheless, there was enough concern that in 2016, the Centers for Medicare and Medicaid Services eliminated all pain-related questions in patient

Danjuro

I've practiced EM for over 20 years and lost several contracts for refusing to ply opioid scripts to drug-seeking patients. Peers and ER heads would jușt tell me to give them a Percocet six pack and get them out so they won't file a "patient" complaint! Too many hospital CEO's worried more about patient satisfaction scores than ethical medicine! I wish I had never gone into emergency medicine!

satisfaction surveys. However, Press Ganey continues to ask questions related to pain management, and there is little doubt that this influences clinicians' practices. To again quote Dr. Sonnenberg, "The mandate is simple: Never deny a request for an antibiotic, an opioid pain medication, a scan, or an admission." He believes Press Ganey "has become a bigger threat to the practice of good medicine than trial lawyers" (Fig. 22.2) [3].

Notably, some patients and healthcare delivery models are more susceptible than others to the patient satisfaction error. VIP patients may be especially vulnerable. When clinicians proclaim they treat "every patient the same," they usually mean they strive to give the poor and disenfranchised the same care they provide to the wealthy, famous, and well-connected. However, while it may be counter-intuitive, VIPs may receive worse care than the average patient. With VIPs, there may be a temptation to deviate from standard procedures, order extra tests, or avoid unpleasant tests that may cause discomfort. Shoa Clarke, an internist and pediatrician, expressed this sentiment by writing, "many doctors worry that VIPs receive *worse* care. I've heard many stories of elite patients who underwent unnecessary tests or were treated with medications unlikely to be helpful because the physician felt pressured to appease them" [17]. I have also seen many VIPs receive unnecessary, "million-dollar" workups for common conditions. There is little doubt that if they were an immigrant treated at the public hospital, they would have received more appropriate care. Notably, VIP patients include not just the famous, the rich, or those with ties to the hospital administration. Other VIPs may be fellow clinicians, emergency responders, and even long-standing patients who are well-known and liked at a particular hospital.

I also suspect that clinicians who practice concierge medicine are highly vulnerable to the patient satisfaction error. In this healthcare delivery model, patients can pay tens of thousands of dollars per year to have round-the-clock access to boutique doctors, who will make house calls, facilitate appointments with other clinicians, and even fly with patients across the country to attend these appointments. I imagine it must be extremely difficult to deny unneeded tests and treatments to patients who pay $80,000 a year [18]. Such enormous fees can't help but distort the clinician-patient relationship, potentially turning the clinician from an independent professional into an employee whose job is to satisfy the boss.

The internet as also changed the practice of medicine as clinicians may feel compelled to satisfy patients to avoid poor scores on online doctor-rating sites. Such reviews can have profound consequences for clinicians, especially those in private practice who likely depend on patients finding them online. While giving patients a public voice in rating their clinicians may seem empowering, it can serve as a disincentive for clinicians to provide their patients with proper care. One clinician, who responded reasonably to a patient's inappropriate demands, relayed the following story on social media:

> I was about 30–40 minutes late to see a new patient in clinic. As I entered the room, the patient boasted to me that he was a CEO of a major company. He then said that if he was ever 30–40 minutes late to a board meeting, they would fire him or demote him. He told me that he found my tardiness unacceptable. I apologized and explained to him that I see a lot of patients with cancer and I always extend them the courtesy to explain everything to them and their families. Sometimes, trying to answer all of their questions isn't possible to do in the allotted time. I promised him that I would always extend him the same courtesy to explain and answer everything. He then proceeded to give me an ultimatum. He said he could either stand up, tear up his paperwork, and walk out, or I could apologize and promise him that I would never be late with him again. I chose to politely respect his first demand and told him that our relationship was too incompatible and I showed him the door. I told my office manager to make sure he doesn't get a bill, and to make sure he gets a letter of termination from our office. Of course, he goes around the websites and rates me with one star, complaining about how rude I am.... sigh, I pray he will find someone who will be able to help him [19].

Clinicians who treat patients so as to avoid negative reviews online or in patient surveys are unlikely to be doing the best for their patients' health. Whenever I see a clinician with pages of pages of glowing patient reviews online, I wonder if that clinician might be telling patients what they want to hear, rather than what they need to hear. Moreover, at present, clinicians have little recourse to combat negative reviews online, other than to grow thick skin. Because of patient privacy laws, clinicians are powerless to defend themselves against malicious or misleading online reviews. Any response at all risks acknowledging that the patient saw the clinician, which is a violation of these laws. As such, clinicians should do their best to know themselves and understand how negative online reviews may affect their practice.

Additionally, a hospital's concern over its patient satisfaction score may also disempower its clinicians in the face of abusive, threatening behavior by patients and their family members. Farshad Farnejad, a trauma surgeon, wrote about the time a mother of a critically ill patient made racist comments towards him and threatened to deport him [20]. Though she had to be escorted out of the hospital multiple times, there was little the hospital staff could do to defend themselves against her tirades. As Dr. Farnejad wrote:

> *If being subject to verbal abuse and threats of violence is accepted as "part of the job" because there is more concern about patient satisfaction, than the safety and well-being of physicians, nurses and other hospital staff, there is something really wrong with the system.*

From a patient's perspective, it is important to note there is no evidence clinicians' ratings are an indicator of their competency. Many aspects of patient satisfaction are beyond the control of the individual clinician who is being rated. One study of 49 doctors who work at both hospitals and freestanding ERs found that patient satisfaction scores were higher when the doctor worked at freestanding facilities, possibly because the wait time is shorter [21]. A study by Kanu Okike and colleagues examined 614 surgeons in five states and found 590 of them had been rated by patients on the internet. There was no correlation between their online rating and the risk-adjusted mortality rate [22]. Some of the surgeons with the highest mortality rates also had the highest online ratings. The authors concluded that "Patients using online rating websites to guide their choice of physician should recognize that these ratings may not reflect actual quality of care as defined by accepted metrics."

Conclusion

Clinicians should remember that the goal of medicine is to care for patients, not please them. Clinicians who sugarcoat bad news or avoid uncomfortable conversations to satisfy their patients aren't doing them any favors. Clinicians with lower patient satisfaction scores may, at times, actually be providing superior care than those with higher scores. Tying clinician compensation to their patient satisfaction scores is extremely problematic, as clinicians may face a conflict between providing proper care for their patients or care that will earn them more money.

Clinicians must also be careful not to give worse care to VIP patients, as more studies and procedures do not equate to better care. Jorge Guzman and colleagues suggested nine principles when dealing with VIPs. These include "resist changing time-honored, effective clinical practices and overriding one's clinical judgment," and having the most senior faculty care for the patient if they are the most appropriate person for their care [23].

Of course, clinicians should not ignore patient satisfaction scores and what their patients say about them online. If a pattern emerges where patients point to a flaw in the clinician's care, then all efforts should be made to rectify this. Perhaps a clinician could improve their communication skills in telling patients why a particular test or treatment is not indicated. Additionally, clinicians should pick their battles. If a patient requests an unneeded blood test, this may be relatively harmless and arguing about this might weaken the clinician-patient relationship. In contrast, acceding to their demand for an inappropriate MRI may set off a cascade of unnecessary and potentially harmful interventions. However, not even the best clinician can convince every patient in every situation, and clinicians need to get used to unsatisfied patients at times. There is also a lesson for patients, who would be wise to avoid clinicians who seem more interested in pleasing them than treating them.

References

1. Falkenberg K. (2013, Jan 2). Why rating your doctor is bad for your health. Forbes. Retrieved from https://www.forbes.com/sites/kaifalkenberg/2013/01/02/why-rating-your-doctor-is-bad-for-your-health/.
2. Health Services Advisory Group. (2017, Mar). HCAHPS survey [PDF file]. Retrieved from https://hcahpsonline.org/globalassets/hcahps/survey-instruments/mail/through-december-31-2017-discharges/click-here-to-view-or-download-the-english-survey-materials..pdf.
3. Sonnenberg W. (2014, Mar 6). Patient satisfaction is overrated. Medscape. Retrieved from https://www.medscape.com/viewarticle/821288#vp_1.
4. Fenton JJ, Jerant AF, Bertakis KD, Franks P. The cost of satisfaction: a national study of patient satisfaction, health care utilization, expenditures, and mortality. Arch Intern Med. 2012;172(5):405–11. https://doi.org/10.1001/archinternmed.2011.1662.
5. Tesser A, Rosen S. The reluctance to transmit bad news. Adv Exp Soc Psychol. 1975;8:193–232. https://doi.org/10.1016/S0065-2601(08)60251-8.
6. O'Neal E, Levine D, Frank J. Reluctance to transmit bad news when the recipient is unknown: experiments in five nations. Soc Behav Personal Int J. 1979;7(1):39–47. https://doi.org/10.2224/sbp.1979.7.1.39.
7. Allison MA, Hurley LP, Markowitz L, Crane LA, Brtnikova M, Beaty BL, Snow M, Cory J, Stokley S, Roark J, Kempe A. Primary care physicians' perspectives about HPV vaccine. Pediatrics. 2016;137(2):e20152488. https://doi.org/10.1542/peds.2015-2488.
8. Rucoba RJ. (2016, Aug 29). How to address vaccine hesitancy: new AAP report says dismissal a last resort. AAP News. Retrieved from http://www.aappublications.org/news/2016/08/29/vaccinehesitancy082916.
9. Haelle T. (2015, Nov 2). What kind of doctor fires vaccine-refusing patients? Forbes. Retrieved from https://www.forbes.com/sites/tarahaelle/2015/11/02/what-kind-of-doctor-fires-vaccine-refusing-patients/.
10. 2008: Measles in Dr. Bob Sears' waiting room. (2011, April 2). [Blog post]. Just the Vax. Retrieved from http://justthevax.blogspot.com/2011/04/2008-measles-in-dr-bob-sears-waiting.html.
11. Hope K, Boyd R, Conaty S, Maywood P. Measles transmission in health care waiting rooms: implications for public health response. Western Pac Surveill Response J. 2012;3(4):33–8. https://doi.org/10.5365/WPSAR.2012.3.3.009.
12. Washington State Department of Health. (2015, July 2). Measles led to death of Clallam Co. woman, first in US in a dozen years [News Release 15–119]. In: Internet Archive Wayback Machine. Retrieved 15 Sept 2018 from https://web.archive.org/web/20171204160652/https://www.doh.wa.gov/Newsroom/2015NewsReleases/15119WAMeaslesRelatedDeath.
13. O'Leary ST, Allison MA, Fisher A, Crane L, Beaty B, Hurley L, Brtnikova M, Jimenez-Zambrano A, Stokley S, Kempe A. Characteristics of physicians who dismiss families for refusing vaccines. Pediatrics. 2015;136(6):1103–11. https://doi.org/10.1542/peds.2015-2086.
14. Ashworth M, White P, Jongsma H, Schofield P, Armstrong D. Antibiotic prescribing and patient satisfaction in primary care in England: cross-sectional analysis of national patient survey data and prescribing data. Br J Gen Pract. 2015;6(642):e40–6. https://doi.org/10.3399/bjgp15X688105.
15. Hoffman J, Tavernise S. (2016, Aug 4). Vexing question on patient surveys: did we ease your pain? The New York Times. Retrieved from https://www.nytimes.com/2016/08/05/health/pain-treatment-hospitals-emergency-rooms-surveys.html.
16. Vaske EO. (Elise Ostwald). (ca. 2016). In: Facebook [KevinMD.com blog page]. Retrieved 15 Sept 2018 from https://www.facebook.com/kevinmdblog/posts/10154096093629886?comment_id=10154096234289886.
17. Clarke S. (2015, Oct 26). How hospitals coddle the rich. The New York Times. Retrieved from https://www.nytimes.com/2015/10/26/opinion/hospitals-red-blanket-problem.html.
18. Schwartz ND. (2017, June 3). The doctor is in. Co-pay? $40,000. The New York Times. Retrieved from https://www.nytimes.com/2017/06/03/business/economy/high-end-medical-care.html.

19. Tsai W. (Wilson). (ca. 2017). In: Facebook [KevinMD.com blog page]. Retrieved 15 Sept 2018 from https://www.facebook.com/kevinmdblog/posts/10154749832094886?comment_id=10155790592519886&notif_id=1506467498680957&notif_t=comment_mention.
20. Farnejad F. (2017, Aug 15). Physicians should not tolerate racism from patients [Blog post]. KevinMD.com. Retrieved from https://www.kevinmd.com/blog/2017/08/physicians-not-tolerate-racism-patients.html?pop=0&ba=1&xid=fb-md-cardio-azb&rt=rtc2220.
21. Salamon M. (2017, Nov 6). Same doctor, different site: lower patient satisfaction. Medscape. Retrieved from https://www.medscape.com/viewarticle/888067.
22. Okike K, Peter-Bibb TK, Xie KC, Okike ON. Association between physician online rating and quality of care. J Med Internet Res. 2016;18(12):e324. https://doi.org/10.2196/jmir.6612.
23. Guzman JA, Sasidhar M, Stoller JK. Caring for VIPs: nine principles. Cleve Clin J Med. 2011;78(2):90–4. https://doi.org/10.3949/ccjm.78a.10113.

Premature Closure: Anchoring Bias, Occam's Error, Availability Bias, Search Satisficing, Yin-Yang Error, Diagnosis Momentum, Triage Cueing, and Unpacking Failure

Introduction

Premature closure is the mistake of accepting a diagnosis before it has been fully verified. Its consequences are reflected in the maxim: "When the diagnosis is made, the thinking stops." It is a powerful factor accounting for a high proportion of missed diagnoses. Several specific errors are discussed here. These are: the anchoring bias, a form of the anchoring bias called Occam's error, the availability bias, search satisficing, the yin-yang error, diagnosis momentum, triage cueing, and unpacking failure. The last section in this chapter will discuss the inverse of premature closure, the failure-to-close error.

Anchoring Bias

Case

Luisa was a 45-year-old woman who presented with the acute onset of difficulty speaking. She was out to dinner with a friend, when she "could not find the right words." On examination, she was able to name most simple objects, but occasionally made errors, calling a "ring" a "bracelet," for example. She was extremely tearful, and her friend said that Luisa's husband had filed for divorce the week prior. A head CT was normal, and the patient was sent home after being treated with an anti-anxiety medication and a referral to a psychiatrist. She presented to another hospital the next day where an MRI revealed a stroke in her left frontal lobe.

What Dr. Martin Was Thinking

This would have been a much easier case had Luisa been celebrating a promotion rather than mourning the end of her marriage. If she did not have such a significant stressor in her life, there is no doubt I would not have rushed to attribute her condition to her psychological state. If she had been older, I would have considered a stroke as well. Instead, the fact that she was tearful blinded me to her serious

J. Howard, *Cognitive Errors and Diagnostic Mistakes*,
https://doi.org/10.1007/978-3-319-93224-8_23

medical condition. I allowed one piece of information to completely distract me from the relevant factors in her case.

Case

Joe was a 56-year-old homeless man who presented in the middle of the night with a headache and high blood pressure. He had a history of HIV, which was well-controlled on medications. He also had a history of opiate abuse, but was in a methadone program. He was uncomfortable, but a neurological exam was normal. A CT scan of his head was normal and a spinal tap was performed to evaluate for either meningitis or a subarachnoid hemorrhage. This was also normal, and the patient was going to be discharged.

However, prior to discharge, Joe reported significant pain in his lower back and weakness in his legs. A CT of his lumbar spine was normal at that time. A repeat neurological consult was called. Examination at that time revealed leg weakness, but the patient was felt not to give full effort, possibly due to his pain.

He spent 20 hours in the ER where he needed several doses of morphine to control his pain. He was finally discharged though a friend had to pick him up as he could not walk. He went to another ER the next day, where an MRI of his lumbar spine revealed blood in his spinal canal, compressing his lower nerve roots. He underwent emergent neurosurgical evacuation of the hematoma and made a good recovery.

What Dr. Feldstein Was Thinking

By the time I met Joe, he had been in the hospital for nearly 18 hours. I had already heard about his case from a medical student, a nurse, the ER physician, and one of the neurology interns. Each time his case was discussed, he was essentially presented to me as "a homeless guy with HIV and substance use who claimed not to be able to walk after getting a spinal tap." Although no one actually said it, the underlying subtext in each presentation was "this guy is faking his symptoms either because he doesn't want to go back to the streets or because he wants pain medications."

So, not surprisingly, when I went and saw Joe, I saw what I was primed to see: a homeless guy who was faking his symptoms either because he didn't want to go back to the streets or because he wanted pain medications. Before I had laid eyes on him, I "knew" exactly what I was going to see. Once Joe had been deemed a faker, it was extremely difficult to remove this label and objectively evaluate him.

Discussion

The anchoring bias occurs when clinicians prematurely establish a diagnosis based on an early, memorable piece of information. It leads clinicians to cling to their initial diagnosis even when the clinical picture changes or additional information is discovered. It is a powerful factor in premature closure. The anchoring bias is partially explained by a phenomenon known as the serial position effect. This shows that information recollection is a U-function: people tend to remember information discussed at the start or the end of a presentation, forgetting information discussed in the middle. The tendency to remember information that is presented early is known as the primacy effect, while the tendency to remember information presented

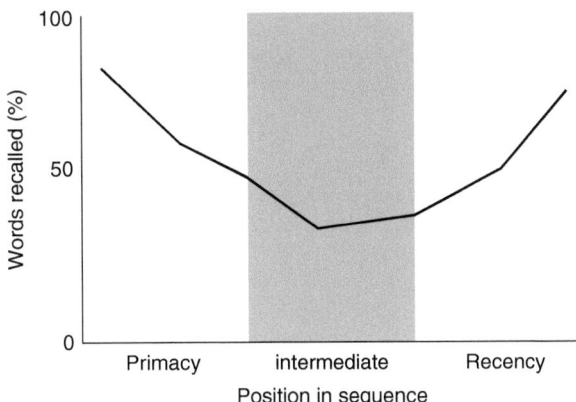

Fig. 23.1 The percentage of words recalled as a function of time

late is known as the recency effect. This is most easily demonstrated by asking people to remember a list of words. The word at the beginning and end are remembered, while those in the middle are forgotten (Fig. 23.1).

The order in which material is presented influences not just our recollection of it, but also our emotional reaction to it. Information is weighted more strongly when it appears early in a series, even when the order is unimportant. The psychologist Solomon Asch found that a person described as "envious, stubborn, critical, impulsive, industrious and intelligent" was rated less favorably than someone described as "intelligent, industrious, impulsive, critical, stubborn and envious" [1].

When experiencing an event, rather than just receiving information, the sequence of events matters as well. People are subject to what is known as the peak–end rule, in which people's judgment of an experience is based largely on how they felt at its most intense point (the peak) and at its end, rather than whole of the experience. If you go on a vacation and lose your wallet on the way home from the airport, that trip will recalled differently than if you had lost your wallet in the middle of the vacation. This has been studied with medical procedures in particular. Donald Redelmeier and Daniel Kahneman surveyed patients who had undergone either a colonoscopy or a lithotripsy (a procedure that uses high energy shock waves to treat kidney stones) [2]. Patients' judgments of total pain were strongly correlated with the peak intensity of pain and with the intensity of pain recorded during the last 3 minutes of the procedure.

In addition to the serial position effect, another powerful factor in the anchoring bias is the priming effect, which occurs when exposure to one stimulus influences the response to subsequent stimuli. For example, look at the two pictures below. How would you fill in the missing letter? (Fig. 23.2).

In the first example, the mosque and crucifix likely primed you to spell "pray," while in the second example, the swings and jungle gym likely primed you to spell "play." Or consider the middle item in the figure below, a demonstration created by Kahneman (Fig. 23.3). Is it the letter "B" or the number "13?" How you are primed is everything.

Here's another demonstration. Quickly spell the word "pots" out loud. Now, what do you do at a green light? Many people will say "stop," having been primed by pots. However, of course, when the light is green, you go.

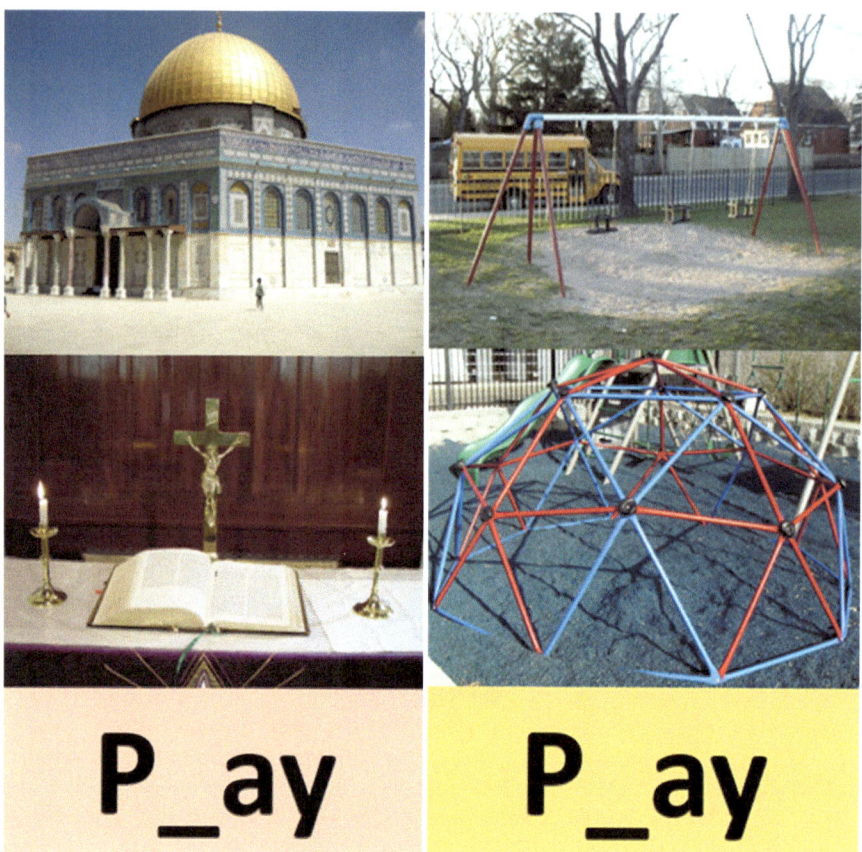

Fig. 23.2 How you fill in the missing letter depends on how you are primed. (**Clockwise from upper left**: The Dome of the Rock); Aarchiba. A set of baby swings [Image file]. In: Wikimedia commons. 2004. Retrieved from https://commons.wikimedia.org/wiki/Category:Swings#/media/File:Baby-swings-2.jpg; GreenGlass1972. A home-use dome climber [Image file]. In: Wikipedia. (n.d.). Retrieved from https://en.wikipedia.org/wiki/Jungle_gym#/media/File:Climberdome.JPG; Brooks L. (Leon). Altar and bible St. Johns Lutheran [Image file]. In: Wikimedia commons. (n.d.). Retrieved from https://commons.wikimedia.org/wiki/Category:Crucifixes#/media/File:Altar_and_bible_st_Johns_Lutheran.jpg.)

A related phenomenon is known as the von Restorff effect (also known as the isolation effect), named after psychiatrist Hedwig von Restorff. She found that in homogenous group of stimuli, an outlier is likely to be more easily recalled. For example, look at the following list of words: green, yellow, blue, hyena, red, yellow, white. The word hyena obviously stands out and will be better remembered for that reason. If a surprising piece of information is presented about a patient, perhaps they are a notorious local criminal or celebrity, this is likely to be remembered, even though that information may be irrelevant to their case (Fig. 23.4).

Fig. 23.3 How you perceive in the middle figure depends on how you are primed. (Kahneman D. Maps of bounded rationality: a perspective on intuitive judgment and choice (Figure 4) [PDF file]. 2002. Retrieved from https://assets.nobelprize.org/uploads/2018/06/kahnemann-lecture.pdf.)

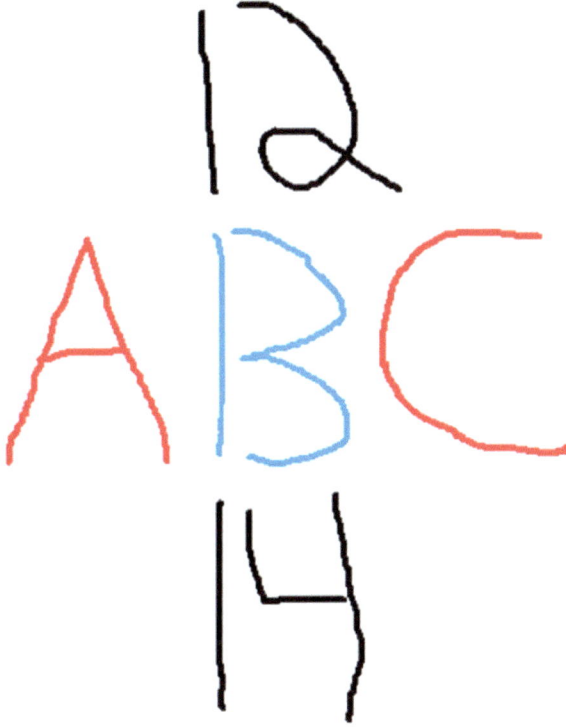

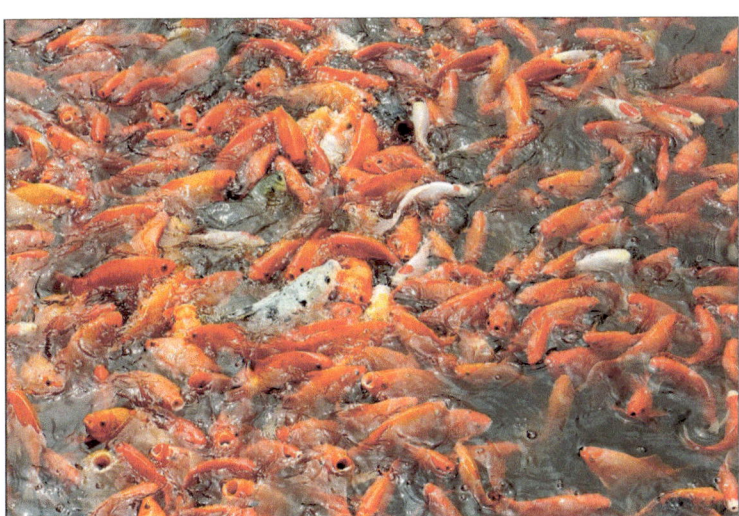

Fig. 23.4 The von Restorff effect. The few white fish stand out and are more easily perceived and recalled. (Kevinmcgill. Quanfu Temple, Zhouzhuang [Image file]. In: Wikimedia commons. 2011. Retrieved from https://commons.wikimedia.org/wiki/Category:Carassius_auratus#/media/File:Feeding_Time_(5695795534).jpg.)

To see how the priming and the von Restorff effect might influence a clinician's judgment consider the following cases:

- David was a 34-year-old gang member who presented from prison with a headache and photophobia. He refused to be examined in a room with bright lights and only said a few words, saying he was in too much pain.
- David was a 34-year-old opiate addict who presented with a headache and photophobia. He refused to be examined in a room with bright lights and only said a few words, saying he was in too much pain.
- David was a 34-year-old cardiologist who presented with a headache and photophobia. He refused to be examined in a room with bright lights and only said a few words, saying he was in too much pain.

In each case, the extra-symptom information does not provide useful data to help determine which of these patients may have a life-threatening disorder and which has a bad migraine. However, the information that the patient is a prisoner and gang member may prime the clinician to believe the patient is feigning symptoms to avoid prison. Similarly, the information that the patient in an opiate addict may prime the clinician to believe the patient is drug-seeking. In contrast, the scenario where the patient is a cardiologist may prime the clinician to trust and identify with the patient, causing them to overlook warning signs that the patient may be drug-seeking.

The fact that a patient is a prisoner in a gang or that he's an opiate addict *might* be highly relevant to the case. Social history such as this is often crucial and certainly should not be omitted. However, it is unlikely to be the most important aspect of the case and has the potential to mislead as much as to clarify. After all, fundamentally, in each of these three cases, the patient is a 34-year-old man with a headache and photophobia. Importantly, once potentially biasing information is presented, it cannot be unheard.

Silvia Mamede and colleagues performed an experiment demonstrating how distracting information can lead clinicians astray. They presented 72 internal medicine residents with six simple and six complex clinical cases. Distracting information was presented at the start of the case, at the end of the case, or not at all [3]. They found that distracting information presented at the start of complex cases significantly increased the rate of misdiagnoses, a demonstration of the priming effect.

The potential for extra-symptom information to bias clinicians was also demonstrated by Lauri Brannon and Kimi Carson [4]. They provided nurses and nursing students with two descriptions of hypothetical patients. In the first case, the patient had chest pain and some subjects were told that he had recently lost his job. In the second case, the patient had symptoms of a stroke and some subjects were told he smelled of alcohol. The subjects were then asked to make a diagnosis, which was then coded as either physical or situational (due to intoxication or stress). In the first scenario, 26% of subjects who were told the patient had lost his job attributed his symptoms to a stress reaction, while none of the subjects who were given the scenario without this information did so. In the second scenario, 74% of subjects who were told the patient smelled of alcohol attributed the symptoms to intoxication, while only 2% did when this information was not given. Of course, people who have undergone a stressful life event are not protected from heart attacks, and intoxicated patients are not protected from strokes. However, this extra piece of information served as an anchor and primed the nurses such that they were less likely to consider serious medical illnesses.

Medical students are correctly taught to present a case by starting out with a patient's chief complaint, which is a concise statement of the patient's presenting symptom and its duration, ideally in the patient's own words. This is then followed by the history of the *present* illness, which in turn is followed by their medical/surgical history and social background. However, once on the wards, many students invert this order and begin their presentation with a recounting of the patient's past medical or surgical history. I believe this to be a mistake, due to its potential to add bias. The first few sentences of a presentation will affect how the listener hears every other aspect of the case. By presenting such history at the start of the presentation, potentially irrelevant information might then have a significant impact on the patient's care. As such, it is important for the core facts of a case to be presented first, without potentially biasing details.

A study by Peter Bytzer showed that even the perception of a normal gastroscopy can be influenced by a patient's history [5]. In his study, he showed 129 endoscopists the same two-minute video, though accompanied by two different histories (reflux-like symptoms and epigastric pain in an elderly woman.) Only 23% of the endoscopists arrived at the same diagnosis for the identical video, and the given history greatly affected their suggested diagnosis. Note, this does not imply that history is irrelevant when looking at images. A normal brain MRI for a 90-year-old would be extremely pathologic for a 20-year-old.

In addition to how we process facts and information, studies have demonstrated that priming can impact our attitudes and behaviors. John Bargh and colleagues performed several such experiments [6]. They found that subjects primed with words relating to rudeness were more likely to interrupt the experimenter compared to subjects primed with polite-related stimuli. Similarly, study subjects exposed to words related to elderly people walked slower when leaving the experiment compared to a control group. Finally, they found that "participants for whom the African American stereotype was primed subliminally reacted with more hostility to a vexatious request of the experimenter." Importantly, other investigators have failed to replicate these findings showing that more research is needed [7]. In a related study, Lawrence Williams and Bargh showed that sensations of physical warmth (or coldness) increased feelings of interpersonal warmth (or coldness), in ways in which the person was unaware. Subjects who briefly held a cup of hot coffee judged a target person as having a "warmer" personality (generous, caring) compared to those who held an iced coffee. Similarly, subjects who held a hot therapeutic pad were more likely to choose a gift for a friend, while those who held a cold pad were more likely to choose a gift for themselves [8]. Other researchers have replicated these results [9].

Given the potential for extraneous factors to serve as an anchor and influence their judgment, clinicians should try to be aware of how they may be primed by their environment when interacting with patients. It's worth considering, for example, how treating patients on the hospital prison ward at Bellevue Hospital may influence clinicians' thinking. In contrast to a normal ward, there are guards, bars, and metal detectors. Patients wear bright orange jumpsuits and shackles when leaving or entering the ward. Those who are too ill to be kept on a routine medical floor are often handcuffed to the bed, with guards stationed nearby. It can be a challenge to ignore these factors when providing care to the patients there, especially for newcomers to the unit. In the same way that being warm can make people behave warmly, it is likely that such hostile, dehumanizing environments can influence clinicians in ways in which they are unaware.

Conclusion

The anchoring bias occurs when one or two pieces of information, often presented at the start or end of a patient's case, creates a lens through which every aspect of the case is then viewed. Clinicians should be aware of how another person's presentation may prime them to have an inappropriate opinion of a case. When presenting patients on rounds or in transitions of care, precautions should be taken to give due consideration to all information, regardless of the order in which it was presented. Clinicians should be aware of the serial position effect and when presenting cases to others, taking care to present the most relevant and important information at the beginning or end of the presentation. They should also be aware of the von Restorff effect, knowing that adding an attention-grabbing detail to the presentation of a case can radically change how the entirety of the case will be heard. Finally, clinicians should be aware that their environment might affect their behavior as well.

Occam's Error

Case

Jerry was a 38-year-old man who presented with two weeks of leg weakness. His symptoms had started in his right leg, but quickly spread to his left leg. He also had numbness below his chest. He had fallen several times, and was bruised on his right hip and flank after a particularly bad fall. His symptoms were confirmed on physical examination, and he had brisk reflexes and upgoing toes, which are signs of neurological dysfunction of the brain or spinal cord. An MRI revealed several enhancing lesions in his cervical spine consistent with multiple sclerosis (MS). A brain MRI was consistent with this diagnosis as well. The patient was treated with five days of steroids with improvement in his strength and sensory function. However, he still had significant pain on his right side. He was discharged to a rehabilitation facility where imaging revealed a right hip fracture.

What Dr. Powers Was Thinking

To me, this was a fairly clear cut case of MS. Once the MRI was done, I pretty much went on autopilot. We had an explanation for his symptoms and the treatment was clear: five days of steroids. Except we didn't have an explanation for all of his symptoms, or at least we didn't search for it. He had pretty bad pain in his hip, and we were more concerned with the reason he was falling, not with the consequences of the fall. As such, we missed a fracture. Probably any first year medical student, unencumbered by what their knowledge of MS symptoms "should" be, would have been more likely than myself to make the correct diagnosis.

Case

Taylor, a 66-year-old woman, presented to the ER with a severe headache, confusion, and visual disturbances. Her blood pressure on arrival was 220/100 mmHg. On examination, she did not know the day of the week, the year, or the mayor of the city. An MRI revealed hyperintense lesions in the occipital lobes of the brain. She was diagnosed with posterior reversible encephalopathy syndrome, which occurs in the setting of rapid, severe increases in blood pressure. It presents with a combination of visual loss, seizures, headaches, and altered mental status (Fig. 23.5).

She said that she had been in too much pain to get out of bed recently and her right leg hurt as well. She added that she had recently returned from visiting her grandson in another state. A urine toxicology screen was positive for cocaine, and the patient revealed she had been using it for the past few days with him. She was treated aggressively with medications to lower her blood pressure. A repeat MRI showed marked resolution of the lesions and the patient's vision and mental status gradually improved. Several days after admission, she developed the acute onset of chest pain, rapid heart rate, and shortness of breath. She was found to have a pulmonary embolism, a blood clot in her lungs. In her initial assessment, the intern had noted swelling of her right calf, and a blood clot had traveled to her lung.

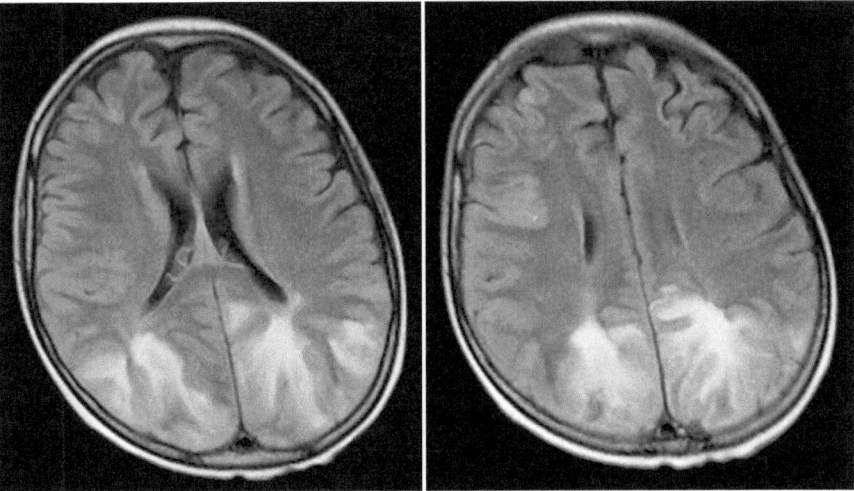

Fig. 23.5 FLAIR MRIs showing hyperintense lesions in the occipital lobes of the brain

What Dr. Banks Was Thinking

Several features made this case unique. She had extremely elevated blood pressure and she had a very interesting physical exam and MRI. Also, let's face it, you don't meet too many grandmothers who do cocaine with their grandchildren. The intern did mention her swollen leg to me, but I neglected it. Had the case been presented to me as a woman with leg pain after taking a long trip and then lying in bed for a few days, there is no doubt I would have immediately ordered tests to evaluate for a deep vein thrombosis (blood clot) in her leg. However, this information was sandwiched in between her neurological symptoms and her use of cocaine. As such, it didn't have the same salience.

Discussion

In the fourteenth century, William of Occam famously stated, "Plurality must not be posited without necessity." There is a natural, and often correct, tendency to invoke Occam's razor, also known as the law of parsimony, in medical diagnosis. It states that the best explanation of any event is the one that requires the fewest possible assumptions. If I were to notice my wallet missing from my pocket, the simplest explanation would be that it fell out. A more complicated explanation, which should be rejected unless compelling evidence emerges, is that invisible aliens extracted my wallet using a powerful tractor beam. Similarly in medicine, clinicians naturally prefer to invoke a single diagnosis to explain a patient's symptoms. If a patient who is admitted to the hospital with severe migraines continues to have headaches, for example, the law of parsimony dictates that her continued symptoms be attributed to this, rather than to her also having an intracranial bleed.

Occam's error occurs when a clinician assumes that a single diagnosis explains all of a patient's symptoms and fails to consider the possibility of multiple diagnoses. It is a variant of the anchoring bias, where an initial disease serves as the "anchor," precluding consideration of other conditions.

Of course, many patients have two or more diseases and the law of parsimony might actually favor invoking several diseases to explain a patient's symptoms. As neurologist Steven Novella wrote:

> In fact, Occam's razor may prefer that we explain a patient's presentation with three or four common or related disorders, rather than one extremely rare disease. The rare disease is introducing a giant new assumption, while the four common conditions to which the patient is at high risk are not really introducing anything new [10].

In other words, a forgetful older man with white spots on his brain MRI is more likely to have two common diseases, such as hypertension and Alzheimer's disease, than a single rare one, such as cerebral autosomal dominant arteriopathy with subcortical infarcts and leukoencephalopathy.

Hickam's dictum, attributed to the doctor John Hickam, is contrasted with Occam's razor. The dictum says: "Patients can have as many diseases as they damn well please" [11]. Charles Frederick Morris Saint, a surgeon, coined Saint's triad to demonstrate this point. It consists of gallstones, hiatal hernia, and diverticulosis of colon. Unlike most medical triads, these conditions were chosen precisely because they are unrelated, and connecting them together emphasizes that patients may have more than one condition. Studies have demonstrated the existence of Occam's error in clinicians. For example, Anja Thormann and colleagues found that in patients with MS and a preexisting chronic disease, the diagnosis of MS was delayed by up to 10 years [12].

Patients with a complex, chronic condition are particularly vulnerable to Occam's error. In discussing such cases, clinicians often lead with this condition. For example, a patient will be described as a "34-year-old man with MS who has had pain in his left leg for three days," instead of simply a "34-year-old man with pain in his left leg for three days." The diagnosis of MS thus serves as an anchor, which may mislead the clinician into assuming that all of the patient's symptoms are due to this disease, inappropriately narrowing the differential diagnosis. Yet patients with MS are susceptible to heart attacks, cancers, and strokes just like everyone else. Indeed this "34-year-old man with pain in his left leg for three days" was a patient of mine who was treated with steroids for MS for nearly a week before it was recognized he had a blood clot in his leg. Had he not had MS, I suspect the correct diagnosis would have been made much sooner. Early in my career, an older woman with MS developed trouble walking, coming to the hospital after a fall. I was completely blinded by her MS and failed to realize that she had fractured her hip.

Obviously, at some point, clinical investigations must stop for every patient. Many patients with MS who develop leg weakness and pain are having a relapse and treatment with steroids is appropriate. Investigating all patients with a never-ending myriad of tests and procedures often leads to the discovery of incidental findings and potentially harmful interventions. However, before concluding that no further diagnostic tests are indicated, clinicians should do their best to ensure that a single diagnosis can explain all of their patient's symptoms. This is difficult to do though, and some of my patients with MS have learned this through experience. As a result, they do not immediately disclose their disease when in an ER to discourage the staff from attributing all of their symptoms to this diagnosis.

Conclusion

There are times when not all of a patient's symptoms can be attributed to a single condition. The same way surgeons take a "time out" before operating to make sure they are performing the right operation on the right patient, clinicians making a diagnosis should pause and consider whether a patient may have more than one disease.

Availability Heuristic

Case

Adam was 28-year-old man who presented to the ER with a headache of 24 hours duration. The headache was described as "throbbing" and was mostly over his right eye. He had some mild nausea and photophobia. He appeared uncomfortable, but otherwise had a normal examination. A non-contrast head CT was normal and a neurology consult was called to advise the ER on treating a migraine. The neurologist insisted on an MR venogram to rule-out sinus venous thrombosis, a serious but uncommon condition where there are blots clots in the venous system of the brain. The neurologist continued this pattern of ordering MR venograms the next month until the head of the neuroradiology department admonished the neurologist for his overuse of the test.

What Dr. Gang Was Thinking

A doctor I know used to joke, "I'm guided by my decades of clinical experience, especially my last case." That is a perfect example of what happened to me. Several weeks before Adam arrived, we had a morbidity and mortality conference about a young woman who presented with a "migraine." She was sent home from the ER, only to return the next day with a seizure and frontal lobe hemorrhage. Only then was she diagnosed with sinus venous thrombosis. The ER doctor who sent her home felt horrible, and the patient ended up not doing well. This case was certainly on my mind every time I saw a patient with a headache after that. The only way to definitively rule out sinus venous thrombosis is an MR venogram or a similar imaging test. In retrospect it was not an appropriate test to order on every patient with a headache, and to be honest, I was unaware that I was doing this until it was brought to my attention.

Case

Lucas was a 28-year-old homeless man who was found unconscious in an abandoned house, with two people by his side, one of whom was dead, the other of whom was also unconscious. On examination, Lucas was obtunded, responding only to painful stimuli. He was given both naloxone and flumazenil, which are antidotes to poisoning by opiates and a class of sedatives called benzodiapines (medications such as Valium™ and Xanax™). He was given several repeat doses when he failed to improve. An MRI done the next day revealed bright lesions in a deep structure of the brain known as the globus pallidus consistent with carbon monoxide poisoning. When the police went back to the house, a space heater was found in a poorly ventilated room (Fig. 23.6).

What Dr. Mehta Was Thinking

There had been several cases at our hospital of patients with severe opiate overdoses, and many more cases in the news of people who never made it to the hospital because they had died. These were amplified in the media after the deaths of celebrities such as Philip Seymour Hoffman and Prince. As such, when Lucas and his companions arrived in the ER, I was primed to treat them as overdose cases. This was not a bad thing on its own. Heroin overdoses were common, they are obviously dangerous, and they are treatable. The respiratory depression caused by heroin can be multiplied when combined with alcohol or benzos like Valium™ or Xanax™. However, in my haste and eagerness to treat him for the overdose, which I was sure he had, I neglected to take a step back and think what else this could be. Had Lucas and his friends been someone who didn't fit my stereotype of a drug user—an older person or a clergyman, for example—I likely would have considered other causes of their presentation. Similarly, had the news and my e-mail not been full of warning

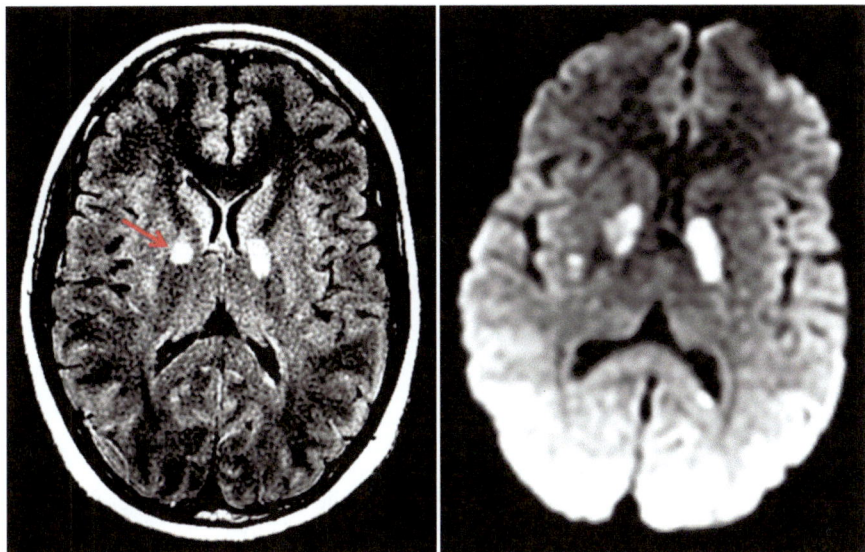

Fig. 23.6 FLAIR and diffusion-weighted MRIs showing hyperintensity in the globus pallidus, due to carbon monoxide poisoning (*red arrow*)

about the crisis of opiate overdoses, I almost certainly would have considered an overdose as my top differential, but not to the exclusion of other conditions. It is important to remember that just because a condition is in the news, this does not mean other conditions don't exist. Ironically, after word of this case spread throughout the hospital, the next dozen or so patients with similar presentations were all evaluated for having carbon monoxide poisoning.

Discussion

The availability heuristic is the tendency to judge things as being more likely, or frequently occurring, if they readily come to mind. It was coined by psychologists Amos Tversky and Daniel Kahneman who explained the heuristic by saying, "If you can think of it, it must be important" [13]. They performed a simple experiment to demonstrate the availability heuristic. They asked subjects the following question: "If a random word is taken from an English text, is it more likely that the word starts with a K, or that K is the third letter?" It is relatively easy to think of words that begin with K, compared to those that have K in the third position. As a result, subjects underestimated the number of words that have K as the third letter, despite the fact that there are more than three times as many such words (Fig. 23.7).

The availability heuristic also causes people to dramatically over or under estimate various risks based on how frequently they occur in the media. Deaths by extremely rare but dramatic events, such as Ebola, may cause a great panic, whereas deaths from causes perceived as mundane and common, such as influenza or traffic accidents, do not generate either the same headlines or concerns. Prominent media

Fig. 23.7 As a consequence of the availability bias, what we think is influenced by what we can recall. (I fucking hate pseudoscience. The availability heuristic subconsciously judges the probability of events by the ease in which examples come to mind. Like all mental heuristics [Image file, Facebook status update]. 2017. Retrieved from https://www.facebook.com/hatepseudoscience/posts/933747793439750.)

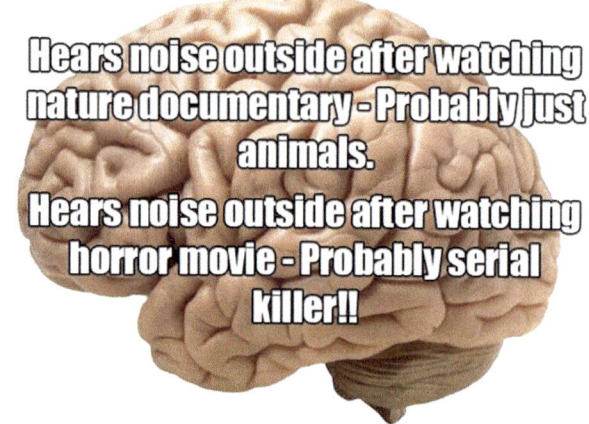

coverage of crimes may lead people to think that the crime rate is higher than it has been in the past, even when the crime rate is at a historic low.

People can behave in incredibly illogical ways as a result of the availability bias. For example, from 2005 to 2015 jihadists killed 94 people in the US, while 301,797 people were killed with guns during this time [14]. Despite this, a 2016 survey of 1,500 Americans found that terrorist attacks were the second most common fear after "corruption of government officials" [15]. In one sense this is not entirely irrational. After all, terrorists may kill thousands of people in one year and none the next (in statistics, such risks are called long-tailed). In contrast, deaths from accidents and diseases are unlikely to fluctuate greatly from year to year (infectious diseases being an important exception to this generalization). Moreover, deaths from terrorist attacks may be low precisely because our fear leads us to protect ourselves against them. However, because of the availability bias, what people fear the most often reflects what the media reports, not what is actually dangerous to them. As Max Bazerman, a business professor, said, "We over-react to visible threats. When there is someone out to get you, it is more visible than when you are silently dying in a hospital." When the availability bias affects risk assessment, people can die. For example, Gerd Gigerenzer, a risk specialist, estimated that an extra 1,595 Americans died in car accidents in the year after the 9/11 terrorist attacks because they chose to drive rather than fly [16].

Our minds naturally filter information that has relevance to us, weeding out seemingly extraneous information. The availability heuristic is similar to a psychological phenomenon known as the frequency illusion (also known as the Baader-Meinhof phenomenon), which occurs when people who learn or notice something novel begin to see it everywhere. For example, if someone buys a new red car, they may start to see that same car wherever they go. While these cars were always there, they previously lacked emotional salience and so went unnoticed. In medicine, recent exposure to a disease, especially in a personal or emotional way, will increase the likelihood of it being considered. Conversely, if a disease has not been encountered, its availability diminishes, and it may be underdiagnosed.

It is only natural that exposure to a disease, either personally or in the media, will increase awareness of it. This is often appropriate, as many conditions do occur in clusters. Clinicians should be aware of outbreaks of infectious diseases or drug epidemics in their area of practice. However, it becomes potentially harmful when other, less available diseases are not considered or when the probability of a certain diagnosis is inappropriately inflated because it was recently seen. At times, a rare diagnosis or bad outcome can garner significant attention within a hospital, affecting the behavior of everyone who learns about it. If a woman presents with confusion and is found to have Creutzfeldt-Jakob disease (CJD), it is likely that her case will be widely discussed and trainees will be brought in to meet her. As a result, this literally one-in-a-million diagnosis may lead the next several patients who present with confusion to be tested for CJD. Obviously, that a rare diagnosis is identified in a particular hospital does not mean the prevalence of that disease has then increased.

Henk Schmidt and colleagues conducted a study demonstrating evidence of the availability heuristic in medicine. In their study, 38 internal medicine residents read a Wikipedia entry about one of two diseases [17]. In a seemingly unrelated study, they were later given eight cases, two that superficially resembled the disease they had read about, two that resembled the other disease they did not read about, and four filler cases. Their diagnostic accuracy was lowest on the two cases that resembled the disease they read about in Wikipedia, showing the impact of the availability heuristic.

I suspect that specialists in particular may be prone to the availability bias. By definition, they see only a small number of conditions and, as such, may be especially prone to diagnose the conditions they treat. One hip specialist told my mother that she had trochanteric bursitis and explained his conclusion in part by telling her "I see it all the time." I also suspect that many complementary and alternative medicine (CAM) practitioners are highly vulnerable to the availability bias. Many CAM practitioners have a small number of go-to explanations as the cause for a diverse range of symptoms. Consider the case of "Lyme literate" clinicians. Such clinicians embrace the concept of chronic Lyme disease, a diagnosis rejected by mainstream medical practitioners. Such clinicians use tests whose sensitivity and specificity have never been validated, believing that "the standard recommended tests… miss 80–90% of cases" [18]. Even when the tests are negative, some clinicians believe that "over time, doctors who see a lot of Lyme patients can consistently pick them out from other fatiguing conditions by just reviewing the patient's history and review of systems (signs and symptoms)." Many "checklists" have been used to screen for chronic Lyme disease. Looking at these lists, it can be hard to think of a symptom that is *not* present. Moreover, I am sure that many otherwise healthy people have several of these symptoms. Who doesn't feel forgetful from time to time or have a headache or trouble sleeping? (Fig. 23.8).

According to Caravan Sonnet, an author who it active in the Lyme community:

The symptoms of Lyme Disease vary but most people struggle from many of the following symptoms: debilitating fatigue, heart issues, heart palpitations, arthritis, facial numbness, blood pressure problems, extreme pain, autoimmune disorders, malnutrition, hair loss, vision problems, skin issues, rashes, panic attacks, adrenal failure (or fatigue), memory

Head, Face, Neck:
Headache
Facial paralysis (like Bell's palsy)
Tingling of nose, cheek, or face
Stiff neck
Sore throat, swollen glands
Heightened allergic sensitivities
Twitching of facial/other muscles
Jaw pain/stiffness (like TMJ)
Change in smell, taste
Digestive/excretory System:
Upset stomach (nausea, vomiting)
Irritable bladder
Unexplained weight loss or gain
Loss of appetite, anorexia

Respiratory/Circulatory Systems:
Difficulty breathing
Night sweats or unexplained chills
Heart palpitations
Diminished exercise tolerance
Heart block, murmur
Chest pain or rib soreness

Psychiatric Symptoms:
Mood swings, irritability, agitation
Depression and anxiety
Personality changes
Malaise
Aggressive behavior / impulsiveness
Suicidal thoughts (rare cases of suicide)
Overemotional reactions, crying easily
Disturbed sleep: too much, too little, difficulty
falling or staying asleep
Suspiciousness, paranoia, hallucinations
Feeling as though you are losing your mind
Obsessive-compulsive behavior
Bipolar disorder/manic behavior
Schizophrenic-like state, including hallucinations

Cognitive Symptoms:
Dementia
Forgetfulness, memory loss (short or long term)
Poor school or work performance
Attention deficit problems, distractibility
Confusion, difficulty thinking
Difficulty with concentration, reading, spelling
Disorientation: getting or feeling lost

Reproduction and Sexuality:

Females:
Unexplained menstrual pain, irregularity
Reproduction problems, miscarriage, stillbirth,
premature birth, neonatal
Death, congenital Lyme disease
Extreme PMS symptoms

Males:
Testicular or pelvic pain
Eye, Vision:
Double or blurry vision, vision changes
Wandering or lazy eye
Conjunctivitis (pink eye)
Oversensitivity to light
Eye pain or swelling around eyes
Floaters/spots in the line of sight
Red eyes

Ears/Hearing:
Decreased hearing
Ringing or buzzing in ears
Sound sensitivity
Pain in ears
Musculoskeletal System:
Joint pain, swelling, or stiffness
Shifting joint pains
Muscle pain or cramps
Poor muscle coordination, loss of reflexes
Loss of muscle tone, muscle weakness

Neurologic System:
Numbness in body, tingling, pinpricks
Burning/stabbing sensations in the body
Burning in feet
Weakness or paralysis of limbs
Tremors or unexplained shaking
Seizures, stroke
Poor balance, dizziness, difficulty walking
Increased motion sickness, wooziness
Lightheadedness, fainting
Encephalopathy (cognitive impairment
from brain involvement)
Encephalitis (inflammation of the brain)
Meningitis (inflammation of the protective
membrane around the brain)
Encephalomyelitis (inflammation of the
brain and spinal cord)
Academic or vocational decline
Difficulty with multitasking
Difficulty with organization and planning
Auditory processing problems
Word finding problems
Slowed speed of processing

Skin Problems:
Benign tumor-like nodules
Erethyma Migrans (rash)

General Well-being:
Decreased interest in play (children)
Extreme fatigue, tiredness, exhaustion
Unexplained fevers (high or low grade)
Flu-like symptoms (early in the illness)
Symptoms seem to change, come and go

Other Organ Problems:
Dysfunction of the thyroid (under or over active
thyroid glands)
Liver inflammation
Bladder & Kidney problems (including bed wetting)

Fig. 23.8 A typical Lyme disease symptom checklist. How many symptoms do you have? (Rebecca. What is lyme disease? [Image file, Blog post]. In Caravan Sonnet. 2018. Retrieved from http://www.caravansonnet.com/2014/05/what-is-lyme-disease.html.)

issues, food allergies, unexplained allergic reactions, insomnia, inability to absorb vita-mins and nutrition, hormonal issues, circulation issues, dizziness, seizures, body numbness, blindness, migraines, paralysis in extremities, heart attacks, inability to handle temperature change, lung function, shortness of breath, menstrual issues, and the list goes on and on and on. I have just listed a few but here are hundreds more.

Moreover, Lyme disease is said to mimic multiple other diseases. As Ms. Sonnet explains:

Lyme is considered the "Great Imitator" and is known to imitate over four hundred different diseases including CFS/ME (Chronic Fatigue Syndrome), Fibromyalgia, IBS, Lupus, MS, Autoimmune Disorders, Alzheimer's, ALS, Migraines, Depression, Meningitis, Lou Gehrig's Disease, and hundreds of others. (Fig. 23.9)

I have often wondered what would happen if 100 healthy people went to a "Lyme literate" clinician. I suspect that many of them, suffering only the aches, pains, and fatigue of aging and everyday life, would be diagnosed with chronic Lyme disease as it the main, and possibly only diagnosis available to these clinicians. This consequences of this are especially important given that patients diagnosed with chronic Lyme disease are treated with antibiotics for months or even years, despite studies showing that this is ineffective [19].

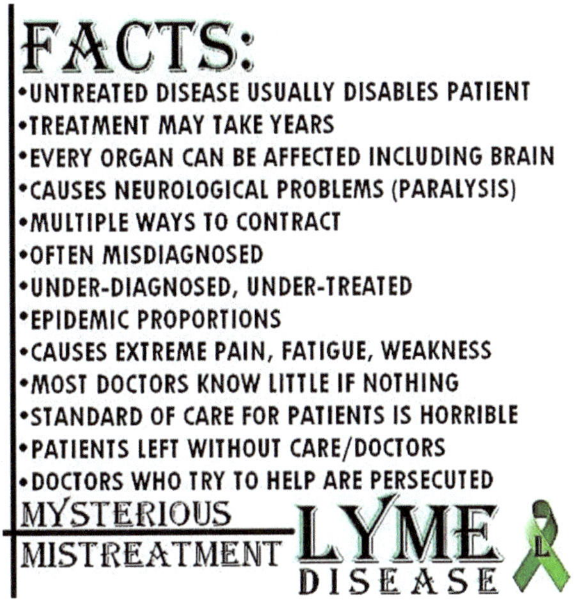

Fig. 23.9 A meme from a Lyme disease awareness page

FACTS:
- UNTREATED DISEASE USUALLY DISABLES PATIENT
- TREATMENT MAY TAKE YEARS
- EVERY ORGAN CAN BE AFFECTED INCLUDING BRAIN
- CAUSES NEUROLOGICAL PROBLEMS (PARALYSIS)
- MULTIPLE WAYS TO CONTRACT
- OFTEN MISDIAGNOSED
- UNDER-DIAGNOSED, UNDER-TREATED
- EPIDEMIC PROPORTIONS
- CAUSES EXTREME PAIN, FATIGUE, WEAKNESS
- MOST DOCTORS KNOW LITTLE IF NOTHING
- STANDARD OF CARE FOR PATIENTS IS HORRIBLE
- PATIENTS LEFT WITHOUT CARE/DOCTORS
- DOCTORS WHO TRY TO HELP ARE PERSECUTED

MYSTERIOUS
MISTREATMENT   LYME
DISEASE

The availability heuristic can also impair the perception of a treatment's risks and benefits. If a clinician has had success or failure with a treatment, it is likely to influence their future use of this treatment, even though their particular experience is unlikely to impact its overall risks/benefit ratio. In my own practice, I routinely use a medication that can rarely cause significant infections, even leading to death. After I cared for a patient with such an infection, I became much more conservative with my use of this medication. Objectively, this makes no sense. Yes, I treated a patient who experienced a bad outcome with this treatment. However, my individual experience this should not dissuade me from its use any more than if I had read about this bad outcome happening to a patient on a different continent. The risks and benefits of this medication did not change just because I happened to personally witness a bad outcome.

Conclusion

Clinicians should be aware that their experience is distorted by recent or memorable, the experiences of their colleagues, and the news. While it is not possible to control what comes to one's mind, clinicians should strive to approach each case as an independent entity, likely completely unrelated to the ones that came before. As Mark Crislip, an infectious disease specialist, said, the three most dangerous words in medicine are "in my experience" [20]. Similarly, clinicians should know that a good or bad outcome with a treatment while under that clinician's care does not affect the overall risk/benefit profile of that treatment.

Search Satisficing

Case

Arnold was a 65-year-old man who presented with leg weakness and numbness for the past six months. Whereas he had previously been an avid golfer, able to walk the entire course without difficulty, he now found it hard to walk more than a couple holes without needing a rest. On examination, his legs were weak and stiff with increased reflexes, indicating a problem in his spinal cord. An MRI revealed a large signal abnormality in the lumbar spine (Fig. 23.10).

He was diagnosed with transverse myelitis, which is a general term for an inflammatory disorder of the spinal cord. He was treated with intravenous steroids without improvement. Arnold sought a second opinion, and the second neurologist noted an

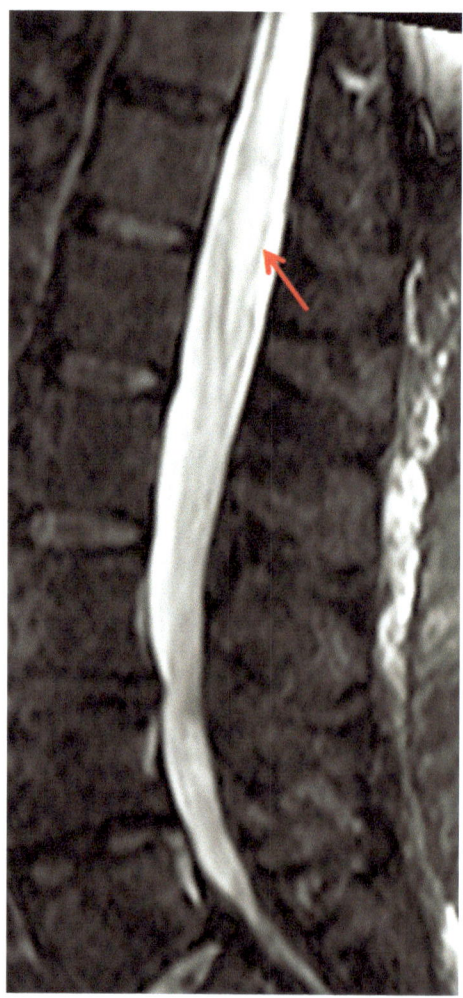

Fig. 23.10 A T2-weighted image shows a bright lesion (*red arrow*) throughout the lumbar spinal cord

abnormal blood vessel in the lumbar spine. He was diagnosed with a vascular malformation of his spinal cord, which was successfully treated with surgery.

What Dr. Deepti Was Thinking

There are few worse feelings as a radiologist than missing a treatable diagnosis. There isn't too much to say about this case, except I didn't see the abnormal blood vessel. Once it was pointed out to me, it was pretty obvious, of course. I am still not sure exactly how I missed this. It wasn't the first time I missed something, and unfortunately, it won't be my last. However, I think that had the rest of the spinal cord been normal, ironically, I would have seen the abnormal blood vessel. Once I saw the marked abnormality in the spinal cord, it made it harder for me to see the even more important abnormality. In the same way, a match lit in a dark room is easier to see than a match lit in a bright room, the abnormal signal in the spinal cord (the bright room), blinded me to the abnormal blood vessel (the match) (Fig. 23.11).

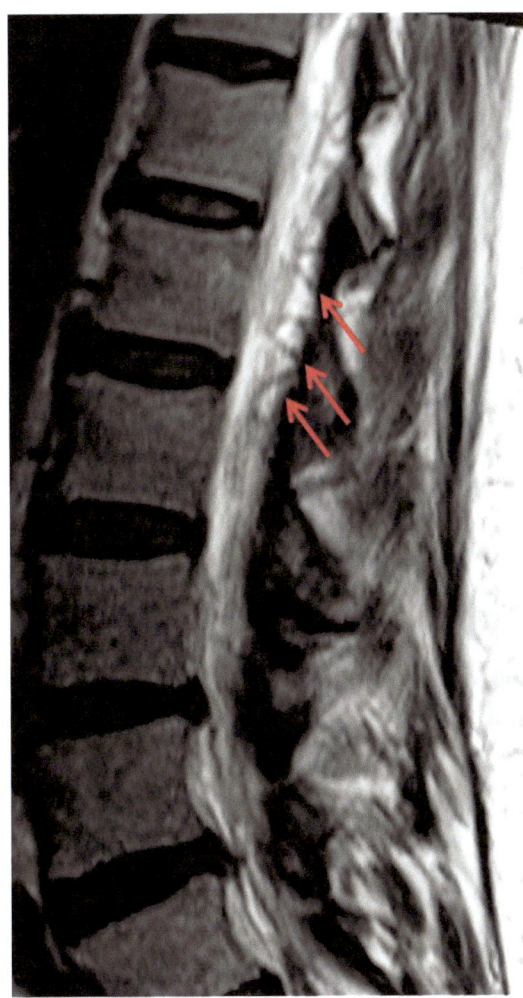

Fig. 23.11 A T2-weighted image shows an abnormal vessel indicated by the red arrows

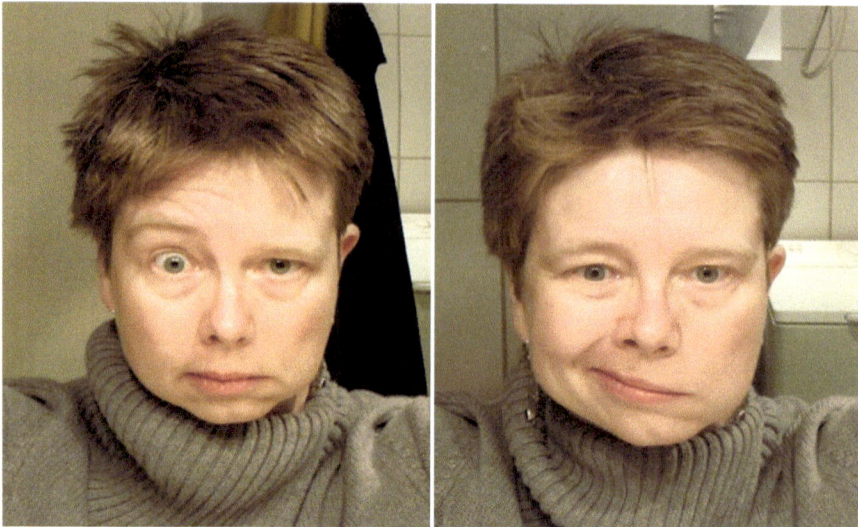

Fig. 23.12 Nancy. (**Left:** Kamphuis A. (Andrea). Self-portrait [Image file]. In: Wikimedia commons. 2012. Retrieved from https://commons.wikimedia.org/wiki/File:Fazialisl%C3%A4hmung_Tag_02_Stirn_1000.jpg; **Right:** Kamphuis A. (Andrea). Bell's palsy [Image file]. In: Wikimedia commons. 2012. Retrieved from https://commons.wikimedia.org/wiki/Category:Bell%27s_palsy#/media/File:Fazialisl%C3%A4hmung_Tag_03_500.jpg.)

Case

Nancy was a 45-year-old woman who awoke with weakness of the facial muscles on the left side of her face. As seen in Fig. 23.12, she could not raise her eyebrow, she had facial droop, and could not fully close her eyes on the left.

An MRI revealed abnormal enhancement of the facial nerve, the nerve that innervates the muscles of facial expression on the left. There was also an abnormal mass in the ethmoid sinus, thought to be due to chronic sinusitis (Fig. 23.13).

She was diagnosed with Bell's palsy, a relatively benign and temporarily form of facial paralysis. She was treated with steroids and antiviral medications. She returned two months later with double vision, nasal congestion, and proptosis (bulging of the eye from the orbit). An MRI at that time revealed a large sinus mass, which was found to be a sinonasal malignant neoplasm on pathological examination (Fig. 23.14).

What Dr. Jacobson Was Thinking

This seemed like a fairly straightforward case of Bell's palsy at the time. I initially thought that my biggest mistake was ordering an MRI at all. Bell's palsy is a fairly common condition and MRIs almost never add anything to the diagnosis. When the MRI came back, the abnormal signal of the facial nerve supported a diagnosis of Bell's palsy. Sinus disease is quite common as well on MRIs and is rarely of any clinical significance. I am a neurologist, and to be honest, my eyes gloss over sinus disease, both when I read the MRI report and when I look at the image myself. I

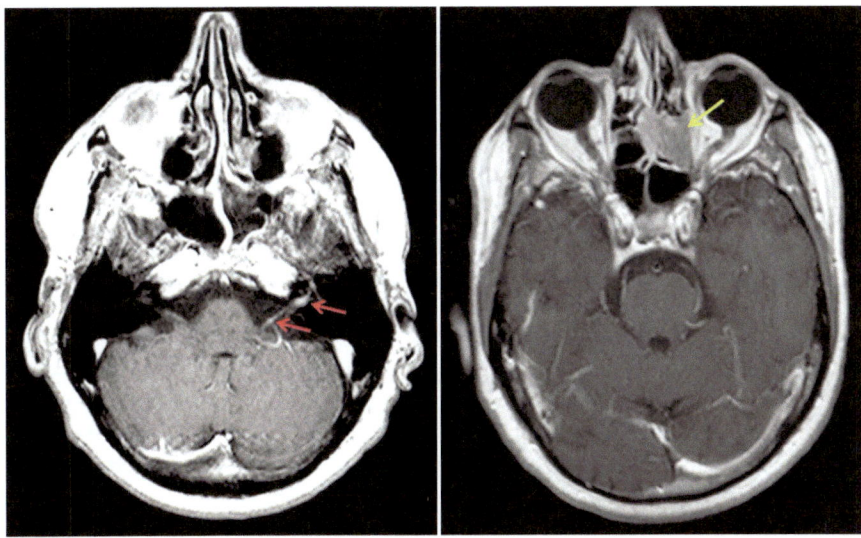

Fig. 23.13 Axial post-contrast T1-weighted images demonstrate enhancement of the facial nerve on the left (red arrows) and a mass in the ethmoid sinus on the left (*yellow arrow*)

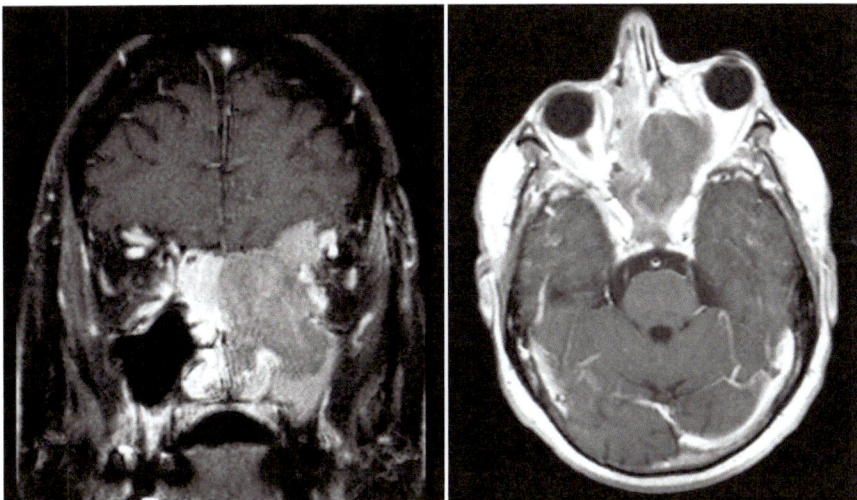

Fig. 23.14 After several months, the mass has grown significantly

don't know too much about ear, nose, and throat pathology, nor do I find it particularly interesting. For me, this was an open and shut case. Obviously, I failed to appreciate the significance of the sinus disease. In retrospect, the cancer had spread to her facial nerve and was the cause of her symptoms. Had I not brushed off the sinus findings, however, her cancer could have been diagnosed earlier, possibly sparing her many of the later symptoms she suffered.

Case

Alex was a 34-year-old man who arrived via ambulance after he was shot several times during a dispute at a picnic. He arrived at the hospital covered in blood, barely conscious, with a pulse of 140 bpm and a low blood pressure of 90/60 mmHg. He was intubated, was given large volumes of intravenous fluid and blood, and was rushed to the operating room. Despite the best efforts of the surgical team, the patient lost a significant amount of blood and suffered devastating, irreversible brain injury. On review of the case, an unrecognized bullet wound in his thigh was found to be responsible for a large amount of his blood loss.

What Dr. Phillips Was Thinking

This was a tragic case. As a trauma surgeon, I am obviously used to seeing young people in horrible situations, but I never get used to it. Alex had several gunshot wounds to his abdomen. These obviously drew our attention and we rushed to repair these. We actually thought he was going to make it. Sadly, no one noticed the wound to his leg until it was too late. Had we caught that in time, Alex might still be alive. I am certain that, had Alex *not* been shot in the abdomen, his leg wound would have been detected.

Discussion

Satisficing (a portmanteau of *satisfy* and *suffice*), a term coined by the economist Herbert Simon, is a decision-making strategy that involves searching through the available alternatives until an acceptability threshold is met. Search satisficing is the natural tendency to stop diagnostic investigations once a presumed cause for a patient's symptoms has been found. It often occurs after a "eureka" moment where a presumed condition is identified, halting all further thinking. It is a version of the premature closure error in which a large and obvious finding on the physical exam or a radiology image draws the attention of the clinician away from a smaller, but still relevant finding. As a consequence of search satisficing, medical comorbidities, second foreign bodies, other fractures, and co-ingestants in poisoning may all be overlooked. It is pervasive and considered one of the most important sources of error in medicine.

A candle lit in a dark room is glaringly obvious. A candle lit in a bright room may not be noticed at all. Similarly, a large and glaring abnormality, such as a tumor, might distract from a smaller, yet more immediately dangerous condition, such as a small intracranial bleed that can grow rapidly with fatal consequences. Additionally, when examining patients, an obvious finding may obscure a subtler, but potentially serious one. A trauma victim may scream in pain about a crushed foot, naturally attracting the attention of the clinician. However, a more serious threat to their life may come from a relatively small penetrating abdominal injury that may be overlooked while their foot is being treated. Not surprisingly, studies have found that patients with severe traumatic injuries were more likely to have missed injuries [21]. For this reason, one of the core tenants of trauma medicine is that the patient's entire body must completely exposed and examined.

The ability of one finding to divert attention from another finding has been demonstrated several times in radiologists. Two studies by Kevin Berbaum and colleagues found that a subtle fracture on a radiograph was likely to be missed when paired with an additional, distracting fracture [22, 23]. Another study by S. Samuel and colleagues found that radiologists missed lung nodules on chest images when another finding was present [24]. Using eye-tracking devices, they found that only in otherwise normal images did the lung nodules receive prolonged visual attention.

On a perceptual level, the relevant psychological phenomenon is known as inattentional or change blindness, a term coined by Arien Mack and Irvin Rock [25]. It occurs when someone is unable to perceive an unexpected stimulus, even when it is plain sight, because it is overshadowed by a stronger, more obvious stimulus. No one can attend to all the stimuli in a complex situation, and people are effectively blind to large swaths of their environment. Inattentional blindness is more likely to occur with unexpected stimuli. We all see what we expect to see and are often blind to unexpected stimuli. Yet occasionally something unexpected can be of great significance.

Inattentional blindness is not a cognitive bias *per se*, but rather a feature of our perceptual systems that blinds us to a great deal of our surroundings. However, from a cognitive perspective, we are blind to our own blindness. Numerous similar studies have shown that people are very poor at predicting how they would have performed in various tasks of attention, often wildly overestimating their own ability. If you have not seen it yet, I strongly encourage you to watch the *Selective Attention Test* video by Daniel Simons [26]. Imagine watching a group of people toss around a basketball. Would you notice if a person in a gorilla costume stepped into the center of the scene, beat his chest a few times, and walked off? Of course you would! However, in a now classic demonstration of inattentional blindness, only half of test subjects saw the gorilla. As Dr. Simons put it, "This experiment reveals two things: that we are missing a lot of what goes on around us, and that we have no idea that we are missing so much" [27]. In another variant on this phenomenon, the same scenario is presented, but this time, one of the basketball players walks off camera and the color of a background curtain changes from red to gold [28]. In this version, the gorilla is easy to spot, you know he is coming after all, but other dramatic changes go unnoticed.

Want to test yourself further? Stop reading now and go to YouTube to see if you can figure out how Richard Wiseman performs the *Color Changing Card Trick* [29]. In the course of this three-minute long video, which purports to be a simply card trick, two people change their shirts, and a table cloth and backdrop both change color. Would you spot these changes? Of course you would, or so you think. I have shown this video to hundreds of medical students over the past few years. Many do not spot any changes, some spot one or two, and I am not sure if anyone has spotted all four. Another jaw-dropping example of inattentional blindness was provided by the illusionist Derren Brown. In one video, he stands on a street corner, holding a map, asking passersby directions to a church. Suddenly two people carrying a large painting pass in between them, and unbeknownst to the other person,

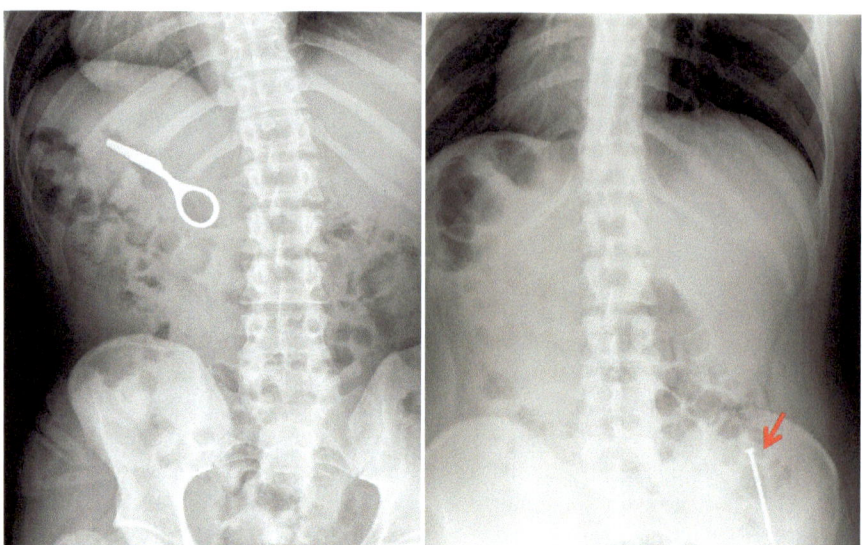

Fig. 23.15 A man who swallowed scissors and a nail

Derren swaps places with one of the people carrying the painting. Shockingly, many people don't notice when Derren, a middle-aged white man with brown hair, is replaced with a black man, a completely bald man, or even a young woman of Asian descent [30]. The clueless pedestrians continue giving directions as if nothing had happened.

Clearly, inattentional blindness is one of the most important tools of any magician. Unfortunately, it can affect clinicians as well. Look, for example, at this image of a woman who swallowed scissors and then later swallowed a nail (Fig. 23.15).

It's subtle, but do you notice anything else wrong? Look at the top of the image. Did you notice her heart is on the right side of her chest and the liver is on the left, a rare finding known as situs inversus? Do you think you would have noticed this had this image been one of hundreds you saw that day, as opposed to being in a discussion about how our perceptions are faulty?

Similarly, look at the head CTs in Fig. 23.16. A large, bright tumor abutting the left temporal lobe distracted the radiologist from a small amount of blood on the right side. However, the tumor is likely benign, and has probably been there for many years. In contrast, the small amount of blood was new and had the potential to expand, posing a much greater threat to the patient.

Inattentional blindness has been demonstrated in radiologists. Trafton Drew and colleagues examined 24 radiologists while performing a common lung nodule detection task. In their study, "a gorilla, 48 times larger than the average nodule, was inserted in the last case" [31]. They found that 83% of radiologists did not see the gorilla, and "eye-tracking revealed that the majority of those who missed the gorilla looked directly at the location of the gorilla." Is it really so scary (or surprising) that radiologists failed to see a gorilla while looking for lung nodules? As long as they saw the lung nodules, it is not clear that they missed something that had no clinical relevance and would never appear on a real image.

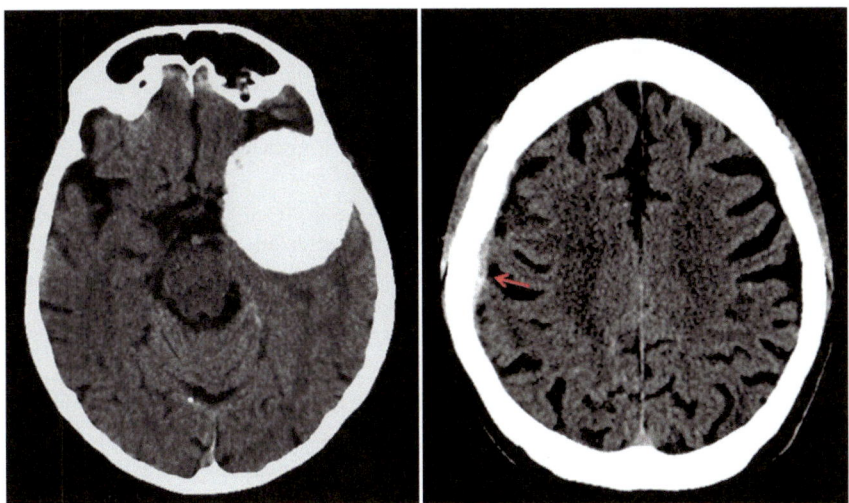

Fig. 23.16 A large tumor distracted from a small bleed (*red arrow*)

Importantly, as with visual images, people may fail to notice important pieces of information with language as well. Answer this question: "How many animals of each kind did Moses take on the ark?" Most people will say two of each animal. While the number is correct, the answer is not. It was Noah, not Moses who took animals on the ark. Many people fail to notice this basic mistake in the question. This phenomenon is known as the Moses illusion [32]. It is one of many types of semantic illusions where people fail to notice errors as long as the incorrect word is semantically related to the sentence's theme.

Inattentional blindness cannot be overcome with thought or effort. Rather, it is lessened by examining patients and images in a systematic way. Various mnemonics may help clinicians minimize the possibility of falling victim to search satisficing by ensuring that investigations are complete and systemic. For example, both trauma medicine and neuroradiology have ABCDE mnemonics to ensure that a thorough, ordered examination of the patient is performed. In trauma, the ABCDE mnemonic is: **a**irway maintenance with cervical spine protection, **b**reathing and ventilation, **c**irculation with hemorrhage control, **d**isability/neurological status, **e**xposure/environmental control). In radiology, the cervical spinal cord is examined according to the following ABCDE mnemonic: **a**lignment, **b**one, **c**ord, **d**isc, **e**verything else.

Another mechanism to minimize inattentional blindness is to have multiple clinicians examine the same patient on multiple occasions. In addition to the primary survey outlined in the ABCDE mnemonic, trauma surgeons are advised to perform a secondary survey and even a tertiary survey, once the patient is stable, to identify lesser injuries that have may have been missed initially. The value of these additional surveys was demonstrated in a study by Adam Brooks and colleagues, who found that in 45 patients with severe trauma, a tertiary survey in the intensive care unit (ICU) identified 12 additional injuries in 10 patients [33]. Most of these missed injuries were orthopedic in nature, and three required an additional surgery. Additionally, a dedicated trauma service and trauma team can reduce the percentage of missed injuries, with one study reporting a 10-fold reduction in such errors after the institution of a designated pediatric trauma response team [34].

Obviously at some point, a diagnosis must be made and treatment rendered. Neither images nor patients can be examined indefinitely. Furthermore, there is a risk that looking at a scan too long can cause radiologists to over-read them, imagining abnormalities that are not there.

Finally, when confronted with an instance of search satisficing, it also important to be aware of the hindsight bias; the tendency after an incident has occurred, to perceive the event as predictable. Every missed radiology or physical exam finding becomes glaringly obvious when it is pointed out.

Conclusion

Just because one obvious diagnosis or finding is found, this does not mean the diagnostic work-up is necessarily complete. Having one fracture, for example, does not mean a patient won't have another. When examining radiology films and performing the physical exam, clinicians should do so in a systematic way to avoid being distracted by obvious findings that obscure subtler, potentially more important ones. In certain situations, such as patients with trauma, multiple clinicians should examine the patient at different intervals to minimize the chances an injury is missed.

Yin-Yang Error

Case

Karen was a 64-year-old woman who presented with six months of unsteady gait and clumsy movements of her arms. She was no longer able to play tennis due to her unsteadiness. She was otherwise healthy, and had not seen a doctor in many years. She denied smoking and drank two glasses of wine per night. She had no family history of any neurological condition. On examination, she was ataxic (clumsy) in both her arms and legs, a sign of dysfunction of the cerebellum. She had seen several different specialists, and this was her second neurology consultation. She arrived to her appointment with the following normal tests:

- Brain MRI and MR angiogram.
- Cervical spine MRI.
- Carotid artery ultrasound.
- CSF analysis.
- EEG.
- Chest CT.
- Mammogram.
- Blood tests: Lyme disease, vitamin deficiencies, celiac disease, syphilis, organ abnormalities (thyroid, liver, kidney), heavy metal toxicities, ceruloplasmin.

The neurologist thought Karen probably was drinking more than she let on, and no further laboratory tests were ordered as her symptoms were attributed to her alcohol use. Over the course of the next few months, her symptoms continued to progress to the point where she had trouble going upstairs and performing fine motor movements. Despite seeing the neurologist two more times over that period, other than a brain MRI, which was normal, no further laboratory tests were ordered. Six months after her initial appointment, she presented with a pelvic mass and was diagnosed with ovarian cancer. She was then diagnosed with paraneoplastic cerebellar degeneration, a neurological disorder caused by antibodies directed against the cerebellum in association with a cancer, most commonly from an underlying pelvic or breast cancers. Karen's mother had died of this cancer as well. Karen was found to carry the BRCA mutation, which is a strong risk for ovarian cancer.

What Dr. Abrahams Was Thinking
I don't think it's ever been formally defined, but every doctor is familiar with the "thick binder sign." When a patient comes to me with a binder full of medical reports and tests from multiple different specialists, my brain involuntarily turns off. The results are invariably normal or only show incidental abnormalities. Karen arrived with many tests already done, none of which revealed anything pathological. While most of these were the appropriate tests, I thought that too many tests had already been ordered, to be honest. In cases like this, I feel the odds are essentially zero that I am going to uncover something that has eluded multiple doctors before me. As such, I feel my main job is to prevent patients from getting unnecessary tests. Had Karen been presented to me as a multiple choice question, I likely would have at least considered a paraneoplastic disorder, though this is a rare condition that I have only seen once before. But the large number of tests that had already been done made me think ordering more tests would be useless.

Discussion
A yin-yang error occurs in patients who have had multiple, unrevealing tests and procedures, leading clinicians to believe that nothing more can be done. Such patients are said to have been "worked up the yin-yang." It is a version of premature closure, though the "diagnosis" is nothing. Of course, it may be perfectly reasonable to conclude that an appropriate diagnostic work-up has been done and no further testing is indicated. Just because a patient is seeing a new clinician, there is no obligation to do "one more test." More testing does not equal better care. Certain tests may be unpleasant and potentially harmful. All tests cost money, and they often reveal incidental findings that are of no clinical significance.

However, when a clinician prematurely decides a patient has been evaluated enough, a yin-yang error occurs. Such an error is likely to happen with patients who have seen multiple prior providers and had multiple unrevealing diagnostic tests. Most clinician are familiar with the patient who arrives with a highly organized binder full of multiple tests and previous clinicians' notes, often from different specialists. The sight of the binder alone may predispose the clinician into thinking no further tests are indicated even before the examination has begun. Such patients may be automatically labeled as having psychiatric conditions such as somatic symptom disorder or conversion disorder. Ultimately, this may be the correct diagnosis. However, these are considered diagnoses of exclusion, meaning that clinicians must ensure they have entirely excluded other conditions.

Although it may annoy some patients, who expect me to have looked over their medical records prior to their arrival, I've learned that, if they have already had a large battery of negative tests, I have difficulty approaching their case with an open mind. Many of these patients have seen clinicians wiser and more experienced than myself, and I may feel I am unlikely to uncover a diagnosis that eluded them. As such, I may reflexively enter the exam room feeling that the patient has a psychiatric condition and that no further tests are indicated. This is a mistake. There is a chance that an important test has not been done or an important piece of information has not been obtained. In the case presented in this chapter, knowing that Karen's mother died of ovarian cancer might have led to the correct diagnosis.

Conclusion

Just because a patient has had an extensive diagnostic evaluation, doesn't necessarily mean they've had a proper one. Clinicians must always consider that a rare diagnosis may have been overlooked. Patients who have had an extensive, negative work-up are not undeserving of thought and potentially more tests.

Diagnosis Momentum

Case

Luisa was a 74-year-old woman on vacation with her husband when he heard her fall in the shower. He found her confused and unable to speak. He told the 911 operator that the ambulance should hurry, as he was sure she was "having a stroke." The operator dispatched an ambulance crew trained in treating strokes and who knew to bring the patient to a specialized stroke center where a team of interventional radiologists were available 24/7. The stroke team was alerted prior to the patient arriving and the EMS workers said, "She's aphasic. I bet she stroked out her left MCA (middle cerebral artery)," referring to the artery that supplies blood to the language areas of the brain in the left hemisphere. The triage nurse confirmed the EMS worker's findings, reporting that the patient was lethargic and had trouble keeping her eyes open. She had trouble naming common objects and was confused about the date and location. She may have had some subtle weakness of her right arm as well, but different examiners did not agree on this.

The patient was placed through the hospital's "stroke pathway," which involved the entire stroke team. A head CT was performed to rule out an intracerebral hemorrhage. When this was normal, the patient was started on tissue plasminogen activator, a medication to dissolve clots in patients with acute strokes. She was then taken to the interventional radiology suite where any clot could be mechanically extracted. However, an examination of her blood vessels was normal as was an MRI done later that evening.

Luisa began to improve several hours later. Upon returning to their hotel room that night, her husband found that she had mixed up her medications while packing, and she had accidently taken her sleeping medication in the middle of the day.

What Dr. Teital Was Thinking

At every step along the way—her husband's report, the 911 operator, the EMS worker, and the ER staff—Luisa was treated as if she was a stroke patient. By the time I saw her, multiple people had been involved in her care to some degree, and all of them were referring to her as "a patient with an acute stroke." No one took a step back and said, "What else could this be?" In retrospect, there were some clues that she did not have an acute stroke. Even acute stroke patients who have trouble speaking are usually wide awake and alert.

Having said that, it's not entirely clear that anything was done wrong in this case. After all, acute strokes are an emergency where every second matters. I would rather over-treat a stroke mimic on occasion than fail to treat an actual stroke. However from the moment her husband placed the 911 call, no one questioned for a moment that she was having an acute stroke. Even though Luisa did well, she was given a medication and placed through a procedure, which did put her at real risk. I suspect that had her husband simply said, "My wife fell in the shower and doesn't seem right," when calling the 911 operator, Luisa would not have been exposed to risky treatments.

Discussion

Diagnosis momentum refers to the fact that once diagnostic labels are attached to patients they tend to become stickier and stickier. It is a form of the availability bias that occurs through intermediaries, including paramedics, nurses, physicians, and patients themselves. What might have started as a possibility gathers increasing momentum until it becomes definite and all other possibilities are excluded. It is particularly likely to occur in hospitals where multiple different clinicians treat the patient in a short period of time. Consider the example of Raymond Donovan, the Secretary of Labor under Ronald Reagan, who was indicted for larceny and fraud. When acquitted, he famously asked, "Which office do I go to get my reputation back?" [35] All too often, patients might find themselves asking the same question. Once a patient is labeled as having a certain disease, it is all too easy to mesh new data to fit that initial diagnosis, instead of reevaluating the diagnosis to see if it fits with the new data.

The underlying process behind diagnosis momentum is known as an availability cascade, a term coined by Timur Kuran and Cass Sunstein. They define an availability cascade as "a self-reinforcing process of collective belief formation by which an expressed perception triggers a chain reaction that gives the perception increasing plausibility through its rising availability in public discourse" [36]. It is a self-reinforcing process that explains the spread of a belief within a group of people and is therefore highly related to the bandwagon effect. As the belief becomes more popular, it triggers a chain reaction such that people adopt the belief because others around them have done so. With the use of social media, ideas that might never have gained traction may become widespread. As a desire for social acceptance overwhelms critical-thinking faculties, implausible conspiracy theories arise and may be widely accepted. Influential people, known as availability entrepreneurs, may seek to exploit this phenomenon to spread an idea or to market a product.

A related phenomenon is known as the illusory truth effect, a term coined by psychologist Lynn Hasher. It refers to the fact that people are likely to believe a statement simply because they have heard it many times. As Dr. Hasher said,

"Repetition makes things seem more plausible, and the effect is likely more power-ful when people are tired or distracted by other information" [37]. It is well-known to politicians who repeat the same talking points to drive home their "message," true or not. It is also the reason behind cultural myths, such as that people use only 10% of their brain or that the Great Wall of China is the only manmade object visible from outer space. Danielle Polange conducted a study showing the power of the illusory truth effect. In her study, subjects were exposed to false new stories that were portrayed by the investigator as true. Five weeks later, "participants who had read the false experimental stories rated them as more truthful and more plausible than participants who had not been exposed to the stories" [38]. Perhaps even more surprising is that subjects who had previously read the fake news stories often believed they had encountered them outside of the experiment.

Often in the medical field, an initially tentative diagnosis is repeated multiple times by different clinicians, until *Voila*, it becomes fact. Multiple times patients have come to me with a diagnosis of MS, for example. They sincerely believe it and many have been treated for it many years. Early in my career, I would almost never question a diagnosis made by other doctors, who were almost always more experienced than myself. Though it is certainly the exception, over the years I have seen many cases where I do not feel a diagnosis of MS was properly made. When a patient comes to me with a diagnosis already provided, my attitude is to "trust, but verify."

Conclusion

Diagnosis momentum occurs when a diagnosis is subject to an availability cascade. Although it is impossible to "unhear" information about a patient, and this would be undesirable, clinicians should do their best to approach each patient as if they were the first person to treat them. Though it may be annoying to patients, who have to repeat their story several times, clinicians should take their own history and conduct their own physical exam of each patient. Avoiding diagnosis momentum requires independently obtaining information and "forgetting" a presumed diagnosis.

Triage Cueing

Case

Carlos was a 68-year-old man presented to the ER with the acute onset of right arm numbness and weakness. He said that he had been typing on the computer at home when he suddenly realized his right arm "did not work." He took a nap hoping that his symptoms would improve, but came to the hospital several hours later when they did not. On examination he had decreased sensation to all modalities from his shoulder down and was quite weak, barely able to lift his arm off the bed. He had no weakness of his arm and face. A head CT was normal and the patient was admit-ted to the neurology service. He spent the night on the neurology service and woke the next morning with severe pain and weakness of his right arm. On examination at that time, his arm was cold and pale. No pulse could be felt in his radial artery and Carlos was taken for an emergent ultrasound, which revealed a clot in his bra-chial artery. He was rushed to surgery and, the clot was removed.

What Dr. Jackson Was Thinking

I had just started my neurology residency when I met Carlos. As such, I figured all patients admitted to the neurology would have a neurological problem. This was obviously not the case. Furthermore, I thought all patients admitted to the neurology service should have a neurological examination. This seems so obvious, it hardly warrants mention. However, with a bit more experience, I realize that this is not the correct way to approach a patient. A patient should not have an examination tailored to what service they are admitted to, but rather they should be examined based on their presenting symptoms.

Ironically, had I met Carlos three months prior, when I was a medical intern, there is little doubt I would have made the correct diagnosis. This is because feeling the radial pulse was often part of the medical examination, though is not considered a part of the neurological examination. Basically, I examined Carlos based on where I was and what medical specialty I was practicing at that moment, not based on his symptoms. I do my best now to *not* think like a neurologist when I first meet a patient. Instead, I try to think like a doctor, and only think like a neurologist once I am confident the patient has a neurological problem.

Case

Tabitha was a 34-year-old woman with no medical or psychiatric history who was brought into the ER by her family, who said that she had not been sleeping and had been "acting crazy" for the past week. Her husband had left her two months prior. She had been very depressed since then, stating "I have been feeling the pain in my body like I felt then, and feeling all the pain it caused everyone else through my body." The week prior to admission she had to plan an event at work and she said she entered "this super epic creative phase," which was "the first time I've ever really been in my body." She stated she was a "Cherokee goddess" with healing powers, and she planned to open a museum which will lead to "a phoenix rising." She reported during the car ride to the hospital she "experienced" being her mother and giving birth to herself. She then "experienced" being a Native American medicine healer and "had all the knowledge and healed everyone." She stated she hasn't been sleeping well the past three nights. She had been cleaning her apartment excessively and her "wardrobe has exploded" recently as she has bought expensive handcrafted garments that represented the kind of clothing line she planned on making for all of her friends. A head CT in the ER was normal, as were basic labs and a urine toxicology screen.

She was admitted to a psychiatric unit and diagnosed with bipolar disorder. She was started on both an antipsychotic and a mood stabilizer, but continued to deteriorate. Within several days, she stopped speaking and getting out of bed. She was diagnosed with presumed catatonia, a condition sometimes seen in patients with bipolar disorder that is characterized by lack of movement and responsiveness to internal stimuli. She was given benzodiazipines, the standard treatment for catatonia, with no improvement. She developed a fever and was started on antibiotics for presumed pneumonia.

She was transferred to the neurology service the next day when she had a generalized seizure. An MRI at that time revealed abnormal signal in the hippocampi, the part of the brain responsible for forming new memories (Fig. 23.17).

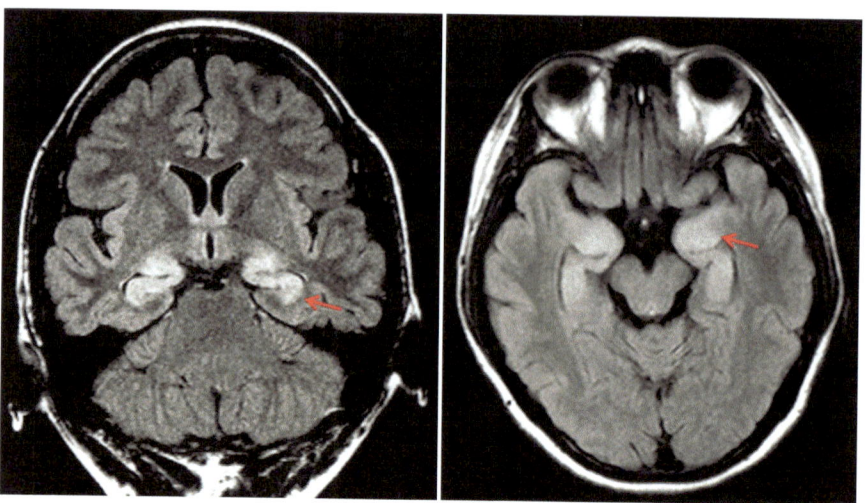

Fig. 23.17 FLAIR MRIs showing abnormal signal in the hippocampi (*red arrows*) bilaterally

Lab work further revealed the presence of antibodies known to cause brain inflammation, and the patient was diagnosed with limbic encephalitis, an inflammatory disorder of the limbic system. Patients present with a combination of memory loss, psychiatric symptoms, sleep disturbance, involuntary movements, autonomic dysfunction, and seizures. The onset of these symptoms can be abrupt or develop over several weeks. In young women, it is often associated with benign, ovarian tumors called teratomas.

What Dr. Patel Was Thinking

When Tabitha first arrived to the psychiatric unit, she seemed to be a textbook case of bipolar disorder. Her symptoms had started shortly after a stressor, and it was hard to find a symptom of mania she did not have. She was not sleeping, she was grandiose, she had increased goal-directed activities, and she was psychotic. I was convinced that she had been "medically cleared" in the ER. However, all too often, psychiatrists such as myself fall under some illusion that the words "medically cleared" mean all medical and neurological diagnoses have been eliminated. Most patients with bipolar disorder respond to the appropriate treatment fairly rapidly. When she worsened, it should have been a clue that her symptoms might be neurological in nature and further testing may be required. Certainly, not every patient who presents with mania needs a battery of neurological tests, but had this patient been admitted primarily to the neurological service rather than the psychiatric ward, there is little doubt her diagnostic work-up would have been expedited.

This case also shows that medicine is not a static field, and conditions that were once thought to be uncommon, might be more common than we think. Although limbic encephalitis was barely taught to us in medical school, I have seen since nearly a dozen cases such as this.

Case

Maya was a 17-year-old girl who presented with severe nausea and vomiting for the past three weeks, along with intractable hiccups for the past five days. She had a large battery of examinations, including a pregnancy test, upper endoscopy, and a CT of her abdomen, all of which were normal. As no cause was found, she was diagnosed with cyclic vomiting syndrome, which is a condition of unclear cause characterized by episode of severe nausea and vomiting. She was placed on anti-nausea medications with minimal relief of her symptoms.

Her mother sought a second opinion from a neurologist who suspected a brain disorder. An MRI revealed a lesion in her brainstem known as the area postrema, which is the vomiting center of the brain.

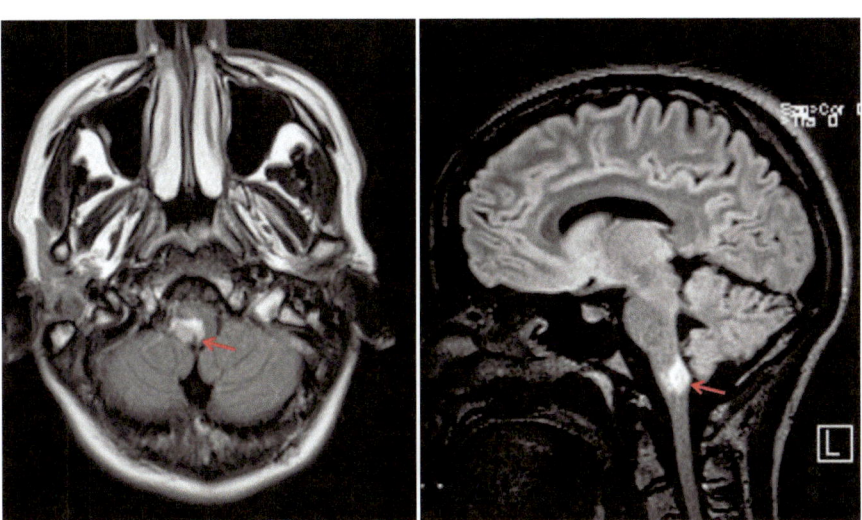

What Dr. Patel Was Thinking

I am the gastroenterologist who first met Maya. Patients with unexplained gastrointestinal distress are rather common. When Maya presented with common complaints, such as nausea and vomiting, I did the standard work-up and stopped when these tests were normal. Had you asked me to describe the neurological pathways that trigger nausea and vomiting, I could have drawn a basic diagram. Yet, when faced with a patient with standard gastrointestinal symptoms, I did not consider that this could be a neurological disorder.

Discussion

Triage cueing is the process by which patients are admitted to different services in the hospital or referred to various specialties for diagnosis and treatment. It is expressed in the maxim: "geography is destiny." Obviously, it makes sense that different clinicians care for patients with diseases relevant to their expertise. Patients with appendicitis should not be admitted to the psychiatric service, and patients with schizophrenia should not be admitted to the surgical service. However, errors can be made if a patient is triaged to the inappropriate specialty or a clinician fails to consider conditions outside of their specialty. After all, patients with gastrointestinal symptoms may have a primary neurological disease, and patients with neurological symptoms might have a vitamin deficiency due to an underlying gastrointestinal disease.

Additionally, errors can occur when a single disease affects multiple different organ systems, while the clinician only concentrates on one. Though the medical world is divided into separate fields primarily based on different organ systems, patients often resist such easy categorization. Consider the case of limbic encephalitis above. Is it a psychiatric, neurological, or obstetrical disease? It is all three and is difficult to classify into standard medical categories.

The unfortunate case of Migdalia Soto demonstrates the power and potential harms of triage cueing. According to news accounts, 47-year-old Ms. Soto presented with the inability to form words, numbness on her right side, and weakness such that she could not stand [39]. Though she had no history of mental illness, she was diagnosed with conversion disorder (a psychiatric condition) and admitted to the psychiatric ward. Once there, the diagnosis stuck. The clinicians on the unit believed only patients with psychiatric disorders were under their care. As such, she was treated with antipsychotics, and the staff wrote that Ms. Soto "believes she cannot walk" and was "delusional that she cannot use the right side of her body." It took five days until the neurological nature of her disease was appreciated and a CT scan was ordered, revealing a stroke.

Triage cueing is similar to the streetlight effect, a term coined by science journalist David Freedman, which occurs when people search where it is easiest, not where it is most appropriate. It is derived from the following parable:

> A policeman sees a man searching for his keys under a streetlight without success. After a few minutes the policeman asks if he is sure he lost them here, and the man replies, no, and that he lost them in the park. The policeman asks why he is searching here, and the man replies, "this is where the light is."

Like the man searching for his keys, clinicians order investigations where they feel the "light" is. For neurologists, the nervous system is the "light." They will order EEGs, spinal taps, nerve conduction studies, and MRIs of the brain and spinal cord. For gastroenterologists, the gastrointestinal tract is the "light." They will order abdominal images, endoscopies, and colonoscopies. Of course, where a clinician looks determines what they see, and if they fail to look in the right spot, they will not make the correct diagnosis. Triage cueing was demonstrated in a study by Ahmad Hashem and colleagues, in which 32 doctors were given four challenging patient cases [40]. The study found that there was a tendency for clinicians to judge a case as being within their own specialty, even when it was not. Specialists generated more diagnostic hypotheses within their domain and assigned higher probabilities to them compared to diagnoses outside their domain.

Triage cueing is evident to me almost every day working with medical students on their neurology rotation. The students I supervise almost always automatically perform the same neurological examination, suggest investigations of the nervous system, and posit a neurological diagnosis for every patient they see. When an older woman recently presented with a sharp stabbing pain in her back, they robotically performed a neurological exam and suspected a spinal cord disorder. I imagine that had they encountered the exact same patient while on their surgical rotation, they would have felt her pulses, ordered a chest CT, and diagnosed an aortic dissection, a life-threatening condition. An interesting study would be to give medical students a vague case, such as a 30-year-old woman with sharp abdominal pain beneath her ribs. They would be asked to propose diagnostic tests and posit the most likely diagnosis. I predict their answers would largely reflect whatever rotation they were on at the moment. Students on their obstetrics rotation would diagnose an ectopic pregnancy, students on their surgery rotation would diagnose appendicitis, and students on their psychiatry rotation would diagnose an anxiety disorder.

I tell medical students, that the first question they should ask when seeing a patient on their neurology rotation is, "does this patient have a neurological problem?" They should not assume that all patients admitted to the neurology service have a neurological problem, a mistake I have seen multiple times. Furthermore, even if they correctly determine that a patient has a neurological problem, there is not a one-size-fits-all neurological examination. For example, Parkinson's disease and myasthenia gravis (MG), a disease in which communication between the nerves and muscles is disrupted, are both diseases of the nervous system. Nonetheless, they are utterly different diseases that affect completely different parts of the nervous system and pose different threats to the patient. Patients with MG can have "crises" in which they develop respiratory fatigue, a life-threatening situation. They need careful assessment and monitoring of their pulmonary function and often need monitoring in the ICU. A clinician who evaluates such a patient by checking for tremor and rigidity, the classic signs of Parkinson's disease, is wasting valuable time.

Patients themselves may also cue clinicians to prematurely jump to an incorrect diagnosis. It is not uncommon for well-meaning patients to announce their perceived diagnosis, potentially biasing the clinician. Certainly, a patient with a headache who says they are having a migraine may very well be correct. However, it is the clinician's job to consider and rule-out more urgent conditions before accepting the patient's diagnosis. Larry Nichols, in describing a case where a patient misdiagnosed herself leading to a cascade of fatal errors, termed this type of error patient cueing [41].

Triage cueing can also occur with regards to the perceived acuity of a patient's condition. A patient who calls 911 with a focal neurological symptom, such as trouble getting out the right words, will certainly get evaluated on emergent basis for a stroke. In contrast, the same patient who walks to the ER with these symptoms is unlikely to provoke the same level of concern.

Finally, triage cueing can occur not with what diagnosis is made, but with what treatment is suggested. For several conditions, different treatment modalities exist, and so-called "turf wars" may occur where each specialty feel their treatment is superior for a given condition. A study of doctors in the US, found 79% of urologists suggested radical surgery for localized prostate cancer, while 92% of radiation oncologists suggested radiation treatment [42]. What often drives treatment recommendations is not a clinician's objective evaluation of the evidence, but the specialty to which the patient is referred.

Conclusion

Diagnostic errors are likely to occur if a clinician automatically assumes that a patient has a problem in their area of expertise and unthinkingly orders diagnostic tests within their field. As psychologist Abraham Maslow said, "I suppose it is tempting, if the only tool you have is a hammer, to treat everything as if it were a nail." Though any individual can only master a small sliver of medicine, they should do their best to think like generalists, not specialists, at least when they first meet a patient. Clearly, gastroenterologists need not be experts in neurological diseases or vice versa. However, a gastroenterologist should at least consider the possibility that a patient with gastrointestinal symptoms might have an underlying neurological problem, and the neurologist should at least consider that a patient with symptoms that seem neurological might have a vascular problem. ER clinicians, who determine the service to which patients are admitted when they enter the hospital, should be aware that by admitting a patient to a certain specialty, they are greatly influencing the care that patient will receive.

Unpacking Failure

Case

Allison was a 26-year-old woman who presented to a neurologist's office with left-sided neck pain. She said that she had gone to a yoga class the week before, and though it was not strenuous, she blamed this for her pain. She said that she was "very health conscious" and routinely did "juice cleanses and detoxes." She was otherwise healthy and had a normal neurological examination. She did not want to take any pain medications that were not "natural." She was advised that her symptoms were most likely musculoskeletal in nature and was told to return if her symptoms were not better.

She returned a three days later saying that her pain was worse. Additionally, she was now numb on the right side of her face, was off balance, slurred her speech, and had trouble swallowing. These findings were confirmed on physical examination and the patient also had a Horner's syndrome. This is the triad of ptiosis (droopy eyelid), miosis (a constricted pupil), and anhydrosis (lack of sweating) (Fig. 23.18).

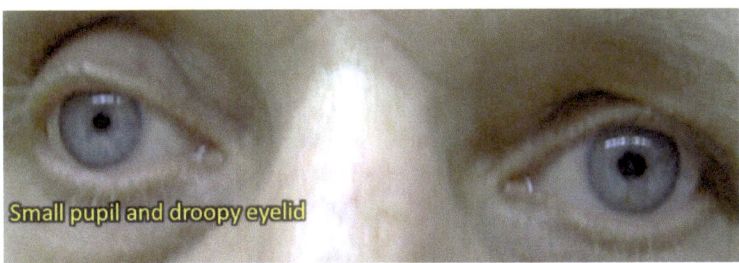

Fig. 23.18 Horner's syndrome. (Bosnjak R, Bacovnik U, Podnar S, Benedicic, M. T1-nerve root neuroma presenting with apical mass and Horner's syndrome [Figure 2]. In Open-i. 2007. Retrieved from https://openi.nlm.nih.gov/detailedresult.php?img=PMC1831774_1749-7221-2-7-2&query=Horner%26rsquo%3Bs+syndrome&req=4&npos=6.)

Horner's syndrome is commonly seen with carotid and vertebral artery dissections, a condition where blood flows in between a tear in blood vessel walls. During this second visit, Allison revealed she had been getting regular chiropractic adjustments, a known risk factor for vertebral artery dissections. An MRI revealed a dissection and a small stroke in the lateral part of her medulla oblongata.

What Dr. Borens Was Thinking

Patients presenting with neck pain are quite common. The vast majority of these are benign and resolve on their own in a short time. Certainly, getting an MRI or CT on every patient with such a complaint would not be feasible or beneficial. Sometimes, there are pathologies, such as a herniated disc, that cause neck pain, but these are not emergencies. In rare instances, however, seemingly mundane complaints can signal dangerous conditions.

Allison blamed her symptoms on her yoga class. While I did ask the patient about neck trauma, she denied it. To her, going to a chiropractor was not trauma. She did not see this as relevant to her condition and saw no reason to mention it. Certainly, it is not my usual practice to ask every patient whether they have seen a chiropractor recently. But that one simple question would likely have led me to diagnosis her condition correctly on the first visit and may have prevented her from having a stroke.

Additionally, I did not examine her eyes during her first visit. I obviously cannot be sure of this, but it is possible that she had Horner's syndrome at that time. Had I detected this physical exam finding, there is no question I would have recognized she had a neurological emergency and would have sent her to the ER.

Discussion

An unpacking failure occurs when patients fail to provide or clinicians fail to elicit or all of the relevant information in their history. As Pat Croskerry wrote:

Failure to elicit all relevant information (unpacking) in establishing a differential diagnosis might result in significant possibilities being missed. If patients are allowed to limit their history giving, or physicians otherwise limit their history taking, unspecified possibilities might be discounted [43].

Taking a patient history is where clinicians practice the art of medicine, and clinicians are taught that nothing is more important than the history. William Osler (1849–1919), often called the Father of Modern Medicine, extolled the value of the patient's history, famously advising clinicians to "Listen to your patient, he is telling you the diagnosis."

Yes, simply listening to patients can often be more difficult than it sounds. Even in ideal circumstances, many symptoms are difficult for patients to put into words. In some instances, a patient may not reveal an important piece of information out of embarrassment. A good clinician will have the ability to make patients feel comfortable talking about sensitive issues and draw out history from reticent patients. At other times, a patient may be unaware that an aspect of their history has great relevance to their present illness. A good clinician will have the ability to uncover relevant historical information without going on a "fishing expedition," obtaining irrelevant details.

At other times, clinicians must glean the important points from patients who present with a laundry list of symptoms. Patients are often instructed to tell their doctor "everything," and indeed some patients report innumerable aches and pains, which may be unrelated to their primary problem. Some patients may over-report symptoms, hoping to ensure the clinician does not "miss anything." Additionally, in many cases, clinicians simply do not have the time to take a detailed history, especially in loud, busy ERs. Finally, many clinicians learn not to trust all of their patients. Medicine has informal rules that demonstrate this skepticism, as clinicians are taught to automatically double the amount of alcohol a patient says they drink. Patients who lie can have a deleterious effect on clinicians. When clinicians do not trust their patients, the history becomes useless.

Conclusion

A patient's history is the core of any medical diagnosis. However, a poorly obtained history may obscure the diagnosis as much as elucidate it. Clinicians who limit their patient's history are guaranteed to occasionally miss an important piece of information that may instantly reveal the diagnosis to them. Having said this, asking taking a history is analogous to any diagnostic test; there is a sensitivity and a specificity. In the same way that performing more tests without a clear indication will lead to overdiagnosis and misdiagnosis, asking a battery of questions to be "complete" often leads to false positive responses. Clinicians may pursue fruitless diagnostic pathways if irrelevant history is valued. As much as possible, clinicians should strive to get their patients simply to describe their symptoms without leading them.

Failure-To-Close Error

Case

Natasha was a 63-year-old woman who presented with the following list of symptoms (Fig. 23.19):

A brain MRI showed several non-specific lesions, a common finding in older patients (Fig. 23.20).

Chronology:

Time Frame	Subject	Note
Halloween 2010	Low Back Pain & Doc notes	• Walking down street lower back is thrown out after weeks of coughing. • Pain intensifies over days, lower back spasming; sometimes cannot turn in bed etc. • Sports doctor refers me to physical therapist. Notes: palpation "tender LS ps"
January 2011	Low Back & Doc Notes	• Xray – No revealing results ("very mild levoscoliosis") • "pain localized to R LB no LE pain or paresthsias
2010 and some 2011	Low Back & Phys Therapy	• Go to physical therapy. • Myofascial release eases pain. Exercises sometimes makes things worse. • Left leg weak. Intense pain gone. Still often low back hurts – can't jog.
April-August 2012	Alexander Technique	• Alexander Technique seemed to help low back.
April 2012	Shingles	• Shingles on right side of face-not painful just exhaustion for a month
July 2012	Low Back & Doc Notes	• "Getting some tingling in LLE sometimes in thigh, others in calf. Started after a long car ride about 3-4 weeks ago. Some LBP w bending lifting." • "Range of motion: pain w lumbar flexion" • "Palpation: tender L LS ps"
Aug 2012	Home Upstate	• Purchase weekend home upstate-lots of ticks on property
December 2012	Shingles	• Shingles on right shoulder blade; exhaustion; some post-herpetic neuralgia-tingling and itching.
Jan 2013-Aug 2013	Physical Therapy	• Physical Therapy once a week-progress on and off till August; want to be able to jog; some exercises cause leg tingling but tingling does not remain.
Feb 2013-present	Coccyx Pain	• Actually not sure when coccyx pain started-perhaps earlier than this, perhaps later; continues to present
March 2013	Low back & Doc Notes	• "Low back pain with prolonged standing…no leg..paresthesia..some upper body exercises but dev an exacerbation of shingles on the L upper shoulder area"
May 2013	Low back & Doc Notes	• "was doing better but was doing some ex in PT and got a flare of the low back pain – pain across the low back and into right buttock. Gets some tingling in front of the left thigh. "
June 2013	Husband Lyme	• Husband: rash plus extreme fever; lyme test came back negative; course of 28 days of antibiotics and no further symptoms.
July 2013	Dead tick test neg	• Found numerous lyme ticks on me crawling, removed. Found one dead in hair-tested negative.
July 2013	Coccyx pain & Doc notes	• "has been doing well in PT – still needs more strength in core and LE strengthening. Strength has improved. Able to do dishes without pain. Able to do more housework. Getting pain in coccyx-has had for a long time-pain is always present in coccyx when sits a certain way" (First time I have mentioned to doctor but have had for months) • "palpation +TTP coccyx"

August 8, 2013 forward	Left leg tingling and intermittent intense pain	• After PT one night, tingling which started after a hard exercise, never went away and since then many different symptoms but for the first month after that mostly tingling in left leg and intermittent acute pain in left buttock
		   o Pain was positional- sitting maybe but especially lying down; standing and walking I always felt better
		   o Many seated positions would cause leg tingling
		   o Lying down in any position would often cause pain in left hip-sometimes keeping me up at night
		   o Car riding always problematic: tingling

August 2013	Eye Doctor	• Eye doctor notices potential risk for Glaucoma-2007: "opening within 40% nerve size"; 2013: "opening with 55% nerve size" – Monitor for glaucoma
Sept 2013	Low back MRI	• Report and image available-apparently does not show anything
Sept 18/19	2 Sick Days	• Sore throat and generally feel under the weather
Mid Sept 2013 ?	Tingling in other parts	• Started noticing slight tingling in left arm when hold phone up and maybe some tingling in right leg/foot
Sept 23, 2013	Annual	• Bloods and urine available

Fig. 23.19 Natasha's symptoms

	Physical	• Lyme test negative
Oct 14 2013 forward	Osteopath-Heel Lift	• 7 mm heel lift in right shoe prescribed • Lots and lots of bodily sensations including roving tingling and pain • Car rides become painful-construct flatter seat which helps to an extent; pain more severe in left hip; numerous very difficult nights
Nov 6 2013	Heel lift removed	• Sensations and pain continue
Nov 15 2013	Hand-purple	• Left hand somewhat numb and slight slight pain-overall more sensation than usual • Purplish – alarming looking to me
Nov 16, 2013	Intense pain –left hip	• Not positional; pain also above hip and in morning after painful night-in front

Differences Between Pre-Heel Lift and Post-Heel Lift
  • Obviously unclear what of this is attributable to heel lift

	Before (i.e. until Oct x 2013)	After (i.e. after Oct x 2013)
Tailbone	• Hurts for about a year	• Still hurts
Hiking	• Most weekends would take "Strenuous" hike listed as 3 ½ hours and do in 2 hrs 45 mins • Hiking always made me feel better	• No longer possible-feel awful afterwards and hard to do
Walking	• Always made me feel better • Best position	• Makes me feel worse-legs and lb and left buttock and tingling bottom of feet
Car riding-bucket seats	• Tingling, but not much or no pain	• Tingling and pain in left buttock • Constructed flatter seat but still get pain/tingling
Sleeping	• Some nights getting to sleep difficult since pain in left buttock • If I sleep, buttock does not hurt on waking	• More nights sleeping difficult because of increased pain in left buttock • Some very severe pain that no position helps
Legs		• Off and on stiffness in legs • Heaviness in legs • Lots of sensations in legs after walking
Pains	• Lower back • Left buttock positional-lying down mostly	• Pains pop up all over body briefly • Left buttock more often; not just lying down; increasingly severe seated and walking • Low back some times too-work chair best, other chairs problematic
Sensations	• Nothing beyond tingling	• Hot cold freezing in legs • Fireworks in legs (lots of sensations) remember esp when lying down • See hand on 11/15/2013 • Muscle twitching-vaginal and other-have also had in past • 11/15-collar bone buzzing sensation • tingling bottom of both feet; tingling in left toes

As of last week realize that walking up stairs increases pain, my bicycle commute increases pain and walking more than a little creates sensations and pain throughout legs and feet.

Reaction to Drugs
  • Cannot tolerate numerous drugs I was prescribed for chronic insomnia (insomnia better post-menopause)

Fig. 23.19 (continued)

A spine MRI showed several bulging discs in her cervical spine, which are also common. The neurologist ordered an electroencephalogram, nerve conduction studies, a spinal tap, an ultrasound of her carotid arteries, as well as a large battery of blood tests, none of which revealed a clear cause for her symptoms. Natasha was referred to a gastroenterologist, pulmonologist, rheumatologist, and cardiologist all of whom ordered their own battery of diagnostic tests, some of them invasive. Several of these tests revealed minor abnormalities, though most of her symptoms went unexplained. Natasha spent a large amount of time undergoing these tests before she was finally diagnosed with somatic symptom disorder by a different neurologist.

What Dr. Orish Was Thinking
Patients like Natasha have always been a challenge for me. Somatic symptom disorder is a psychiatric condition where patients have multiple, unexplained physical

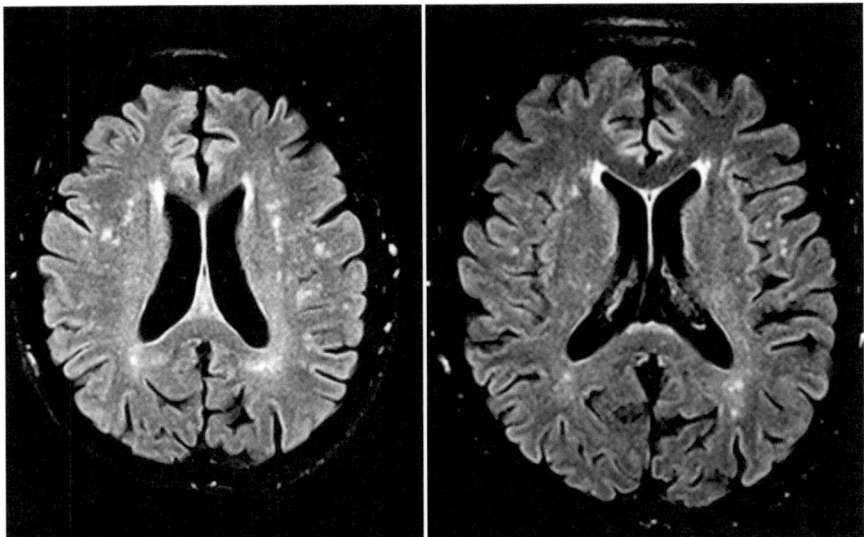

Fig. 23.20 A FLAIR MRI showing nonspecific white matter lesions

symptoms that cause them emotional distress and impair their function. Importantly, it is a diagnosis of exclusion. This means it can only be diagnosed once all other diagnoses have been eliminated. Unfortunately, there is rarely a point where a clinician can definitely say, "I've ruled out *everything*." There is always one more test that can be done. I am never comfortable when I diagnosis someone with somatic symptom disorder. I always have nagging suspicion I am missing something.

Additionally, no patient wants to hear that they have somatic symptom disorder. Several patients have become quite upset with me when I suggested this diagnosis. Natasha was fixated on the abnormalities on her brain MRI and the bulging discs in her neck. I was not able to convince her that such findings are more common than not in people her age. Though I suspected she had somatic symptom disorder, I didn't feel comfortable telling her that.

I realize my job is not to please patients, but to tell them their diagnosis as accurately as possible. But by not revealing my suspected diagnosis and by ordering as many tests and referrals as I did, I did not do Natasha any favors.

Discussion

The failure-to-close error occurs when clinicians are unable to put the brakes on an unrevealing diagnostic work-up, leading to unnecessary tests and procedures. It is a subset of the commission bias, which results from the belief that harm to patients can best be prevented by active intervention. It is the opposite of premature closure, specifically the yin-yang error, which occurs when clinicians assume that because an extensive diagnostic work-up has already been done, there is nothing left to do.

Stories of a heroic clinician making a life-changing diagnosis on a patient whose symptoms have stumped other unimaginative clinicians are a staple of medical literature. For example, Jerome Groopman begins his book *How Doctors Think* with the case of a woman who had unexplained weight loss and stomach pain [44]. She had been seen by multiple clinicians and subject to multiple medical tests over the course of many years to no avail. Without a definitive diagnosis, she was thought to have a psychiatric disorder. It wasn't until an independent thinker approached her case with an open mind that she was finally diagnosed with celiac disease. She was restored to health by eliminating gluten from her diet.

However in reality, patients with a panoply of unexplained symptoms, characteristic of the psychiatric condition somatic symptom disorder, are too often subject to an endless cycle of diagnostic tests, procedures, and referrals to specialists, all of whom order a battery of tests within their domain. A clinician who refuses to order unnecessary medical tests is unlikely to find themselves portrayed as a hero in a medical book. Yet, a clinician who prevents unnecessary tests and procedures may easily do as much good as the heroic doctor in Dr. Groopman's book. There are some patients who seemingly spend their lives going from one clinician to another. They accumulate multiple questionable diagnoses, which are likely artifacts of over-testing. Figure 23.21 shows the "problem list" from a 30-year-old patient of mine who has a mild case of MS as well as somatic symptom disorder.

⚕ ▴   Diagnosis

> MS (multiple sclerosis)
> Depression
> Bipolar disorder
> Hypertension
> Multiple sclerosis
> Ataxia
> Right hemiparesis
> Lumbar strain
> Left foot drop
> Tinnitus
> Epistaxis
> TMJ arthralgia
> Snoring
> Hearing loss d/t noise
> Hearing loss of both ears
> Bipolar affective
> Right foot drop
> HTN (hypertension)
> Bipolar 1 disorder
> SOB (shortness of breath)
> Gait disorder
> Difficulty with activities of daily living
> Chest pain of pericarditis
> Chest pain
> Pericarditis
> Obstructive lung disease
> Restrictive lung disease
> Essential hypertension
> Anxiety
> Costochondritis

Fig. 23.21 The "problem list" from a patient with somatic symptom disorder

US DUPLEX VENOUS LOWER EXTREMITY BILATERAL	PULMONARY FUNCTION TEST
US DUPLEX CAROTID ARTERIES BILATERAL	ECHOCARDIOGRAM TRANSTHORACIC COMPLETE
US DUPLEX VENOUS LOWER EXTREMITY RIGHT	OXYGEN VIA DEVICE TO KEEP O2 SATURATION ABO...
US BREAST LIMITED RIGHT	OXYGEN VIA DEVICE TO KEEP O2 SATURATION ABO...
CT CHEST WITHOUT IV CONTRAST	UPPER GI ENDOSCOPY, W OR W/O BIOPSY
CT CHEST WITHOUT IV CONTRAST	COLONOSCOPY W OR W/O BIOPSY
MAMMO DIGITAL DIAGNOSTIC BILATERAL	COLONOSCOPY W OR W/O BIOPSY
XR CHEST PA AND LATERAL	UPPER GI ENDOSCOPY, W OR W/O BIOPSY
MAMMO DIAGNOSTIC BILATERAL	AUTONOMIC TESTING
US NECK	CARDIAC EP PROCEDURE
MRI SPINE OUTSIDE FILM COMPARISON NEURO	OXYGEN VIA DEVICE TO KEEP O2 SATURATION ABO...
MRI NEURO OUTSIDE FILM COMPARISON	PULMONARY FUNCTION TEST
MRI CERVICAL SPINE WITHOUT IV CONTRAST BONE	PULMONARY FUNCTION TEST
MRI BRAIN WITH AND WITHOUT IV CONTRAST	STRESS TEST, EXERCISE
MRI CERVICAL SPINE WITH AND WITHOUT IV CONTRAST	COMPREHENSIVE HEARING TEST
US ANKLE LIMITED LEFT	
US BREAST OUTSIDE FILM COMPARISON	MRI LUMBAR SPINE WITHOUT IV CONTRAST NEURO
MAMMO OUTSIDE FILM COMPARISON	MRI THORACIC SPINE WITHOUT IV CONTRAST NEURO
MAMMO OUTSIDE FILM COMPARISON	MRI CERVICAL SPINE WITH IV CONTRAST NEURO
US BREAST LIMITED BILATERAL	MRI BRAIN WITH AND WITHOUT IV CONTRAST
MAMMO DIAGNOSTIC BILATERAL	MRI CERVICAL SPINE WITHOUT IV CONTRAST NEURO
XR FOOT AP LATERAL AND OBLIQUE LEFT	MRI BRAIN WITHOUT IV CONTRAST
IR LUMBAR PUNCTURE FLUORO GUIDED	

Fig. 23.22 The multiple tests ordered on a patient with somatic symptom disorder

Figure 23.22 shows how she has been subject to multiple tests and procedures. She also has had an enormous number of laboratory tests. Most importantly, there is scant evidence that these investigations and the treatments they have engendered have improved her health in a meaningful way.

The consequences of over-testing can be physical, psychological, and economic. Many diagnostic tests carry risks or are unpleasant. All can provoke anxiety. None of them are free. Simply put, more testing is not synonymous with better testing, a topic covered in more detail in the chapter on the commission bias.

Conclusion

It can be difficult, if not impossible, to know exactly when is the appropriate time to put the brakes on a diagnostic work-up and say, "enough is enough." It can be similarly difficult for a clinician to tell a patient "no further tests are indicated" than to order yet one more test. Additionally, clinicians are understandably fearful that they will "miss something." When a clinician feels trapped between a failure-to-close and a yin-yang error, it is appropriate to seek a second opinion from a colleague who can hopefully evaluate the patient with a fresh pair of eyes and decide if any further tests are needed.

References

1. Asch SE. Forming impressions of personality. J Abnorm Soc Psychol. 1946;41:258–90.
2. Redelmeier DA, Kahneman D. Patients' memories of painful medical treatments: real-time and retrospective evaluations of two minimally invasive procedures. Pain. 1996;66(1):3–8. https://doi.org/10.1016/0304-3959(96)02994-6.

3. Mamede S, Van Gog T, Van Den Berge K, Van Saase JL, Schmidt HG. Why do doctors make mistakes? A study of the role of salient distracting clinical features. Acad Med. 2014;89(1):114–20. https://doi.org/10.1097/ACM.0000000000000077.

4. Brannon LA, Carson KL. The representativeness heuristic: influence on nurses' decision making. Appl Nurs Res. 2003;16(3):201–4.

5. Bytzer P. Information bias in endoscopic assessment. Am J Gastroenterol. 2007;102:1585–7. https://doi.org/10.1111/j.1572-0241.2006.00911.x.

6. Bargh JA, Chen M, Burrows L. Automaticity of social behavior: direct effects of trait construct and stereotype activation on action. J Pers Soc Psychol. 1996;71(2):230.

7. Yong E. (2012, Mar 10). A failed replication draws a scathing personal attack from a psychology professor [Blog post]. Discover Magazine. Retrieved from http://blogs.discovermagazine.com/notrocketscience/2012/03/10/failed-replication-bargh-psychology-study-doyen/.

8. Williams LE, Bargh JA. Experiencing physical warmth promotes interpersonal warmth. Science. 2008;322(5901):606–7. https://doi.org/10.1126/science.1162548.

9. Lynott D, Corker KS, Wortman J, Connell L, Donnellan MB, Lucas RE, O'Brien K. Replicating "Experiencing physical warmth promotes interpersonal warmth". Soc Psychol. 2014;45:216–22. https://doi.org/10.1027/1864-9335/a000187.

10. Novella S. (2014, Jan 28). Occam's razor vs Hickam's dictum [Blog entry]. Neurologica Blog. Retrieved from https://theness.com/neurologicablog/index.php/occams-razor-vs-hickams-dictum/.

11. Borden N, Linklater D. Hickam's dictum. West J Emerg Med. 2013;14(2):164. https://doi.org/10.5811/westjem.2012.10.12164.

12. Thormann A, Sørensen PS, Koch-Henriksen N, Laursen B, Magyari M. Comorbidity in multiple sclerosis is associated with diagnostic delays and increased mortality. Neurology. 2017;89(16):1668–75. https://doi.org/10.1212/WNL.0000000000004508.

13. Tversky A, Kahneman D. Availability: a heuristic for judging frequency and probability. Cogn Psychol. 1973;5(2):207–32. https://doi.org/10.1016/0010-0285(73)90033-9.

14. Anderson J. (2017, Jan 31). The psychology of why 94 deaths from terrorism are scarier than 301,797 deaths from guns. Quartz. Retrieved from https://qz.com/898207/the-psychology-of-why-americans-are-more-scared-of-terrorism-than-guns-though-guns-are-3210-times-likelier-to-kill-them/.

15. Chapman University. (2016, Oct 12). What do Americans fear? Science Daily. Retrieved from https://www.sciencedaily.com/releases/2016/10/161012160030.htm.

16. Ball J. (2011, Sept 5). September 11's indirect toll: road deaths linked to fearful flyers. The Guardian. https://www.theguardian.com/world/2011/sep/05/september-11-road-deaths.

17. Schmidt HG, Mamede S, van den Berge K, van Gog T, van Saase JLCM, Rikers RMJP. Exposure to media information about a disease can cause doctors to misdiagnose similar-looking clinical cases. Acad Med. 2014;89(2):285–91. https://doi.org/10.1097/ACM.0000000000000107.

18. Holtorf Medical Group. (n.d.). What to look for in a LLMD (Lyme literate medical doctor). Retrieved 15 Sept 2018 from https://www.holtorfmed.com/what-to-look-for-in-a-llmd-lyme-literate-medical-doctor/.

19. Berende A, ter Hofstede HJM, Vos FJ, van Middendrop H, Vogelaar ML, Tromp M, van den Hoogen FH, Donders AR, Evers AW, Kullberg BJ. Randomized trial of longer-term therapy for symptoms attributed to Lyme disease. N Engl J Med. 2016;374(13):1209–20. https://doi.org/10.1056/NEJMoa1505425.

20. Hall H. (2011, Apr 12). The role of experience in science-based medicine. Science-Based Medicine. Retrieved from https://sciencebasedmedicine.org/the-role-of-experience-in-science-based-medicine/.

21. Williams BG, Hlaing T, Aaland MO. Ten-year retrospective study of delayed diagnosis of injury in pediatric trauma patients at a level II trauma center. Pediatr Emerg Care. 2009;25(8):489–93. https://doi.org/10.1097/PEC.0b013e3181b0a07d.

22. Berbaum KS, El-Khoury GY, Ohashi K, Schartz KM, Caldwell RT, Madsen M, Franken EA. Satisfaction of search in multitrauma patients: severity of detected fractures. Acad Radiol. 2007;14(6):711–22. https://doi.org/10.1016/j.acra.2007.02.016.

23. Berbaum KS, El-Khoury GY, Franken EA, Kuehn DM, Meis DM, Dorfman DD, Warnock NG, Thompson BH, SCS K, Kathol MH. Missed fractures resulting from satisfaction of search effect. Emerg Radiol. 1994;1(5):242–9. https://doi.org/10.1007/BF02614935.

24. Samuel S, Kundel HL, Nodine CF, Toto LC. Mechanism of satisfaction of search: eye position recordings in the reading of chest radiographs. Radiology. 1995;194(3):895–902. https://doi.org/10.1148/radiology.194.3.7862998.

25. Mack A, Rock I. Inattentional blindness. PSYCHE. 1999;5:3.

26. Simons D. (2010, Mar 10). Selective attention test [Video file]. Retrieved from https://www.youtube.com/watch?v=vJG698U2Mvo.

27. Chabris C, Simons D. (2010). The invisible gorilla. Retrieved 15 Sept 2018 from http://www.theinvisiblegorilla.com/gorilla_experiment.html.

28. Simons D. (2010, Apr 28). The monkey business illusion [Video file]. Retrieved from https://www.youtube.com/watch?v=IGQmdoK_ZfY.

29. Quirkology. (2012, Nov 21). Colour changing card trick [Video file]. Retrieved from https://www.youtube.com/watch?annotation_id=annotation_262395&feature=iv&src_vid=voAntzB7EwE&v=v3iPrBrGSJM.

30. 777Skeptic. (2007, Aug 26). Derren Brown – person swap [Video file]. Retrieved from https://www.youtube.com/watch?v=vBPG_OBgTWg.

31. Drew T, Vo MLH, Wolfe JM. The invisible gorilla strikes again: sustained inattentional blindness in expert observers. Psychol Sci. 2013;24(9):1848–53. https://doi.org/10.1177/0956797613479386.

32. Erickson T, Mattson ME. From words to meaning: a semantic illusion. J Verbal Learn Verbal Behav. 1981;20(5):540–51. https://doi.org/10.1016/S0022-5371(81)90165-1.

33. Brooks A, Holroyd B, Riley B. Missed injury in major trauma patients. Injury. 2004;35(4):407–10. https://doi.org/10.1016/S0020-1383(03)00219-5.

34. Perno JF, Schunk JE, Hansen KW, Furnival RA. Significant reduction in delayed diagnosis of injury with implementation of a pediatric trauma service. Pediatr Emerg Care. 2005;21(6):367–71. https://doi.org/10.1097/01.pec.0000166726.84308.cf.

35. Raab S. (1987, May 26). Donovan cleared of fraud charges by jury in Bronx. The New York Times. Retrieved from https://www.nytimes.com/1987/05/26/nyregion/donovan-cleared-of-fraud-charges-by-jury-in-bronx.html?pagewanted=all.

36. Kuran T, Sunstein CR. Availability cascades and risk regulation. Stan L Rev. 1998;51:683.

37. Dreyfus E. (2017, Feb 11). Want to make a lie seem true? Say it again. And again. And again. Wired. Retrieved from https://www.wired.com/2017/02/dont-believe-lies-just-people-repeat/.

38. Polage DC. Making up history: false memories of fake news stories. Eur J Psychol. 2012;8(2):245–50. https://doi.org/10.5964/ejop.v8i2.456.

39. Moore T. (2009, July28). Error at Lincoln hospital emergency room leaves woman a shadow of self. New York Daily News. Retrieved from http://www.nydailynews.com/new-york/error-lincoln-hospital-emergency-room-leaves-woman-shadow-article-1.431065#.

40. Hashem A, Chi MT, Friedman CP. Medical errors as a result of specialization. J Biomed Inform. 2003;36(1–2):61–9.

41. Nichols L. Patient cueing, a type of diagnostic error. Autops Case Rep. 2016;6(10):27–31. https://doi.org/10.4322/acr.2016.023.

42. Wennberg JE, Cooper MM. (Eds.) (1996). The Dartmouth atlas of health care in the United States [PDF file]. Retrieved from http://www.dartmouthatlas.org/downloads/atlases/96Atlas.pdf.

43. Nickson C. (2016, May 17). Cognitive dispositions to respond. Lifeinthefastlane.com. Retrieved from https://lifeinthefastlane.com/ccc/cognitive-dispositions-to-respond/.

44. Groopman J. How doctors think. New York: Houghton Mufflin Company; 2007.

Case

Joseph was a 34-year-old man who presented with a seizure. He had been complaining of a headache for five days prior to admission, and his wife noticed he had trouble "getting out certain words." He was a member of the Hasidic Jewish community in Brooklyn, New York. He was otherwise healthy and had some mild weakness of his right arm on examination. An MRI revealed a ring-enhancing mass in the left frontal lobe with swelling. The radiologist gave a large differential of what the lesion could be, including tumors and infections. He underwent a biopsy, which revealed neurocysticercosis, which is an infection with *Taenia solium*, a pork tapeworm. He was treated with an anti-parasitic medication with a good outcome (Fig. 24.1).

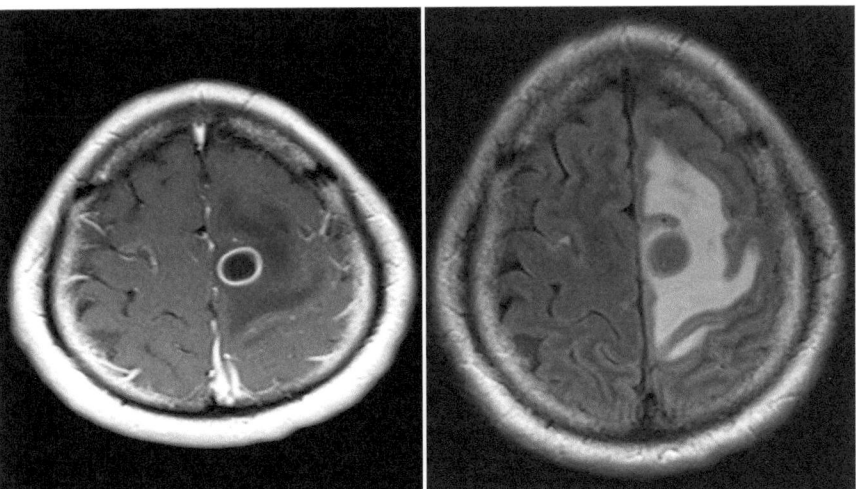

Fig. 24.1 Post-contrast T1WI and FLAIR MRI demonstrate a ring-enhancing lesion with edema in the left frontal lobe

© Springer International Publishing AG, part of Springer Nature 2019   425
J. Howard, *Cognitive Errors and Diagnostic Mistakes*,
https://doi.org/10.1007/978-3-319-93224-8_24

What Dr. White Was Thinking

Neurocysticercosis is the most common parasitic infection of the central nervous system and is common in India, Mexico and South America, as well as parts of Asia, Africa, and Eastern Europe. Initial human infection occurs due to the consumption of infected pork. The cystericerci embed in the stomach and the eggs are excreted in the feces. Ingestion of *T. solium* eggs then occurs via the fecal-oral route. The larvae attach to and invade the intestine where they migrate throughout the body.

Had the patient been Carlos from Mexico rather than Joseph from Brooklyn, there is little question I would have made the correct diagnosis the moment he walked in the door. In every single multiple-choice question on patients with neurocysticercosis, the patient is from Mexico or South America.

But Joseph did not fit my preconceptions a patient with neurocysticercosis. In order to become infected with *T. solium*, it is not necessary to eat pork. Rather, one only needs to eat food prepared by someone who ate pork and then did not properly wash their hands. Fortunately, Joseph did well, but the biopsy was not necessary. It exposed him to anxiety, discomfort, and some risk of serious complications. Brain biopsies should be done only when they are absolutely necessary. Also, his treatment neurocysticercosis was delayed by nearly a week while he waited for the biopsy and its results.

Case

James was a 47-year-old African-American man who presented with three days of difficulty speaking and weakness of his right arm. On examination, he had errors in his spontaneous speech and difficulty naming certain objects. An MRI revealed a large, enhancing lesion in his right frontal lobe and well as several other bright lesions in both frontal lobes (Fig. 24.2).

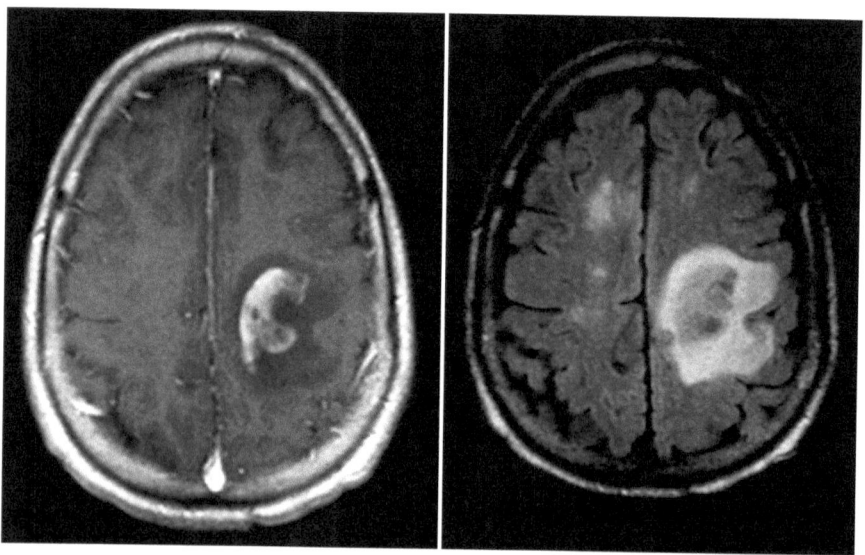

Fig. 24.2 Post-contrast T1WI and FLAIR MRI demonstrate a large, enhancing lesion with edema in the left frontal lobe

As James had smoked one pack of cigarettes daily since he was a teenager, a chest CT was performed that revealed no evidence of malignancy. The neurologist still thought cancer was the most likely diagnosis, and a brain biopsy was performed, which revealed demyelination consistent with multiple sclerosis (MS).

What Dr. Walsh Was Thinking

James caught me off guard. I did not even consider MS. Most patients with MS are females between the ages of 20–40 years who present with numbness, weakness, or visual disturbances. Most of the time, the MRI in patients with MS will show multiple, small, round lesions near the fluid-filled spaces in the center of the brain. Despite this, some patients with MS will be men. Some will be older than 50. Some will present with the loss of higher brain function, such as language deficits. Some will present with a large lesion that might be virtually indistinguishable from a tumor. I have a mental image of what patients with MS look like, and it is basically the opposite of James. He did fine in the end. Yet, had I considered this diagnosis, it is possible I would have been able to spare him the brain biopsy.

Discussion

The representativeness bias is a force that drives the diagnostician towards looking for prototypical manifestations of disease: if it looks like a duck, walks like a duck, quacks like a duck, then it is a duck. Certainly, by definition, most diseases will appear in prototypical patients (or else they would not be prototypical). Yet, restraining decision-making along these pattern-recognition lines leads to atypical variants being missed. Errors can also occur when there is an over-reliance on a patient's demographic factors or behaviors, as opposed to their clinical presentation. A 30-year-old white woman is likely to be over-diagnosed with MS because she fits the demographic profile of someone with this disease. In contrast, MS might not be considered in a 50-year-old black man, because he does not fit the demographic profile. Errors can also occur when clinicians focus on classic presentations of a rare disease, while neglecting to consider atypical presentations of a common disease. This is called base-rate neglect and will be discussed in the next section.

We can all create vivid portraits of people based on relatively little information. If I told you to imagine a star basketball player, a billionaire hedge fund manager, a Republican congressman from Kansas, or the winner of a high school math competition, whether you wanted to or not, a stereotypical image popped into your mind for each of these people. You can likely create vivid portrait of what they look like, how they dress, their background, family life, and beliefs. Similarly, many medical diagnoses create an instantaneous, involuntary image in a clinician's mind. Simply saying a disease, such as sarcoidosis, MS, anorexia, or heart attack, will create an image of a stereotypical patient based on a clinician's experience and the textbook descriptions of these cases.

Of course, such disease stereotypes are often correct. While many diseases seem to affect people randomly, many others cluster in different populations based on their age, race, sex, country of origin, and a multitude of other factors in a patient's history. Clinicians often spend a large amount of time collecting a patient's demographic information and learning about their behaviors to help narrow the differential diagnosis. It is crucial that this information be taken into account when making many medical diagnoses. After all, most patients with lung cancer are older people with a long smoking history.

However, just like with all stereotypes, there will be many exceptions to proto-typical presentations of diseases. Though most patients with lung cancer will be older smokers, some will be younger people who never smoked. Though neurocys-ticercosis most commonly occurs in people from South America and India who eat pork, there have been outbreaks of the disease in Orthodox Jewish communities [1]. We can all imagine a stereotypical stroke patient: an older, obese man with hyper-tension and a long history of smoking. But this does not mean younger, healthy patients without these risk factors are therefore immune from strokes. Clinicians can make mistakes when real patients differ from the stereotypical patients they encounter in textbooks and on multiple-choice exams.

Finally, stereotypes can be simply wrong. Does the man pictured below match your stereotype of a star basketball player? Probably not. But that's Steve Nash. He was an eight-time NBA All-Star, a seven-time All-NBA selection, and two-time winner of the NBA Most Valuable Player award (Fig. 24.3).

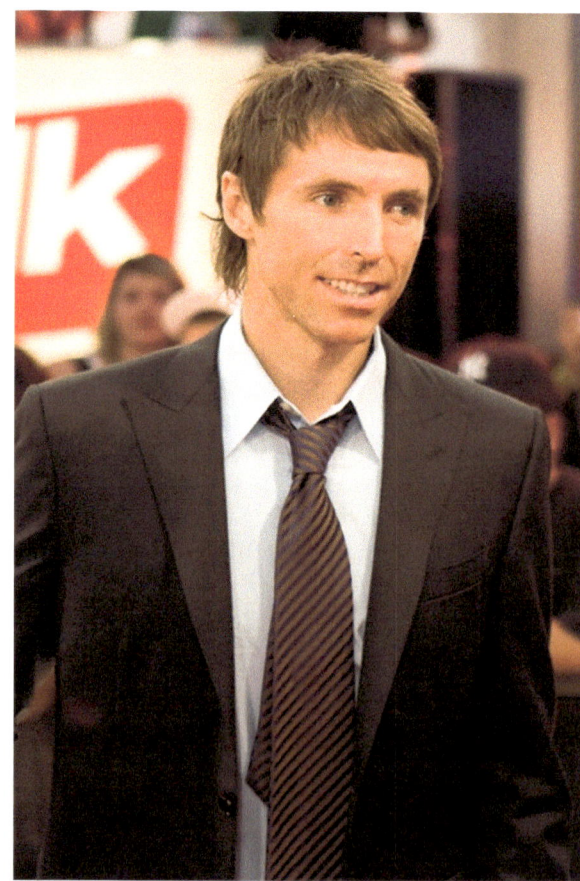

Fig. 24.3 Steve Nash. (Burdett R. (Richard). Steve Nash at the eTalk Festival Party, during the Toronto International Film Festival [Image file]. In: Wikimedia commons. 2008. Retrieved from https://commons. wikimedia.org/wiki/ Category:Steve_Nash#/ media/File:ETalk2008-Steve_Nash.jpg)

Stereotypes can be wrong with more weighty matters as well. For example, there is evidence that white people both use and sell drugs more often than African-Americans, though African-Americans are more likely to be arrested for this crime [2].

The potential of stereotypes to mislead clinicians was demonstrated in a study by Ronald Triplet [3]. Subjects were provided with a patient with vague symptoms, such as fatigue and recurrent infections. They were given descriptions of five diseases: influenza, leukemia, AIDS, meningitis, and appendicitis, which were chosen in part because their symptoms often overlap. They were asked to determine the most likely diagnosis. When told that a female patient was a homosexual, subjects rated her as being more likely to have AIDS than a heterosexual woman with identical symptoms. Although lesbians are in fact less likely to contract AIDS than heterosexual women, because they were broadly categorized in the higher risk group of "homosexuals," they were inappropriately judged to be at higher risk than heterosexual women.

Conclusion

Extra-symptom characteristics can strongly bias a diagnostician. Clinicians should do their best not let the "textbook" example of a disease distract them from potentially atypical presentations. Though the typical case of MS is a 30-year-old white woman, this does not mean that an older black man is protected from the disease.

Base Rate Neglect

Case

Keisha was a 38-year-old woman who presented with a headache and photophobia for two days. She had some mild nausea, but no vomiting. She was otherwise healthy and did not have a history of headaches. She said her entire head hurt and the pain was throbbing. She had a temperature of 100.4°F, but her vital signs were otherwise normal. She appeared uncomfortable in the ER and had a difficult time participating in the neurological examination as she did not want to get off the stretcher. However, as best as could be determined, she had a normal examination. A head CT and routine laboratory work were normal as well. A lumbar puncture revealed 15 red blood cells. As there was a concern for herpes encephalitis, she was started on acyclovir, and the patient suffered minor renal failure as a result. She was not permanently injured, but had to remain in the hospital for a week getting intravenous fluids, while her renal function normalized. In the meantime, definitive studies of her spinal fluid were negative for herpes encephalitis.

What Dr. Polly Was Thinking

There is an informal rule in medicine that says one should treat herpes encephalitis the moment one considers the diagnosis. It is a horrible disease with severe consequences if left untreated. Several years ago, a patient was sent home from the ER who turned out to have herpes encephalitis. Unfortunately, this has led to numerous patients with migraine and other benign headache disorders being treated for herpes encephalitis until it is ruled out. We probably admit one patient per week to rule-out herpes encephalitis. The definitive test can take several days to come back, and once patients are started on acyclovir in the ER, they are basically committed to staying on it for the next couple of days until the test results come back. Yet, herpes encephalitis is a rare disease, affecting approximately two in a million people.

Case
Kelly was a 35-year-old woman presented for medical clearance for bariatric surgery. Aside from her obesity, she had no medical complaints or history. She smoked for a few years as a teenager, but had not smoked for 15 years. As part of her preoperative evaluation, a routine chest X-ray was performed, revealing a small lesion in the right upper lobe. This was confirmed on chest CT, and the radiologist wrote that "a neoplasm cannot be excluded." She was taken for a bronchoscopy in order to obtain a biopsy, which revealed non-specific granulomatous disease. She was grateful to the doctor for having ruled-out cancer.

What Dr. Gutenstein Was Thinking
The patient understandably anxious about the possibility that she might have lung cancer, and so was I. It was pretty startling to read a radiologists report saying the word neoplasm. I also know that CT scans almost never miss lung cancers- they are very sensitive tests. However, in a woman her age, especially a non-smoker, the odds that she had lung cancer are vanishingly small. In retrospect, the best course of action would have been to simply repeat the chest X-ray in a few months. CT scans are a source of radiation, and though her bronchoscopy and biopsy went fine, these tests are not without complications. She was certainly relieved to not have cancer, and was happy the biopsy was done. However, refusing to perform a test or procedure for which there is no indication, even if it upsets the patient, is part of a doctor's job.

Discussion
Base-rate neglect refers the tendency to ignore the true prevalence of a disease in making a diagnosis. The base rate of a disease can be either inflated or deflated, leading to faulty diagnostic reasoning or misinterpretation of test results. Consider the following statistics:

1. 66% drivers who die in car crashes are sober.
2. 90% of people who get cancer are right-handed.
3. In a recent outbreak of whooping cough, 54% of children had been vaccinated against it.

So, do you now believe that it is safe to drive while intoxicated? Do you believe that being left-handed protects you from cancer? Do you believe the whooping cough vaccine is useless? Of course not. You probably recognize that drunk drivers represent a small fraction of the overall drivers, that most people are right-handed, and that most children are vaccinated. You successfully recognized that the base-rate matters. Yet, in other scenarios, accounting for the base-rate can be much more difficult.

A simple scenario created by Daniel Kahneman and Amos Tversky showed how ignoring the base-rate lead to faulty conclusion. Consider the following scenario:

> Steve is very shy and withdrawn, invariably helpful, but with little interested in people, or in the world of reality. A meek and tidy soul, he has a need for order and structure, and a passion for detail. Is Steve more likely to be a librarian or a school teacher?

Most people would answer that Steve is more likely to be a librarian. Certainly, he sounds like one. However, there are many more school teachers than there are librarians. Therefore, the odds are higher that Steve is an unusual school teacher than a typical librarian.

Another of their studies demonstrated how the representativeness bias and neglecting the base-rate can lead to erroneous conclusions [4]. They divided study subjects into three groups.

1. The "**base-rate group**" was given nine fields of graduate studies and asked to write down their best guess for the percentage of first year students in the field. The nine fields were business administration, computer science, engineering, humanities/education, law, library science, medicine, physical/life sciences, and social science/social work.
2. The "**similarity group**" was given the following personality sketch:

> Tom W. is of high intelligence, although lacking in true creativity. He has a need for order and clarity, and for neat and tidy systems in which every detail finds its appropriate place. His writing is rather dull and mechanical, occasionally enlivened by somewhat corny puns and by flashes of imagination of the sci-fi type. He has a strong drive for competence. He seems to feel little sympathy for other people and does not enjoy interacting with others. Self-centered, he nonetheless has a deep moral sense."

They were then provided the nine fields above and ask to determine how similar Tom W. was to a prototypical student in that field.

3. The "**prediction group**" was also given the description of Tom W. and told he was a graduate student. They were then asked to rank which of the nine fields he was most likely to study.

The base-rate group believed there were more students studying education and humanities than computer science. The similarity group felt that Tom W. best fit the prototype of someone studying computer science. Demonstrating a neglect of the base-rate, the estimates in the prediction group were much closer to the similarity group than to the base-rate group. Almost all of the participants in the prediction group thought that Tom W. would be more likely to study computer science than education or humanities. This shows how the prediction group undervalued the base-rate of the nine fields, overvalued the stereotype of a typical computer science student, and thus fell victim to the representativeness bias.

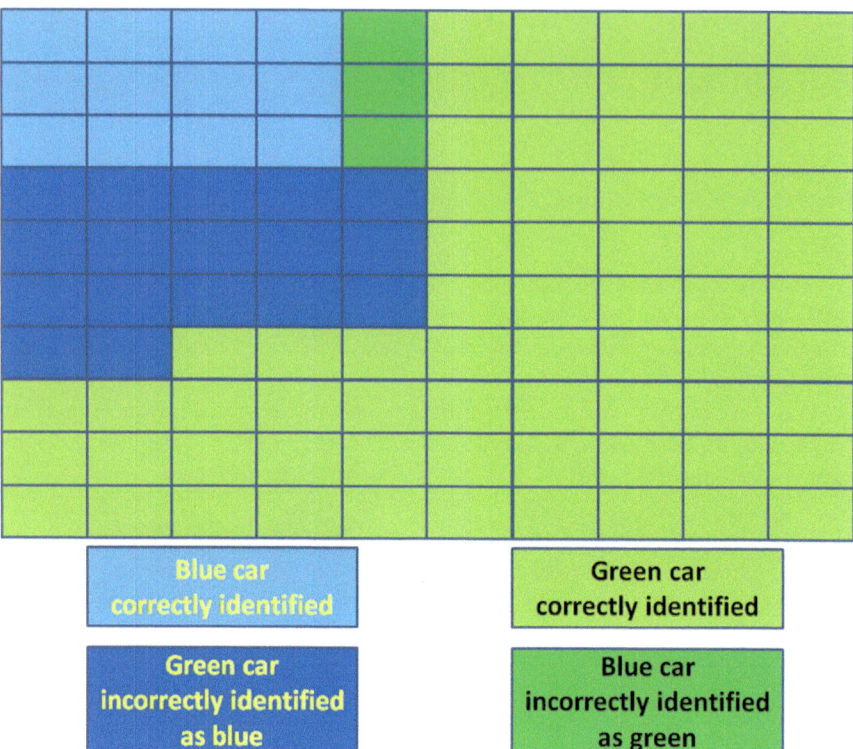

Fig. 24.4 The taxi cab problem. The witness was right 80% of the time, but out of the 29 cars he said were blue, only 12 (41%) actually were blue

Another example by Kahneman and Tversky showed how much trouble people have taking into account the base-rate in solving problems:

> *A cab was involved in a hit and run accident at night. Two cab companies, Green and Blue, operate in the city. You are given the following data:*
>
> * *85% of the cabs in the city are green and 15% are blue.*
> * *A witness identified the cab as blue.*
> * *The court tested the reliability of the witness under the circumstances that existed on the night of the accident, and concluded that the witness correctly identified each one of the two colors 80% of the time and failed 20% of the time.*
>
> *What is the probability that the cab involved in the accident was blue rather than green?*

Most people estimate that the likelihood the cab was blue is about 80%. However, when the numbers are crunched, the likelihood that cab is blue is only 41% (Fig. 24.4).

This shows that when the base-rates are greatly uneven, even an accurate witness (or diagnostic test) can be wrong more often than he is right. Yet another classic example by Kahneman and Tversky showed that, at times, people are more likely to judge multiple specific conditions to be true rather than a single general one, an error known as the conjunction fallacy [5]. Consider the following problem:

Linda is 31-years-old, single, outspoken, and very bright. She majored in philosophy. As a student, she was deeply concerned with issues of discrimination and social justice, and also participated in anti-nuclear demonstrations. Which is more probable?

    1. *Linda is a bank teller.*
    2. *Linda is a bank teller and is active in the feminist movement.*

While it's certainly tempting to say that number two is correct, it is not. The likelihood that Linda is a bank teller alone is higher than the likelihood she is a bank teller and *anything* else.

A related cognitive bias is known as insensitivity to sample size, which occurs when people judge the probability of as event without taking into account the sample size. In a demonstration of this, Kahneman and Tversky gave subjects the following problem [6]:

A certain town is served by two hospitals. In the larger hospital about 45 babies are born each day, and in the smaller hospital about 15 babies are born each day. As you know, about 50% of all babies are boys. However, the exact percentage varies from day to day. Sometimes it may be higher than 50%, sometimes lower.

*   For a period of one year, each hospital recorded the days on which more than 60% of the babies born were boys. Which hospital do you think recorded more such days?*

    1. *The larger hospital.*
    2. *The smaller hospital.*
    3. *About the same (that is, within 5% of each other).*

Fifty-six percent of subjects chose option three, and 22% of subjects chose options 1 or 2. However, the hospital with 45 births is much more likely to have similar numbers of boys and girls born on a given day than the hospital with 15 births. Though it is not intuitively obvious, small sample sizes are likely to have more variation than larger ones. This becomes trivially easy to understand when asking, "Who is more likely to flip only heads; someone who tosses a coin twice or someone who tosses it 100 times?"

It's easy to see how these cognitive errors might trip up a clinician. For example, a 60-year-old man with the rapid progression of memory loss is a classic presentation for Creutzfeldt-Jakob disease. Yet this patient is still more likely to have an unusual form of Alzheimer's disease, which affects around 200,000 Americans under the age of 65, than Creutzfeldt-Jakob disease, which is literally a one-in-a-million disease.

Consideration of the disease base-rate is especially crucial when interpreting diagnostic tests. When evaluating any test result, clinicians should strive to use Bayesian reasoning, which is a mathematical formula and reasoning strategy that describes the probability of an event based on prior knowledge of conditions related to the event. Let's do a test.

A powerful new CT scanner never fails to detect a case of breast cancer. However, it reveals a false diagnosis of breast cancer in 5% of healthy women.

In women younger than 50 years-old, the rate of breast cancer is one in a thousand. If this scan comes back abnormal in Robin, a 45-year-old woman, what is the probability she actually has cancer? It sure sounds like Robin likely has breast cancer. After all, the test never misses a breast cancer in sick women and is accurate 95% of the time in healthy ones. [In statistics, how certain someone is that a positive test result is in fact a true positive is called the positive predictive value (PPV). PPV = True Positives/ (True Positives + False Positives)].

Let's do the math with a sample of 1,000 women. In this group, we can expect that one woman will have breast cancer, and there is a 100% certainty that the test will be abnormal for her- a true positive test result. The other 999 women will not have breast cancer, but with a 5% error rate there will be 50 false positive test results. Therefore, the odds that Robin actually has breast cancer are only one in 51, or about 2%.

Test result	Yes cancer	No cancer	Interpretation
Positive	1	50	1 out of 51 patients who tests positive will actually have cancer.
Negative	0	849	

This does not mean the new CT scanner is necessarily a useless test. It is flawless in ruling-out cancer. If a woman comes in with extreme anxiety because she is worried she has breast cancer, it may be worth doing this test to reassure her. However, if a woman tests positive, and the results of that test are not properly understood, she is likely to suffer unnecessary anxiety and testing.

What if we change the scenario to a 70-year-old woman and the rate of breast cancer to one in 10? In 1,000 women from this group, 100 of them will have breast cancer, while 900 won't. The PPV Positive predictive value (PPV) jumps to 100/145, or 69%. Even with a very high base-rate of 10%, 30% of patients with a positive test will still be healthy.

Test result	Yes cancer	No cancer	Interpretation
Positive	100	45	100 out of 145 patients who tests positive will actually have cancer.
Negative	0	755	

Unfortunately, doctors often perform very poorly on tasks that require understanding of the base-rate. Risk specialist Gerd Gigerenzer created the following scenario:

A 50-year-old woman, no symptoms, participates in routine mammography screening. She tests positive, is alarmed, and wants to know from you whether she has breast cancer for certain or what the chances are. Apart from the screening results, you know nothing else about this woman. How many women who test positive actually have breast cancer? What is the best answer?

1. *9 in 10.*
2. *8 in 10.*
3. *1 in 10.*
4. *1 in 100.*

Given:

- *The probability that a woman has breast cancer is 1% ("prevalence").*
- *If a woman has breast cancer, the probability that she tests positive is 90% ("sensitivity").*
- *If a woman does not have breast cancer, the probability that she nevertheless tests positive is 9% ("false alarm rate").*

In a group of 160 gynecologists, nearly half answered that the patient's odd of having cancer was nine in 10, while only 21% correctly answered that her odds were one in 10 [7]. They would have done better had they guessed randomly. A study by Britta Anderson and colleagues tested 4,713 gynecology residents with a multiple-choice question, similar to the one above, asking them to identify the positive predictive value of a positive screening mammogram [8]. Only 26% picked the correct answer, which is basically what would have happened had they randomly guessed the answer. Another interesting finding from Dr. Anderson's study was that responders who correctly answered the question rated their statistical literacy training as worse than those who got it wrong. Consistent with the Dunning-Kruger effect, "residents who need additional statistical literacy training may be the least likely to recognize the inadequacy of their training."

Dr. Gigerenzer has found that clinicians do much better on these problems when they are presented as natural frequencies as follows [7]:

Assume you conduct breast cancer screening using mammography in a certain region. You know the following information about the women in this region:

- *10 out of every 1,000 women have breast cancer.*
- *Of these 10 women with breast cancer, 9 test positive.*
- *Of the 990 women without cancer, about 89 nevertheless test positive.*

When presented this way, 87% of gynecologists answered correctly. Despite this, few medical journals present statistics in a way to maximize the probability they will be correctly understood by their readers.

Importantly, these scenarios differ from most clinical practice in that the base-rate of the disease is provided for the clinician. ER clinicians may encounter dozens of different diagnoses daily, and unless they know the base-rate for each disease, even the most statistically savvy clinician will have a hard time interpreting tests. Unfortunately, research has shown that there is a great deal of variability when clinicians attempt to estimate the base-rate of various diseases [9].

In addition to this, presenting risks in relative, rather than absolute terms, can particularly distort the perception of risk (or benefit) of a treatment if the base-rate is not taken into account. The **absolute risk** of a disease is the risk of developing a disease over a time period. In contrast, the **relative risk** of a disease compares the risks in two groups. The clinical relevance of the relative risk cannot be interpreted without considering the absolute risk. For example, women have about a 12% lifetime chance of developing breast cancer, while men have a 0.1% risk. A medication that lowered the risk of breast cancer by 20% would be a miracle for women and close to useless for most men, given that women get breast cancer at 120 times the rate of men. People are just not intuitively good at grasping risk when it is expressed numerically. When given the statement "Cancer kills 2,414 people out of 10,000" people believe cancer is more dangerous than those who are told "Cancer kills 24.14 people out of 100." The influence of the size of the numerator and denominator on how people perceive numbers is called the ratio bias [10].

It is also easy for people to get confused between quantities and proportionality. For example, a medication that decreased one's risk of cancer by 1% would still be extremely valuable even if it raised one's risk of a serious but rare event, say being eaten by a shark, by 500%. Obviously, this is because only a handful of humans are eaten by sharks around the world annually, while cancer is extremely common. However when confronted with these possibilities, it is difficult to objectively grasp the risks and benefits posed by the treatment. There is a natural tendency to prefer large decreases in small risks to small decreases in large risks, even though the small decrease in the larger risk offers the greatest overall benefit.

Journalists often exploit base-rate neglect to create sensational headlines. Consider this headline from the Daily Mail: "Child's Risk of Brain Cancer Triples After Just Two CT Scans" [11]. Scary right? Yet, because the absolute risk of brain cancer is low, about 10,000 head CT scans would have to be given to children younger than 10 years to cause one additional brain tumor. Similarly, an article in The Sun warned of the dangers of eating processed meats by declaring "Careless Pork Costs Lives." It went on to say that people who ate large quantities of processed meat had a 20% increased risk of colon cancer. However, given that the lifetime risk of colon cancer is 5%, the absolute risk only jumped to 6% [12].

Another headline in the Telegraph was "Newer Contraceptive Pills Raise Risk of Blood Clot Four Fold" [13]. The article begins by saying, "More than 1 million women are at increased risk of developing a dangerous blood clot because they are using new forms of the contraceptive pill, a study shows." A tragic anecdote then followed, "The research was published just weeks after the death of Tamworth teaching assistant Fallan Kurek, 21, who collapsed after taking the pill, albeit an older less dangerous form." However, later in the article, the lead author of the research, Yana Vinogradova, explained that the use of new generation contraceptive pills would be expected to cause about 14 additional blood clots per year in the entire country of England. As John Guillebaud, a contraception expert explained, "The death rate of it is low but if you have got millions of people taking the pill, one or two people will have a bad outcome like this."

The consequences of fearmongering headlines that take advantage of the base-rate neglect are real. In 1995, England suffered an unfortunate event known as the "pill scare" [14]. A letter was sent out by the UK Committee on Safety of Medicines warning about the risk of blood clots due to third generation oral contraceptives. Nearly 200,000 clinicians received a letter warning them that oral contraceptives increased the risk of a dangerous clot by 100%. Yet the actual risk for any individual woman increased from one in 7,000 to two in 7,000. This shows how small absolute risks can

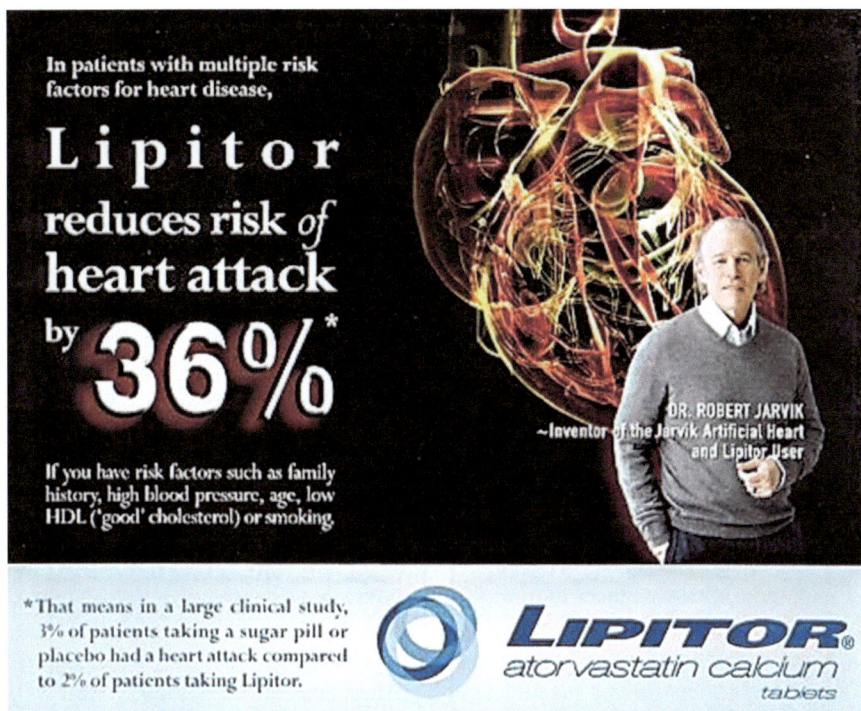

Fig. 24.5 Lipitor™ reduces the risk of a heart attack by 36%! But read the fine print. (Eades MR. Absolute risk versus relative risk: Why you need to know the difference [Image file, Blog post]. The Blog of Michael R. Eades, MD. 2013. Retrieved from https://proteinpower.com/drmike/2013/12/30/absolute-risk-versus-relative-risk-need-know-difference/.)

translate into large relative risks when the base-rate is low. Not surprisingly the "dear doctor" warning letters garnered significant media attention at the time, needlessly scaring many women. As a result of the ensuing panic, the use of these oral contraceptives predictably plummeted. After several years of falling abortion rates, there was an equally predictable increase in the number of conceptions and abortions, particularly in young women [15]. In 1996, there were 13,500 more abortions than in 1995, an increase of 8.3%. This increase correlated with the warning letter about the pill. In contrast, the rate of blood clots was unchanged over this time span [16].

Pharmaceutical companies also frequently use relative risk to extol the benefits of their products. By proclaiming that a medication improves the rate of some condition without giving the absolute improvement, they can make relatively improvements seem major. The advertisement for Lipitor™ boasts in big letters that it reduces the risk of heart attack by 36% (Fig. 24.5).

However, by reading the fine print, one learns that in the study that 3% of patients on placebo had a heart attack, while 2% of patients taking Lipitor did. On a population level, this reduction in heart attacks can translate into big numbers. However, the chances that any one individual will benefit are still rather low, at 1%. As Mark Twain said, "There are lies, damned lies, and statistics."

Conclusion

Obviously, rare diseases exist in medicine and, taken together, rare diseases are quite common. However, an individual rare disease is just that—rare—and all things being equal, clinicians should presume a patient has a common disease before diagnosing a rare one. The base-rate of a disease must be considered when making a diagnosis. The classic presentation of an unusual disease is often less common than an uncommon presentation of a typical one. As such, when taking into account a characteristic of a patient's case, rather than consider how *typical* that characteristic may be for a disease, clinicians should focus on how *predictive* that characteristic is.

Additionally, the base-rate of any disease must be taken into account when interpreting diagnostic tests. If told about a diagnostic test that never misses a case of breast cancer and only has a false diagnostic rate of 5%, one's gut instinct says that if a woman tests positive for breast cancer using this test, then she is likely to have the disease. However, as shown in this chapter, one cannot interpret such diagnostic studies without taking into account the base-rate of the disease. A failure to understand Bayesian reasoning explains why many doctors over-screen for many cancers. Indeed, mammograms in women between the ages of 40–59 years have been found to not reduce breast cancer mortality, though they have been shown to lead to over-diagnosis and potentially harmful treatments.

The website understandinguncertainty.org calculated that there are "2,845 different ways of expressing the effect on the risk of an event of an intervention" [10]. Given this, it is easy to see how statistics can confuse people and how those with an agenda can use statistics to mislead. If I were to redesign medical school, courses in statistics would be as prominent as gross anatomy and physiology. While statistics are taught at every medical school, it is often treated as an afterthought. Yet, medical statistics is the one course every clinician needs to understand no matter in what field they practice. I agree with Dr. Gigerenzer who wrote, "It's not a problem of the medical mind. It's a problem of training at the universities, in the medical departments where young doctors are trained in everything except statistical thinking" [17].

Zebra Retreat

Case

Steven was a 45-year-old man who awoke with left-sided numbness. He was otherwise healthy, but his wife said that he had become forgetful recently. His father had died at age 60 from a stroke, and his family always suspected that he had MS, as he was wheelchair-bound for several years prior to his death. Steven's MRI showed multiple white matter lesions and several darker lesions, termed "black holes," which can be seen in MS (Fig. 24.6). A spinal tap was negative for oligoclonal bands, a marker of inflammation found in about 90% of patients with MS.

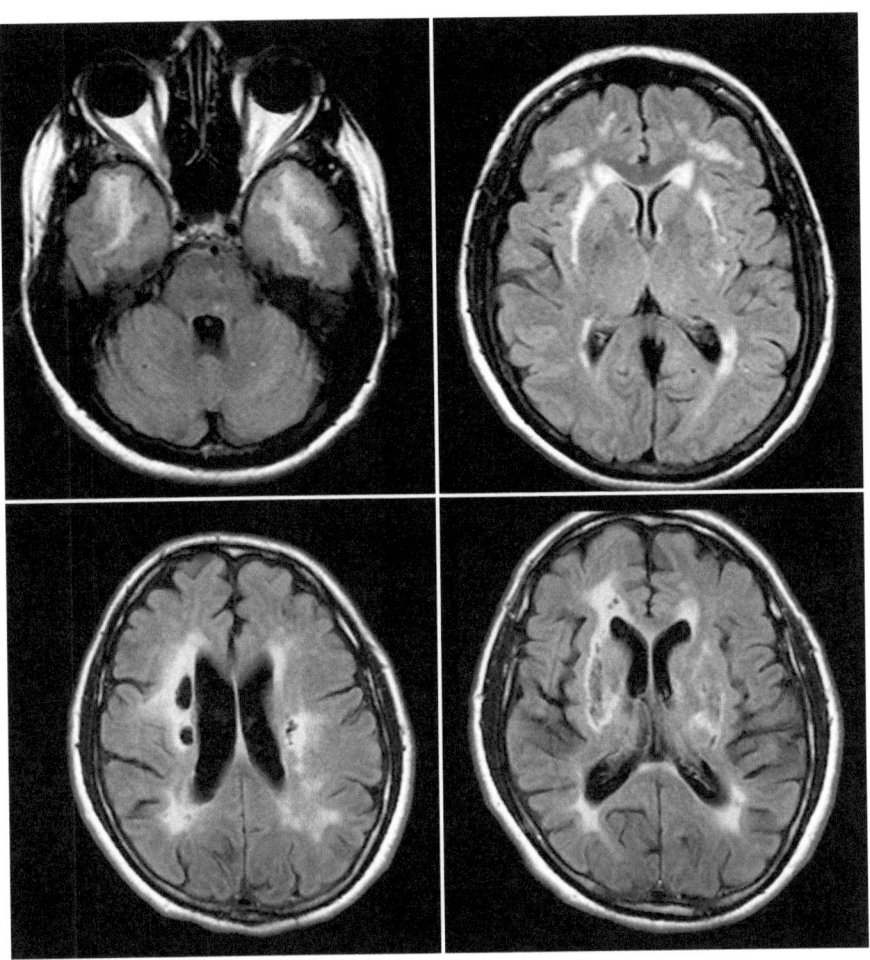

Fig. 24.6 FLAIR MRIs showing extensive white matter disease and dark areas of severe brain injury

Based on his clinical presentation and imaging, Steven was diagnosed with MS. Despite being placed on an effective treatment, he continued to have relapses and progression of disability. He also responded poorly to steroids, which are used to decrease inflammation in active MS and usually result in rapid symptomatic improvement. He became progressively demented and needed a wheelchair within three years. His wife felt that his family history, the lack of oligoclonal bands, and his poor response to treatment justified pursuing a more thorough diagnostic work-up. However, the neurologist refused, saying that she didn't want to go on a "fishing expedition."

Steven's wife sought a second opinion from another neurologist who suspected a genetic condition. Steven was eventually diagnosed with cerebral autosomal dominant arteriopathy with subcortical infarcts and leukoencephalopathy (CADASIL), a rare hereditary stroke disorder.

What Dr. Gross Was Thinking

There was no question that Steven was an atypical case in many ways. His spinal tap was normal, but that can be the case in 10% of patients with MS. His father may have had MS, but no one knew for sure, and a positive family history occurs in approximately 1% of patients with MS. So that did not particularly bother me either. He had a rapid progression of disability despite being on an effective medication. But this medication is far from a cure. It doesn't work for everyone. MS is a common disease, and I thought that he just had a severe, atypical case.

I was taught to be judicious with the use of medical tests. I was taught to consider the pre-test probability of each test, the likelihood that it will change treatment, as well as the cost and risks of the test. Several of my peers who did "million-dollar work-ups" on many of their patients were criticized (and snickered at) for wasting money and subjecting their patients to unnecessary, unpleasant, and even potentially harmful tests. Though his wife wanted to pursue other diagnostic tests, I didn't want to be one of *those* doctors.

Additionally, I practice in a small-town and it is not easy to refer patients for neurogenetic testing. Given the potential implications for his family, it imperative that a diagnosis such as CADASIL be made only by a qualified specialist who can help him and his family understand the implications of this diagnosis.

Discussion

Clinicians often like to invoke the law of parsimony: the simplest explanation is usually the correct one. Common diseases are by definition common, and rare diseases (informally called "zebras") are by definition rare. Medical students are taught that "common things are common," and as such, common diseases should first be considered before entertaining more obscure diagnoses. This is captured in the time-honored medical aphorism that "When you hear hoof beats, think of horses not zebras," attributed to Theodore Woodward. This is sometimes referred to as Sutton's law, which states clinicians should first investigate the most likely diagnosis before considering rare diseases. It is named after the bank robber Willie Sutton, who reportedly told a journalist that he robbed banks "because that's where the money is."

A rare disease is formally defined as one that affects less than 200,000 individuals in the US. When considered in totality, rare diseases are quite common. According to the National Human Genome Research Institute, there are nearly 6,800 rare diseases, affecting 25–30 million Americans [18]. The vast majority of these are genetic disorders, and many of them have neurological manifestations. Although it varies by specialty, some clinicians see a wide variety of rare diseases every day. In some instances, clinicians may over-estimate the likelihood of a zebra, so as not to "miss something," or because diagnosing an obscure disease can be gratifying. However, in other instances, clinicians may reject pursuing a rare diagnosis, a phenomenon termed a zebra retreat. A zebra retreat occurs when a rare diagnosis is rejected for various reasons. As Pat Crokerry wrote, these reasons include:

- Self-consciousness and under-confidence about entertaining a remote and unusual diagnosis, and gaining a reputation for being esoteric.
- Perceived inertia in the system and barriers to obtaining special or costly tests.
- The fear of being seen as unrealistic and wasteful of resources.
- Underestimating or overestimating the base-rate for the diagnosis.
- Team members may exert coercive pressure to avoid wasting the team's time.
- The clinical environment may be very busy and the anticipated time and effort to pursue the diagnosis might dilute the physician's conviction.
- Inconvenience of the time of day or weekend and difficulty getting access to specialists.
- Unfamiliarity with the diagnosis might make the physician less likely to go down an unfamiliar road.
- Fatigue, sleep deprivation, or other distractions may tip the physician toward retreat.

Many forces work against a clinician who invokes a zebra. Clinicians are rightfully discouraged from going on so-called "fishing expeditions" or giving their patients a "million-dollar work-up." The harms of medical over-testing are well documented. Over-testing can lead to a cascade of further tests, which reveal abnormal, though not necessarily pathological, findings. Tests can be costly and many are unpleasant or risky.

Moreover, invoking a zebra often puts clinicians on uncomfortable terrain. When I see patients with common conditions, there is a sense of comfort, at least in terms of the diagnosis and management of their condition. Although it can be a devastating disease, I feel at home treating MS. I am comfortable making the diagnosis, have a sense of its prognosis, and am comfortable advising patients about their treatment options. It's like walking around my own neighborhood. In this sense, common diseases trigger the mere-exposure effect, the psychological phenomenon where people develop a preference for familiar things because they are familiar.

In contrast, patients with zebras trigger a sense of uncertainty, like being in a foreign country. This is how I feel on those rare occasions I treat patients with neurosarcoidosis or neuro-Behçet's disease. A clinician who diagnoses a zebra may doubt themselves, and they are unlikely to be familiar with its management. It may require them to use unfamiliar medications. There is rarely a large evidence base to guide treatment with rare diseases, forcing the clinician to deal with uncertainty.

Invoking a zebra may also necessitate the involvement of other clinicians to perform procedures and diagnostic tests. As no clinician wants to develop a reputation as someone who "cries wolf," they may resist requesting invasive procedures needed to make a diagnosis. For example, if I feel one of my patients needs a biopsy, I have to request this from a neurosurgeon. Hopefully, they feel that when I make this request, it is because they trust my judgment that other, less invasive diagnostic options have proved fruitless. I'm also fortunate that excellent neurosurgeons are available whenever I need them. For neurologists working in more remote areas, a great deal of effort may be required to get a patient to see a neurosurgeon. As such, the consequences of "crying wolf" may be perceived as greater, leading to further reluctance to summon a neurosurgeon when one is needed.

Finally, zebras are almost never good news. Rather, they are often serious, poorly understood diseases with few treatment options. Clinicians may be reluctant to pursue diagnoses for which little is known and little can be done, furthering a zebra retreat.

Conclusion

The decision as to whether or not it is appropriate to chase a zebra must be made on a case-to-case basis. It is a delicate balancing act between not being afraid to pursue obscure diagnoses, while at the same time not subjecting patients to unnecessary tests. However, zebras exist, and a clinician who never chases a zebra won't ever catch one.

References

1. Schantz PM, Moore AC, Muñoz JL, Hartman BJ, Schaefer JA, Aron AM, Persaud D, Sarti E, Wilson M, Flisser A. Neurocysticercosis in an Orthodox Jewish community in New York City. N Engl J Med. 1992;327(10):692–5. https://doi.org/10.1056/NEJM199209033271004.
2. Ingraham C. (2017, Sept 30). White people are more likely to deal drugs, but black people are more likely to get arrested for it. The Washington Post. https://www.washingtonpost.com/news/wonk/wp/2014/09/30/white-people-are-more-likely-to-deal-drugs-but-black-people-are-more-likely-to-get-arrested-for-it.
3. Triplet RG. Discriminatory biases in the perception of illness: the application of availability and representativeness heuristics to the AIDS crisis. Basic Appl Soc Psychol. 1992;13(3):303–22.
4. Kahneman D, Tversky A. On the psychology of prediction. Psychol Rev. 1973;80(4):237–51. https://doi.org/10.1037/h0034747.
5. Tversky A, Kahneman D. Judgments of and by representativeness. In: Kahneman D, Slovic P, Tversky A, editors. Judgement under uncertainty: heuristics and biases. Cambridge: Cambridge University Press; 1982. p. 84–98.
6. Tversky A, Kahneman D. Judgment under uncertainty: heuristics and biases. Science. 1974;185(4157):1124–31. https://doi.org/10.1126/science.185.4157.1124.
7. Gigerenzer G, Gaissmaier W, Kurz-Milcke E, Schwartz LM, Woloshin S. Helping doctors and patients make sense of health statistics. Psychol Sci Public Interest. 2008;8(2):53–96.
8. Anderson BL, Williams S, Schulkin J. Statistical literacy of obstetrics-gynecology residents. J Grad Med Educ. 2013;5(2):272–5. https://doi.org/10.4300/JGME-D-12-00161.1.
9. Phelps MA, Levitt MA. Pretest probability estimates: a pitfall to the clinical utility of evidence-based medicine? Acad Emerg Med. 2004;11(6):692–4.
10. gmp26. (2009, Feb 23). 2845 ways to spin the risk [Blog post]. Understanding Uncertainty. https://understandinguncertainty.org/node/233.
11. Hope J. (2012, June 6). Child's risk of brain cancer triples after just two CT scans. DailyMail. com. Retrieved from https://www.dailymail.co.uk/health/article-2155678/Childs-risk-brain-cancer-tripled-head-CT-scans.html.

12. Riesch H, Spiegelhalter DJ. 'Careless pork costs lives': risk stories from science to press release to media. Health Risk Soc. 2011;13(1):47–64. https://doi.org/10.1080/13698575.2010.540645.
13. Knapton S. (2015, May 26). Newer contraceptive pills raise risk of blood clot four fold. The Telegraph. Retrieved from https://www.telegraph.co.uk/news/science/science-news/11630581/Newer-contraceptive-pills-raise-risk-of-blood-clot-four-fold.html.
14. Furedi A. The public health implications of the 1995 'pill scare. Hum Reprod Update. 1999;5(6):621–6.
15. Wood R, Botting B, Dunnell K. Trends in conceptions before and after the 1995 pill scare. Popul Trends. 1997;89:5–12.
16. Farmer RD, Williams TJ, Simpson EL, Nightingale AL. Effect of 1995 pill scare on rates of venous thromboembolism among women taking combined oral contraceptives: analysis of general practice research database. BMJ. 2000;321(7259):477–9.
17. Kremer W. (2014). Do doctors understand test results? BBC News Magazine. Retrieved from https://www.bbc.com/news/magazine-28166019.
18. U.S. Department of Health & Human Services, National Institutes of Health, National Genome Research Institute. (2012, Feb 27). Frequently asked questions about rare diseases. Retrieved from https://www.genome.gov/27531963/faq-about-rare-diseases/.

Case

Sylvia was a 65-year-old woman who presented to her doctor for a routine visit. She was healthy and, other than some "aches and pains," felt well. She requested a thyroid ultrasound, as a good friend of hers had recently died from thyroid cancer. Her doctor agreed and a small pre-cancerous nodule was found, requiring Sylvia to have her thyroid gland removed as a precaution. She sustained a nerve injury during the procedure, which left her with a hoarse voice. However, she expressed gratitude to her doctor and credited him with saving her life.

What Dr. Jiang Was Thinking

Although Sylvia sustained a minor injury during the surgery, we were both thrilled that her cancer was detected early. As a primary care doctor, I am a big advocate of cancer-screening. Obviously, I am never happy when a screening test is abnormal. But I know that, in the long run, they save lives and prevent suffering. Early detection makes so much sense; the earlier a cancer is found, the less likely it is to spread and the easier it is to treat. A whole generation of doctors were raised with this mantra. However, many screening tests don't seem to be doing nearly as much good as I thought. I'm glad that this subject has continued to be researched. There are a lot of unanswered questions.

Discussion

A screening error occurs due to the overly zealous use of screening tests. Given the ubiquity of screening tests, it is important to understand the biases inherent in such tests. Clinicians and patients alike have a strong, intuitive sense that screening can detect diseases, particularly cancer, prior to symptom onset. In turn, this can allow for the early initiation of treatment, preventing suffering and saving lives.

The World Health Organization published guidelines in 1968 called the *Principles and Practice of Screening for Disease*, in which they proposed criteria for a screening program based on the disease, the test itself, and characteristic of the screened population [1]. In essence they are:

© Springer International Publishing AG, part of Springer Nature 2019
J. Howard, *Cognitive Errors and Diagnostic Mistakes*,
https://doi.org/10.1007/978-3-319-93224-8_25

Disease
- The condition should be an important health problem.
- There should be a latent stage of the disease.
- The disease should be common, but not universal.
- The natural history of the disease should be adequately understood.
- There should be a treatment for the condition.

Test
- The test should have high sensitivity to detect asymptomatic disease and a reasonable specificity to avoid false positive results.
- The test should be safe and well-tolerated.
- The test detects disease early enough to treat.

Population
- Facilities for diagnosis and treatment should be available.
- There should be an agreed policy on whom to treat.
- The total cost of finding a case should be economically balanced in relation to medical expenditure as a whole.
- Case-finding should be a continuous process, not just a "once and for all" project.

Importantly, only certain types of cancers can have their natural history meaningfully altered by a screening test. Some cancers progress too quickly for a screening test to be of use. An aggressive cancer that kills a patient in a few months is unlikely to be detected on a screening test early enough that it can be effectively treated. Other cancers progress very slowly, and most people will die of another disease before the cancer causes symptoms. For example, most elderly men die with prostate cancer, not of prostate cancer. Detecting these indolent cancers leads to overdiagnosis and overtreatment. As such, screening tests are only valuable for those cancers that progress at an intermediate rate. Such cancers can be detected in a pre-symptomatic state *and* will eventually cause symptoms in most patients (Fig. 25.1).

Moreover, only certain patients are reasonable candidates for screening tests. Elderly people, or those very ill with other diseases, are much more likely to die before a screen-detected cancer can become symptomatic. By some estimates, it takes nearly a decade before the benefits of screening tests can be seen. As Cary Gross, an internist, said, "In patients well into their 80s, with other chronic conditions, it's highly unlikely that they will receive any benefit from screening, and more likely that the harms will outweigh the benefits" [2]. Despite this, many older people still receive screening tests. According to one study, more than half of men at high-risk to die over the next decade received a prostate specific antigen (PSA) test [3]. The study also found that people with short life expectancies also received screening for breast, cervical, and colorectal cancers. Another study found that 18%

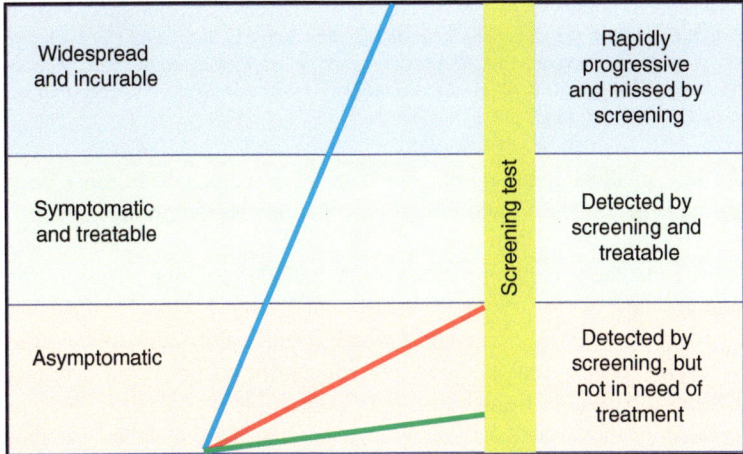

Fig. 25.1 The blue line represents a rapidly progressive cancer that will be missed by a screening test. The red line represents a soon-to-be symptomatic cancer that will be detected by a screening test. The green line represents a harmless cancer that will be detected by a screening test. Only those cancers represented by the red line will be improved by screening tests

of women with severe cognitive impairment who were older than the age of 70 years received regular mammograms, though the test is highly unlikely to benefit them [4].

While well-intentioned and intuitively appealing, the common-sense notion that "earlier is better" when it comes to cancer detection has often not been borne out by the evidence. Screening tests that were universally recommended only a few years ago have been scaled back or even abandoned in the face of evidence they do more harm than good.

For example, in 2009 the US Preventive Services Task Force (USPSTF) revised its guidelines to suggest that annual mammography begin at age 50, not 40, and that they be done every other year, not annually [5]. Additionally, breast self-examination is actively discouraged. In 2014, the results of The Canadian National Breast Screening Study were published supporting this change [6]. This study, which began in 1980, tracked nearly 90,000 women ages 40–59 years old over a 25-year period. The women were divided into two groups. One received an annual mammogram for five years and the other did not. The study found that the death rates from breast cancer were essentially the same for both groups. It also found that 22% of the women who had breast cancer diagnosed via mammogram were overdiagnosed. This means they had been diagnosed with a breast cancer that never would have caused symptoms had it remained undetected. These women were nonetheless treated with surgery, chemotherapy, and radiation.

More dramatically, in 2012, the USPSTF gave a strong recommendation against the use of the PSA test to screen for prostate cancer [7]. Previously, the PSA test had been recommended as an annual test for millions of American men. Richard Ablin, who discovered PSA, laid out the case against this test by writing:

Men lucky enough to reach old age are much more likely to die with prostate cancer than to die of it. Even then, the test is hardly more effective than a coin toss. As I've been trying to make clear for many years now, PSA testing can't detect prostate cancer and, more important, it can't distinguish between the two types of prostate cancer — the one that will kill you and the one that won't [8].

Like any medical intervention, the risks of screening tests must be weighed against the benefits. Harms and limitations of screening programs include:

- Harms from the screening process itself include radiation exposure, pain, and anxiety.
- Screening tests have the potential for both overdiagnosis and misdiagnosis, turning healthy people into patients. Overdiagnosis occurs when a test correctly identifies a "disease," though one that never would have caused problems if left untreated in the expected lifetime of a patient. This is called pseudodisease. Misdiagnosis occurs when a test is misread or an incidental finding is interpreted as pathological. False positive results can set off a cascade of further diagnostic tests and treatments that have the potential to harm and are unnecessary in retrospect. The treatment for prostate cancer, for example, commonly causes incontinence and urinary dysfunction. Rarely, it can kill patients. Overdiagnosis and misdiagnosis are not uncommon. By some estimates two-thirds of prostate cancers and one-third of breast cancers are overdiagnosed [9a, b].
- False negative results may give false comfort and delay the final diagnosis.
- Performing tests when the majority of people do not have the disease is costly and time consuming. In 2009, for example, $20 billion dollars were spent on prostate and breast cancer screening [10].

Several biases may predispose clinicians into thinking that screening tests are beneficial, though often they are not. Suppose, for example, that men who were diagnosed with prostate cancer after having a PSA as a screening test lived seven years after their diagnosis. In contrast, men with prostate cancer who had not undergone PSA screening and presented due to clinical symptoms lived only two years after the diagnosis of their cancer. Similarly, suppose a group of women underwent mammography, and the majority of these women who were then diagnosed with breast cancer were still alive after five years. In contrast, another group of women with breast cancer did not undergo mammography, and a minority of them were still alive after five years. It seems like these screening tests are of enormous value, allowing for earlier diagnosis and earlier treatment of the cancer. But several biases show that this is not necessarily the case.

Lead Time Bias Lead time is the amount of time between when a disease is detected using a screening test and when it normally becomes clinically apparent. It can make screening tests seem more effective than they actually are. If a man is diagnosed with prostate cancer based on screening at age 55 and dies as age 62, he has survived seven years with the disease. In contrast, a man who develops symptoms of prostate cancer at age 60 and dies at age 62 has survived only two years with the disease. It is true that the man whose cancer was diagnosed with screening survived with the cancer five years longer than the man who did not get screened. However, the test did not prolong his life at all, as both men died at age 62. As such, the screening test increases survival rates, but not mortality rates. In fact, the 55-year-old man lived for an extra five years with the potentially burdensome knowledge and may have endured treatments with highly unpleasant side effects that did not prolong his life. The patient, unaware of the lead time bias, may nonetheless feel that the screening test has granted him extra years of life compared to the man who did not get screened (Fig. 25.2).

Length Bias The length bias occurs because screening tests are more likely to detect slowly-progressing cancers, which have a relatively favorable prognosis. The probability that a screening test will detect a pre-symptomatic cancer is inversely proportional to its rate of progression. A highly aggressive cancer, which kills someone in several months is very unlikely to be detected by a screening test. In contrast, a cancer that progresses over the course of many years is highly likely to be detected. As such, screening may not cause cancers to be less dangerous, rather less dangerous cancers are more likely to be detected by screening. This again gives the illusion that screening prolongs survival. The ideal screening test will detect cancers that grow slowly enough to be detected, but rapidly enough so that they would cause symptoms if left untreated (Fig. 25.3).

Fig. 25.2 Because of the lead time bias, the screened patient survives longer with cancer than the unscreened patient. Yet, both die at the same age

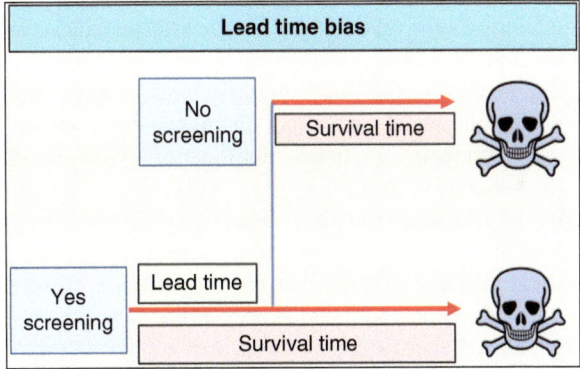

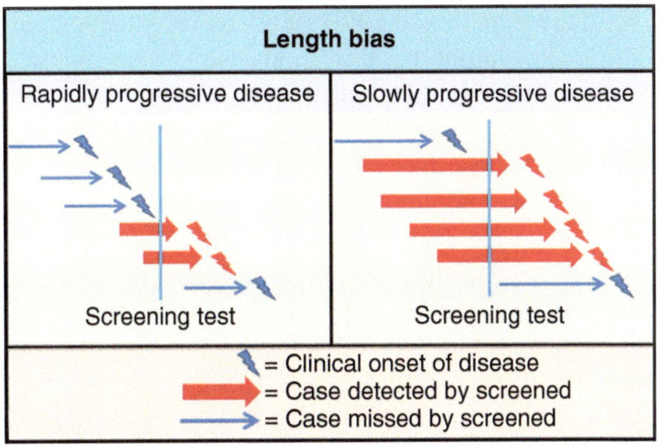

Fig. 25.3 Because of the length bias, slowly progressive cancers are much more likely to be detected than rapidly progressive cancers. Out of 12 cancers, the screening test below will detect 6

Fig. 25.4 Because of overdiagnosis, people falsely labeled with a lethal cancer increase the survival time in the screened group

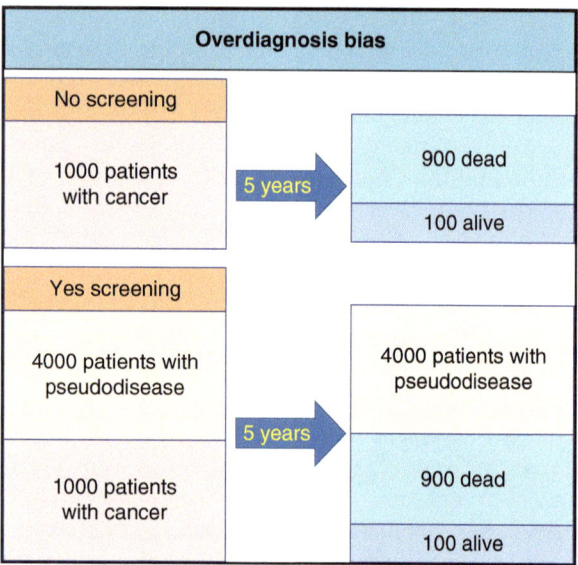

Overdiagnosis In addition to detecting potentially fatal cases of cancer, screening tests also detect pseudodisease, which refers to a sliect "disease" that would not present in a patient's lifetime. Once a screening program has begun, the incidence of cancer will naturally increase. As a result of pseudodisease, there is an overestimation of survival time among screen-detected cases. For example, consider a cancer that has a benign form and a lethal form that kills 90% of people after five years. The benign form is four-times as common as the lethal form. A screening test can detect this cancer, but cannot distinguish between the benign and lethal forms.

If a screening test detected this cancer in 5,000 people, 1,000 of them would have the lethal form. After five years, 4,1000 (82%) people in the screened group would be alive. In contrast, only 100 out of 1,000 (10%) unscreened patients with the lethal form of the cancer would be alive after five years. A naïve statistician could use these numbers to claim that screened patients survived at an eight-fold higher rate than unscreened patients. However, the fact that survival is dramatically improved in the screened group is an artifact of the screening test failing to discriminate between benign and lethal cancers. In each group, 90% of people with the lethal form die from it, and 100% of people with the benign form are still alive. The main difference might be that thousands of people with a benign cancer received "treatment" they didn't need (Fig. 25.4).

A real-life example of this occurred after South Korea instituted a screening program for thyroid cancer in 1999. In 2011, over 40,000 new cases of thyroid cancer were diagnosed, which is about 100 times greater than the number of people who die of the disease [11]. This represented a 15-fold increase from 1993, and it quickly became the most prevalent cancer in South Korea. However, when mortality from thyroid cancer was studied, the program turned out not to have made any

Fig. 25.5 Because of selection bias, people at risk for a disease may be more eager to participate in a screening program

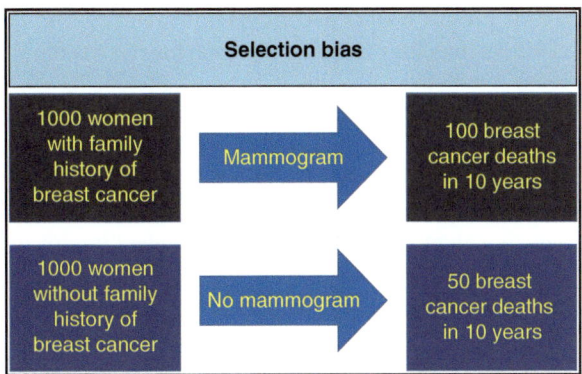

difference at all, though tens of thousands of people were treated for it. Moreover, complications from the surgery were not rare, with 11% developing hypoparathyroidism and 2% developing vocal-cord paralysis. In March 2014, eight physicians from South Korea formed the Physician Coalition for Prevention of Overdiagnosis of Thyroid Cancer, and within several months, there was a large decline of 35% in the number of thyroid surgeries performed [12].

Selection Bias The selection bias occurs because participants in screening programs are unlikely to be representative of the general population. They may be less healthy than the general population, thus underestimating the value of the screening test. For example, if women with a strong family history of breast cancer were more likely to participate in a mammography program, the screened group would likely have worse outcomes. This would make the screening test appear less effective than if it were applied to the general population (Fig. 25.5).

Conversely, when participants in a screening program are healthier than the general population, the value of the screening test will be overestimated. People who care little for their own health are unlikely to be motivated to participate in a screening program. In contrast, people who care greatly for their health maybe eager to do so. Rather than keeping people healthy, a screening program may select for healthy people.

Will Rogers Phenomenon
Will Rogers is reported to have said, "When the Okies left Oklahoma and moved to California, they raised the average intelligence level in both states." The Will Rogers phenomenon occurs when an element is moved from one category to another and the following is true:

- The moved element is less than the average for the group it is leaving. Removing it will therefore increase the average of the starting group.
- The moved element is greater than the average of the group it is entering. Adding it to the new group will increase its average.

As a result of the Will Rogers phenomenon, screening tests may appear more effective than they actually are. Imagine, for example, a group of students in classroom A with the following test scores: 56, 65, 76, 89, 90. The average for class A is 75.2. Another group of students in class B had the following test scores: 23, 34, 45, 46. The average for class B is 37. Now, suppose the student who scored 56 is moved from class A to class B. The average score for classroom A increases to 80, and the average score for class B increases to 40.8. Both classes have improved their average, though obviously no individual student improved their score.

The same can occur with cancer screening. When a screening test detects cancer in asymptomatic people, they are moved from the "healthy" group to the "ill" group. Because they do have some form of cancer, removing them for the "healthy" group increases the life expectancy of the group. Yet, because they have an early, asymptomatic case of cancer, they are healthier than the "ill" group. Therefore, the life expectancy of the "ill" group is raised as well. This is similar to moving the student from classroom A to classroom B. As the lifespans of both the "healthy" and "ill" groups are both increased, this can make a screening program appear to be beneficial, even when detecting the cancer early does not actually allow any individual to live longer.

What to Do?
Whether or not a given screening program is effective at preventing suffering and saving lives can only be determined with rigorous scientific studies where the above biases are accounted for. Even then, the question of which screening tests are beneficial in which populations can be incredible difficult to answer. Different clinicians looking at the same raw data can come to different conclusions. Indeed, after the USPSTF recommendation against PSA screening, many clinicians believed the pendulum had swung too far in the opposite direction. The number of men diagnosed with prostate cancer in the US decreased from 213,562 in 2011 to 180,043 in 2012. By some estimates, this will lead to an increase of 1,241 deaths from prostate cancer [13].

Clearly, there is often not a one-size-fits-all approach for which screening tests are valuable in which patients. Imagine a woman considering mammography. Based on her age and family history, there is a 1% chance the mammogram will detect a cancer, which left untreated will claim her life. However, there is a 10% chance an indolent cancer will be found that will not cause her any symptoms if left untreated. As there is no way to distinguish between lethal and harmless cancers, they all will be treated with surgery, radiation, and medications. Should the woman get this mammogram? There is no single, right answer. Clinicians should do their best to provide patients with information so that they can make a decision that best fits with their values and preferences.

Note that criticisms of screening tests, which are very common amongst practitioners of complementary and alternative medicine (CAM), can be easy to make in retrospect, once the results of large studies are known. When a study in the *New England Journal of Medicine* concluded that mammograms had only a "small effect on the rate of death from breast cancer," CAM advocates celebrated this conclusion [14]. Mike Adams, founder of the website Natural News, wrote a typical CAM-style essay titled *Shock Study: Mammograms A Medical Hoax, Over One Million American Women Maimed By Unnecessary 'Treatment' For Cancer They Never Had* [15]. It stated:

> *Mammography is a cruel medical hoax. As I have described here on Natural News many times, the primary purpose of mammography is not to "save" women from cancer, but to recruit women into false positives that scare them into expensive, toxic treatments like chemotherapy, radiation and surgery.*
> *The "dirty little secret" of the cancer industry is that the very same oncologists who scare women into falsely believing they have breast cancer are also the ones pocketing huge profits from selling those women chemotherapy drugs. The conflicts of interest and abandonment of ethics across the cancer industry is breathtaking.*

Similarly, Sayer Ji, founder of the website Greenmedinfo, wrote an essay titled *30 Years of Breast Screening: 1.3 Million Wrongly Treated* [16]. Had large studies come to the conclusion that screening tests save more lives than clinicians thought, it would be easy to criticize mainstream medicine for undervaluing them and failing to treat cancers while they were in their earliest stages. Let's be clear, many screening tests, including mammograms, certainly do save lives. Due to a combination of better treatments and screening programs, a study by Carol Desantis and colleagues found that deaths from breast cancer fell almost 40% between 1989 and 2015, equating to 322,600 lives saved in the US [17].

Moreover, CAM practitioners often advocate for dubious screening tests that have the potential for all of the same errors as those suggested by mainstream medicine. For example, digital infrared thermal imaging, better known as thermography, is a technique that measures differences in body temperature as a means of cancer screening. In an article extolling its benefits, CAM practitioner Christiane Northrup correctly discussed the potential of mammograms to lead to overdiagnosis and overtreatment. However, she then proceeded to suggest thermography because it is supposedly more *sensitive* than mammography, writing, "The most promising aspect of thermography is its ability to spot anomalies years before mammography" [18]. Similarly, an article on greenmedinfo.com declared that:

> *Thermography offers the opportunity for much earlier breast disease detection than is possible through self-examination, doctor examination or mammography alone because the procedure can detect the subtlest of physiologic changes that accompany breast pathology, whether it is cancer, fibrocystic disease, an infection or a vascular disease* [19].

While the potential for mammograms to lead to overtreatment is correctly lamented, the issue is not considered with a test deemed more powerful than mammography. As is usually the case, CAM practitioners embrace tests that conventional medicine rejects, primarily because conventional medicine rejects them. Indeed, formal studies of thermography have found it is not clinically useful as a screening test for breast cancer [20].

Conclusion

While it "makes sense" that detecting a cancer earlier will lead to better outcomes, this intuitive belief is often wrong. Several biases may make screening programs more effective than they actually are. Screening tests come with the potential to harm patients, and these harms must be balanced against the benefits.

Patient advocacy groups, medical societies, and governmental agencies have long promoted screening as a necessary tool in the fight against cancer and are often resistant to suggestions that screening tests may be useless or even harmful. In contrast, CAM practitioners profit by spreading fear and doubt about screening tests.

Well-designed scientific studies can best assess the benefits and risks of screening tests. However, just like there is no "right" amount of money we all should save for retirement, different people can come to different conclusions about the value of same screening test.

References

1. Wilson JMG, Jungner G. (1968). Principles and practices of screening for disease. World Health Organization: Institute Repository for Information Sharing. Retrieved from http://www.who.int/iris/handle/10665/37650.
2. Szabo L. (2017, Dec 19). Too many older patients get cancer screenings. The New York Times. https://www.nytimes.com/2017/12/19/well/live/cancer-screening-tests-seniors-older-patients-harms-overdiagnosis-overtreatment.html.
3. Royce TJ, Hendrix LH, Stokes WA, Allen IM, Chen RC. Cancer screening rates in individuals with different life expectancies. JAMA Intern Med. 2017;174(10):1558–65. https://doi.org/10.1001/jamainternmed.2014.3895.
4. Mehta KM, Zung KZ, Kistler CE, Chang A, Walter LC. Impact of cognitive impairment on screening mammography use in older US women. Am J Public Health. 2010;100(10):1917–23. https://doi.org/10.2105/AJPH.2008.158485.
5. U.S. Preventative Services Task Force. (2013). Final recommendation statement: breast cancer: screening [Archived version]. Retrieved from https://www.uspreventiveservicestaskforce.org/Page/Document/RecommendationStatementFinal/breast-cancer-screening.
6. Miller AB, Wall C, Baines CJ, Sun P, To T, Narod SA. Twenty five year follow-up for breast cancer incidence and mortality of the Canadian National Breast Screening Study: randomised screening trial. BMJ. 2014;348:g366. https://doi.org/10.1136/bmj.g366.
7. U.S. Preventative Services Task Force. (2013). Final recommendation statement: prostate cancer: screening [Archived version]. Retrieved from https://www.uspreventiveservicestaskforce.org/Page/Document/RecommendationStatementFinal/prostate-cancer-screening.
8. Ablin RJ. (2010, May 10). The great prostate mistake. The New York Times. Retrieved from https://www.nytimes.com/2010/03/10/opinion/10Ablin.html.
9a. Loeb S, Bjurlin MA, Nicholson J, Tammela TL, Penson DF, Carter HB, Carroll P, Etzioni R. Overdiagnosis and overtreatment of prostate cancer. Eur Urol. 2014;65(6):1046–55. https://doi.org/10.1016/j.eururo.2013.12.062.
9b. Jørgensen KJ, Gøtzsche PC, Kalager M, Zahl P. Breast cancer screening in Denmark: a cohort study of tumor size and overdiagnosis. Ann Intern Med. 2017;166(5):313–23. https://doi.org/10.7326/M16-0270.
10. Esserman L, Shieh Y, Thompson I. Rethinking screening for breast cancer and prostate cancer. JAMA. 2009;302(15):1685–92. https://doi.org/10.1001/jama.2009.1498.
11. Ahn HS, Kim HJ, Welch HG. Korea's thyroid-cancer "epidemic" – screening and overdiagnosis. N Engl J Med. 2014;371(19):1765–7. https://doi.org/10.1056/NEJMp1409841.

12. Ahn HS, Welch HG. South Korea's thyroid-cancer "epidemic" – turning the tide. N Engl J Med. 2015;373(24):2389–90. https://doi.org/10.1056/NEJMc1507622.
13. Penson DF. The pendulum of prostate cancer screening. JAMA. 2015;314(19):2031–3. https://doi.org/10.1001/jama.2015.13775.
14. Bleyer A, Welch HG. Effect of three decades of screening mammography on breast-cancer incidence. N Engl J Med. 2012;367(21):1998–2005. https://doi.org/10.1056/NEJMoa1206809.
15. Adams M. (2012, Nov 27). Shock study: mammograms a medical hoax, over one million American women maimed by unnecessary 'treatment' for cancer they never had. NaturalNews. https://www.naturalnews.com/038099_mammograms_false_positives_overdiagnosis.html#.
16. Ji S. (2012, Nov 22). 30 years of breast screening: 13 million wrongly treated. GreenMedInfo. Retrieved from http://www.greenmedinfo.com/blog/30-years-breast-screening-13-million-wrongly-treated.
17. DeSantis CE, Ma J, Goding Sauer A, Newman LA, Jemal A. Breast cancer statistics, 2017, racial disparity in mortality by state. CA Cancer J Clin. 2017;64:439–48. https://doi.org/10.3322/caac.21412.
18. Northrup C. (2017, Oct 9). The best breast cancer screening tests: 5 more reasons not to get a mammogram. ChristianeNorthrupMD. Retrieved from https://www.drnorthrup.com/best-breast-cancer-screening-tests/.
19. Desaulniers V. (2015, Mar 21). Thermography is key for early detection of breast cancer. GreenMedInfo. Retrieved from http://www.greenmedinfo.com/blog/thermography-key-early-detection-breast-cancer.
20. Kontos M, Wilson R, Fentiman I. Digital infrared thermal imaging (DITI) of breast lesions: sensitivity and specificity of detection of primary breast cancers. Clin Radiol. 2011;66(6):536–9. https://doi.org/10.1016/j.crad.2011.01.009.

Selection Bias and Endowment Effect

Case

Natalie was a 26-year-old woman who suffered from depression. She was not sui-cidal and was still able to go to work. However, she was tired much of the time and found little joy in activities she formerly found pleasurable. She wanted to treat her condition "naturally," and found a practitioner of holistic medicine whose blogs she admired. She wrote to the doctor and was sent a long questionnaire, shown below, about her symptoms, beliefs, and willingness to change her lifestyle.

Introduction

Consultations are $4,497 which includes a two-hour consultation *and* a one-hour follow-up. Follow-ups thereafter are $570 for 45 minutes. Dr. Woo typically orders extensive blood work, which is usually covered by insurance. In addition, he may ask you complete a stool and saliva test, which ranges between $100 and $400 each, and are not typically eligible for reimbursement from insurance. As part of your comprehensive plan, Dr. Woo may recommend a monthly supplement regimen. Cost of supplements is not included in the session fee and are purchased through an outside vendor.

Application Steps

Step 1

Are you familiar with Dr. Woo's blog? Have you read his book, *Owning Your Mind?* It is highly recommended that you take some time to read both to fully understand his approach to psychiatric treatment and general wellness. Many of your questions regarding his experience treating specific conditions can be answered there.

© Springer International Publishing AG, part of Springer Nature 2019   457
J. Howard, *Cognitive Errors and Diagnostic Mistakes*,
https://doi.org/10.1007/978-3-319-93224-8_26

Step 2

Please fill out the following questionnaire and email it back to our office.

1. What is your age?
2. What are you seeking help with? Please provide details.
3. Have you ever been hospitalized for these issues?
4. Are you interested in tapering psychiatric medication?
5. Do you have any fear around tapering your medication?
6. Have you already tapered medication or attempting to taper? If so, are you experiencing withdrawal symptoms? What are the symptoms?
7. Please list your past and current medications, including duration of treatment. Please indicate which medications you are currently taking.
8. In Dr. Woo's consideration of all applications, it's important that he feels patients share his beliefs not just about psychiatric medications, but all pharmaceutical products, including vaccines, antibiotics, birth control, and over the counter products. Please take some time to read this article, "How to Live Without Medications" and tell us about how you share this belief.
9. Have you read his blog and book, *Owning Your Mind*? Have you completed the 30-day program in his book?
10. Do you believe that pharmaceutical medication is necessary in your treatment?
11. Do you have diagnosed medical problems? Please list them.
12. Have you consulted with a functional medicine/holistic provider about these issues?
13. Why are you seeking a holistic approach to your mental health and wellness? Please provide details.
14. Do you plan to continue seeing any conventional doctors while a patient?
15. Please discuss your motivation for achieving optimal wellness with this treatment. Are you currently ready to begin implementing radical lifestyle and dietary changes?
16. Dr. Woo requires that all patients eliminate gluten and dairy from their diet after the first consultation. Are you willing to eliminate both without exceptions?
17. Generally describe your daily diet including meals, snacks, and beverages.
18. Do you eat red meat? There is no vegetarian or vegan version of this diet, so consuming red meat will be a requirement.
19. Dr. Woo may recommend that patients personally perform daily coffee enemas. If this is recommended to you, it would be required in your treatment. If you are not familiar with this detox protocol, please take a moment to learn more about it from his website. Are you willing to do this yourself?
20. Do you have a spiritual practice? Do you meditate, sit, pray?
21. Who is a part of your support system? Are your parents, siblings, or partner supportive of your choice for this type of treatment?
22. How much do you believe that pharmaceutical products are necessary for daily issues like headaches, reflux, cramps? For acute issues? For emergencies? Do you get flu shots?

23. Do you give pharmaceutical products to your children, including vaccinations?
24. Are you willing/able to take dietary supplements when indicated?
25. Are you available for monthly follow-ups in the first 6 months of treatment?
26. Are you able to pay for your own sessions or will someone else be covering the cost? Are you able to pay for the monthly cost of supplements recommended by Dr. Woo?
27. All patient communication, appointment scheduling and appointment summaries can be done on our online patient portal. Will you be able to access this on a computer?
28. What is your phone number?
29. Please confirm that you have reviewed our fee structure as noted above in this email. Our fees are subject to change and may have already changed if you were asked to fill out an updated application after a prior request. The fee quoted above in this message is guaranteed for your session.
30. If your application is initially accepted, the next step involves scheduling a brief call with office staff before Dr. Woo's final review. Due to such a high volume of application submissions, kindly note that we are only able to schedule calls with those who are ready to begin as a patient in the next few weeks. If you still need to confirm insurance coverage, we ask that this is done prior to this call. Thank you.

Natalie received an appointment twelve weeks later. After her initial consultation, she was advised to stop eating gluten, dairy, sugar, and genetically modified foods. She was advised to avoid all pharmaceutical products, including vaccines. Lab work, which cost $350, was also ordered during the initial visit. On her second visit, she was told to drink turmeric tea twice daily and start each morning with a coffee enema to remove "toxins." She was started on a supplement regimen based on her lab results, which cost $440 per month. She also started meditating for at least one hour every morning. After four weeks, Natalie reported feeling more energetic, and she began volunteering at an animal shelter again. With her permission, Dr. Woo posted Natalie's success story on social media to market his treatment and book.

What Dr. Woo Was Thinking
I purposefully run a selective clinic. Patients have to fill out an application before their first visit. I have to make sure that the patient can adhere to my protocol, and obviously they have to feel that the treatment is right for them. I estimate I reject almost half of the patients who apply to see me. I can tell from the application process that some patients just aren't ready to make the changes I require, and I wouldn't be doing them any favors by seeing them. I know my protocol isn't easy, and I want patients to be really dedicated to making profound changes in their lives. An initial consultation with me lasts two hours and I take a very detailed history of the patient's symptoms and current lifestyle. I also perform a complete laboratory evaluation, including stool samples. I realize my protocol is not easy to follow, and not everyone is ready to make the necessary changes in their lives. However, for those who are ready to make real changes, the treatment is highly effective.

Discussion

The selection bias refers to a situation where individuals select themselves into a group, thus creating an unrepresentative sample of the general population. It is most commonly encountered in clinical research where it confounds study results by creating unequal comparisons between two groups. For example, if an observational study found that people who exercise regularly are less depressed, it would be inappropriate to then conclude that exercise prevents depression. Other possible explanations are that depression prevents people from being able to exercise in the first place or that some people have a condition that both causes depression and prevents them from exercising. Only a study where some subjects are randomized to an exercise regimen while others are not could accurately determine the relationship between exercise and depression. The selection bias affects clinicians as well, because patients chose their clinicians and, to varying degrees, clinicians chose their patients. It can be considered a variant of the availability bias that occurs because clinicians are only aware of patients who seek medical attention from them.

To see how the selection bias might mislead a clinician, consider a woman who develops a mild case of optic neuritis, a condition characterized by visual loss and eye pain. Most patients recover well, though it is often the first symptom of multiple sclerosis (MS). Let's pretend our patient attributes her optic neuritis to "eye strain," does not seek medical attention and recovers in a few days. If nothing happens to her again, a neurologist like me will never know this patient existed. In contrast, patients with optic neuritis who have other symptoms suggestive of MS are much more likely to seek further care. Having primarily encountered those patients who return with a second attack, it may be easy for me to have an overly negative perspective on the overall prognosis of isolated optic neuritis. On the other end of the spectrum, homecare nurses have told me about a large number of bedbound patients with MS who can only leave their house with great difficulty. Sadly, there is little for a neurologist to do in these cases. Since few of these patients come to my office, there is a large group of patients with devastating disease, to whose existence I am largely blind.

The selection bias occurs not only because patients chose when to seek treatment, but also because, to varying degrees, clinicians choose which patients they will see. The more a clinician screens potential patients, the more likely they are to be affected by the selection bias. Clinicians who charge expensive fees will never see poor patients. Clinicians with a long wait time will never see acutely ill patients. Clinicians who offer alternative treatments will see only patients who are highly predisposed to believe in their efficacy. Clinicians who work in ERs are likely to only see patients whose treatments are *not* working. For example, a patient with epilepsy whose seizures are well-controlled is unlikely to go the ER.

A psychiatrist like the one in the case, who only sees highly screened patients, in a cash-only, outpatient practice with a long waiting list, will be shielded from treating floridly psychotic patients or those who are imminently suicidal. The questionnaire in this case (which is from an actual psychiatrist) basically guarantees that no patient with major depression will ever make it through the screening process. Patients with major depression barely have the energy to get out of bed, much less

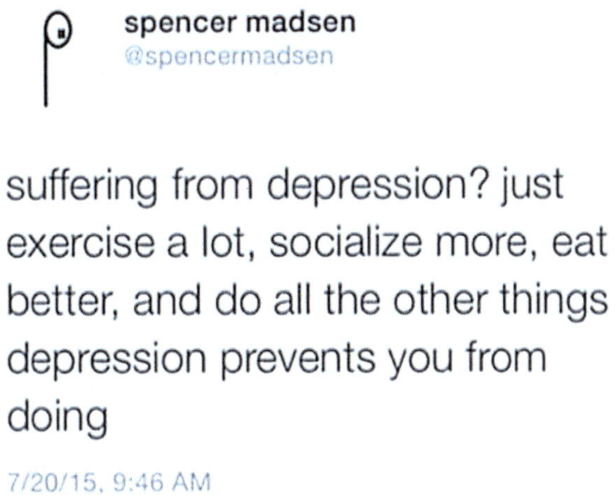

Fig. 26.1 The problem with treating depression with treatments depressed people can't do. (Spencer madsen. Suffering from depression? Just exercise a lot, socialize more, eat, better, and do [Twitter moment]. 2015. Retrieved from https://twitter.com/spencermadsen.)

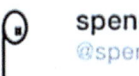

spencer madsen
@spencermadsen

suffering from depression? just exercise a lot, socialize more, eat better, and do all the other things depression prevents you from doing

7/20/15, 9:46 AM

commit to meditation, daily coffee enemas, and "radical lifestyle and dietary changes." Many depressed patients would find it difficult even fill out this survey. As the nature of his practice shields him from this population, he may develop a distorted perception of psychiatric illnesses. While wealth does not protect against mental illness, a psychiatrist who charges $4,497 for an initial visit will not treat patients dealing with the stressors that accompany poverty (Fig. 26.1).

Furthermore, as a result of this thorough screening process, the psychiatrist is guaranteed to encounter only patients who are philosophically inclined to believe in the efficacy of his treatments. A patient who scoffs at the notion of coffee enemas to cure his depression will not pass the screening process. This creates a highly biased sample, and will distort the psychiatrist's ability to objectively evaluate the efficacy of his treatments. If this psychiatrist boasts about the efficacy of his treatment for depression, it is likely because no one who passed the screening process was suffering from major depression in the first place. I suspect that if the psychiatrist required patients to perform almost *any* task that required a significant amount of energy, time, and devotion, the results would be the same; patients with mild depression would eventually feel better, while people with severe depression would never be able to start treatment.

The selection bias is one of the many reasons why the efficacy of treatments can only be properly judged through formal clinical trials, not selected anecdotes from "highly satisfied" patients. Importantly, a similar bias can affect clinical research, where it is called the healthy user bias. It occurs as the type of person that generally agrees to participate in medical research is often not representative of the general population. Study subjects are generally healthier and motivated to take the advice of clinicians, thus limiting the generalizability of some clinical studies.

Psychiatrist Kelly Brogan, who uses coffee enemas and other unscientific methods to treat mental illnesses, actually boasts that she screens for patients who she thinks will respond to her treatments. In an essay entitle "Holistic Medicine: Do You Believe?" she wrote, "I do a preliminary assessment to establish how willing a given patient is to shed their fear. And how much faith they bring to the healing process, to the unpredictability and complexity of their journey, and to their intuition" [1]. When asked in an interview if her dietary changes for psychiatric disorders ever failed, she replied, "Not in a long time, because I screen for readiness. I screen for a mindset. If you are ready, and you believe that a whole radical next chapter in your life is forthcoming, then I'm just part of the ritual." She went on to say, "If you don't believe that this is going to do anything for you and you're a skeptic, it won't" [2]. There is a grain of truth in this, of course. There is evidence that, for some conditions, a patient's expectation of a treatment's value will influence its success. However, this is certainly not the case for many conditions, and if it were, all treatments of children, demented patients, or unconscious patients would be futile.

Let's consider the results I might achieve if I screened my patients similarly to the psychiatrist in this chapter. I could be the most successful neurologist in history (at least in my own mind). This is because I have developed the Howard Protocol™ to treat MS. The core principle of the Howard Protocol™ is simple; patients have to jog one mile per day, eat gluten and genetically modified foods, and make sure they are up-to-date on their vaccines. I realize that the Howard Protocol™ is not for everyone, but I guarantee that any MS patient who adheres to the Howard Protocol™ will never need a wheelchair or even a cane! If you go to my website, you'll find multiple testimonials of people who swear the Howard Protocol™ worked for them. Most of them were able to completely stop their medications. Before a patient gets an appointment with me, they have to show their willingness to shed their fear by adhering to my protocol for one month. While this means I have to turn some patients away, my treatment would not work for them anyway; they are simply not ready for it.

So, have I discovered the cure for MS? Will I get a Nobel Prize? Of course not. Similar to Dr. Woo's screening questions in the case, my "protocol" screens out patients with enough disability to prevent them from jogging a mile. This leaves only the healthiest patients as my "success stories." I suspect that the selection bias largely accounts for the genuine belief many practitioners of complementary and alternative medicine (CAM) have in their treatments. They screen out patients who are unlikely to respond and primarily accept patients who are likely to improve.

The selection bias affects patients as well. Patient reports of a treatment's efficacy are likely to be positively influenced by treatments that require a great deal of cost, both in terms of money and lifestyle modifications. Patients who have to undergo a rigorous selection process are likely to judge the treatment more favorably than treatments that require minimal effort to obtain. The notion that a difficult initiation process leads to greater liking was first described by Eliot Aronson and Judson Mills [3]. In their study, subjects were randomly assigned to three initiation scenarios; mild, medium, and severe. They found that subjects who underwent a severe initiation to join a group perceived it as being significantly more attractive than did those who underwent a mild initiation or no initiation at all. Their work has

Fig. 26.2 An American soldier being hazed, 1904. (Unknown. American soldier being hazed by being thrown high in the air [Image file]. In: Wikimedia commons. 1904. Retrieved from https://commons.wikimedia.org/wiki/File:Soldier_being_initiated_(1904).jpg.)

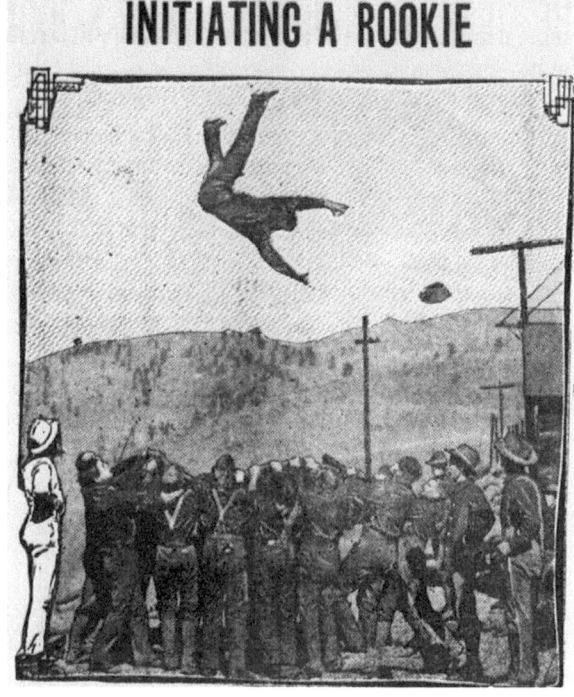

been replicated and is known as the "suffering-leading-to-liking" phenomenon [4]. It posits that the more a person suffers to obtain something, the more they will value it. The suffering-leading-to-liking phenomenon is the basis behind group initiations and rites of passage. It explains why hazing is common in fraternities/sororities, military units, sports teams, and gangs. It helps build group solidary and cohesion. Powerful initiation rites can partially explain why soldiers bond together strongly enough to kill and die for one another (Fig. 26.2).

Additionally, the price of a treatment alone may bias patients. Research has shown that, in the absence of other indicators, people use the price of an item as a measure of its value, though there is usually a poor correlation between the price of an item and objective measures of its quality [5]. Donald Lichtenstein and Scot Burton showed that consumers commonly perceive the association between price and quality to be higher than it actually is [6]. For example, people drinking wine enjoy it more if they believe they are drinking an expensive vintage [6]. Pranksters at a food convention can get experts to gush over food from McDonald's, as long as it is arranged properly and they are led to believe it is organic [7].

Research has shown the association between cost and perceived quality can specifically affect patients' perceptions of medical treatments. Alberto Epsay and colleagues conducted a study of 12 patients with moderately advanced Parkinson's disease who were told that they were being given one of two treatments that were identical except for a manufacturing difference, which made one treatment 15 times more expensive than the other. Though both pills were placebo, the response to the more "expensive" placebo was slightly more robust compared to the cheap pill, leading the authors to conclude that, "perception of cost is capable of influencing motor function and brain activation in Parkinson disease" [8]. In a similar study, Dan Ariely and colleagues gave a light electric shock to 82 study subjects [9]. They rated their pain before and after getting a placebo medication for pain. Some subjects were told the medication was new and cost $2.50 per pill. Eighty-five percent of these subjects said the medication reduced the pain. The other subjects were told the medication cost 10 cents. At this low price, only 61% of patients said the pain was diminished. Before you consider yourself immune to this cognitive error, however, imagine whether or not you would feel comfortable going to a surgeon who boasted of the "lowest prices in town."

Another important concept related to the selection bias is a phenomenon known as the endowment effect, which posits that once someone has acquired an item, this ownership alone increases its value in their eyes. This is specifically the case for something that is difficult to obtain. Psychologist Daniel Ariely provided a demonstration of the endowment effect by studying students who had won tickets to an important basketball game at Duke University [10]. Winning such tickets requires luck, but only those who put forth substantial effort by camping out for days are eligible. He asked the winners how much they would be willing to sell their tickets for, and the average response was $2,400. He then asked the losers how much they would be willing to spend to buy tickets, and the average response was $175. Out of a hundred students, not one loser was willing to pay the price proposed by one winner. The winners imagined that the basketball game would be a once-in-a-lifetime experience and had a hard time putting a monetary value on this. The losers, meanwhile, imagined all the other things they could do with the money other than attend one basketball game.

A related concept is appropriately called the snob effect. This term describes the phenomenon of wealthy people valuing expensive objects precisely because they are expensive and unavailable to poor people. Certain items, such as designer clothes, fine wine, and "detox" retreats are status symbols that signal the owner is wealthy. The object itself may not outperform similar objects that cost substantially less money. For example, a Rolex watch that costs $30,000 does not tell time any better than a $20 watch. Economists call such objects Veblen goods. In contrast to most objects, Veblen goods become more desirable as the price increases, something that violates the normal law of supply and demand.

In many ways, patients who have made it through an arduous selection process to consult with an expensive, exclusive clinician are the like the winners of exclusive basketball tickets or the owners of a Rolex watch. Patients come to "own" their treatment the way they would an exclusive ticket or expensive object. They are likely to perceive costly, time-consuming treatments as valuable, precisely because they are expensive and time-consuming. A patient who pays large sums of money for a "detoxification" treatment at a "boutique" clinic is likely to be predisposed by that high fee alone to judge the treatment as powerful and successful. This is likely particularly to be the case for CAM treatments, which often require patients to the identity with the general worldview of the clinician.

Other biases, discussed in other chapters, are also likely to affect how patients who have undergone an arduous selection process perceive treatment efficacy. One of these is the sunk cost error, which is the tendency to continue a suboptimal course of action because substantial resources have already been devoted to it. Another is the choice-supportive bias, which is the tendency to recall positive attributes of a chosen option, while ascribing negative attributes to a rejected option.

Finally, it should be noted that it is appropriate for most clinicians to screen potential patients to some degree. If someone with a brain tumor wishes to consult with a Parkinson's disease specialist, it is eminently appropriate for that clinician to screen that patient and refer them to a neuro-oncologist.

Conclusion

Clinicians who heavily screen their patients should be aware that their selection process will skew their patient population and limit their ability to evaluate the natural history of the disease they treat and the efficacy of their treatments. Clinicians who screen out the most ill patients will necessarily be blind to the most challenging cases.

A rigorous selection process may also influence patients. In Mark Twain's novel, Tom Sawyer is made to whitewash a fence as punishment for skipping school. By pretending that this chore is in fact an honor, he cleverly persuades several friends not only to do the work, but to pay him for the privilege. As Twain wrote:

> Tom said to himself that it was not such a hollow world, after all. He had discovered a great law of human action, without knowing it – namely, that in order to make a man or a boy covet a thing, it is only necessary to make the thing difficult to attain [11].

Similarly, patients' perceptions of treatment efficacy are likely to be positively influenced by a rigorous selection process and high cost. This may lead to a feedback loop where clinicians who perform expensive, time-consuming, or invasive procedures are systematically mislead about their efficacy by the reports of their patients. As such, patient testimonials should be viewed with strong skepticism. The selection bias shows that only by studying treatments in large, randomized, blinded, controlled trials can the efficacy of a treatment truly be measured.

References

1. Brogan K. (n.d.). Holistic medicine: do you believe? Kelly Brogan MD. Retrieved 15 Sept 2018 from https://kellybroganmd.com/do-you-believe/.
2. Holiday J. (2017, July 19). Deconstructing Kelly Brogan ep. 3: medicine is religion [Video file]. Retrieved from https://www.youtube.com/watch?v=7o9RUtdTczM.
3. Aronson E, Mills J. The effect of severity of initiation on liking for a group [PDF file]. J Abnorm Soc Psychol. 1959;59(2):177. Retrieved from http://faculty.uncfsu.edu/tvancantfort/Syllabi/Gresearch/Readings/A_Aronson.pdf.
4. Gerard HB, Mathewson GC. The effects of severity of initiation on liking for a group: a replication. J Exp Soc Psychol. 1966;2(3):278–87. https://doi.org/10.1016/0022-1031(66)90084-9.
5. Boyle PJ, Lathrop ES. Are consumers' perceptions of price-quality relationships well calibrated? Int J Consum Stud. 2009;33(1):58–63. https://doi.org/10.1111/j.1470-6431.2008.00722.x.

6. Lichtenstein DR, Burton S. The relationship between perceived and objective price-quality. J Mark Res. 1989;26(4):429–43. https://doi.org/10.2307/3172763.

7. Anderson LV. (2014). What happens when you serve McDonald's to food snobs and tell them it's organic. SLATE. Retrieved from http://www.slate.com/blogs/browbeat/2014/10/23/mcdonald_s_organic_prank_for_foodies_two_dutch_pranksters_play_trick_at.html.

8. Espay AJ, Norris MM, Eliassen JC, Dwivedi A, Smith MS, Banks C, Allendorfer JB, Lang AE, Fleck DE, Linke MJ, Szaflarski JP. Placebo effect of medication cost in Parkinson disease. Neurology. 2015;10 https://doi.org/10.1212/WNL.0000000000001282.

9. Duke University. (2008, Mar 5). You get what you pay for? Costly placebo works better than cheap one. ScienceDaily. https://www.sciencedaily.com/releases/2008/03/080304173339.htm.

10. Kolbert E. (2008). What was I thinking? The New Yorker. Retrieved from https://www.newyorker.com/magazine/2008/02/25/what-was-i-thinking.

11. Duncan D, Ward GC (Writers), Burns K (Director). Mark Twain [Television series episode]. In: Duncan D, Burns K (Producers). American Lives. Walpole: Florentine Films; 2001

Case

Jane was 56-year-old woman who presented with fever, diarrhea, nausea, and abdominal pain several weeks after she completed several courses of antibiotics for a persistent upper respiratory infection. She was diagnosed with *Clostridium difficile (C. diff)* colitis, a bacterial infection that often occurs after the use of systemic antibiotics that alter normal bowel bacterial flora. It is typically treated with further antibiotics, however this treatment is not always effective, and Jane continued to have severe symptoms despite this treatment. She had read about an investigative treatment where feces from a healthy individual are placed in the colon of the infected patient to restore the balance of normal bacterial flora. Her gastroenterologist, Dr. Jordan, strongly advised her not do this treatment, saying there was no evidence it was effective and the person offering it to her was probably a "quack looking to make a quick buck." After suffering for three more months, Jane travelled to a different state to have the procedure done. Her symptoms vanished within one week.

What Dr. Jordan Was Thinking

I consider myself a pretty skeptical doctor. I resist trends and fads, especially those supposed "miracle cures your doctor doesn't want you to know about." Our knowledge of the microbiome—the immense number of microorganisms that live in and on our bodies—is a new science. I have no doubt that as our understanding of it increases, treatments will emerge. However, at present, the claim made by some—that "all health begins in the gut," and that various diets and "detoxes" can cure almost any disease—vastly outstrip the evidence to support this.

When Jane first told me that she had read on the internet about fecal transplantation for treatment-resistant *C. diff* infections, my skeptical radar went off immediately. It didn't make sense to me from a mechanistic standpoint, as if she had told me that counting backwards while eating blueberries was going to cure her. It seemed like she was about to give a large sum of money away to a quack. I view it is as my job to protect my patients, many of whom are desperate for a cure, against

© Springer International Publishing AG, part of Springer Nature 2019
J. Howard, *Cognitive Errors and Diagnostic Mistakes*,
https://doi.org/10.1007/978-3-319-93224-8_27

unscrupulous practitioners whose treatments may threaten their health and definitely threaten their wallets. When I read about fecal transplantation, I saw that there were a large number of testimonials on the internet, and those always make me very suspicious. And, in my defense, large studies confirming the benefits of fecal transplantation for *C. diff* infections still had not yet been done. So I was not wrong when I told her that it had not yet been tested.

However, I was wrong in dismissing the entire idea as completely implausible without at least reviewing the scientific literature on the subject thus far. Just because a lot of my "red flags" went up, this doesn't mean I should have dismissed the treatment right away. Fecal transplants are now the standard of care for patients with treatment-resistant *C. diff* infection, and they are effective in nearly 90% of patients for whom antibiotics have failed [1].

Discussion

The history of medicine is tragically filled with discoveries of great significance that were initially ridiculed and dismissed. The Semmelweis reflex is the tendency to reject new evidence or new knowledge because it contradicts established norms, beliefs, or scientific paradigms. It takes its name from the reaction of the medical community to the findings of Ignaz Semmelweiss (1818–1865), a Hungarian doctor who showed that handwashing dramatically reduced the incidence of a common and often fatal obstetrical infection known as puerperal fever.

Semmelweiss first noticed that women who gave birth attended by doctors and medical students died nearly five times more often than women attended by midwives. After some failed attempts to explain this finding, he considered that perhaps one difference between the groups was that doctors and medical students performed autopsies, often of women who had recently died of puerperal fever, prior to delivering babies. In contrast, midwives did not perform autopsies. Although he knew nothing of germ theory, he reasoned that some "morbid poison" was being spread from the dead women to the living via the medical staff. He subsequently instructed staff members to wash their hands and equipment with a chlorine solution. The result was a near complete elimination of puerperal fever.

Instead of being lauded as a hero, he was dismissed as a quack. His ideas contradicted established scientific and medical thought of the time, which was still dominated by the ancient notion of diseases being caused by an imbalance in one of four humors. Many of his contemporaries felt that he was blaming the doctors for the death of their patients. Semmelweis did not help his cause. He didn't publish his work for 13 years and rudely berated anyone who questioned him. His behavior continued to deteriorate to such an extent that he lost his job and was eventually placed in an asylum, where he was beaten by the guards and died two weeks later. After his death and the discoveries of germ theory by Louis Pasteur and antisepsis, by Joseph Lister, his ideas gained universal acceptance. Today, he is largely revered for his lonely, determined quest to save the lives of women in childbirth (Fig. 27.1). Predictably, Lister's discoveries were also initially rejected and mocked when he first published them in 1867. In 1873, The Lancet, even went as far as to warn surgeons against using his sterilization technique.

Fig. 27.1 I agree. (The Logic of Science. [Image file, Facebook status update]. 2015. Retrieved from https://www.facebook.com/thelogicofscience/posts/1701754906722572.)

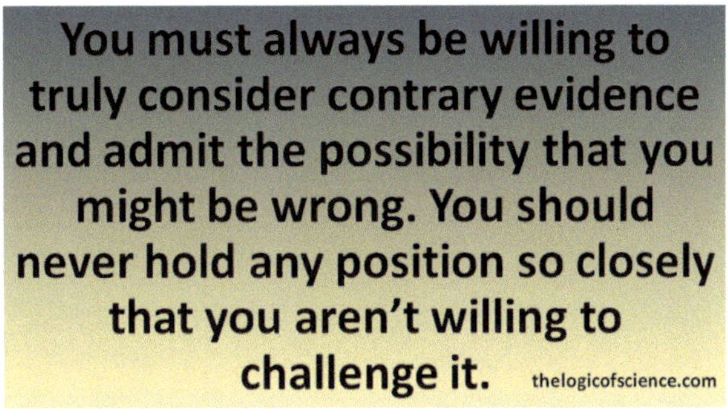

You must always be willing to truly consider contrary evidence and admit the possibility that you might be wrong. You should never hold any position so closely that you aren't willing to challenge it. thelogicofscience.com

Similar examples are not hard to find. Scurvy, which is caused by a deficiency of vitamin C, was a common cause of death in sailors for many centuries. It is characterized by loose teeth, bleeding gums, infections, and hemorrhages. In 1601, Captain James Lancaster placed the crew of one of his four ships on daily doses of lemon juice. By the midway point of the trip, 110 of 278 sailors who received no lemon juice had died, while no man who drank it died.

In 1747, 146 years later, James Lind, a doctor in the Scottish navy, conducted the first controlled trial in the history of medicine. He selected 12 sailors suffering from scurvy and divided them into six pairs. Two were given citrus fruits, while the rest were given other foods in addition to a regular diet. Those fed oranges and lemons made a rapid and full recovery, while the others did not. While the importance of his finding seems to have been recognized at the time, it took the British Navy another 48 years to require citrus fruits for its sailors. It took another 70 years after Lind's experiment until the British Board of Trade adopted this dietary requirement for all of its sailors, thus eliminating scurvy in British sailors. (It was the use of limes to fulfill the requirement that gave rise to the name "limeys" for British sailors) [2]. Overall, it took 264 years from Lancaster's discovery of how to prevent scurvy until it was adopted throughout the British Empire.

Similarly, the power of vaccination to prevent smallpox was known for several decades before the seminal work of Edward Jenner. In 1765, John Fewster, an English surgeon, presented a paper titled *Cow Pox and Its Ability to Prevent Smallpox* to the London medical society. No one seemed to recognize its potential, including Dr. Fewster, who reportedly "let the matter drop" [3]. The first documented instance of vaccination was by an English farmer named Benjamin Jesty, who vaccinated his family during a smallpox outbreak in 1774. Like many before him, he was punished for his wisdom and courage. According to accounts from the time, he was "hooted at, reviled and pelted whenever he attended markets in the neighbourhood" [4]. That milkmaids exposed to cowpox were subsequently immune from smallpox was relatively common knowledge amongst English doctors at the time and vaccination was a common practice amongst farmers even prior to Jesty. Nonetheless, Jesty was assaulted for this "inhumane act" and his neighbors "feared their metamorphosis into horned beasts" [5]. Of course, Jesty was right, and his family was later protected from the disease when exposed to it. In 1798, over 20 years after Jesty's vaccine,

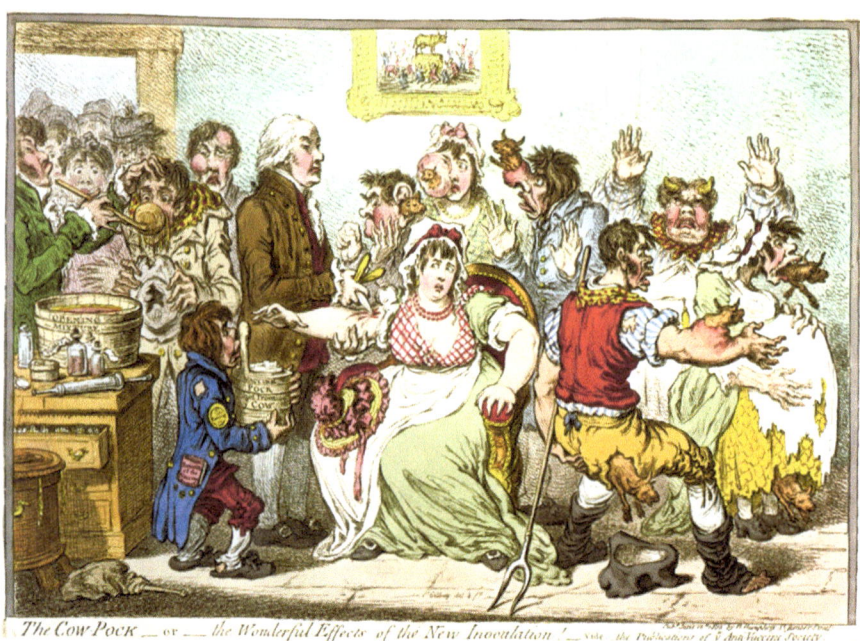

Fig. 27.2 James Gillray's 1802 caricature of Edward Jenner vaccinating fearful patients. (Gillray J. (JamesThe cow pock [Image file]. In: Wikimedia commons. 1802. Retrieved from https://commons.wikimedia.org/wiki/File:The_cow_pock.jpg.)

Edward Jenner introduced vaccination to the world, saving countless of millions of lives and paving the way for the eradication of smallpox. Not surprisingly, fearful objections to Jenner's work were common as well. As a caricature from 1802 shows, many patients feared vaccination would make them sprout cowlike appendages (Fig. 27.2).

In more recent times, Barry Marshall and Robin Warren cultured an unknown bacterium, later named *Helicobacter pylori*, from patients with gastric ulcers and theorized that the bacteria was the causative agent. Their hypothesis contradicted accepted medical dogma at the time, which held that the gastric environment was too acidic to support bacterial life. The only way to prove their theory was to experiment on a human. And so in 1984, Dr. Marshall bravely drank *H. pylori* himself. He developed gastritis eight days later, the rapid response surprising even him. A subsequent biopsy showed *H. pylori* had colonized his stomach, demonstrating that it was the cause of gastric ulcers.

Their work reversed established medical doctrine that gastric ulcers were caused by stress, excess gastric acid, and spicy foods. It was also a direct blow to the pharmaceutical industry, which profited from the mistaken belief that gastric ulcers could only be treated by antacids that needed to be taken daily for years, rather than a short course of antibiotics. "Everyone was against me, but I knew I was right," Dr. Marshall said upon being honored by the American Academy of Achievement [6]. "I think I've always just gone my own way," he said in a later interview. "As I often say, in science, you've got to be pretty thick-skinned and ready to take the blows." Drs. Marshall and Warren were awarded the Nobel Prize for their work in 2005.

In contrast to the pervasive myth of the ignored genius whose work lies dormant for decades or longer, medicine does generally utilize new treatments when there is sufficient evidence of their efficacy. Fecal transplants are actually a perfect example of the willingness of medicine to adapt to new evidence. The treatment, which has now become standard of care for *C. diff* infections that do not respond to antibiotics, was hardly on the radar of most clinicians only a decade ago. Currently, it is being explored as a treatment for a wide range of other diseases, including Parkinson's and multiple sclerosis (MS). There is little doubt that if rigorous studies demonstrate that fecal transplants are effective for these conditions, clinicians will not hesitate to use it. Additionally, when the evidence suggests an accepted medical practice is ineffective, the medical community does alter its practices, albeit sometimes not as rapidly as desired. Many practices that were routine only a few years ago, such as the use of coronary stents in patients with stable coronary artery disease, have decreased dramatically as evidence accumulated that the harms outweighed the benefits.

Many complementary and alternative medicine (CAM) practitioners point to ridiculed treatments that are now widely accepted, or treatments that were widely accepted but are now ridiculed, as evidence that mainstream medicine is fundamentally flawed. Precisely the opposite is true. The willingness of mainstream medicine to investigate its own practices and change them according to new evidence is its great strength. It would be much worse if mainstream medicine refused to investigate its most cherished practices and admit its mistakes when new evidence emerged. From dietary recommendations, to cancer screenings, and the use of hormone replacement in post-menopausal women, mainstream medicine has reversed itself in dramatic and significant ways in modern times.

However, just because mainstream medicine was once wrong about some treatments, it does not follow that it is currently wrong about most treatments, as many CAM practitioners suggest. Undoubtedly many medical practices that are accepted as effective today will be discarded in the future. This is in marked contrast to the "detoxes" and "natural" supplements of CAM, which will persist in one form or another as long as people are willing to pay for them. Similarly, there is some ridiculed, fringe belief that will one day become widespread. Once its value is recognized, it will be easy to look back and scoff at those who initially dismissed it. Again, this is in marked contrast to CAM, which often rejects treatments, such as vaccines, which are hundreds of years old and have been investigated in literally hundreds of thousands of studies.

Clinical procedure	Landmark trial	Current rate of use
Flu vaccination	1968 [7]	55% [8]
Thrombolytic therapy	1971 [9]	20% [10]
Pneumococcal vaccination	1977 [11]	35.6% [8]
Diabetic eye exam	1981 [4]	38.4% [6]
Beta blockers after MI	1982 [12]	61.9% [6]
Mammography	1982 [13]	70.4% [6]
Cholesterol screening	1984 [14]	65% [15]
Fecal occult blood test	1986 [16]	17% [17]
Diabetic foot care	1993 [18]	20% [19]

Fig. 27.3 Even many decades after certain treatments were validated, they remained woefully underused in the year 2000

Certainly, there is room for improvement. E. Andrew Balas and Suzanne Boren calculated in 2000, that it takes 17 years on average before a significant discovery is adopted into routine patient care [7]. The benefit of the pneumococcal vaccine was demonstrated in 1977, for example, but by 2000 it was used only 35.6% of the time (Fig. 27.3) [8].

Not all of this is due to the stubbornness of clinicians. The sheer volume of new medical information is overwhelming. Brian Alper and colleagues estimated that "Physicians trained in epidemiology would take an estimated 627.5 hours per month to evaluate these articles" [9]. Considering there are an average of 731 hours per month, this is clearly an impossible task. Moreover, much of this information is filled with dense statistics or basic science that is not geared towards practicing clinicians.

Conclusion
The history of medicine is full of people who proposed ideas that were considered heretical at the time, but are now considered established truths. Clinicians who resist new information because it contradicts established medical dogma run the risk of missing important new discoveries. As Frank Zappa said, "A mind is like a parachute. It doesn't work if it is not open" (Fig. 27.4).

Note that the Semmelweis reflex is opposite of the Galileo fallacy (discussed in the next section), which posits that diagnoses and treatments that are mocked by the mainstream medical establishment are right primarily for that reason. For every clinician like Drs. Marshall and Warren who were initially dismissed for proposing a dramatic, new medical paradigm only later to be proven heroically correct, there are many more mavericks who were dismissed for proposing a dramatic, new medical paradigm, whose theories turned out to be spectacularly and dangerously wrong. In contrast to the now-famous individual who defied medical convention only to be vindicated by history, most of these flawed mavericks are now completely forgotten or are just mere footnotes to history.

Fig. 27.4 Frank Zappa gets it right. (Jean-Luc. Frank Zappa, Records on wheels, Toronto, Sept 24, 1977 [Image file]. In: Wikimedia commons. 2005. Retrieved from https://commons.wikimedia.org/wiki/Frank_Zappa#/media/File:The_famous_mustache_and_goatee.jpg.)

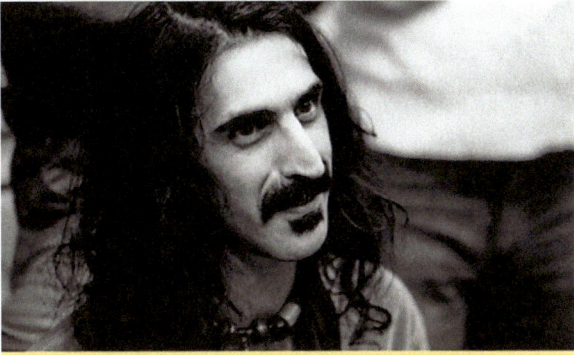

A mind is like a parachute. It doesn't work if it isn't open.

Frank Zappa

Galileo Fallacy

Case

Rebecca was a 45-year-old woman who had been diagnosed with relapsing-remitting multiple sclerosis (MS) 10 years prior. She had had multiple relapses despite treatment and was in need of a walker to walk outside. She read about a new theory called chronic cerebrospinal venous insufficiency (CCSVI) put forth by Paolo Zamboni, a vascular surgeon. His theory posited that the cause of MS was impaired venous drainage and that using an intervention known as angioplasty, the veins could be opened and the cause of MS could be relieved. According to Zamboni, many symptoms of MS abated after an endovascular procedure to open these veins. He was confident enough in it that it was performed on his own wife, who suffers from MS. Dr. Zamboni termed this the "liberation procedure."

While Rebecca's neurologist discouraged her from pursuing the treatment, she found an interventional radiologist, Dr. Sears, who had performed the procedure on multiple patients and was advertising online. She had the procedure done, and though she reported feeling better for the first few weeks, but after two months she was back to her baseline.

What Dr. Sears Was Thinking

Medicine has been wrong so many times before, and the history of medicine is full of so-called "quacks" who were later proven right. I read Zamboni's initial work and found it quite convincing. I knew that a lot of neurologists scoffed at the idea. Doctors can be very closed-minded a lot of the time, and let's be frank, neurologists would have a lot to lose if a cure for MS were found. Similarly, I know that medications for MS make an enormous amount of money for pharmaceutical companies. So when opposition to Zamboni's ideas sprung up from the predictable sources, I was not surprised or concerned. In fact, the intense opposition from so many disparate sources led to me to be more enthusiastic about the procedure. I performed the liberation procedure on nearly 50 patients, all of whom reported feeling better. One woman said that after receiving the treatment:

> The first thing that I noticed was my eyesight – amazing, just incredible. From pre-procedure in the waiting bay, couldn't read the signs on the wall, to coming out and being placed in the same bay and wow, there they were. Everything clear as a bell. This is my mobility scooter that I used to have to use to go out anywhere – shopping, any of those sorts of things, before I had the venoplasty. Happily sitting here gathering dust now [10].

However, as it was subjected to larger, controlled studies, evidence emerged that Zamboni's findings could not be replicated in a larger group of patients. The Multiple Sclerosis Society devoted millions of dollars to study CCSVI, and seven research projects failed to find any evidence for its existence. A study done in 2013 of nearly 2,000 patients flatly declared "CCSVI is not associated with MS" [11]. Not only does the procedure not work, it has the potential to harm. In 2012, the FDA reported cases of "death, stroke, detachment and migration of the stents, damage to the treated vein, blood clots, cranial nerve damage and abdominal bleeding associated with the experimental procedure" [12]. Based on this evidence, I had to concede I was wrong. As neurologist Steven Novella wrote about the liberation procedure:

> There is nothing wrong with coming up with a new and even radical idea in medicine. That is the raw material for scientific investigation. It is unacceptable, however, to refuse to abandon your hypothesis in the face of overwhelmingly negative evidence. That is when you pass from the realm of mainstream science into the realm of the crank. In medicine this has direct implications for patients, and therefore there is also a significant ethical dimension [13].

While I admire Dr. Zamboni for thinking outside the box, I eventually had to abandon the procedure. Dr. Zamboni himself, to his great credit, was the first author on a study in 2017 that showed CCSVI had no benefit in patients with MS compared to a sham procedure [14]. This paper bluntly concluded that CCSVI "cannot be recommended for patients with relapsing-remitting multiple sclerosis."

Despite overwhelming evidence against Dr. Zamboni's liberation procedure, there are patient groups that still advocate for the procedure and doctors willing to perform it, often for high fees. They are convinced that the liberation procedure works, that neurologists and pharmaceutical companies are conspiring to suppress the truth about this, and that history will one day recognize Dr. Zamboni as a persecuted genius.

Fig. 27.5 Different does not mean being useful

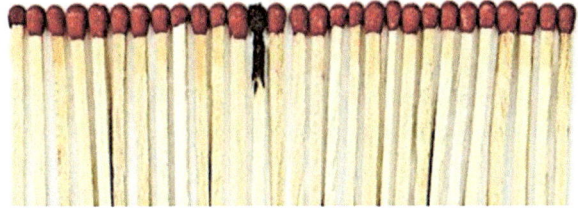

Just because you're different Doesn't mean you're useful

Discussion

The Galileo fallacy occurs when clinicians embrace diseases, tests, and treatments that are dismissed by the mainstream medical establishment precisely because they are dismissed by the mainstream medical establishment. It is named after the Italian astronomer, Galileo Galilei (1564–1642) who was convicted of heresy by the Catholic Church during the Roman Inquisition and placed under house arrest for spreading the doctrine of heliocentrism.

Some clinicians, especially those who practice CAM, are especially prone to the Galileo fallacy. They are drawn to implausible and unproven theories precisely because they are rejected by mainstream medicine. In their view, the fact that Galileo was persecuted for beliefs that are now universally accepted is proof that many currently rejected beliefs will eventually be vindicated. The Galileo fallacy is most likely to occur in overly-confident clinicians with contrarian personalities, whose self-identity is based in part on rebelling against the mainstream (the reactance bias). These clinicians receive an ego-boost by portraying themselves as modern-day Galileos, more knowledgeable and advanced than their unenlightened peers. For such clinicians and their acolytes, opposition to their ideas from mainstream medicine and even formal government sanction is confirmation of their rectitude and evidence of the grave threat they pose to mainstream institutions (Fig. 27.5).

Consider this 2012 TV news piece titled *MS Cure*? about "medical mavericks" who claim that MS is caused by an infection with *Chlamydia pneumoniae* and can therefore be treated with antibiotics [10]. The segment begins with footage of Nobel Prize winner Barry Marshall who overturned medical dogma by demonstrating that bacteria, not stress, causes stomach ulcers.

Narration

Australian scientists, Warren and Marshall, went to extraordinary lengths to prove that stomach ulcers were not caused by stress, but by a bacterial infection. Marshall took the ultimate leap of faith and infected himself with the bug.

Barry Marshall

I said to my wife, 'I took the bacteria, I've got the illness.' And she said, 'You did what?'

Narration

Fortunately a simple course of antibiotics cured him. The pair won a Nobel Prize in 2005. Similarly in 2008, Italian doctor Paolo Zamboni was ridiculed when he proposed a whole new approach to MS. He claimed that instead of treating nerve damage, doctors should be focused on blood vessels. He believed that MS was due to a narrowing of the veins in the neck. Zamboni's theory gave hope to millions of MS sufferers, but many neurologists scoffed at the idea – including Vicki's.

Vicki Robinson

He was very dismissive, just didn't feel that it had anything to do with MS, and that was the end of the conversation.

Dr Maryanne Demasi

How did that make you feel?

Vicki Robinson

I was really angry, actually.

The implication here is very clear: Nobel prize winners were dismissed in the past. Paolo Zamboni and those who claim MS can be treated with antibiotics are being dismissed today. Therefore, their genius will one day be widely recognized.

Undoubtedly, the history of medicine is full of brave, free-thinking mavericks who proposed theories and treatments that were considered laughably implausible at the time, but are now considered established truths. However, there are many more people who proposed theories and treatments that were considered laughably implausible at the time and are still considered laughably implausible today. In contrast to the geniuses we immortalize, these individuals are now historical footnotes because their ideas were indeed, incredibly wrong. Because of the survival bias, there is a tendency to think that an independent thinker who is scoffed at today is likely to be vindicated in the future. Yet, just because an idea is different, doesn't mean it is right. Examples of lone mavericks overturning established medical paradigms are extremely rare. Frank Zappa may have been right when he said that "A mind is like a parachute. It doesn't work if it is not open." However, in the words of Carl Sagan, "It pays to keep an open mind, but not so open your brains fall out (Fig. 27.6)."

Consider the example of Franz Mesmer (1734–1815), a German doctor who proposed that energy transfer occurred between all animated and inanimate objects, something he called animal magnetism. He treated his patients with high doses of iron and then moved magnets over their bodies. Patients would enter a trance-like state and emerge feeling better. He later abandoned the use of iron, believing that his own hands were magnetic and could have the same effect. In 1784, King Louis XVI appointed four members of the

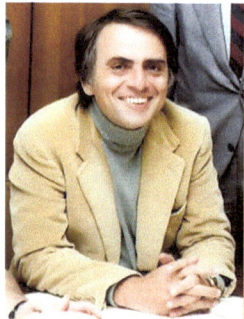

It pays to keep an open mind, but not so open your brains fall out.
Carl Sagan

Fig. 27.6 Carl Sagan gets it right. (NASA/JPL. Carl Sagan [Image file]. In: Wikimedia commons. 1979. Retrieved from https://commons.wikimedia.org/wiki/Carl_Sagan#/media/File:Carl_Sagan_Planetary_Society.JPG.)

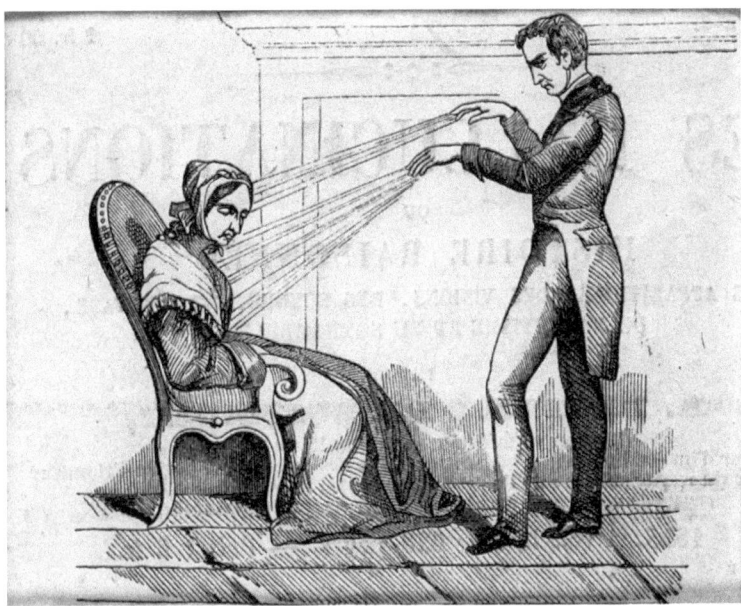

Fig. 27.7 A practitioner of mesmerism using animal magnetism on a woman who responds with convulsions. (Wellcome Collection Gallery. A practitioner of mesmerism using animal magnetism on a woman who responds with convulsions [Image file]. In: Wikimedia commons. 2014. Retrieved from https://commons.wikimedia.org/wiki/Category:Alternative_medicine#/media/File:A_practitioner_of_Mesmerism_using_Animal_Magnetism_Wellcome_V0011094.jpg.)

Faculty of Medicine as commissioners to investigate his treatment. After an extensive investigation, the commission concluded that there was no evidence for animal magnetism. Whatever benefits the treatment produced were correctly attributed to "imagination," which we would now call the placebo effect. Mesmer was driven into exile soon afterwards. Although some people continued to practice his treatment for several years, today he is remembered primarily as the origin of the word "mesmerize" (Fig. 27.7).

German doctor Franz Josef Gall (1758–1828), the founder of phrenology, provides another interesting example of a largely forgotten maverick who promoted ideas that are now confined to the history books. Gall believed that the bumps and indentations on the skull reflected pressure from the brain below. He claimed to have discovered 27 "fundamental faculties" that reflected a person's personality, character, and talents. Gall's ideas were revolutionary, and many scientists, politicians, and organizations, including the Catholic Church, objected to his ideas. Unlike with Galileo, Gall's detractors were largely right. While Gall did hit on a fundamental truth that the brain is the seat of human consciousness and that many of its functions can be localized, phrenology itself is now universally recognized as pseudoscience (Fig. 27.8).

You have also likely never heard of Johann Caspar Spurzheim (1776–1832), a protégé of Gall's who became famous in several European countries for spreading the doctrine of phrenology (Fig. 27.9).

You've probably also never heard of Elisha Perkins (1741–1799), a doctor from Connecticut. He developed "tractors," which were three-inch metal rods with a point at the end. He would touch the sharp ends to the area where they patient was suffering, claiming they would "draw off the noxious electrical fluid that lay at the root of

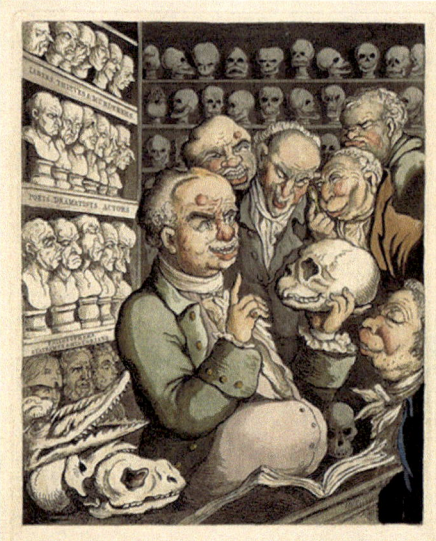
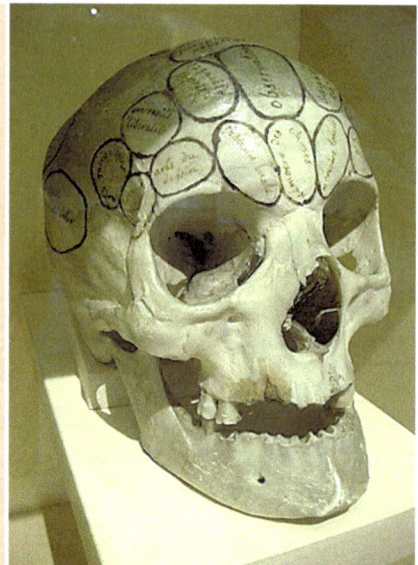

Fig. 27.8 An etching from 1808 showing Franz Joseph Gall leading a discussion on phrenology with five colleagues, among his extensive collection of skulls and model heads. A phrenology skull. (**Left**: Wellcome Collection Gallery. Franz Joseph Gall leading a discussion on phrenology with five colleagues, among his extensive collection of skulls and model heads [Image file]. In: Wikimedia commons. 2014. Retrieved from https://commons.wikimedia.org/wiki/Category:Caricatures_of_physicians#/media/File:Franz_Joseph_Gall_leading_a_discussion_on_phrenology_with_fi_Wellcome_V0011105.jpg.)

Fig. 27.9 Franz Joseph Gall and Johann Caspar Spurzheim examining a patient. (Wellcome Collection Gallery. Franz Joseph Gall and Johann Caspar Spurzheim examining a patient [Image file]. In: Wikimedia commons. 2014. Retrieved from https://commons.wikimedia.org/wiki/Category:Caricatures_of_physicians#/media/File:Franz_Joseph_Gall_and_Johann_Caspar_Spurzheim_examining_a_pa_Wellcome_V0011103.jpg.)

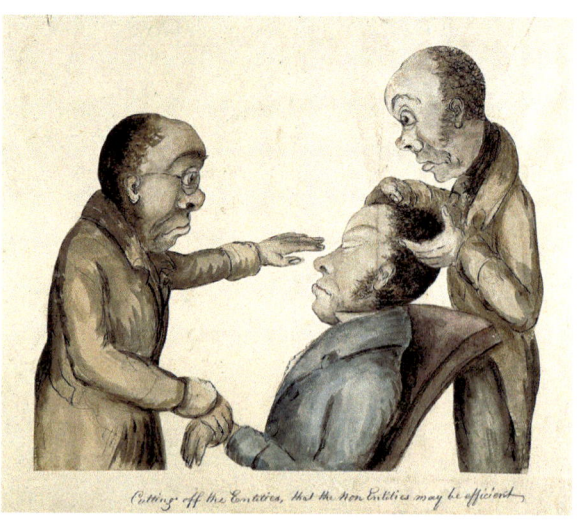

suffering" [15]. He boasted of thousands of patients cured and claimed his treatment could be used on local inflammations, facial and head pain, rheumatism, and multiple similar diseases. George Washington purchased a set of his tractors and for a period his treatment was popular in the US and several European countries. Despite this, his treatment was labeled "delusive quackery" by the Connecticut Medical Society, and he was expelled from this organization as he was considered "a patentee and user of nostrums." Perkins dismissed his critics on the grounds that they were arrogant and elitists (Fig. 27.10).

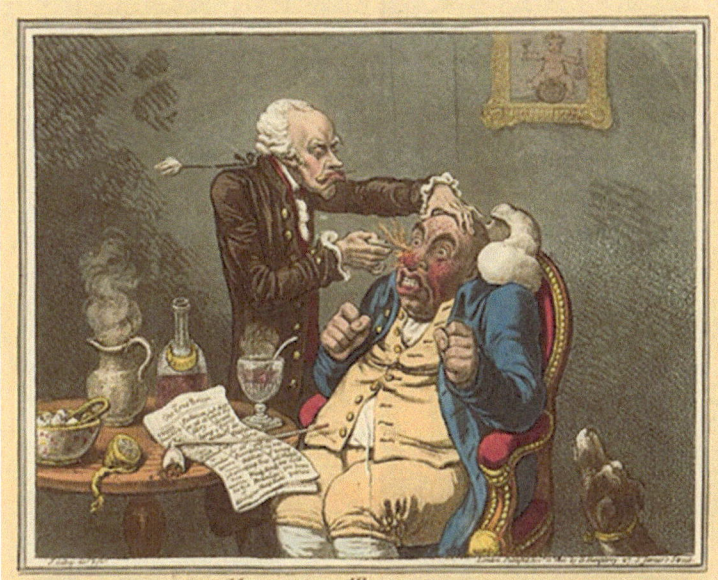

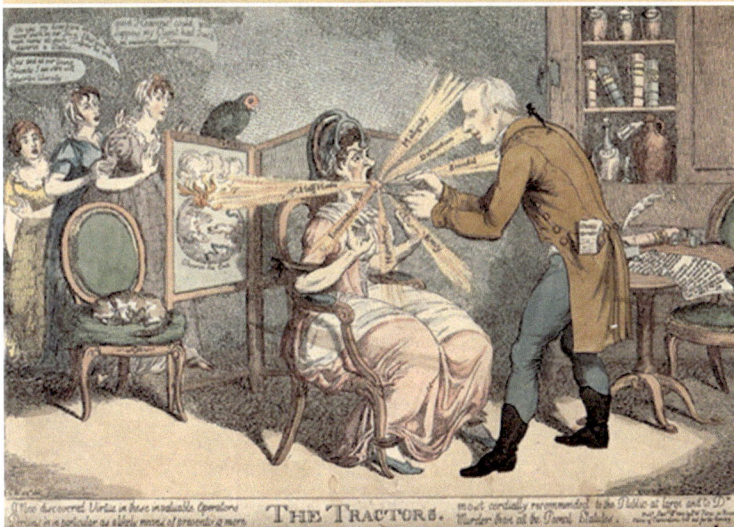

Fig. 27.10 Caricature of a quack treating a patient with Perkins tractors and an operator treating Ann Ford, a society lady, with Perkins tractors, for her venomous tongue. (**Top**: Wellcome Collection Gallery. (Metallic Tractors [Image file]. In: Wikipedia. 2014. Retrieved from https://en.wikipedia.org/wiki/Elisha_Perkins#/media/File:James_Gillray,_%22Metallic_Tractors%22,_showing_Elisha_Perkins_Wellcome_M0010466.jpg; **Bottom**: Wellcome Collection Gallery. An operator treating Ann Ford, a society lady, with "Perkins's tractors", for her venomous tongue [Image file]. In: Wikimedia commons. 2014. Retrieved from https://commons.wikimedia.org/wiki/Category:Quackery#/media/File:An_operator_treating_Ann_Ford,_a_society_lady,_with_%22Perkins_Wellcome_V0011092.jpg.)

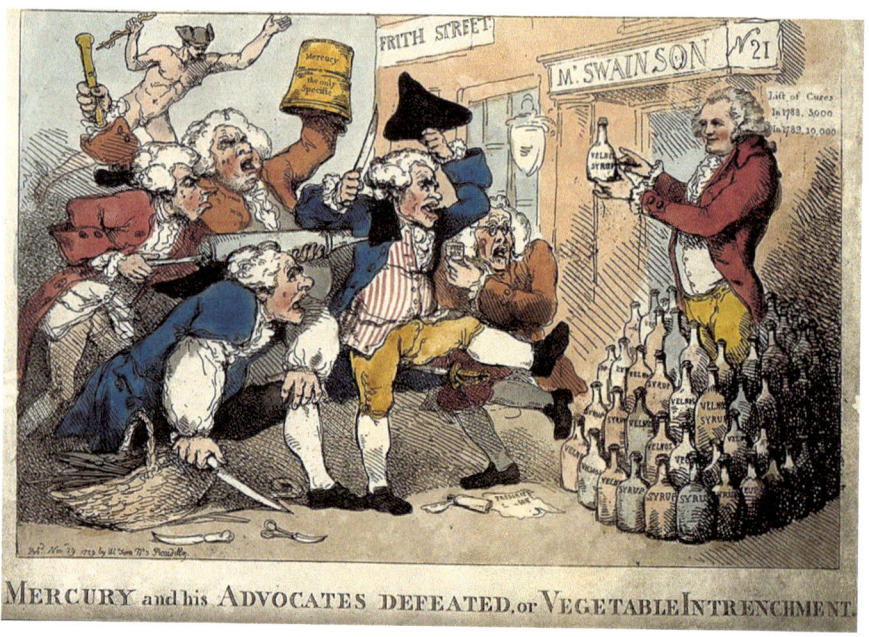

Fig. 27.11 Isaac Swainson promoting his "Velnos' Vegetable Syrup," facing an onslaught of rival practitioners advocating mercury-based treatments. (Wellcome Collection Gallery. Isaac Swainson promoting his 'Velno's Vegetable Syrup', facing an onslaught of rival practitioners advocating mercury [Image file]. In: Wikimedia commons. 2014. Retrieved from https://commons.wikimedia.org/wiki/Category:Quackery#/media/File:Isaac_Swainson_promoting_his_'Velnos_syrup',_facing_an_onsla_Wellcome_V0010912.jpg.)

You've probably never heard of Isaac Swainson (1746–1812) either. Swainson enriched himself with a medicine called "Velnos' Vegetable Syrup." In was purported to treated venereal diseases, including "the pox" and the "French disease," as well as gout, leprosy, dropsy, consumption, scurvy, cancer, diarrhea, scrofula, and tape worms. According to accounts, Swainson complained that charlatans were selling ineffective imitations of his product (Fig. 27.11).

You've probably also never heard of Isaac Lewis (1815–1884), a physicist and inventor who patented an invention called an electric belt in 1853. This belt, and multiple competitors, purported to treat innumerable conditions through the administration of electric shocks. One advertisement claimed it could cure "nervousness, sleeplessness, rheumatism, sciatica, lumbago, torpid liver and kindred ailments." Men would even shock their penises hoping to cure impotence (Fig. 27.12) [16]. Another forgotten Galileo, Francisque Crotte, developed an "electrical remedy" for tuberculosis (Fig. 27.13) [17].

Other Galileos believed that diabetes could be treated with electrotherapy using a vacuum electrode. The text, accompanying Fig. 27.14, says the electrode should be applied to the abdomen and the current turned up as high as the patient can tolerate for 10 then the electrode should be moved to another spot, until the whole abdomen has been treated. The treatment should be repeated every other day. It claims the treatment never fails to lower the blood sugar level [18].

James Morison (1770–1840) is another doctor whose name is largely forgotten today. He was a British doctor who believed that all diseases were caused by impurities of the blood, a theory of disease he called the Hygeian system. Like many modern Galileos, he used his own history as a marketing tool. According to his account, after "thirty-five years' inexpressible suffering" and failure of multiple other treatments, he managed "his own extraordinary cure" by taking vegetable pills of his own compounding. The treatment consisted of "laxative made from aloes, jalap, gamboges, colocynth, cream of tartar, myrrh, and rhubarb" [19]. He called his treatment "vegetable universal medicine," though they were commonly known as "Morison's Pills." Though he tried to give away his pill, he only became successful when he enabled appointed agents to sell it. Letters of recommendation from patients claimed his pill could treat "stomach complaints, cholera, liver complaints, general debility,

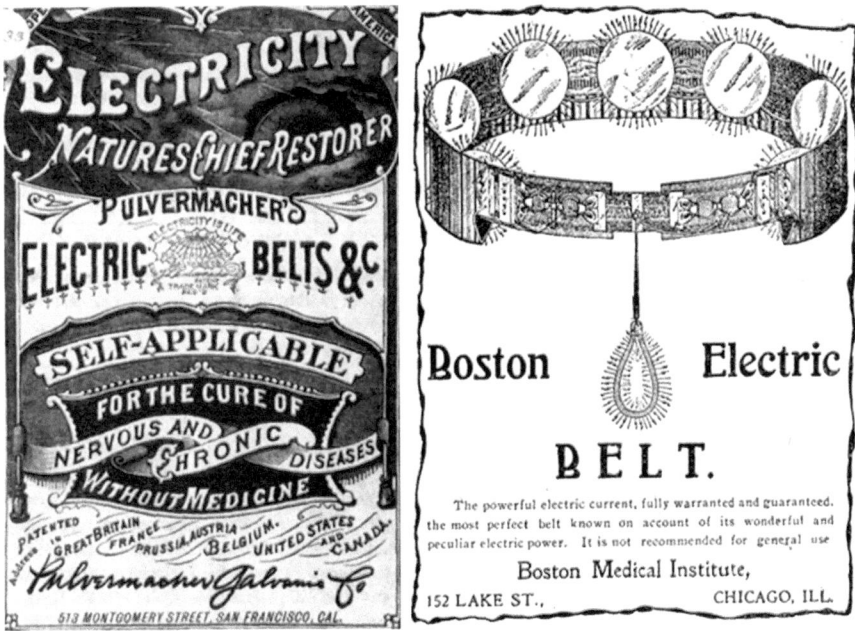

Fig. 27.12 Advertisements for a Pulvermacher electric belt and several competitors. (**Left:** Smerdis of Tlön. Pulvermacher's electric belts [Image file]. In: Wikimedia commons. 2005. Retrieved from https://commons.wikimedia.org/wiki/File:Pulvermacher%27s_Electric_Belts. png; **Right:** Wellcome Collection Gallery. Boston electric belt - 1912 [Image file]. In: Wikimedia Commons. 2018. Retrieved from https://commons.wikimedia.org/wiki/File:Boston_Electric_ Belt._Wellcome_L0003568.jpg; **Continued:** Wellcome Collection Gallery. All in search of health [Image file]. In: Wikimedia commons. 2018. Retrieved from https://commons.wikimedia.org/wiki/ File:All_in_search_of_health_Wellcome_L0074968.jpg.)

Fig. 27.12 (continued)

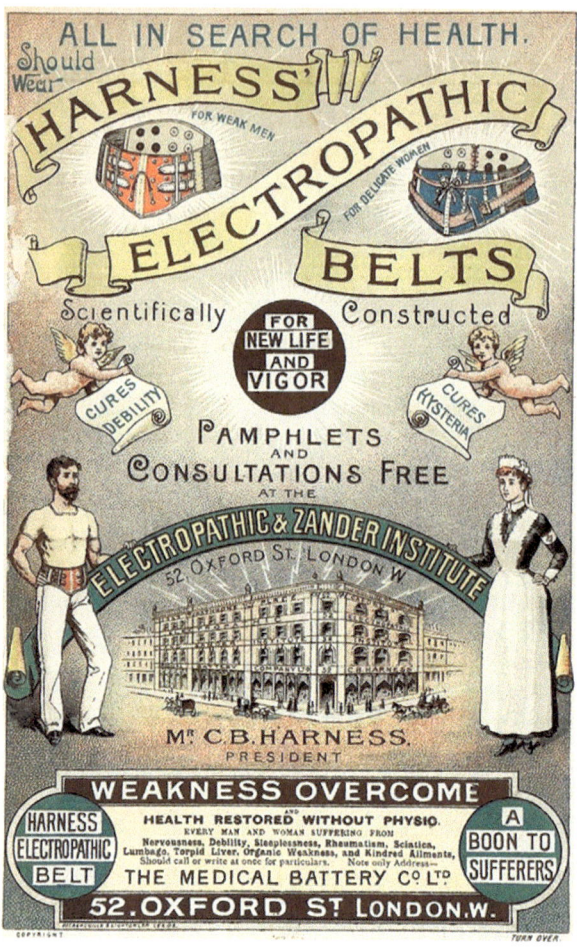

jaundice, worms, gravel, limb pain after falls, and eye problems; they were even being used to treat snake bites and scorpion stings in Madras in 1866" [20]. Other publications went much further than this (Fig. 27.15).

With claims that are eerily similar to modern-day Galileos, "He appealed to the general public because of the missionary-like zeal in which he opposed 'orthodox' medicine; in particular, he attacked physicians' excessive fees and toxic medicine" [19]. He also founded a school with a legitimate-sounding name, The British College of Health, to sell his products. This was described as "one of the cleverest things he ever did…by taking on a sort of corporate philanthropic existence he removed himself from the category of a mere commercial exploiter of a proprietary medicine" and created "a sort of University of Morisonism" (Fig. 27.16) [20].

Morison was vilified by the mainstream medical establishment at this time. He was said to be guilty of "fraud and extortion" and his pills were called "active poison." Several deaths were blamed on his pills and one vendor was convicted of manslaughter. Thomas Wakley, the founding editor of *The Lancet*, spent over 10 years trying to debunk Morison's claims (Fig. 27.17) [19].

Fig. 27.13 Francisque Crotte "curing" tuberculosis with his electrical remedy. (Wellcome Collection Gallery. Francisque Crôtte applying his electrical [Image file]. In: Wikimedia commons. 2018. Retrieved from https://commons.wikimedia.org/wiki/File:Francisque_Cr%C3%B4tte_applying_his_electrical_remedy_for_Wellcome_L0038314.jpg.)

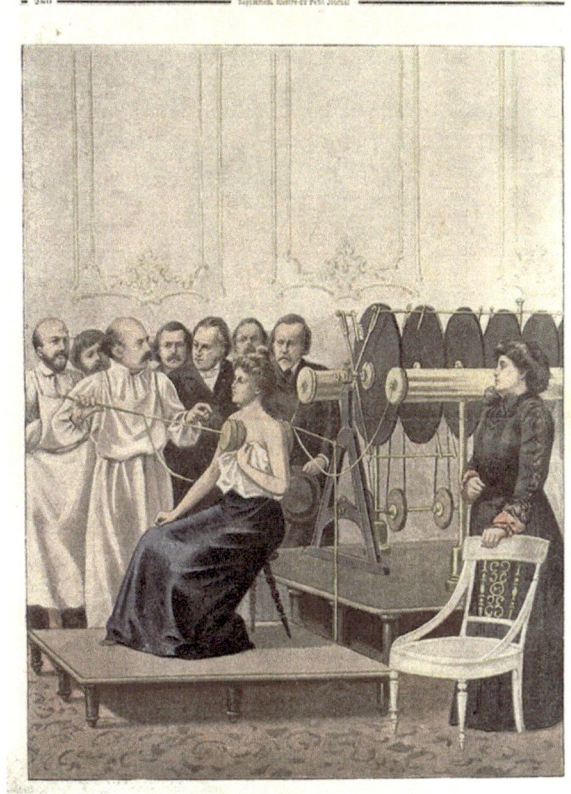

LA CURE DE LA TUBERCULOSE

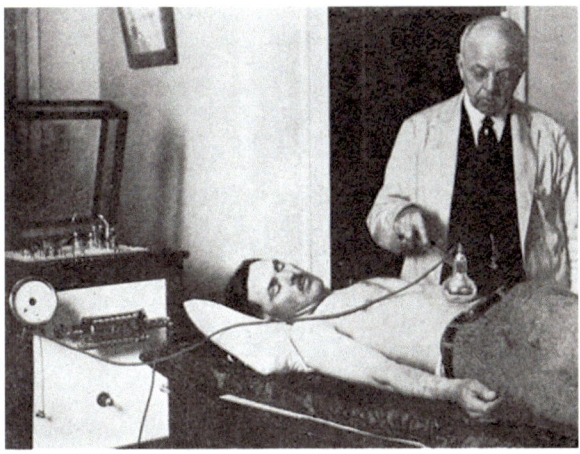

Fig. 27.14 "Treating" diabetes with electricity. (Baker Grover B. (Burton). Treatment of diabetes mellitus in 1922 by electrotherapy using a vacuum electrode. [Image file]. In: Wikimedia commons. 1921. Retrieved from https://commons.wikimedia.org/wiki/Category:Electrotherapy#/media/File:Diabetes_electrotherapy_with_vacuum_electrode_1922.jpg.)

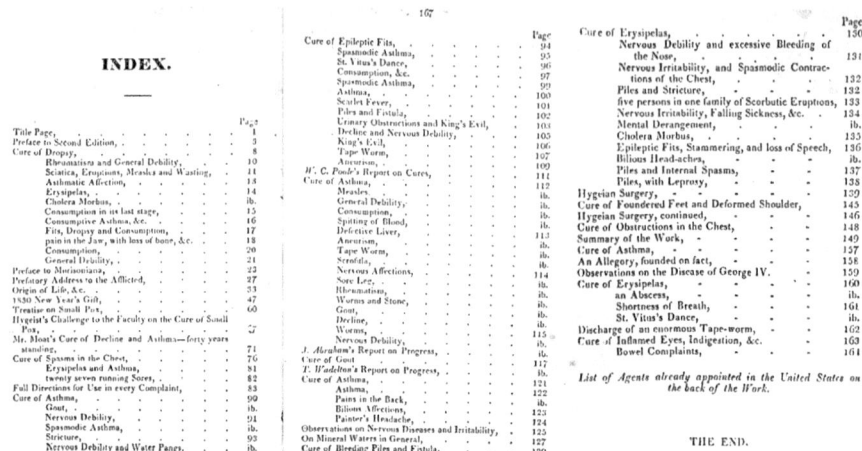

Fig. 27.15 Conditions treated by vegetable universal medicine according to an 1830 publication titled *The Practical Proofs of the Soundness of the Hygeian System of Physiology*. (Moat T. The practical proofs of the soundness of the Hygeian system of physiology: Selected from the appendix of "Morisoniana", as incontrovertible Brooklyn: Self-published. 1831. (Scanned version retrieved from https://archive.org/details/63751640R.nlm.nih.gov.)

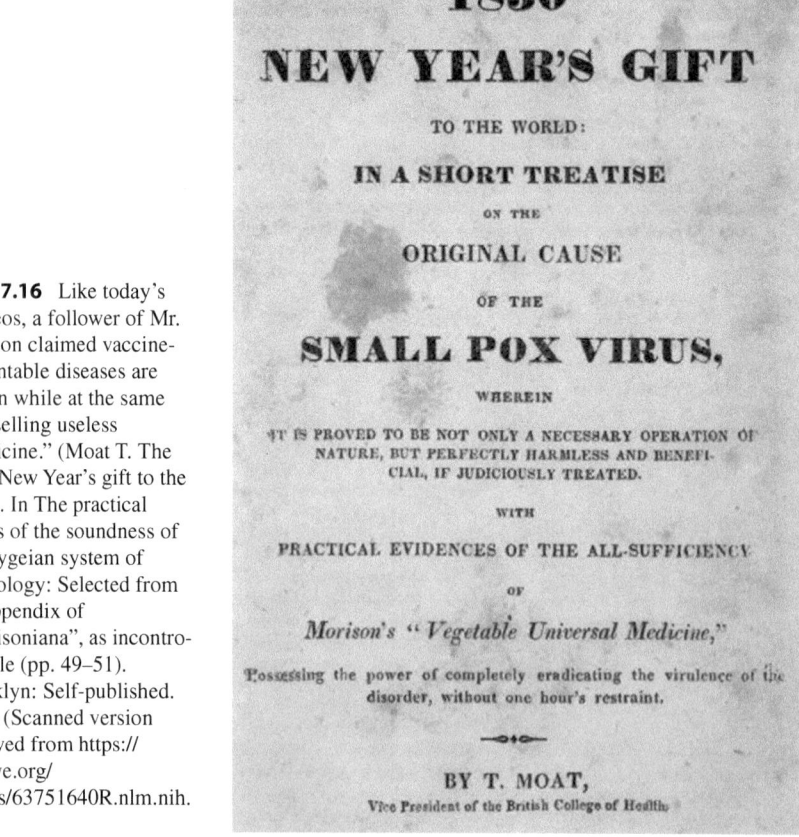

Fig. 27.16 Like today's Galileos, a follower of Mr. Morison claimed vaccine-preventable diseases are benign while at the same time selling useless "medicine." (Moat T. The 1830 New Year's gift to the world. In The practical proofs of the soundness of the Hygeian system of physiology: Selected from the appendix of "Morisoniana", as incontro-vertible (pp. 49–51). Brooklyn: Self-published. 1831. (Scanned version retrieved from https://archive.org/details/63751640R.nlm.nih.gov.)

Fig. 27.17 Lithograph depicting a man who has overdosed on Morison's Vegetable Pills. (Wellcome Collection Gallery. Coloured lithograph (C. J. Grant, 1831) depicting a man who has overdosed on James Morison's Vegetable Pills [Image file]. In: Wikipedia. 2014. Retrieved from https://en.wikipedia.org/wiki/James_Morison_(physician)#/media/File:A_man_in_bed_with_vegetables_sprouting_from_all_parts_of_his_Wellcome_V0011125.jpg)

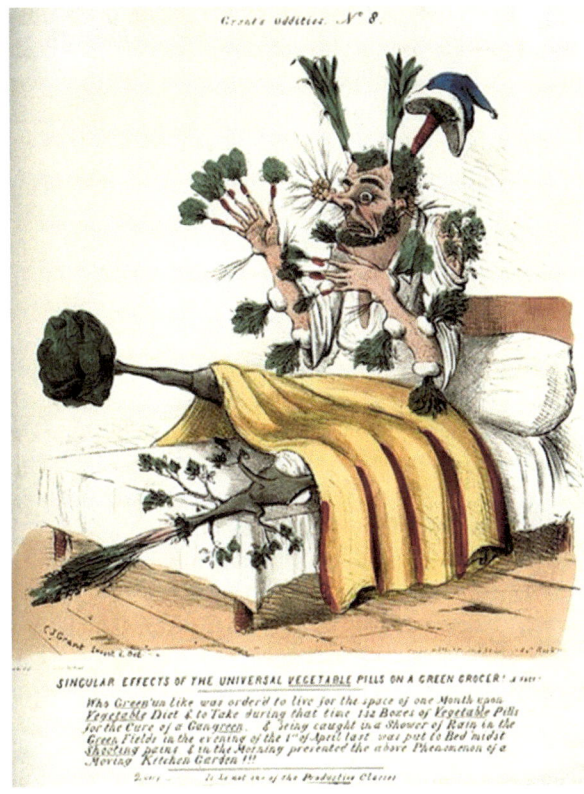

Of course, this small list just scratches the surface, and entire tomes have been written about the history of innumerable, forgotten, treatments that are now recognized as quackery [21]. With the passage of time, it is easy to dismiss Mesmer, Gall, Spurzheim, Perkins, Swainson, Pulvermacher, Morison, and countless others like them as relics of a prescientific era. Yet our time is scarcely different. Variants of Mesmerism are alive and well, though they have been rebranded as energy healing and Reiki. They are offered at "integrative" medical centers, many of them based in the most prestigious medical institutions. Modern-day versions of Velnos' Vegetable Syrup and Morison's vegetable universal medicine abound on the internet and in health food stores. People still rush to embrace scientifically implausibly fad treatments, often pushed by unethical clinicians and celebrity "wellness" gurus. Almost all of them will suffer the same fate as Mesmer, Gall, Spurzheim, Perkins, Swainson, Pulvermacher, and Morison, becoming interesting footnotes to medical history, if they are remembered at all.

There is certainly no shortage today of grandiose clinicians who consider themselves modern-day Galileos. For example, *Radical Cures Your Doctor Thinks are Crazy* was the title of an episode of *The Dr. Oz Show*, featuring CAM luminary Joseph Mercola, an osteopath. From the idea that vaccines are dangerous and unnecessary to the belief that sunscreens cause cancer and that HIV does not cause AIDS, there is hardly a single idea of mainstream medicine that Dr. Mercola does not reject. He boasts on his website, mercola.com, that he is dedicated to "Exposing corporate, government, and mass media hype that diverts you away from what is truly best for your health and often to a path that leads straight into an early grave" [22]. He runs an online business empire, selling a wide variety of products that earns over seven million dollars annually by some estimates [23]. While it is easy to find out how to contact a customer service representative from his website, I could not figure out how a prospective patient might make an appointment. In fact, it is not clear he sees patients at all. Dr. Mercola has run afoul of government regulatory agencies multiple times, most recently because of claims that the tanning beds he sells carry no risk for skin cancers and can "reverse the appearance of aging" [24]. There is little doubt that these warnings only bolster his credentials among his most committed followers.

Examples of "persecuted," alternative doctors who have supposedly discovered "cancer cures" are also plentiful. Dr. Max Gerson (1881–1959), for example, developed a cancer treatment protocol that consisted of dietary changes, innumerable supplements, and "detoxification" with up to five daily coffee enemas. The dietary changes are not trivial. According to the Gerson Institute, which carries on his work, they involve "flooding the body with nutrients from about 15 to 20 pounds of organically grown fruits and vegetables daily" [25]. Dr. Gerson felt that he cured his migraines with this protocol and then used it to treat diabetes and tuberculosis. He came to believe that "toxins" were responsible for cancers and all degenerative illnesses. He used his therapy to treat these diseases as well. There is no evidence that his treatment works beyond patient testimonials and anecdotes.

His protocol is still practiced at several Gerson centers around the world, and he is described as a modern-day Galileo by devotees of CAM. For example, an article in the magazine Organic Lifestyle was titled *Dr. Max Gerson – Persecuted for Curing Cancer Naturally* [26]. The article claims that "As is often the case when alternative treatments prevail, Dr. Gerson became the object of derision and suspicion by critics in the medical community." His grandson titled his biography *Dr. Max Gerson: Healing the Hopeless*. As this is described on the Gerson Institute website, it stresses not the evidence behind his treatment, but rather that he and his followers are persecuted Galileos:

> Dr. Max Gerson: Healing the Hopeless *discusses the development of his world-famous dietary therapy and the struggles this medical pioneer faced as he challenged orthodox medicine with his nutritional protocol. This inspiring and uplifting biography follows Dr. Gerson through Nazi persecution, then persecution in the United States from the medical establishment, the continuation of his work despite the opposition, his questionable death, his daughter Charlotte's work, and finally the present, where the Gerson Institute works to continue his legacy and vision* [27].

Nicholas Gonzalez (1947–2015) is another modern-day Galileo who similarly believed most cancers, as well as completely unrelated conditions, such as Lyme disease and MS, were caused by "toxins." He believed these conditions could be treated by dietary modification, the use of pancreatic enzymes, and other supplements, and twice daily coffee enemas. He required his patients to take up to 175 pills per day. He based his theories on the works of an orthodontist, William Donald Kelley. Consistent with Galileo fallacy, he wrote a book about Dr. Kelley titled, *One Man Alone: An Investigation of Nutrition, Cancer, and William Donald Kelley.* The book includes "50 representative case histories of patients diagnosed with a variety of poor prognosis or terminal malignancies who did well under Dr. Kelley's care, with copies of the actual relevant medical records" [28].

Texas doctor Stanislaw Burzynski is yet another Galileo who claims cancer can be cured with "antineoplastons," which are naturally occurring peptides in blood and urine that Dr. Burzynski discovered in the 1970s. Many CAM advocates extol the virtues of this treatment, with such articles as *Antineoplastons: A Cure for Cancer Ignored For 45 Years,* which appeared on the website greenmedinfo.com [29]. He has been the subject of several flattering documentaries as well. However, despite his claims, there is no scientific evidence that antineoplastons treat cancer.

Like many others, Dr. Burzynski exhibits the Galileo fallacy, saying, "The idea of fighting people in authority became natural to me. I learned that you must never let them defeat you in your own core" [30]. Dr. Burzynski's method is to establish clinical trials, which desperate patients have to pay hundreds of thousands of dollars to enter. After decades failing to publish results from almost all of these "trials," he was formally sanctioned by Texas Medical Board in 2017. He was placed on probation, was fined $360,000, was ordered to complete 44 hours of continuing medical education, and was required to pass the board's medical jurisprudence exam. Previously, disciplinary actions dating back several decades failed largely due to sympathetic politicians and the activism of some patients, who were convinced that only he could save them. There is little doubt that this latest punishment will only confirm their belief that he is a persecuted genius. It should be noted that for every "miracle patient" who swears by his treatment, there are an equal number of families who have shared their experience of unsuccessful treatments, the heartache, and great financial hardship that resulted (Fig. 27.18) [31].

Like a religious convert, many CAM Galileos feel compelled to share stories of their "transformation" from the darkness of conventional medicine to the light of CAM. In an homage to her own glory, anti-vaccine doctor Suzanne Humphries titled her autobiography *Rising From the Dead.* The book is described thusly [32]:

This autobiography tells the intricate and personal story one doctor's path through medical school and out into academia, specialty medicine, and practice, having to conform to the system's standards. Like many doctors, she was on the way to becoming one of the walking dead. Then, one day she realized that policy was harming her patients, and she took a stand. This resulted in hostility and ostracism by the authorities and her peers in the system. In 2011, depressed and deflated, life was difficult in all directions … until she found peace through an unexpected path and a new friend. The co-author of Dissolving Illusions: Disease, Vaccines, and the Forgotten History brings you her entertaining autobiography, which will surprise you and have you wondering if your own doctor could be inadvertently threatening your health.

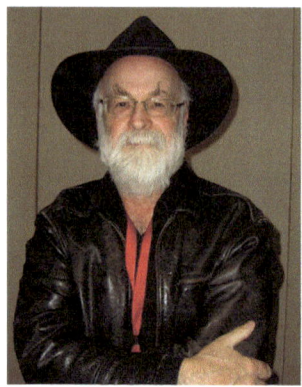

The problem with having an open mind, of course, is that people will insist on coming along and putting things in it.
Terry Pratchett

Fig. 27.18 Terry Pratchett gets it right. (Novi L. (Luigi). Novelist Terry Pratchett on day 2 of the 2012 New York Comic Con [Image file]. In: Wikimedia commons. 2012. Retrieved from https://commons.wikimedia.org/wiki/Category:Terry_Pratchett#/media/File:10.12.12TerryPratchettByLuigiNovi1.jpg.)

In a similar example of self-glorification, ironically titled *Sacred Activism: Moving Beyond the Ego,* self-proclaimed Galileo Kelly Brogan, a psychiatrist, wrote about how she realized her own intuition and personal experience were more powerful and trustworthy than the scientific method:

I began to understand science as a tool rather than a doctrine. In the wrong hands, it was a weapon of destruction, and I had to make room to integrate this. The room that I had constructed to keep myself safe was blown out with the bellows of my rage and indignation. I put myself $200K in debt, spent years of my life traumatized by the indentured servitude of medical school and residency to learn what?! A pile of lies and convenient 'truths' that serve an autocratic machine of human oppression?

I felt an ancient fire kindle inside me that churned and twisted with my own native force. I held my sword aloft. I began writing, speaking, lecturing. I changed my practice. And, of course, I was given the gift of my own health challenge to initiate me into the realm of self-healing and the power of food as information. Now I had proof – my recovery, and then the recovery of dozens of my patients as I began to arm them with what they intuitively knew to be the reason they had been stuck: our systems are making us sick and then profiting off of our ongoing illness" [33].

Steven Gundry, a contributor to Gwyneth Paltrow's website Goop, is another interesting example of a self-proclaimed Galileo. He has impeccable credentials as a former professor and chairman of cardiothoracic surgery at Loma Linda University Medical Center. He has published over 300 articles and holds several patents for medical devices. However, believing himself to be a medical Galileo, he abandoned this in 2002 to open The Center for Restorative Medicine. As he wrote on his website [34]:

I believe I've discovered some unconventional truths about human nutrition. The Gundry MD philosophy is a radical departure from the traditional dietary "wisdom" which has failed so many Americans over the past few decades... I have spent the last 14 years study-

ing the human microbiome – and developing the principles of Holobiotics that have since changed the lives of countless men and women. My center – based in Palm Springs, CA – is devoted to teaching patients how to live healthier lives through diet and lifestyle choices. My ultimate vision is to help them avoid the kind of surgeries I performed for over three decades. And the rest of the medical world is still catching up.

Like many Galileos, Dr. Gundry uses himself as evidence, saying about his treatment "And I know… because it worked for me." I am sure it will surprise no one to learn that he is peddling a book, as well as a large array of skincare products and expensive supplements. As with many Galileos, it's trivially easy to figure out how to buy his products or contact a customer service representative. However, I could not figure out how a prospective patient might make an appointment.

At their most extreme, CAM Galileos and their devotees embrace extraordinarily dark conspiracy theories. For example, Erin Elizabeth, the partner of Dr. Mercola, promulgated the notion that Dr. Gonzalez, who died suddenly in 2015, was a victim of worldwide plot to murder "holistic" doctors. She wrote after his death:

Again, just because I've written articles on these doctors doesn't mean I know or believe they're connected. I don't know. But I can't say with certainty that they aren't. I know many family members believe their deaths weren't 'natural' or accidental and want answers and investigations opened now (if they aren't already) and I hope they get the answers they deserve very soon!" [35].

She has published a collection of 60 "holistic" doctors whom she feels may have been murdered to suppress their treatments [36]. The fear is genuine. Dr. Brogan said in an interview that she felt her life was in danger after the publication of her book, which strongly discourages the use of pharmaceutical products, such that she took out a larger life insurance policy [37]. While it must be terrifying to feel one's life is in danger, the corollary to this is the fantasy that, similar to Galileo, one is so important and threatening that drug companies are willing to murder you (Fig. 27.19).

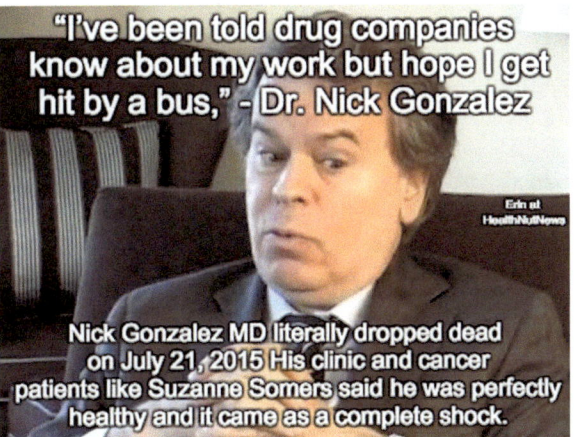

Fig. 27.19 A conspiracy meme suggesting that holistic doctors are being murdered because they threaten drug companies. (Nick Gonzalez MD. Image file. In: HealthNutNews. 2015. Retrieved from https://www.healthnutnews.com/wp-content/uploads/2015/08/nickgonzalez.png.)

In the same way that that the villain of the Galileo story is the Catholic Church, the modern-day Galileo fallacy is invariably coupled with vilification of the pharmaceutical industry, regulatory agencies, and mainstream medical institutions. CAM Galileos routinely posit that mainstream acceptance of their ideas is lacking only because "Big Pharma," a corrupt government, and a brainwashed medical community are suppressing their miracle cures. They believe that mainstream medical doctors and regulatory agencies are closed-minded at best and hopelessly corrupt and enmeshed with the pharmaceutical industry at worst. They frequently share a litany of grievances against these institutions as part of the marketing of their products.

Not all of their criticisms of pharmaceutical companies and mainstream medicine are incorrect, of course. However, those criticisms that have a shred of legitimacy are the same ones largely shared by mainstream clinicians. CAM Galileos cannot explain why their criticisms of the pharmaceutical industry earn them ridicule and threats from "Big Pharma" assassins, while mainstream critics of the pharmaceutical industry remain not only unscathed, but lauded. For example, Ben Goldacre, author of *Bad Pharma: How Drug Companies Mislead Doctors and Harm Patients*, is highly respected, not despite this book, but because of it. Similarly, Marcia Angell, author of T*he Truth About the Drug Companies: How They Deceive Us and What to Do About It*, remains a highly respected faculty member at Harvard University. Adriane Fugh-Berman runs an organization known as PharmedOut at Georgetown University Medical Center. Its goals are to "document and disseminate information about how pharmaceutical companies influence prescribing, foster access to unbiased information about drugs, and encourage physicians to choose pharma-free CME" [38]. Dr. Fugh-Berman is highly respected for this work. Multiple chapters in this book are highly critical of the pharmaceutical industry. I do not think I will die an untimely death at the hands of pharmaceutical assassins.

The tendency of CAM Galileos to exploit the failings of mainstream medicine is an example of the Texas sharpshooter fallacy. This fallacy is based on the parable of a person who randomly shoots holes in the side of a barn and afterwards paints a bullseye around each hole. Many CAM practitioners criticize essentially every aspect of mainstream medicine and gleefully celebrate when occasionally one of their critiques turns out to be right. For example, many anti-vaccine advocates delighted in a study sponsored by The CDC showing that baboons vaccinated against pertussis could still spread the disease, even if they did not show any symptoms. However, the willingness of mainstream medicine to study its most cherished beliefs and alter them when new evidence emerges is not a failure, but rather its greatest strength.

Additionally, pointing out that mainstream medicine has been wrong in the past and regulatory agencies have failed to protect the public at times, does not prove that any CAM treatment is valid and will one day be widely accepted. Similarly, the fact that pharmaceutical companies try to maximize their profits and are sometimes guilty of unethical behavior does not mean CAM treatments work. As Dr. Goldacre memorably said, "Pharma being shit does not mean magic beans cure cancer." Additionally, when clinicians such as myself castigate CAM, this does not imply an endorsement of pharmaceutical companies or that we are on their payroll (Fig. 27.20).

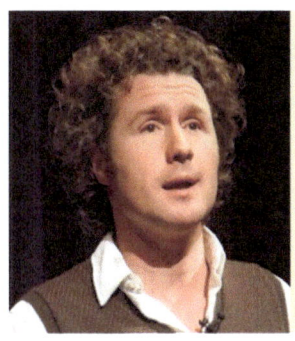

Pharma being shit does not mean magic beans cure cancer.
Ben Goldacre

Fig. 27.20 Ben Goldacre gets it right. (Cornelius G. (Gaius). Ben Goldacre speaking at TAM London Oct 2009 [Image file]. In: Wikimedia commons. 2009. Retrieved from https://commons.wikimedia.org/wiki/Category:Ben_Goldacre#/media/File:Ben_Goldacre_TAM_London_2009.JPG.)

In part because of this mistrust, CAM Galileos reject the standard agencies and methods that vet mainstream medical science. As Dr. Mercola says on his website:

> Clinical trials conducted by heavily biased 'researchers,' advertisements, and news stories carefully scripted to scare you into belief, highly polished corporate offices and corporate websites, and an extreme focus on whatever has the most profit potential – not lifesaving or life-enhancing potential – are not qualifications. They are scams [22].

Given these beliefs, it should not be a surprise that when CAM treatments fail in clinical trials, this dissuades neither the Galileos themselves nor their devotees. Much like cult members who remain unmoved when their leader's prediction of the end of the word fails to materialize, failed scientific studies of CAM treatments only reinvigorates their faith in the treatment and cast further suspicion on the mainstream science. Often, CAM Galileos claim that the scientific method simply is not equipped to study their treatments at all (Fig. 27.21).

When clinicians tout themselves as modern-day Galileos, many patients are eager to embrace the personas these doctors create. Indeed, Americans spent $34 billion dollars on alternative medicine in 2009, a number that has certainly increased since then [39]. Much of this is out-of-pocket payments, as most insurers do not pay for unproven treatments [40]. Patients turn to CAM Galileos for many reasons. Many are understandably desperate when mainstream medicine has no answers or cures for their illness. Others distrust large medical institutions and pharmaceutical companies. Many have a self-identity based on a "natural" lifestyle.

At first glance, it may seem surprising that adherents of CAM are eager to simultaneous embrace the cancer treatments of Galileos like Drs. Burzynski and Gonzalez; after all, the proposed treatments have nothing in common. One uses "antineoplastons," while the other involves hundreds of pills of pancreatic enzymes and daily coffee enemas. Additionally, it may seem baffling that these protocols are popular in the "natural" health community, as there is nothing natural about injecting coffee into one's rectum or taking hundreds of supplements every day.

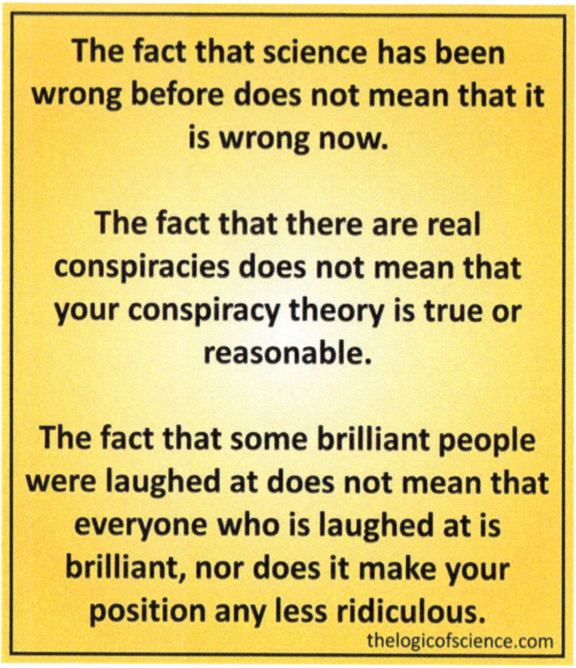

Fig. 27.21 I agree. (The Logic of Science. [Image file, Facebook status update]. 2015. Retrieved from https://www.facebook.com/thelogicofscience/posts/1789191471312248:0.)

Yet, what they both offer is the mystique of Galileo; a persecuted individual who bravely rejects core tenets of stodgy medical dogma and who persists in the face of ridicule from their peers and threats from the government. As such, Galileos are not selling a specific treatment, as much as they are promoting a lifestyle and identity. At some level, Galileos are fundamentally selling themselves. Not surprisingly, the websites of many Galileos often feature glamor shots of the Galileo (often doing yoga on a beach or mountaintop) and information about their personal life, such as what they eat, how they exercise, and products they endorse.

Galileos succeed not by convincing their patients with science and evidence, but through identifying with them and gaining their trust. Dr. Mercola, for example, flatters visitors to his website and creates mistrust about mainstream medicine. He writes:

> You are wise to question who you can trust when it comes to maintaining, enhancing, or rebuilding your health. With all websites, newspapers, magazines, and other publications offering health advice, with every new multi-million dollar TV ad for another proclaimed miracle drug, with any recommendation offered by traditional and natural physicians, it is essential to answer this question above all others: what is their real motivation? (Fig. 27.22) [22].

This personal identification with the Galileo explains why devotees of CAM practitioners defend them the way a cult member defends their guru. For example, look at the way J. B. Handley, co-founder of the anti-vaccine group Generation

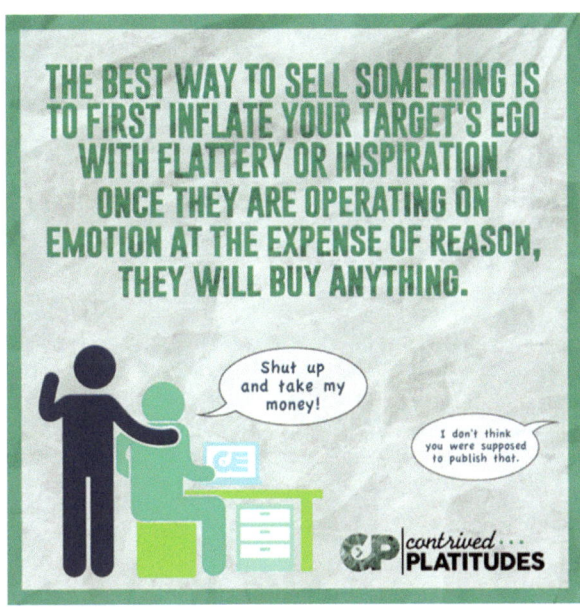

Fig. 27.22 Anti-vaccine doctor and self-proclaimed Galileo Dr. Toni Bark using herself to sell her philosophy. (Contrived Platitudes. [Image file, Facebook status update]. 2015. Retrieved from https://www.facebook.com/contrivedplatitudes/photos/a.1388700168115128/1390209207964224/?type=3.)

Rescue, described the father of the modern-day anti-vaccine movement, "To our community, Andrew Wakefield is Nelson Mandela and Jesus Christ rolled up into one. He's a symbol of how all of us feel" [41].

Yet another technique of many Galileos is the use of pseudo-profound bullshit. This term (really!) was coined by Gordon Pennycook and colleagues, who defined as it "seemingly impressive assertions that are presented as true and meaningful but are actually vacuous" [42]. In their study, they gave subjects bullshit statements "consisting of buzzwords randomly organized into statements with syntactic structure but no discernible meaning (e.g., "Wholeness quiets infinite phenomena")." Many of the bullshit statements were derived from tweets by the new age guru Deepak Chopra. He is known to produce statements such as "Freedom is knowing you are not a person" [43]. Others came from the websites the *New Age Bullshit Generator* and the *Wisdom of Chopra,* which produce random statements such as "Infinity gives rise to nonlocal chaos" and "Hidden meaning is in the midst of ephemeral potentiality (Fig. 27.23)."

While many subjects recognized these statements as meaningless, the 27% who thought they were profound were more likely to believe in paranormal phenomenon, conspiracy theories, and CAM. In contrast, those who recognized the statements as bullshit scored higher on measures of intelligence, skepticism, and rationality.

Fig. 27.23 I agree. (Contrived Platitudes. [Image file, Facebook status update]. 2015. Retrieved from https://www.facebook.com/contrivedplatitudes/photos/a.1388700168115128/1401873190131159/?type=3.)

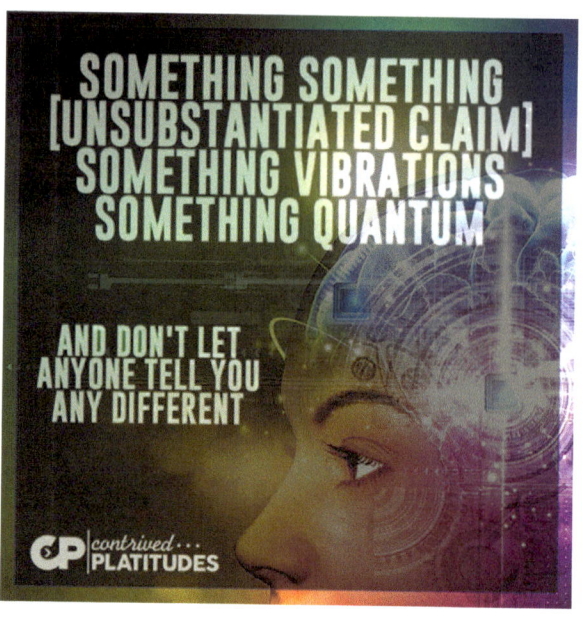

Pseudo-profound bullshit is similar to a phenomenon called the Dr. Fox effect. In a classic demonstration conducted by Donald Naftulin and colleagues in the 1970s, psychiatrists, psychologists, educational administrators, and social workers heard a lecture titled *Mathematical Game Theory and its Application to Physician Education* [44]. The lecture was given by Dr. Myron L. Fox, who was described as a highly accomplished expert on game theory and mathematics. Contrary to a stereotypical mathematician, Dr. Fox was engaging, warm, and humorous. Three separate audiences rated his talk favorably. A video of his lecture is available on YouTube if you want to watch it [45].

However, in reality, Dr. Fox was an actor whose talk was purposely filled "with an excessive use of double-talk, neologisms, non-sequiturs, and contradicting statements." His lively presentation and winning personality, "seduced" the audience into believing he was knowledgeable and that his lecture was meaningful. Replications of this study have shown that perhaps the situation is not so dire. When shown the original Dr. Fox video, audiences continue to rate him as an effective, engaging speaker [46]. However, when queried further, many students felt they didn't learn anything from him.

Not surprisingly, pseudo-profound bullshit and the Dr. Fox effect are common with CAM practitioners. Consider this statement from Dr. Brogan, "based on our growing knowledge of the microbiome, some theorize that illness is simply a resonant activation of *internal* microorganisms when detox and recalibration are needed" [47]. Here's another, "in order to live life in the ever-coveted flow, we need to push ourselves beyond the comfort zones of our mind, shed layers of story, and Ego in order to become all that much more ourselves" [47]. Don't feel bad if you don't understand these. They're meaningless. They're pseudo-profound bullshit.

Fig. 27.24 Satirical pseudo-profound bullshit. (Brogan K. [Kelly Brogan MD]. Are you ready? Do you feel the unsuspecting power of the lunar feminine [Facebook status update]. 2017. Retrieved from https://www.facebook.com/KellyBroganMD/posts/738070219733162.)

Kelly Brogan MD - Holistic Psychiatrist ⋯
· 21 August 2017 · 🌐

Are you ready? Do you feel the unsuspecting power of the lunar feminine coming into union with the fiery masculine? These polarities, in this auspicious balance, help us to see that there is no good/bad, no right/wrong…only perspectives, orientation, and moments that dissolve the divides. Here's to our healing, our transformation, and our expansion as a collective 🙏

Cognitive scientist Dan Sperber coined a term, the guru effect, which helps explain how pseudo-profound bullshit can be very useful for CAM Galileos. He defined the guru effect as the tendency for people to "judge profound what they have failed to grasp" [48]. He argued that "obscure texts and their authors come to be overestimated, often ridiculously so, not in spite but because of their very obscurity" (Fig. 27.24).

Unfortunately, pseudo-profound bullshit seems to work. One study found that by using technology and jargon, the so-called "the trappings of science," people were more likely to view paranormal investigators as "scientific and credible" [49]. Another paper found that using "scientific or scientific-related terms" was common in advertisements for skin-care products. It concluded that a "combination of the conceptual complexity and the Greco-Latin etymology of most of these terms is a guarantee of significant persuasion to the layperson" [50]. Through the use of pseudo-profound bullshit, many CAM Galileos are able to pursuade people they are misunderstood geniuses, convincing them to buy their books and products.

Sadly, when desperate patients put themselves in the care of CAM Galileos, the consequences can be devastating. Real people get hurt and die. The website whatstheharm.net has a collection of tragic stories of people harmed by CAM. It's sobering to read. These harms have been formally documented multiple times as well. One study examined 840 patients diagnosed with breast, prostate, lung, or colorectal cancer from 2004 to 2013. 280 patients received alternative treatments while 560 patients received conventional treatments such as chemotherapy, surgery, and radiation [51]. James Yu, an oncologist, said "we became interested in this topic after seeing too many patients present in our clinics with advanced cancers that were treated with ineffective and unproven alternative therapies alone" [52]. The results of the study backed up his experience, finding that cancer patients who used CAM significantly were more likely to die than those who chose conventional treatments. As the US Public Health Service poster from 1938 shows, the tendency for desperate people to be taken advantage of by quacks is, sadly, an old one (Fig. 27.25).

Fig. 27.25 Pseudo-
profound bullshit (Works
Project Administration
Poster Collection. Beware
the cancer quack [Image
file]. In: Wikimedia
commons. (ca. 1937).
Retrieved from https://
commons.wikimedia.org/
wiki/File:Beware_the_can-
cer_quack_LCCN98518641.
tif.)

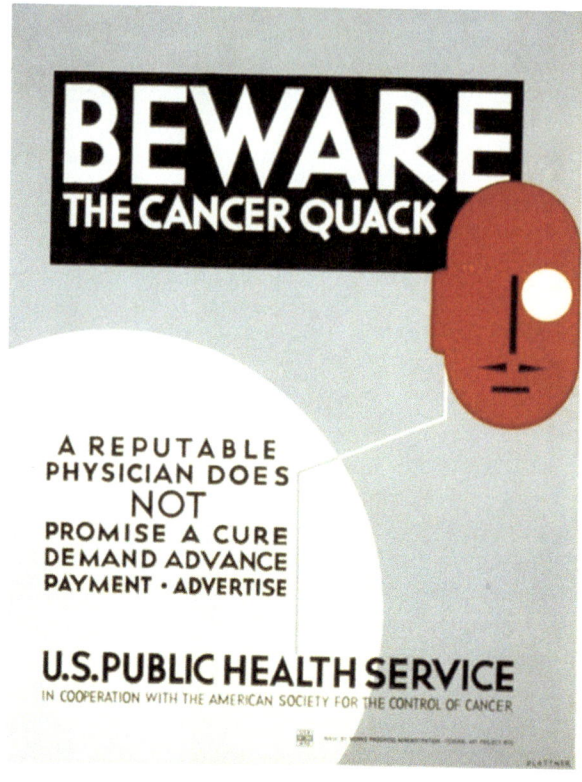

Conclusion

When confronted with a radical new theory of disease or a radical treatment, clinicians should strive to keep an open mind, while simultaneously recognizing that
sudden, dramatic shifts in medical paradigms are quite rare. Some treatments or
theories of disease that are now considered implausible may one day be widely
accepted by mainstream medicine. However, this does not mean that all implausible
theories are deserving of respect. When a clinician proposes a radical new scientific
theory or treatment, it must be studied in large numbers of people and replicated by
others in rigorous scientific trials before it can overturn established medical knowledge. As Carl Sagan said, "The fact that some geniuses were laughed at does not
imply that all who are laughed at are geniuses. They laughed at Columbus, they
laughed at Fulton, they laughed at the Wright brothers. But they also laughed at Bozo
the Clown" (Fig. 27.26).

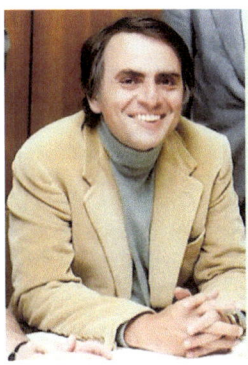
The fact that some geniuses were laughed at does not imply that all who are laughed at are geniuses. They laughed at Columbus, they laughed at Fulton, they laughed at the Wright brothers. But they also laughed at Bozo the Clown.
Carl Sagan

Fig. 27.26 Cancer quacks have always been around and probably always will be. (NASA/JPL. Carl Sagan [Image file]. In: Wikimedia commons. 1979. Retrieved from https://commons.wikimedia.org/wiki/Carl_Sagan#/media/File:Carl_Sagan_Planetary_Society.JPG.)

References

1. Rohlke F, Stollman N. Fecal microbiota transplantation in relapsing *Clostridium difficile* infection. Ther Adv Gastroenterol. 2012;5(6):403–20. https://doi.org/10.1177/1756283X12453637.
2. Syed M. Black box thinking: marginal gains and the secrets of high performance [Google Books version]. London: John Murray – Carmelite House; 2015.
3. Hopkins DR. The greatest killer: smallpox in history [Google Books version]. Chicago: The University of Chicago Press; 2002.
4. Hancock M, Tomlin A. The rough guide to Dorset, Hampshire & the Isle of Wight. [[Google Books version]. London: Rough Guides Publishing Company; 2010.
5. Bartholomew RE, Radford B. The Martians have landed! A history of media-driven panics and hoaxes [Google Books version]. Jefferson: McFarland & Company, Inc; 2012.
6. Beattie-Moss M. (2008, Feb 4). Gut instincts: a profile of Nobel laureate Barry Marshall. Penn State News. Retrieved from https://news.psu.edu/story/140921/2008/02/04/research/gut-instincts-profile-nobel-laureate-barry-marshall.
7. Morris ZS, Wooding S, Grant J. The answer is 17 years, what is the question: understanding time lags in translational research. J R Soc Med. 2011;104(12):510–20. https://doi.org/10.1258/jrsm.2011.110180.
8. Balas EA, Boren SA. Managing clinical knowledge for health care improvement. In: McCray BJ, editor. Yearbook of medical informatics 2000: patient-centered systems. Stuttgart: Schattauer Verlagsgesellschaft; 2000. p. 65–70.
9. Alper BS, Hand JA, Elliott SG, Kinkade S, Hauan MJ, Onion DK, Sklar BM. How much effort is needed to keep up with the literature relevant for primary care. J Med Libr Assoc. 2004;92(4):429–37.
10. ABC Catalyst. (2012, Aug 23). MS cure? [Video file]. Retrieved from http://www.abc.net.au/catalyst/stories/3572695.htm.

11. Comi C, Battaglia MA, Bertolotto A, Del Sette M, Ghezzi A, Malferrari G, Salvetti M, Sormani MP, Tesio L, Stolz E, Zaratin P, Mancardi G, the CoSMo Collaborative Study Group. Observational case-control study of the prevalence of chronic cerebrospinal venous insufficiency in multiple sclerosis: results from the CoSMo study. Mult Scler J. 2013;19(11):1508–17. https://doi.org/10.1177/1352458513501231.

12. FDA issues alert on potential dangers of unproven treatment for multiple sclerosis. (2012, May 11). VascularNews. Retrieved 15 Sept 2018 from https://vascularnews.com/fda-issues-alert-on-potential-dangers-of-unproven-treatment-for-multiple-sclerosis/.

13. Novella S. (2016, Oct 26). Update on CCSVI and multiple sclerosis. Science-Based Medicine. Retrieved from https://sciencebasedmedicine.org/update-on-ccsvi-and-multiple-sclerosis/.

14. Zamboni P, Tesio L, Galimberti S, Massacesi L, Salvi F, D'Alessandro R, Cenni P, Galeotti R, Papini D, D'Amico R, Simi S, Valsecchi MG, Filippini G. Efficacy and safety of extracranial vein angioplasty in multiple sclerosis. JAMA Neurol. 2018;75(1):35–43. https://doi.org/10.1001/jamaneurol.2017.3825.

15. Watts G. (2005, Jan 5). Histories: Elisha Perkins and his 'medical tractors'. New Scientist Retrieved from https://www.newscientist.com/article/mg18524815-200-histories-elisha-perkins-and-his-medical-tractors/.

16. Aran I. (2016, May 9). Men used to subject their penises to electric shocks to treat impotence. Splinter News. Retrieved from https://splinternews.com/men-used-to-subject-their-penises-to-electric-shocks-to-1793855289.

17. Salivas A. Report on the treatment of tuberculosis by Francisque Crôtte's method. In: MacKenzie H, Beevor HR, Perkins JJ, editors. Transactions of the British Congress on Tuberculosis for the prevention of consumption, vol. III. London: William Clowes and Sons, Limited; 1902. p. 477–9.) [Google Books version].

18. Diabetes electrotherapy with vacuum electrode [Image file]. (n.d.). In: Wikimedia Commons. Retrieved 15 Sept 2018 from https://commons.wikimedia.org/wiki/File:Diabetes_electrotherapy_with_vacuum_electrode_1922.jpg.

19. University of Virginia. (n.d.). English caricature: Quacks & nostrums [Online image exhibit]. Retrieved from http://exhibits.hsl.virginia.edu/caricatures/en4-quacks/.

20. UCL Bloomsbury Project. (2011, Apr 13). British College of Health: also known as Society of Hygeists. Retrieved from http://www.ucl.ac.uk/bloomsbury-project/institutions/british_college_of_health.htm.

21. Harris RF. Rigor mortis: how sloppy science creates worthless cures, crushes hope, and wastes billions. New York: Hachette Book Group; 2017.

22. About Dr. Mercola. (n.d.). Mercola. Retrieved 15 Sept 2018 from http://www.mercola.com/forms/background.htm.

23. Smith B. (2012, Jan 31). Dr. Mercola: Visionary or quack? Chicago Magazine. Retrieved from http://www.chicagomag.com/Chicago-Magazine/February-2012/Dr-Joseph-Mercola-Visionary-or-Quack/.

24. Federal Trade Commission. (2016, Apr 14). Marketers of indoor tanning systems to pay refunds to consumers. Retrieved from https://www.ftc.gov/news-events/press-releases/2016/04/marketers-indoor-tanning-systems-pay-refunds-consumers.

25. The Gerson Therapy. (2011). The Gerson therapy. Gerson Institute. Retrieved 15 Sept 2018 from https://gerson.org/gerpress/the-gerson-therapy/.

26. Edwards M. (2016, May 20). Dr. Max Gerson – persecuted for curing cancer naturally. Organic Lifestyle. Retrieved from https://www.organiclifestylemagazine.com/issue/13-dr-max-gerson.

27. The Gerson Institute. (n.d.). Dr. Max Gerson. Retrieved 15 Sept 2018 from https://gerson.org/gerpress/dr-max-gerson/.

28. New Spring Press. (n.d.). Review of the book One man alone: an investigation of nutrition, cancer, and William Donald Kelley. Retrieved 15 Sept 2018 from https://www.newspringpress.com/oneman.html.

29. Ji, S. (2012, Apr 22). Antineoplastons: a cure for cancer ignored for 45 years? GreenMedInfo. http://www.greenmedinfo.com/blog/antineoplastons-cure-cancer-ignored-45-years.
30. Gorski DH. Stanislaw Burzynski: four decades of an unproven cancer cure. Skept Inq. 2014;38(2). Retrieved from https://www.csicop.org/si/show/stanislaw_burzynski_four_decades_of_an_unproven_cancer_cure.
31. The OTHER Burzynski Patient Group. (n.d.). About TOBPG. Retrieved 15 Sept 2018 from https://theotherburzynskipatientgroup.wordpress.com/about/.
32. Humprhies S. (n.d.). Rising from the dead. Suzanne Humphries, MD. Retrieved 15 Sept 2018 from http://drsuzanne.net/rising-from-the-dead/.
33. Brogan K. (n.d.). Sacred activism: moving beyond the ego. Kelly Brogan MD. Retrieved 15 Sept 2018 from https://kellybroganmd.com/sacred-activism-moving-beyond-ego/.
34. Gundry S. (n.d.). A letter from Steven Gundry, MD. GundryMD. Retrieved 15 Sept 2018 from https://gundrymd.com/gundry-md/.
35. Elizabeth E. (2015, Aug 21). Holistic MD Nick Gonzalez, who died suddenly, said he'd heard big pharma hoped he'd get hit by a bus. HealthNutNews. Retrieved from https://www.healthnutnews.com/holistic-md-nick-gonzalez-who-died-suddenly-said-hed-heard-big-pharma-hopes-he-gets-hit-by-a-bus/.
36. Elizabeth E. (2016, Mar 12). Unintended holistic doctor death series: over 90 dead. HealthNutNews. Retrieved from https://www.healthnutnews.com/recap-on-my-unintended-series-the-holistic-doctor-deaths/.
37. Holiday J. (2017, July 24). Deconstructing Kelly Brogan ep 4: all the conspiracies (Re-upload) [Video file]. Retrieved from https://www.youtube.com/watch?v=t_mfXzwheTM.
38. PharmedOut. (n.d.). About us. Retrieved 15 Sept 2018 from http://www.pharmedout.org/aboutus.html.
39. U.S. Department of Health & Human Services, National Institutes of Health, National Center for Complementary and Integrative Health. (2009, July 30). Americans spent $33.9 billion out-of-pocket on complementary and alternative medicine. Retrieved from https://nccih.nih.gov/news/2009/073009.htm.
40. Nahin RL, Barns PM, Stussman BJ. (2016). Expenditures on complementary health approaches: United States, 2012. National Health Statistics Report, 95. Retrieved from https://www.cdc.gov/nchs/data/nhsr/nhsr095.pdf.
41. Dominus S. (2011, Apr 24). The crash and burn of an autism guru. The New York Times Magazine. Retrieved from https://www.nytimes.com/2011/04/24/magazine/mag-24Autism-t.html.
42. Pennycook G, Cheyne JA, Barr N, Koehler DJ, Fugelsang JA. On the reception and detection of pseudo-profound bullshit [PDF file]. Judgm Decis Mak. 2015;10(6):549–63. Retrieved from http://journal.sjdm.org/15/15923a/jdm15923a.pdf.
43. Chopra D. [Deepak Chopra]. (2018, Jan 4). Freedom is knowing you are not a person [Twitter moment]. Retrieved from https://twitter.com/DeepakChopra/status/949001781232717825.
44. Naftulin DH, Ware JE, Donnelly FA. The Doctor Fox lecture: a paradigm of educational seduction. J Med Educ. 1973;48(7):630–5.
45. Kreuter D. (2012, June 15). Doctor Fox lecture [Video file]. Retrieved from https://www.youtube.com/watch?v=Rcr6UJwaPlQ.
46. Peer E, Babad E. The Doctor Fox research (1973) rerevisited: "Educational seduction" ruled out. J Educ Psychol. 2014;106(1):36–45. https://doi.org/10.1037/a0033827.
47. Brogan K. (n.d.). Holistic medicine: a life without fear. Kelly Brogan MD. Retrieved 15 Sept 2018 from https://kellybroganmd.com/holistic-medicine-a-life-without-fear/.
48. Sperber D. The guru effect. Rev Philos Psychol. 2010;1(4):583–92. https://doi.org/10.1007/s13164-010-0025-0.
49. Brewer PR. The trappings of science: media messages, scientific authority, and beliefs about paranormal investigators. Sci Commun. 2012;35(3):311–33. https://doi.org/10.1177/1075547012454599.

50. Arroyo MD. Scientific language in skin-care advertising: persuading through opacity [PDF version]. Revista española de lingüística aplicada. 2013;26:197–214. Retrieved from https://pdfs.semanticscholar.org/8ab7/7c858da5299ddeead1bfe64486a8698c0a26.pdf.
51. Johnson SB, Park HS, Gross CP, Yu JB. Use of alternative medicine for cancer and its impact on survival. JNCI: J Natl Cancer Inst. 2018;110(1):121–4. https://doi.org/10.1093/jnci/djx145.
52. Doerr A. (2017, Aug 10). Using only alternative medicine for cancer linked to lower survival rate. Yale News. Retrieved from https://news.yale.edu/2017/08/10/using-only-alternative-medicine-cancer-linked-lower-survival-rate.

28

This chapter discusses several aspects of clinical care that are not intrinsic cognitive biases, but rather features of modern medicine that profoundly affect clinicians' decision-making processes, at times forcing them to provide suboptimal care to their patients. These are:

- **Alarm Fatigue:** Alarm fatigue occurs when clinicians become immune to warnings about their patients due to repeated false alarms.
- **Defensive Medicine:** Defensive medicine occurs when care is driven not by what is in the best interest of the patient, but rather what is likely to protect the clinician from a malpractice suit.
- **Graded Clinician Error:** The graded clinician error occurs when clinicians who are graded on their patients' outcome respond to this incentive by refusing to treat the sickest patients or by exaggerating their problems to make them appear more ill than they really are.
- **Electronic Medical Record Error:** The electronic medical record (EMR) error occurs when clinicians are forced to slavishly click buttons on a computer to give the appearance of providing care to their patients at the expense of actually taking care of their patients.

While clinicians cannot always change their behavior to avoid these errors, they should be aware of them and how they might affect patient care. The solution to these problems are technical, administrative, and political.

Alarm Fatigue

Case
Richard was a 70-year-old man who presented with trouble swallowing. He was diagnosed with myasthenia gravis (MG), a disease in which disordered communication between the muscle and nerves causes weakness. He was admitted to the

© Springer International Publishing AG, part of Springer Nature 2019   501
J. Howard, *Cognitive Errors and Diagnostic Mistakes*,
https://doi.org/10.1007/978-3-319-93224-8_28

hospital and started on pyridostigmine, a medication that improves neuromuscular communication in patients with MG. Seven hours after arrival, he was found in severe respiratory distress. He needed to be intubated, but had suffered from significant cerebral anoxia. A review of his case by the hospital administration revealed that respiratory alarms had been going off in his room for 5 minutes before anyone arrived, and that the intern had walked by the room during that time without paying any attention to the alarm.

What Dr. Dickson Was Thinking

I can sure see how this case looks horrible to an outsider. It would be easy to say that I ignored the alarm that said he wasn't breathing, which I guess I did. However, it neglects the fact that alarms are constantly going off in the intensive care unit (ICU). If a patient's connection to a monitor gets disrupted in any way, it will beep, and most patients have several different monitors. So, there are innumerable false alarms, and it is not uncommon for multiple doctors and nurses to walk past a beeping monitor. When I was a student, I would sprint to every beeping monitor for the first few days. But I soon realized this was a waste 99.9% of the time, and it significantly interfered with caring for patients. I obviously can't distinguish a real alarm from a false one. So, I am not sure what to do.

Discussion

Alarm fatigue occurs when clinicians become immune to warnings about their patients due to repeated false alarms. In Ivan Pavlov's classic experiment, his dog started salivating to the sound of a bell alone after the bell had been previously paired with food. However, the dog stopped salivating once the bell was rung several times, but no food was given. In classical conditioning, this behavior is known as extinction. It occurs when a conditioned stimulus (a bell) is presented alone, so that it no longer predicts the coming of the unconditioned stimulus (food). This causes the conditioned response (salivation) to disappear. In this chapter's case, the conditioned stimulus (the alarm) was no longer paired with the unconditioned stimulus (a patient in distress), causing extinction of the conditioned response (checking on the patient) (Fig. 28.1).

Unfortunately, many of the systems designed to alert clinicians to problems are overly sensitive and have the effect of desensitizing them. The Emergency Care Research Institute (ERCI) puts out an annual list of Top Ten Health Technology Hazards, and every year, alarm fatigue and other alarm malfunctions are at the top of the list [1]. As Maria Cvach, the assistant director of nursing, clinical standards at Johns Hopkins said:

> In hospitals today, we have too many alarming devices. The alarm default settings are not set to actionable levels, and the alarm limits are set too tight. Monitor alarm systems are very sensitive and unlikely to miss a true event; however, this results in too many false positives. We have moved to large clinical units with unclear alarm system accountability; private rooms with doors closed that make it hard to hear alarm signals; and duplicate alarm conditions which desensitize staff [2].

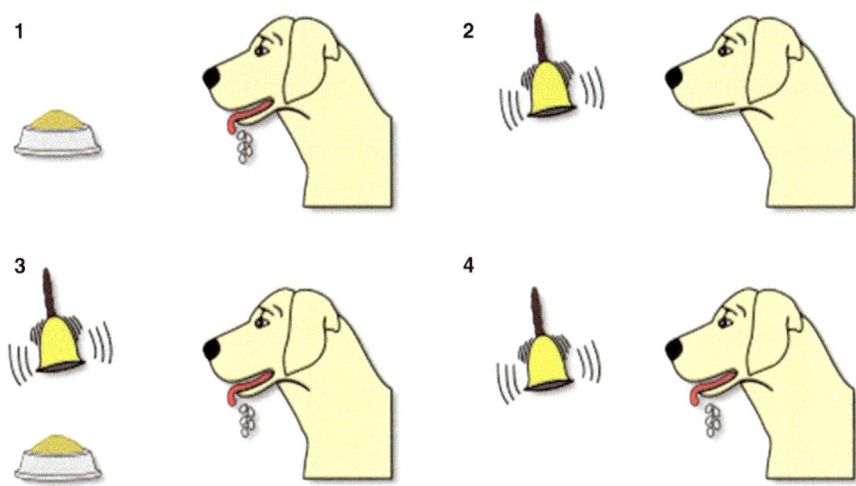

Fig. 28.1 Pavlov's dog started salivating to the sound of a bell along, after the bell had been paired with food. (Maxxl². Pavlov's dog conditioning [Image file]. In: Wikimedia commons. 2014. Retrieved from https://commons.wikimedia.org/wiki/File:Pavlov%27s_dog_conditioning.svg.)

A student or intern, new to the hospital, might be tempted to pay attention to every alarm. They will soon learn this is impossible. Barbara Drew and colleagues studied 461 adults in ICUs at the University of California, San Francisco Medical Center over a thirty one day period in 2014 [3]. They found that 2,558,760 unique alarms were recorded. 381,560 were audible, averaging almost 200 such alarms per patient per day. Another study found that in a twelve day period at Johns Hopkins Hospital, there were 58,764 alarms, which averaged out to 350 alarms per bed per day. The pediatric ICU had 20,158 auditory alarms in eight days for 17 beds [2]. Things were even noisier in one ICU, where there were an average of 771 alarm conditions per bed per day. Intensivist Adam Sapirstein noted, "It could have been one full-time person's sole job to just respond to all of those alarms" [2].

Even more concerning is that almost all of these are false alarms. Overall, estimates of false positives range from 72% to 99% [4]. In the San Francisco Medical Center ICU, 88.8% of the nearly 13,000 arrhythmia alarms were false positives. At Johns Hopkins, of 157 apnea alarm conditions, 90% were thought to be false. Given this, it is tempting for clinicians to simply silence oversensitive alarms, and patient deaths have resulted from this [1]. In a survey of 1,327 clinicians, 77% felt that alarms disrupted patient care, while 78% felt decreased trust in alarms can cause caregivers to disable them [5]. Combined with the psychological phenomenon of diffusion of responsibility, alarms can be rendered functionally useless. Kathryn Pelczarski, director of ECRI's applied solutions group noted:

> There may be so many alarms going off, it sort of becomes the background noise. We have seen situations where all the nurses are responsible for all alarms within that unit and there is the assumption that someone else will get that alarm. I frequently see alarms turned down to the point of being inaudible [6].

Yet, just because a patient monitor is going off, this doesn't mean the patient is fine. Patients have been killed and injured because of alarm errors. The Joint Commission's Sentinel Event database received 98 reports of alarm-related events from 2009 to 2012 [7]. Eighty patients died and 13 were permanently disabled. In contrast to clinicians who ignore alarms, those who tend to every false alarm will find themselves caring for monitors, possibly to the detriment of the actual patients to which they are attached.

Additionally, ill patients cannot rest when their rooms are a cacophony of beeps and buzzers. Patients are already woken excessively and often needlessly to have their vital signs taken, labs drawn, and to be given medications. Sleep disruption has been linked to negative health outcomes and patient distress [8]. Anything that can be done to allow patients to rest in the hospital is beneficial, and studies have shown that patients who can sleep in the hospital have better outcomes [9].

Several adjustments to alarms have resulted in improvements. Changing the threshold at which an alarm will go off and having a brief time delay of 15 seconds has been shown to meaningfully reduce the number of alarms. At Johns Hopkins, for example, the number of alarms on a medical progressive care unit was decreased from 16,952 to 9,647, a 43% reduction. There was also a 24–74% reduction of alarm conditions on six intensive and intermediate care units [2].

A similar type of alarm fatigue occurs as the computer software designed to catch drug-drug interactions and patient allergies is overly sensitive. As any clinician who has had the unfortunate experience ordering medications using an electronic medical record (EMR) knows, it is essentially impossible to order two medications without the computer flagging *some* interaction between them. Not surprisingly, clinicians quickly learn to ignore these "warnings." A study by Saul Weingert and colleagues found that "physicians overrode 91.2% of drug allergy and 89.4% of high-severity drug interaction alerts" [10]. Computer software that finds an interaction between every medication is no better than software that fails to find an interaction between any medications.

In addition to monitors and computers, doctors are notified about potential problems from multiple sources, including nurses, pharmacists, radiologists, and laboratory technicians. I have worked in environments where nurses were obligated to report "everything" to the doctor. For example, every time a patient had a minimally elevated blood pressure, the doctor was paged, even if the patient had no symptoms and their blood pressure had been elevated for two straight weeks. An unintended consequence of this was that eventually doctors became desensitized to the nurses' calls, and some opportunities were missed to help ill patients. In contrast, laboratory technicians and radiologists would generally call only when there was a "panic value" or significant radiographic abnormality that needed urgent attention. Their calls usually meant something serious was wrong, and were not ignored.

Another related problem occurs when clinicians try to determine whether a patient may be having a side effect from one of their medications. According to a paper by Jon Duke and colleagues, the average drug label lists 70 possible side effects and some list more than 500 [11]. Some side effects, such as nausea, are listed on nearly 75% of drug labels. Medications also commonly list contradictory side effects, such as diarrhea and constipation. Listing these side effects is a means of protecting pharmaceutical companies from potential lawsuits, not informing clinicians in a meaningful way about medication side effects. Like an alarm that goes off constantly for little reason, a drug label that lists hundreds of side effects, which may or may not be related to the drug, is scarcely better than a label that lists no side effects at all.

Any clinician, trying to deal with different alarms, computer notifications, and phone calls quickly enters a state of learned helplessness, a concept developed by the psychologist Martin Seligman. He found that dogs that had received electric shocks that they could not avoid, later did not even try to escape such shocks when avoidance was possible. In contrast, dogs that had not received such shocks immediately tried to escape their situation. Certainly, it is a bit dramatic to compare a clinician receiving excessive alarms to a dog being repeatedly shocked. However, the similarity lies in that both groups soon abandon any attempt to react to the adverse stimulus.

Finally, recognition of alarm fatigue has public health implications, as it can affect the entire populace. When members of the public are constantly bombarded by ceaseless safety warnings, the warnings are all too often ignored. For example, a law in California known as Proposition 65 requires that business warn citizens when they might be exposed to naturally occurring or synthetic chemicals that are known to cause cancer or birth defects or other reproductive harm. There are over 850 chemicals on this list [12]. In order to avoid possible legal ramifications, businesses often put up warning signs, even for chemicals that are not present. The results are predictable. As journalist Mariel Garza wrote:

> The problem is that Proposition 65 warning signs and labels are everywhere you look — office buildings, gas stations, pot shops, just to name a few... Since Californians can't escape the chemicals, or the many signs warning about them, the only rational reaction has been to ignore them. Obviously that was not the intent of the 1986 ballot measure that created the state law to identify and list dangerous chemicals, but it does show that warnings without action or context aren't particularly helpful [13].

Conclusion

Alarm fatigue is a problem beyond the powers of any individual clinician to fix. It is impossible to work in an environment where false alarms are the norm and *not* become desensitized to them. Computer designers should improve monitors and software so that clinicians can be notified of potential problems without an overwhelming number of false alarms. I am sure that this is not an easy task. Alarms have to be set at a threshold where they are sensitive enough to pick up real patient events, without an abundance of false negatives. However, as Johns Hopkins has shown, reducing false alarms is possible. Similar efforts need to be made to ensure computer software flags meaningful drug interactions without flagging an interaction between nearly every drug. Finally, hospital administrators should strive to create an environment where nurses can use their clinical judgment when notifying doctors, calling only when there is a problem they feel warrants the doctor's attention. Nurses should not feel required to document "doctor notified" in the chart for problems they know are trivial.

Defensive Medicine

Case
Richard was a 34-year-old man who presented to the ER after falling off his bike. He had a mild abrasion to his right ear, but otherwise had no evidence of head trauma. He was wearing a helmet and said that he was "barely moving" when he fell. He had a normal exam and no neurological complaints. The ER doctor ordered a head CT just to be sure there was no intracranial bleed. Even though the clinician knew that there was no indication for the CT based on guidelines, a colleague of his had been sued under similar circumstances.

What Dr. Abrams Was Thinking
I knew that Richard had mild head trauma and a CT was not indicated. The indications for a head CT in patients with mild head trauma are posted in the ER. Of these, Joe only had a small abrasion on his ear, and he told me that he got this struggling to get his bike off of him. However, my colleague was really suffering after a patient sued her in similar circumstances. Her patient only had a small amount of blood which was found on a CT scan done by another hospital several days later. The CT didn't change his care at all, but he sued anyway. She's really struggling with this, wondering what it might mean for her future. So, when patients like Joe come around, I know they don't need head CTs. I know that there's nothing I'm going to find anything that will change their care. But the last thing I need is a lawsuit.

Case
Allana was a 43-year-old woman who presented in premature labor. She had used *in vitro* fertilization to get pregnant and was carrying twins. After noticing worrisome findings on the fetal monitors, she was rushed for a cesarean section. Once of the babies suffered from a brain hemorrhage and was left with cerebral palsy. Allana successfully sued the obstetrician who performed the operation.

What Dr. Waters Was Thinking
This was certainly a tragic case. Allana was a high-risk pregnancy and from what I was seeing on the fetal monitors, there was no way this was going to have a happy outcome. Given the circumstances, I think I did the best I could. But of course, Allana was devastated by what happened, and a lawyer in her family encouraged her to sue. The case went on for several years before going to trial. Her lawyer did a masterful job of manipulating the emotions of the jurors. I knew after that, there was no way I was going to treat a patient like Allana again. There's just too much risk.

So now, I do basic gynecological care and still deliver babies of young, low risk mothers. Someone else can take care of the Allanas of the world. I won't be giving any ambulance-chasing lawyer any business.

Discussion

Medicolegal concerns, unfortunately, influence medicine and those who practice it in profound ways. Clinicians often feel obligated to practice defensive medicine, which occurs when care is driven not by what is in the best interest of the patient, but rather what is likely to protect the clinician from a malpractice suit. While it is not a cognitive bias per se, the practice of defensive medicine has become second nature to many clinicians, resulting in thoughtless care and wasted resources as clinicians want to protect themselves against the possibility of a lawsuit. Combined with the significant effect on patients, this makes defensive medicine an important topic for discussion in the context of cognitive biases.

There are two forms of defensive medicine: assurance and avoidance medicine. Assurance medicine involves excessive and unnecessary tests and procedures to prevent medical malpractice claims and demonstrate the clinician is practicing according to the standard of care. Due to malpractice fears, many clinicians feel obligated to order tests or perform procedures that they do not deem clinically necessary. Over-testing has the potential to harm patients both through the risks of the tests themselves and through the discovery of incidental findings. One ER doctor kept a list of patients she saw during one shift and how she felt defensive medicine impacted their care. After describing multiple cases in a single shift where she ordered extra tests to cover herself, she said that had she missed anything:

> I would be spending the next several years listening to a plaintiff's attorney telling everyone how the patient's injury is an example of why I am a bad doctor and why clinical examination alone is simply not good enough. That, my friends, is defensive medicine at work [14].

Avoidance medicine occurs when clinicians refuse to perform high-risk procedures or treat high-risk patients. Some clinicians move to different states or simply quit medicine altogether to avoid malpractice claims.

Though it differs greatly from one specialty to another, malpractice lawsuits are relatively common. A study by Anupam Jena and colleagues found that, each year, 7.4% of doctors had a malpractice claim, though only 22% of these suits resulted in payments to claimants [15]. In high-risk specialties, such as neurosurgery, nearly 20% of doctors faced a malpractice claim each year. In these specialties, almost all doctors will become involved in one or more lawsuits over the course of their careers. Importantly, clinicians can be sued even if no error occurred. Almost all medical procedures carry some risk, and a known complication is not the same thing as an error. A study by David Studdert and colleagues examined almost 1,500 malpractice claims and found that 37% involved no medical error [16]. For 3% of the claims, there was no evidence patients were even injured. Such claims are unlikely to be paid, but can still be costly to defend. Malpractice suits can last 5–7 years, and even when a lawsuit does not result in a claim being paid, fees paid to lawyers, experts, and courts can still total hundreds of thousands of dollars. Having said this, most injured patients do not sue. Approximately 2–3% of patients injured by medical negligence file lawsuits, and only half of them recover money [17].

Given that lawsuits are common, it is not surprising that defensive medicine is also common. A study by David Studdert and colleagues surveyed 824 Pennsylvania doctors in high-risk specialties (emergency medicine, general surgery, orthopedic surgery, neurosurgery, obstetrics/gynecology, and radiology) to determine the prevalence and characteristics of defensive medicine [18]. They found that 92% of doctors ordered imaging tests and other diagnostic measures for assurance, while 42% avoided high risk procedures, patients with significant complications, or patients they perceived as litigious.

Unfortunately, the negative effects of defensive medicine on patients and the healthcare system in general are significant. Anecdotes of clinicians changing their practice due to defensive medicine have been borne out by multiple studies. A study by A. Russell Localio and colleagues, for example, found that Cesarean delivery rates in the US increased from 4.5 to 24.1 per 100 births from 1965 to 1986 in part because of malpractice fears [19]. In 2010 Jackson Healthcare, the third largest healthcare staffing agency in the US, conducted a national survey of over 1,400 doctors [20]. Respondents felt that defensive medicine and fears of malpractice suits:

- Decreased patients' access to healthcare (76%).
- Negatively impacted patient care (72%).
- Has had a negative effect on the way they view patients (71%).
- Came between the doctor and patient (67%).
- Hampered their decision-making ability (57%).
- Delayed the adoption of new techniques/procedures/treatments (53%).

Additionally, defensive medicine is now part of the informal medical school curriculum. In the Jackson Healthcare survey, 83% of doctors ages 25–34 years-old reported being taught in medical school to avoid lawsuits.

Additionally, because of malpractice fears, some clinicians may simply avoid treating high-risk patients or performing high-risk procedures, even though they may feel the patient may benefit. Other studies have found that high liability costs cause clinicians in high-risk specialties to stop practicing or move elsewhere. A study by Michelle Mello and colleagues found the supply of obstetrician-gynecologists in Pennsylvania fell by 8% in the years after a malpractice "crisis" [21]. Similar results were found in New Jersey after malpractice costs increased 128% in 4 years [22]. As a result, many obstetricians stopped delivering babies, and several entire obstetrical practices reported they stopped delivering babies or caring for women with high-risk pregnancies.

Unfortunately, underserved areas are to be the most affected when there are clinician shortages due to high medical malpractice costs [23a, b]. Mark Rosing, the chairman of obstetrics and gynecology at a hospital in the Bronx, New York, has a very difficult time attracting clinicians to work there. He explained:

> Providers are very, very resistant or hesitant to come practice here, because in many cases, it can literally destroy their careers. Making a decision to practice here, taking care of patients that really need quality care — in doing so, you're basically guaranteed within five or 10 years to have a list of malpractice suits that may make you unemployable elsewhere [24].

In addition to this, many clinicians spend many hours documenting their reasoning in the chart, not because it will benefit the patient, but because documentation is a clinician's only defense in a malpractice case. Many clinicians spend significantly more time in front of a computer than with their patients. While there are many factors behind this, one of them is that clinicians often feel the need to protect themselves against a potential lawsuit in every patient encounter. Clinicians are taught that "it if wasn't documented, it didn't happen." One psychiatrist wrote on social media, "I spend 50% of my time documenting for a future lawsuit. I could be with my patients" [25].

A fear of malpractice lawsuits also drives bandwagon behavior. One of the requirements of a medical malpractice suit is that the clinician must practice outside the "medical standard of care." This is defined as "the type and level of care an ordinary, prudent, health care professional, with the same training and experience, would provide under similar circumstances in the same community" [26]. The standard of care threshold may force clinicians to practice medicine as the majority of clinicians in their community practice it, not as they feel is appropriate. As such, there may be a strong disincentive for clinicians to be the first in their community to deviate from "accepted practice," even when such deviation is evidence-based. In focus groups on why cardiologists continue to place coronary artery stents in patients for whom there is no demonstrable benefit, one responded, "In California, if this person had an event within two years, the doctor who didn't intervene would be successfully sued" [27]. Daniel Merenstein, a family medicine doctors who was sued for correctly counselling a patient about the risks and benefits of screening for prostate cancer, wrote the following about his experience:

> It is often claimed that malpractice is a mechanism for holding physicians accountable and improving the quality of care. This case illustrates quite the opposite: punishing the translation of evidence into practice, impeding improvements to care, and ensconcing practices that hurt patients. In our system, the physicians who are slow to change are the winners [28].

Not surprisingly, defensive medicine is very expensive. Although estimates vary, defensive medicine costs tens or even hundreds of billions of dollars per year [29]. Often these costs are born by individual clinicians. According to an analysis by *The New York Times*, insurance for individual obstetricians practicing in high-risk areas can approach nearly $200,000 per year [24].

Malpractice suits can be costly in other ways as well, as they can take an extreme emotional toll on clinicians, most of whom care deeply about their patients. A study by Charles Balch found that lawsuits against surgeons lead to burnout, depression, and even suicidal thoughts [30]. As Dr. Balch said, the stress of a malpractice suit "is right up there with financial distress, serious work-home conflicts and life-and-death circumstances" [31]. Given the length of time malpractice cases take, the stress and energy of dealing with them can occupy a significant amount of time of a clinician's career. Additionally, malpractice information is permanently and publically available in online records and may follow a clinician throughout the rest of their career. Ultimately, this trickles down to patients. Clinicians who are distressed because of a lawsuit are unlikely to be in a mental state where they can optimally care for patients.

States with apology laws

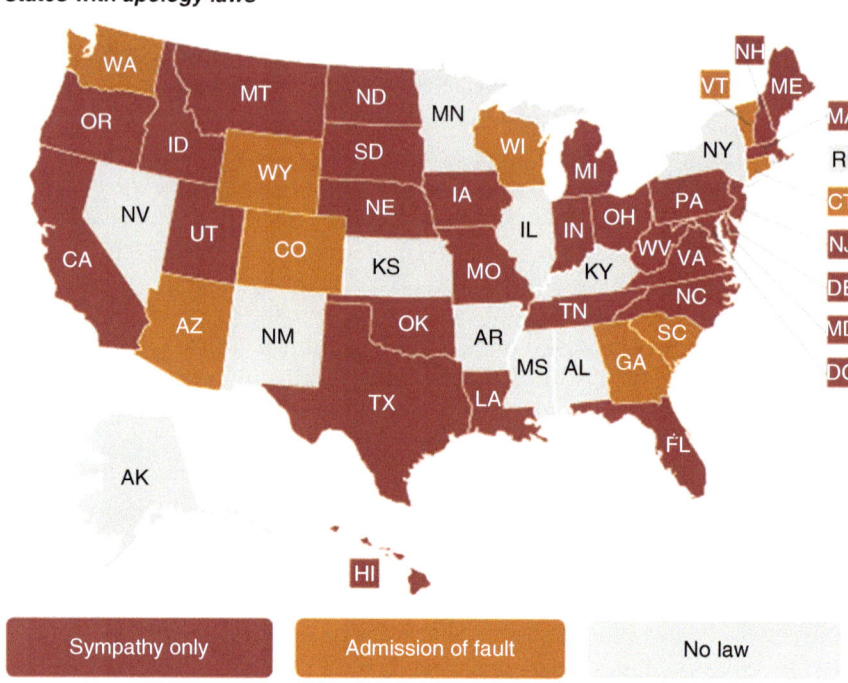

Fig. 28.2 States with apology laws. (Source: *Annals of Internal Medicine*; various news reports. Balancing doctor egos and errors: Page 4 of 4. [Image file]. In: Medical economics. 2016. Retrieved from http://www.medicaleconomics.com/medical-economics-blog/balancing-doctor-egos-and-errors/page/0/3.)

Fortunately, clinicians have some power to limit their likelihood of being sued. Many patients are motivated to sue their clinicians not only when there is a bad outcome, but also when there was insult added to this injury. A paper by two lawyers, Carol Liebmann and Chris Hyman, reported that when patients file a lawsuit, their primary motivations were a perception that the clinician was not honest about the incident and that no one explained what went wrong [32]. The conventional wisdom that apologies are admissions of error that may lead to a lawsuit are completely backwards. While clinicians should always talk to a lawyer if they feel that an error has been made, a majority of states have "apology laws" which prevent apologies from clinicians from being used against them in future lawsuits (Fig. 28.2).

Some states even protect acknowledgements of fault that may accompany any apology. Massachusetts, for example has a policy called "Disclosure, Apology and Offer." Under this policy, when there is a bad outcome, "patients and their families are provided full disclosure of what happened, what it means for the patient medically, and what will be done to prevent the error from recurring" [33]. Moreover, clinicians are not left to fend for themselves under his model, as patient safety coordinators help clinicians throughout the entire process from acknowledging the error to discussing compensation with malpractice insurers. This is especially important as most medical errors do not involve negligence by individual clinicians, as much as systems errors where multiple small mistakes add up to a large one. However, even this policy had little effect on clinicians' practice, with 90% of Massachusetts doctors saying that the policy had no effect on their practice of defensive medicine [29].

Conclusion

Due to malpractice fears, clinicians frequently order tests that they do not deem medically necessary. At other times, clinicians may simply stop caring for patients they perceive as a high risk. If patients get frustrated that their clinician is staring at the computer screen and not them, defensive medicine is partly to blame. The adherence to "standard of care" and a fear of lawsuits has also undoubtedly influenced medical practice as clinicians may be reluctant to be the first in their community to abandon harmful practices or adopt beneficial new ones.

The costs of a lawsuit can be substantial, both financially and emotionally. As such, it is difficult to tell clinicians they should avoid defensive medicine. Clinicians feel an understandable need to protect their careers. However, clinicians should never let defensive medicine interfere with the optimal care of a patient. As defensive medicine is done for the benefit of the clinician, it is a violation of medical ethics. When an error is made, the best way for clinician to avoid lawsuits is to openly acknowledge it and apologize.

Graded Clinician Error

Case

Aviad was a 67-year-old man who presented with chest pain and was found to have severe coronary artery disease placing him at high risk for a heart attack. He had several other medical problems, such as diabetes and hypertension, and prostate cancer. He smoked nearly two packs of cigarettes per day and never exercised. The surgeon felt that he would benefit from a coronary artery bypass grafting but refused to perform the operation. He felt that Aviad was too ill, and if there was a bad outcome it would reflect poorly on the "report card" his state kept on all cardiovascular surgeons. Aviad went to another state where he had a successful operation.

What Dr. Page Was Thinking

I used to operate on patients like Aviad all the time. However, three years ago my state instituted a report card. We all get graded now on how our patients do. Several of my colleagues have received pay cuts because of their "poor performance," and one even lost operating privileges at our hospital. Someone like Aviad is exactly the kind of patient who can really bring down my score. As a result, I won't operate on patients like him. I know it's not the right thing to do, but I really don't see what choice I have.

Discussion

The law of unintended consequences deals with unforeseen and unintended outcomes. It is captured in the expression, "the road to hell is paved with good intentions." An unfortunate demonstration of this has been the effect of grading clinicians based on patient outcomes. This has mostly been done with cardiovascular surgeons and cardiologists performing coronary artery stenting. On the face of it, grading clinicians based on how their patients fare seems to a be common-sense measure. If a surgeon has exceptionally poor outcomes, then this is something patients, hospitals, and even governmental licensing agencies should be aware of. Conversely, if a surgeon has exceptional outcomes, this might be something anyone contemplating cardiac surgery would also want to know.

However, patient outcomes are as likely to reflect the patient as they are the skill of the clinician. The surgeons that treat the sickest patients and perform the most difficult operations will naturally have the worst outcomes. In contrast, surgeons who operate on the healthiest patients and avoid complex operations are going to have the best outcomes. As one surgeon said, "The so-called best surgeons are only doing the most straightforward cases" [34].

Not surprisingly, surgeons who receive grades strive to improve them, and one way they do this is by changing how they select their patients. Predictably, they decline to operate on the sickest, most high-risk patients. One study from Pennsylvania found that after the implementation of report cards, 63% of cardiovascular surgeons said they were less likely to operate on severely ill patients, while none said they were more likely [35]. Fifty-nine percent cardiologists reported trouble finding surgeons who were willing to operate on their patients. Another study compared the rate of coronary artery stenting for acute myocardial infarction (AMI) and cardiogenic shock in Michigan, where there is no public reporting, and New York, where there is public reporting [36]. Predictably, patients in Michigan more frequently underwent coronary artery stenting than those in New York. The authors suggested that, "A propensity in New York toward not intervening on higher-risk patients because of fear of public reporting of high mortality rates is a possible explanation for these differences." Another study found that New York patients with AMIs and cardiogenic shock were less likely to undergo coronary artery stenting and waited significantly longer to have heart surgery compared to their non-New York counterparts [37].

Another study found that surgical report cards in New York and Pennsylvania led to effective surgical techniques being abandoned in favor of less effective medical treatments. Ultimately, patients were hurt. The study concluded that these programs "combined with delays in treatment, led sicker patients to have substantially higher frequencies of heart failure and repeated AMIs and ultimately, higher total costs of care" [38].

In response to these realities, regulators created formulas to try to account for a patient's baseline health so as not to penalize clinicians who treated the sickest patients. More unintended consequences followed. Such formulas encouraged clinicians to game the system by diagnosing their patients with as many conditions as possible in order to make them seem as sick as possible. Surgeons had a clear motivation to make every one of their patients appear to be a high-risk surgical candidate. In New York, for example, there was a dramatic "upcoding" of cardiac risk factors and reporting of medical comorbidities once surgeons' outcomes became public in 1990 [39].

Another version of the graded-clinician error occurs when clinicians are forced to pay attention to metrics that are peripherally related to the care of the patient in front of them, but may be related to their salary. Often times, clinicians' financial compensation is determined in part by whether their patients are up to date on preventative health measures and whether or not patients with diseases, such as diabetes, have maintained adequate control of their blood sugar levels. Again, while this sounds reasonable on the surface, the law of unintended consequences applies. Peter Ubel, a doctor and behavioral scientist, described a particularly egregious example of this, writing:

> She came to the urgent care center with a sprained ankle. The primary care provider gave her excellent care, expertly applying evidence-based evaluation guidelines to her situation, and, thereby, avoiding unnecessary X-rays. By all measures, the provider's care was excellent, but the interaction still ended up reducing his salary. You see, that patient's only medical interaction that year was for this ankle sprain, and the provider was therefore held accountable for all of her primary care needs. Since she had not received a mammogram that year, or received a diabetes screening, he incurred an end-of-the-year penalty for failing to meet these quality standards [40].

Grading clinicians by such metrics, while well-intended and intuitively wise, also leads to unfortunate consequences. Clinicians are not rewarded for giving thoughtful, appropriate care, but for checking off boxes on the EMR to give the appearance of good care.

The law of unintended consequences applies to entire hospitals as well. The Hospital Readmissions Reduction Program, which started in 2012, financially penalizes hospitals that have above average readmission rates for patients with heart failure, heart attacks, and pneumonia [41]. This program was certainly well intended. Prior to this program, hospitals could earn more money if these patients were readmitted to the hospital than by providing appropriate, outpatient care.

While the program succeeded in reducing readmissions, hospitals now had a financial incentive to discharge patients who returned with these conditions, even if they might benefit from being readmitted. A study by Ankur Gupta and colleagues correlated reduced readmissions with a small increase in thirty day and one-year mortality rates in patients with heart failure [42]. In contrast, another study found no such increase in the mortality rate, indicating more research must be done [43].

Additionally, hospitals may stop giving care to the most ill patients in order to improve their ratings. Steven Blum, a hospitalist at a veteran's hospital, said in an interview, "It's a numbers game. The leadership has figured out the hospital can actually do better by seeing less patients. These numbers show up on the director's report card, so it is very important they look good" [44]. Obviously, this hurts patients. One surgeon, Michael Mann, said that he was part of a hospital where he was discouraged from performing high-risk surgeries. In an interview he said, "I'm very ashamed. I colluded. I was told not to operate and pulled back, and at least one of my patients died because of it" [44]. However, when hospital metrics improve, it can mean a pay raise for the hospital director. According to one news account, "By denying veterans care, the ratings climbed rapidly from one star to two in 2016 and the director earned a bonus of $8,120" [44].

Additionally, like individual clinicians, hospitals have perverse incentives to game the system by making their patients seem more ill than they actually are. One study found that hospitals were able to decrease their financial penalties for a readmitted patient if they coded their illness as more severe than it actually was [45].

Conclusion

While measuring a clinician's performance by the outcomes of their patients makes sense on a surface level, the law of unintended consequences may create perverse incentives for clinicians. To a large degree, patient outcomes are not a reflection of the skill and care of the clinician, but rather indicative of the patients they treat and the complexity of the treatments they provide. Clinicians who are graded on their patients' outcome are likely to respond to this incentive by refusing to treat the sickest, most vulnerable patients. Similarly, clinicians may spend time on health measures unrelated to a patient's complaint, simply because they are being graded this way. Instead of focusing on fixing a patient's injured ankle, a clinician may spend time asking about issues that are utterly unrelated to the purpose of the visit in order to satisfy arbitrary metrics on a grading system.

Fixing the graded clinician error is not a clinician's job, but rather the job of government regulators and hospital administrators. However, the importance of these policies, on both individual clinicians and hospitals, should not be underestimated. In the words of Robert Yeh, a cardiologist:

> I find there to be some cognitive dissonance in the way those who call for the absolute highest levels of evidence for treatments such as device and drugs (which I agree with) are often willing to relax those standards in the evaluation of health policy. Bad health policies, like bad drugs, have unanticipated side effects [46].

The Electronic Medical Record Error

Case

Michael was a 69-year-old man who first presented with a laceration on his finger. He was cutting a bagel at home when the knife slipped and cut his finger. Michael said that he was otherwise healthy, that he hadn't seen a doctor in 10 years, and that he still swam a mile every day. The wound was closed without sutures and Michael was given a sterilizing ointment to put on the wound. He returned the next month when his wife found him confused at home and he was found to have a small ischemic stroke of his left temporal lobe affecting his ability to communicate. While in the hospital, Michael developed a urinary tract infection and was placed on an antibiotic to which he had a severe allergic reaction. When Michael improved, he said that he had known about his allergies to "drugs with sulfa in them." However, during his first visit when he cut his finger, the ER clinician, Dr. Plant, had documented that Michael had no allergies.

What Dr. Plant Was Thinking
I am the doctor who saw Michael after he cut his finger. It's true that I documented Michael had no allergies. It's also true that I didn't ask him whether he had any allergies. I only documented that Michael had no allergies because the computer forces me to do it. I also documented that he had no history of disease or prior surgeries, that he wasn't depressed, that he wasn't abused at home, and probably 100 other things. The EMR unfortunately makes the me fill out dozens of different fields and click the mouse 100 times no matter why a patient comes to the hospital. It was a busy night in the ER- they all are- and I admit that I didn't treat Michael's case as a detailed primary care visit. He just had a small little cut on his finger and it took me one minute to take care of it. Had I properly filled out every field of his electronic chart, it would have taken me 30 minutes, and I wouldn't have been able to spend time with the sick people who actually needed my care.

Case
Leslie was a 45-year-old woman who was admitted to the hospital after she developed chest pain. She had been treated for insomnia with lorazepam 2 mg nightly for over 20 years. Lorazepam is a controlled substance requiring a monthly refill. As she travelled frequently, her psychiatrist, Dr. Mullen, wrote the prescription for her to take 8 mg at bedtime. He would then give her 120 pills. The admitting intern read in the EMR that she was prescribed 8 mg of lorazepam at night and ordered this dose for her. Leslie was sedated for nearly 24 hours after taking four-times her usual dose of the medication.

What Dr. Mullen Was Thinking
I had given Leslie 120 tablets of lorazepam every four months for nearly 10 years. Then our hospital shifted from paper to EMRs. Writing a prescription like lorazepam is extremely cumbersome. We have to login to a state database to verify that the patient is not getting controlled substances from other providers. We then get texted a code from this database that we have to type in to our own medical record. I understand that the intention behind this is to prevent patients from getting prescriptions from multiple different doctors. The whole process takes about five minutes, which doesn't sound so bad, except that I have to do it multiple times daily and click dozens of buttons in the process. If I did it properly, it would take me an 30 minutes or so every day. So, both for my sake and for the patients I know well, I often write the prescription so they have a supply lasting several months. For Leslie, I wrote that she would take 8 mg at night, when we both knew she would only take 2 mg.

Moreover, we are expected to verify every patient's medications at every visit and enter them into the EMR. Again, this sounds easy and reasonable. However, for every medication, we are supposed to enter why they take it, for how long they've taken it, the dose they take, and whether they've had adverse side effects from it. For my older patients, some of whom take 10 or more medications, this process takes 15 minutes out of a 20-minute visit. If I were to do it correctly, I would barely have time to say "hello."

Unfortunately, the intern who admitted Leslie trusted the EMR and gave her a much higher dose of lorazepam than she actually takes. The intern is not to blame here. However, I am not sure what I am supposed to do. I can take meticulous care of the EMR, or I can take care of the human in front of me. It's one or the other.

Discussion

The EMR error occurs when clinicians are forced to mindlessly click buttons on a computer to give the appearance of taking care of their patients at the expense of actually taking care of their patients. Unfortunately, clinicians all too often have to choose between taking care of their patients or the EMR and the myriad of paper forms that are still a routine part of health care. Simply put, a clinician who correctly fills out the EMR is unlikely to be doing the best for their patients. Theresa Brown, a registered nurse, illustrated this dilemma by writing:

> A nurse could spend 10 minutes documenting a patient's fall risk, or 10 minutes trying to keep patients from falling. It seems obvious that a computer record of 'fall risk' cannot in and of itself prevent falls, but completing those records is considered essential in hospitals. As a result, real fall-prevention efforts — encouraging patients to use the call light, ordering a bedside commode, having an aide do hourly check-ins — get short shrift" [47]

John Levinson, Bruce H. Price, and Vikas Saini made a similar observation in an article titled *Death by A Thousand Clicks* [48]:

> It happens every day, in exam rooms across the country, something that would have been unthinkable 20 years ago: Doctors and nurses turn away from their patients and focus their attention elsewhere — on their computer screens. By the time the doctor can finally turn back to her patient, she will have spent close to half of the appointment serving not the needs of her patient, but of the electronic medical record.

The anecdotes have been confirmed in several studies. A study of 29 medical interns at Johns Hopkins University by Lauren Block and colleagues in 2013 found that they spent 40% of their time working on a computer and only 12% of their time with patients [49]. As Dr. Block said, "Spending an average of eight minutes a day with each patient just doesn't seem like enough time to me" [50]. She is obviously right. Another study of 57 doctors in the US found they spent 27% of their time directly interacting with patients and 49% of their time working on the computer and doing desk work [51]. Even when they are with patients, 37% of their time is spent staring at a computer screen. A study of 471 primary care doctors found that on an average day, they spent the same amount of time on a computer as with patients. A study of ER doctors, found they spent 43% of their time entering data and only 28% of their time with patients. They clicked the mouse nearly 4,000 times during a 10-hour shift [52]. Another study found that internists lose an average of 48 minutes every day clicking buttons on the computer [53]. Moreover, many doctors work several more hours on the computer when they get home.

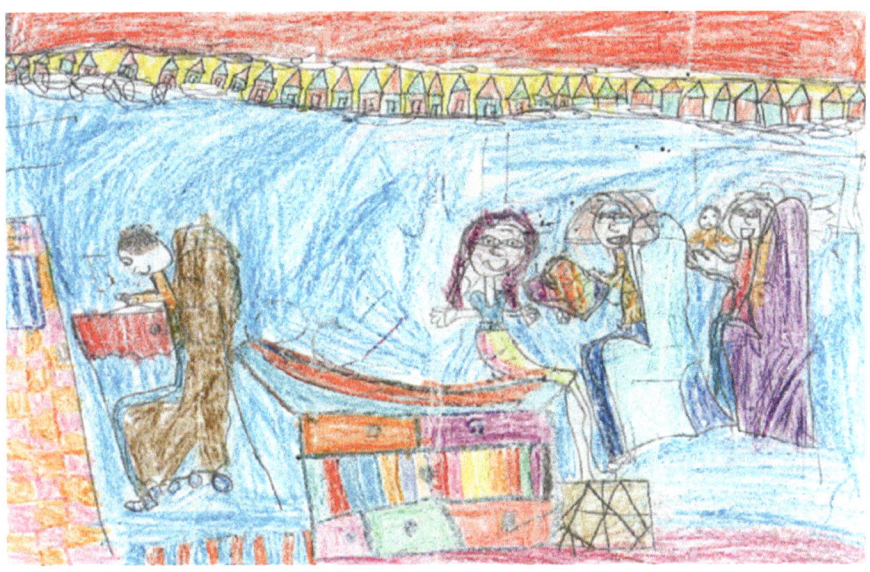

Fig. 28.3 A doctor typing with his back to the patient. (Toll E. The cost of technology [Image file]. JAMA 2012;307(23):2497–2498. https://doi.org/10.1001/jama.2012.4946.)

Additionally, the EMR can significantly degrade the clinician-patient relationship. An article by Elizabeth Toll, a pediatrician, accompanied by a child's picture of her visit to her doctor, demonstrated this well. Dr. Toll wrote:

> *No one was more surprised than the physician himself. The drawing was unmistakable. It showed the artist—a 7-year-old girl—on the examining table. Her older sister was seated nearby in a chair, as was her mother, cradling her baby sister. The doctor sat staring at the computer, his back to the patient—and everyone else. All were smiling. The picture was carefully drawn with beautiful colors and details, and you couldn't miss the message (Fig. 28.3) [54].*

Abrham Verghese, a professor of medicine, has said that clinicians today often don't care for human beings, but "IPatients." He wrote:

> *The patient is still at the center, but more as an icon for another entity clothed in binary garments: the "iPatient." Often, emergency room personnel have already scanned, tested, and diagnosed, so that interns meet a fully formed iPatient long before seeing the real patient. The iPatient's blood counts and emanations are tracked and trended like a Dow Jones Index, and pop-up flags remind caregivers to feed or bleed. iPatients are handily discussed (or "card-flipped") in the bunker, while the real patients keep the beds warm and ensure that the folders bearing their names stay alive on the computer [55].*

In addition to being time consuming and dehumanizing, slavish devotion to the EMR can require clinicians to be dishonest at times. Many EMRs have required fields for every patient encounter. Clinicians are often forced to ask whether their patients smoke, if they are depressed, whether they have been abused, if they are in pain, what diseases run in their families, and innumerable similar questions. While such information can be crucial for many patients and each question sounds reasonable by itself, it is not necessary for every patient to be asked a large panoply of questions that are unrelated to their visit. Consider an otherwise healthy 20-year-old woman who comes to the ER with an abrasion on her elbow after falling off her bike. The ER clinician has the choice between spending precious minutes asking questions completely unrelated to her visit in order to properly fill out the EMR or treating her wound and moving on to the next patient. As clinicians are forced to fill out fields that are irrelevant to the visit, often the only way to see patients efficiently is to incorrectly fill out their chart.

Additionally, such one-size-fits-all records discourages thoughtful care. Working with psychiatry interns, I know they often invariably ask each patient the exact same questions no matter their clinical presentation. A young man may arrive distraught that his girlfriend broke up with him, while another may be brought in by the police after he tried to enter Trump Tower to warn the president about an upcoming alien invasion. In part because the interns have to fill out the exact same medical record on every patient, patients with wildly diverse histories and presentations will be often asked the exact same questions in a thoughtless, robotic manner.

Another error can occur when clinicians enter crucial information in the EMR to the exclusion of verbal communication. An example of such an error occurred with the case of Thomas Eric Duncan. He presented in 2014 to the Texas Health Presbyterian Hospital ER with a fever, headache, abdominal pain, vertigo, and nausea. He was discharged from the ER at that time, though he returned several days later. Two nurses who treated Duncan contracted Ebola, and nearly 100 other people were exposed. An expert panel who reviewed the case partially faulted the over-reliance on the EMR for this potential public health disaster. Although Duncan told a nurse he had recently been in Africa and this information was entered in the EMR, it was not verbally communicated to the doctor in charge of his care. Though the nurse entered his travel history in the EMR, the workflow for the nurse was different from that of the doctor, who did not see this crucial piece of history. "The lessons shared by THR (Texas Health Resources) after the Ebola events also speaks to an over-reliance on the EMR for communication of important clinical information between the key members of the patient's clinical care team," the panel wrote [56].

Many of these errors occur because EMRs are not designed for the benefit of the clinician. They are designed to maximize billing. As a result, even trivial orders such as a blood test require the clinician to click multiple boxes saying where the blood will be drawn, when the blood will be drawn, and to which lab the blood will be sent. If a mistake is made, the clinician must start from scratch and reorder the lab. Ordering imaging tests and medications similarly requires innumerable clicks. For almost every order, multiple "warning" messages occur, which are routinely ignored. My wife described the EMR as a "Choose Your Own Adventure" with 100 choices at every page. Invariably, whenever clinicians start to get used to the EMR, an "upgrade" renders much of their previous knowledge obsolete. Neurologist Steven Novella recognized there is a large gap between the people who design

EMRs and the clinicians who use them, writing, "the problem is in communicating between IT experts and medical experts. IT experts don't understand what health care providers need, and the providers don't necessarily understand what an EMR can and should do" [57].

Not surprisingly, mistakes are common when using an EMR. One error almost all clinicians will make from time to time is to confuse which patients' chart is open. It is trivially easy to order a test for one patient thinking you are ordering it for another. Dennis Bethel, an emergency doctor, wrote an amusing piece about how challenges with the EMR lead him to regularly order pregnancy tests on men [58]. However, he recognizes that "As easy as it is to order a pregnancy test on a man, it is equally as easy to give potassium to someone with hyperkalemia. And causing an iatrogenic life-threatening arrhythmia is nothing to snicker about."

Yet another error is that information can be easily copied from one note to the next. This feature is a time-saving advantage in many ways, as clinicians do not have to type a patient's history from scratch every note. Yet, it leads to errors being propagated in the medical chart. For example, I have seen patient described as a "56-year-old man with hypertension and diabetes" for several years in a row. When a clinician writes that a 60-year-old is 56-years-old, it calls into question almost everything they write.

Another consequence of poorly designed EMRs is clinician burn-out. Anecdotes of clinicians leaving medicine or retiring early due to frustrations with EMRs abound. Keith White, a pediatrician said that after the implementation of EPIC, one of the most common EMRs, there was an exodus of doctors. He said:

> Six doctors have left this year. We were not ready for EPIC and EPIC was not ready for us. As a result, the providers are struggling to provide safe and effective care for 100,000 citizens of the county, many of whom are very ill. We often feel that we are failing. We are very tired … many doctors have left and all are considering leaving [59].

Additionally, EMRs can occasionally malfunction or are taken down for several hours due to upgrades. This can have a deleterious effect on entire hospitals. As Michael Kirsch wrote:

> When our EMR freezes, malfunctions, or simply goes on strike, our office is paralyzed. Although I appear to the patients as a breathing and willing medical practitioner, I might as well be a storefront mannequin who appears lifelike, but cannot function. We cannot access the patients' records, write a prescription or enter a new office visit [60].

Finally, EMRs are expensive. Many hospitals pay tens or even hundreds of millions of dollars to install them. Some cost even more than this. According to Becker's Hospital Review the "Mayo Clinic announced plans to switch to Epic's EMR in early 2015… new reports indicate Mayo expects to spend $1.5 billion on the implementation and infrastructure over the next five years" [61]. Some hospitals even employee medical scribes, whose sole job it is to care for the EMR, while clinicians actually care for patients [62]. Data breaches also contribute to the cost of EMRs. From 2009 to 2015, the health care records of 135 million Americans were compromised, costing an estimated $50.6 billion [63].

Conclusion

Few clinicians lament the days of paper records. Doctors' handwriting was as bad as the stereotypes made it out to be. Though sloppy handwriting was fodder for cartoonists, illegible medical records actually compromised patient care in meaningful ways. Going to the medical records office at 2 AM to search for a patient's paper chart is a chore no young clinician will know. Being able to see labs and images at the click of a button is a miracle. Additionally, a well-designed EMR can help clinicians adhere to evidence-based guidelines and make cost-conscious decisions. There is some evidence that EMRs have helped to reduce medical errors [64].

Despite their advantages and potential to further transform health care, many of the changes wrought by EMRs have been detrimental to patient care and clinician satisfaction. Many clinicians spend large portions of their day clicking the mouse over and over again. Many feel they are little more than glorified data entry clerks. Clinicians often feel at the mercy of the EMR and that they must adjust to it, rather than it adjusting to them.

The fact that most clinicians spend significantly more time in front of a computer than they do in front of their patients is a travesty, in my opinion. A clinician who properly fills out every field in the EMR is be unlikely to properly connect with their patients and may spend valuable time treating the computer, not the patient. A clinician who prioritizes the appearance of good care by meticulously taking care of every aspect of documentation is unlikely to devote sufficient time to actually caring for patients. Finally, clinicians should not assume that because a crucial piece of information is entered in the EMR it will be seen. Busy clinicians cannot review even a small fraction of the EMR for most patients. The EMR should not take the place of verbal communication.

References

1. Keller JP. Clinical alarm hazards: a "top ten" health technology safety concern. J Electrocardiol. 2012;45(6):588–91. https://doi.org/10.1016/j.jelectrocard.2012.08.050.
2. AAMI Foundation & Healthcare Technology Safety Institute. (n.d.). Safety innovations: using data to drive alarm system improvement efforts: The Johns Hopkins hospital experience [PDF file]. Retrieved from http://s3.amazonaws.com/rdcms-aami/files/production/public/FileDownloads/HTSI/Johns_Hopkins_White_Paper.pdf.
3. Drew BJ, Harris P, Zègre-Hemsey JK, Mammone T, Schindler D, Salas-Boni R, Bai Y, Tinoco A, Ding Q, Hu X. Insights into the problem of alarm fatigue with physiologic monitor devices: a comprehensive observational study of consecutive intensive care unit patients. PLoS One. 2014;9(10):e110274. https://doi.org/10.1371/journal.pone.0110274.
4. Sendelbach S, Funk M. Alarm fatigue: a patient safety concern. AACN Adv Crit Care. 2013;24(4):378–86. https://doi.org/10.1097/NCI.0b013e3182a903f9.
5. Korniewicz DM, Clark T, David Y. A national online survey on the effectiveness of clinical alarms. Am J Crit Care. 2008;17(1):36–41.
6. Kowalczyk L. (2010, Feb 21). MGH death spurs review of patient monitors. The Boston Globe. Retrieved from http://archive.boston.com/news/health/articles/2010/02/21/mgh_death_spurs_review_of_patient_monitors/?page=full.

7. The Joint Commission. (2013). Sentinel event alert issue 50: medical device alarm safety in hospitals. Retrieved from https://www.jointcommission.org/sea_issue_50/.
8. Yoder JC, Yuen TC, Churpek MM, Arora VM, Edelson DP. A prospective study of night-time vital sign monitoring frequency and risk of clinical deterioration. JAMA Intern Med. 2013;173(16):1554–5. https://doi.org/10.1001/jamainternmed.2013.7791.
9. Kaiser Health News. (2015, Aug 20). Study shows sleep tied to better patient experience, outcomes. Healthcare Finance. Retrieved from https://www.healthcarefinancenews.com/news/study-shows-sleep-tied-better-patient-experience-outcomes.
10. Weingart SN, Toth M, Sands DZ, Aronson MD, Davis RB, Phillips RS. Physicians' decision to override computerized drug alerts in primary care. Arch Intern Med. 2003;163(21):2625–31. https://doi.org/10.1001/archinte.163.21.2625.
11. Duke J, Friedlin J, Ryan P. A quantitative analysis of adverse events and "overwarning" in drug labeling. JAMA Intern Med. 2011;171(10):941–54. https://doi.org/10.1001/archinternmed.2011.182.
12. California Environmental Protection Agency, Office of Environmental Health Hazard Assessment. (n.d.). The Proposition 65 list. Retrieved 15 Sept 2018 from https://oehha.ca.gov/proposition-65/proposition-65-list.
13. Garza M. (2017, June 29). Adding Roundup to Prop. 65 list is a victory, but will Californians heed the warning? Los Angeles Times. Retrieved from http://www.latimes.com/opinion/opinion-la/la-ol-round-up-proposition-65-story.html.
14. Dr. Whitecoat. (2009, Jan 19). Defensive medicine at work [Blog post]. Dr. Whitecoat. Retrieved from http://drwhitecoat.com/defensive-medicine-at-work/.
15. Jena AB, Seabury S, Lakdawalla D, Chandra A. Malpractice risk according to physician specialty. N Engl J Med. 2011;365(7):629–36. https://doi.org/10.1056/NEJMsa1012370.
16. Studdert DM, Mello MM, Gawande AA, Gandhi TK, Kachalia A, Yoon C, Puopolo AL, Brennan TA. Claims, errors, and compensation payments in medical malpractice litigation. N Engl J Med. 2006;352(19):2024–33. https://doi.org/10.1056/NEJMsa054479.
17. Kachalia A, Mello MM. New directions in medical liability reform. N Engl J Med. 2011;364(16):1564–72. https://doi.org/10.1056/NEJMhpr1012821.
18. Studdert DM, Mello MM, Sage WM, DesRoches CM, Peugh J, Zapert K, Brennan TA. Defensive medicine among high-risk specialist physician in a volatile malpractice environment. JAMA. 2005;293(21):2609–17. https://doi.org/10.1001/jama.293.21.2609.
19. Localio AR, Lawthers AG, Bengtson JM, Hebert LE, Weaver SL, Brennan TA, Landis JR. Relationship between malpractice claims and cesarean delivery. JAMA. 1993;269(3):366–73. https://doi.org/10.1001/jama.1993.03500030064034.
20. Jackson Healthcare. (n.d.). Defensive medicine: impacts beyond costs summary of phase III findings. Retrieved 15 Sept 2018 from https://jacksonhealthcare.com/media-room/surveys/def-med-phase-3-summary/.
21. Mello MM, Studdert DM, Schumi J, Brennan TA, Sage WM. Changes in physician supply and scope of practice during a malpractice crisis: evidence from Pennsylvania. Health Aff. 2007;26(3) https://doi.org/10.1377/hlthaff.26.3.w425.
22. Donlen J, Spicer Puro J. The impact of the medical malpractice crisis on OB-GYNs and patients in southern New Jersey. N J Med. 2003;100(9):12–9.
23a. Rosenblatt RA, Whelan A, Hart LG. Obstetric practice patterns in Washington state after tort reform: has the access problem been solved? Obstet Gynecol. 1990;76(6):1105–10.
23b. Fondren LK, Ricketts TC. The North Carolina obstetrics access and professional liability study: a rural-urban analysis. J Rural Health. 1993;9(2):129–37.
24. Wang V. (2017, Dec 15). In: Bronx, obstetricians may find work inspiring, and careers hindered. The New York Times. Retrieved from https://www.nytimes.com/2017/12/15/nyregion/in-bronx-obstetricians-may-find-work-inspiring-and-careers-hindered.html.
25. Gunther JK. [Jenifer Karine] (n.d.). Post [Facebook]. Retrieved 15 Sept 2018 from https://www.facebook.com/kevinmdblog/posts/10154749832094886?comment_id=10155790592519886&notif_id=1506467498680957&notif_t=comment_mention.

26. NOLO. (n.d.). What is the medical standard of care in a malpractice case? Retrieved 15 Sept 2018 from https://www.nolo.com/legal-encyclopedia/medical-standard-care-malpractice-case.html.
27. Epstein D. (2017, Feb 22). When evidence says no, but doctors say yes. ProPublica. Retrieved from https://www.propublica.org/article/when-evidence-says-no-but-doctors-say-yes.
28. Merenstein D. Winners and losers. JAMA. 2004;291(1):15–6. https://doi.org/10.1001/jama.291.1.15.
29. Scherz H, Oliver W. (2013, Aug 27). Defensive medicine: a cure worse than the disease. Forbes. Retrieved from https://www.forbes.com/sites/realspin/2013/08/27/defensive-medicine-a-cure-worse-than-the-disease.
30. Balch CM, Oreskovich MR, Dyrbye LN, Colaiano JM, Satele DV, Sloan JA, Shanafelt TD. Personal consequences of malpractice lawsuits on American surgeons. J Am Coll Surg. 2011;213(5):657–67. https://doi.org/10.1016/j.jamcollsurg.2011.08.005.
31. Pho K. (2012, Feb 26). Reducing the emotional impact of medical malpractice [Blog post]. KevinMD.com. Retrieved from https://www.kevinmd.com/blog/2012/02/reducing-emotional-impact-medical-malpractice.html.
32. Leibman CB, Stern Hyman C. A mediation skills model to manage disclosure of errors and adverse events to patients. Health Aff. 2004;23(4):22–32. https://doi.org/10.1377/hlthaff.23.4.22.
33. Medical Economics. (2014, June 10). Apology laws: talking to patients about adverse events. Medical Economics. Retrieved from http://www.medicaleconomics.com/medical-economics/content/tags/apology-laws/apology-laws-talking-patients-about-adverse-events?page=full.
34. Jauhar S. (2015, July 22). Giving doctors grades. The New York Times. Retrieved from https://www.nytimes.com/2015/07/22/opinion/giving-doctors-grades.html?
35. Schneider EC, Epstein AM. Influence of cardiac-surgery performance reports on referral practices and access to care – a survey of cardiovascular specialists. N Engl J Med. 1996;335(4):251–6. https://doi.org/10.1056/NEJM199607253350406.
36. Moscucci M, Eagle KA, Share D, Smith D, De Franco AC, O'Donnell M, Kline-Rogers E, Jani SM, Brown DL. Public reporting and case selection for percutaneous coronary interventions: an analysis from two large multicenter percutaneous coronary intervention databases. J Am Coll Cardiol. 2005;45(11):1759–65. https://doi.org/10.1016/j.jacc.2005.01.055.
37. Apolito RA, Greenberg MA, Menegus MA, Lowe AM, Sleeper LA, Goldberger MH, Remick J, Radford MJ, Hochman JS. Impact of the New York State Cardiac Surgery and Percutaneous Coronary Intervention Reporting System on the management of patients with acute myocardial infarction complicated by cardiogenic shock. Am Heart J. 2008;155(2):267–73. https://doi.org/10.1016/j.ahj.2007.10.013.
38. Dranove D, Kessler D, McClellan M, Satterhwaite M. Is more information better? The effects of "report cards" on health care providers. J Polit Econ. 2003;111(3):555–88.
39. Green J, Wintfeld N. Report cards on cardiac surgeons – assessing New York state's approach. N Engl J Med. 1995;332(18):1229–33. https://doi.org/10.1056/NEJM199505043321812.
40. Ubel P. (2015, Nov 23). The joy has been sucked out of medicine. Here's why [Blog post]. KevinMD.com. Retrieved from https://www.kevinmd.com/blog/2015/11/the-joy-has-been-sucked-out-of-medicine-heres-why.html.
41. U.S. Centers for Medicare & Medicaid Services. (2018, Apr 27). Readmissions reduction program (HRRP). Retrieved from https://www.cms.gov/medicare/medicare-fee-for-service-payment/acuteinpatientpps/readmissions-reduction-program.html.
42. Gupta A, Allen LA, Bhatt DL, Cox M, DeVore AD, Heidenreich PA, Hernandez AF, Peterson ED, Matsouaka RA, Yancy CW, Fonarow GC. Association of the hospital readmissions reduction program implementation with readmission and mortality outcomes in heart failure. JAMA Cardiol. 2018;3(1):44–53. https://doi.org/10.1001/jamacardio.2017.4265.
43. Dharmarajan K, Wang Y, Lin Z, Norman ST, Ross JS, Horwitz LI, Desai NR, Suter LG, Drye EE, Bernheim SM, Krumholz HM. Association of changing hospital readmission rates with mortality rates after hospital discharge. JAMA. 2017;318(3):270–8. https://doi.org/10.1001/jama.2017.8444.

44. Philipps D. (2018, Jan 1). At veterans hospital in Oregon, a push for better ratings puts patients at risk, doctors say. The New York Times. Retrieved from https://www.nytimes.com/2018/01/01/us/at-veterans-hospital-in-oregon-a-push-for-better-ratings-puts-patients-at-risk-doctors-say.html.

45. Ibrahim AM, Dimick JB, Sinha SS, Hollingsworth JM, Nuliyalu U, Ryan AM. Assocciation of coded severity with readmission reduction after the hospital readmissions reduction program. JAMA Intern Med. 2018;178(2):290–2. https://doi.org/10.1001/jamainternmed.2017.6148.

46. Ross C. (2017, Dec 11). The data are in, but debate rages: are hospital readmission penalties a good idea? STAT. https://www.statnews.com/2017/12/11/hospital-readmissions-debate/.

47. Brown T. (2015, Dec 20). When hospital paperwork crowds out hospital care. The New York Times. Retrieved from https://www.nytimes.com/2015/12/20/opinion/sunday/when-hospital-paperwork-crowds-out-hospital-care.html.

48. Levinson J, Price BH, Saini V. (2017, May 12). Death by a thousand clicks: leading Boston doctors decry electronic medical records. WBUR. Retrieved from http://www.wbur.org/commonhealth/2017/05/12/boston-electronic-medical-records.

49. Block L, Habicht R, Wu AW, Desai SV, Wang K, Silva KN, Niessen T, Oliver N, Feldman L. In the wake of the 2003 and 2011 duty hours regulations, how do internal medicine interns spend their time. J Gen Intern Med. 2013;28(8):1042–7. https://doi.org/10.1007/s11606-013-2376-6.

50. Johns Hopkins Medicine. (2013, Apr 23). Doctors-in-training spend very little time at patient beside, study finds [News Release]. Retrieved from https://www.hopkinsmedicine.org/news/media/releases/doctors_in_training_spend_very_little_time_at_patient_bedside_study_finds.

51. Sinsky C, Colligan L, Li L, Prgomet M, Reynolds S, Goeders L, Westbrook J, Tutty M, Blike G. Allocation of physician time in ambulatory practice: a time and motion study in 4 specialties. Ann Intern Med. 2016;165(11):753–60. https://doi.org/10.7326/M16.0961.

52. Tai-Seale M, Olson CW, Li J, Chan AS, Morikawa C, Durbin M, Wang W, Luft HS. Electronic health record logs indicate that physicians split time evenly between seeing patients and desktop medicine. Health Aff. 2017;36(4):655–62. https://doi.org/10.1377/hlthaff.2016.0811.

53. McDonald CJ, Callaghan FM, Weissman A, Goodwin RM, Mundkur M, Kuhn T. Use of internist's free time by ambulatory care electronic medical record systems. JAMA Intern Med. 2014;174(11):1860–3. https://doi.org/10.1001/jamainternmed.2014.4506.

54. Toll E. The cost of technology. JAMA. 2012;3017(23):2497–8. https://doi.org/10.1001/jama.2012.4946.

55. Verghese A. Culture shock – patient as icon, icon as patient. N Engl J Med. 2008;359(26):2748–51.

56. Cortese D, Abbott P, Chassin M, Lyon GM, Riley WJ. (n.d.). The expert panel report to Texas Health Resources leadership on the 2014 Ebola events [PDF file]. Retrieved from https://www.texashealth.org/assets/documents/system/public_relations/expert_panel_report_to_thr_on_evd_response.pdf.

57. Novella S. (2017, Dec 13). Medical profession is underutilizing computer technology. Science-Based Medicine. Retrieved from https://sciencebasedmedicine.org/medical-profession-is-underutilizing-computer-technology/.

58. Bethel D. (2016, Mar 27). This doctor orders pregnancy tests on men. You're probably doing it too [Blog post]. KevinMD.com. Retrieved from https://www.kevinmd.com/blog/2016/03/this-doctor-orders-pregnancy-tests-on-men-youre-probably-doing-it-too.html.

59. Gurley RJ. (2014, Mar 10). Whether retiring or fleeing, doctors are leaving health care [Blog post]. Centers for Health Journalism. Retrieved from https://www.centerforhealthjournalism.org/2014/03/10/whether-it%E2%80%99s-retire-or-flee-doctors-are-leaving-health-care.

60. Kirsch M. (2017, Dec 3). When EMRs crash: it's time to push back [Blog post]. KevinMD.com. Retrieved from https://www.kevinmd.com/blog/2017/12/emrs-crash-time-push-back.html.

61. Becker's Health IT & CIO Report. (2016, Mar 8). 5 Epic contracts – and their costs – so far in 2016. Retrieved from https://www.beckershospitalreview.com/healthcare-information-technology/5-epic-contracts-and-their-costs-so-far-in-2016.html.

62. Bailey M. (2016, Apr 25). The pay is low, the typing nonstop, but the medical scribe business is booming. STAT. Retrieved from https://www.statnews.com/2016/04/25/scribes-emergency-room/.
63. O'Neill Hayes T. (2015, Aug 6). Are electronic medical records worth the costs of implementation? American Action Forum. Retrieved from https://www.americanactionforum.org/research/are-electronic-medical-records-worth-the-costs-of-implementation/.
64. Rajasekar H. An evaluation of electronic health records in reducing preventable medical error rates in the United States: a detailed report. J Health Med Info. 2015;6:210. https://doi.org/10.4172/2157-7420.1000210.

Case

Robin was a 41-year-old woman who presented with low-back pain for three days. The pain started after she spent the day bike riding. She was evaluated by the neurology resident in the ER and sent home with muscle relaxers and anti-inflammatory drugs. She returned the next day with a low-grade fever and weakness in her legs. An MRI was done at that time, and Robin was diagnosed with a spinal epidural abscess, a neurosurgical emergency. Further history revealed that she abused heroin. A morbidity and mortality conference was held where the attending doctor discussed several of the cognitive biases that led to the missed diagnosis.

What Dr. Howard Was Thinking

I'd spent several years studying cognitive biases. As such, I am pretty sure that I not only understand them well, but am perfectly capable of detecting them in my own thinking. I'm not going to pretend that I am a robot who is free of biases. But there is also no question that my research awakened me to my own biases and allowed me to eliminate most of them and minimize the others.

By focusing in on her bike riding, the doctors who took care of Robin were guilty of the anchoring bias, a form of premature closure. They also were guilty of the omission bias and zebra retreat. Finally, they did not properly unpack the patient's history, learning that she used drugs. I honestly cannot imagine myself making the same mistakes.

Discussion

Look at the red dot in the picture below with your right-eye covered. At about 10 inches away, the gap in the blue line will disappear, and it will seem continuous.

This is known as the physiological blind spot. It occurs as there are no light receptors in the part of the retina where the optic nerve is located. Your brain automatically fills in the gap created by the optic nerve with what it expects to see, and thus you normally not perceive your blind spot.

In the same way that your visual system fills in the gap created by your blind spot with what it expects, your mind "fill in the gaps" of your knowledge with what you expect or want to be true. And in the same way that you cannot notice your visual blind spot without specifically looking for it, you cannot notice your cognitive blind spots unless something draws your attention to them.

Ask yourself, do you feel you are more or less biased than the average person? Almost everyone feels that cognitive biases are problems for other people. In contrast, almost no one appreciates the degree to which they suffer from cognitive biases. This phenomenon is known as the blind spot bias, a term coined by Emily Pronin. In a study of 661 people by Irene Scopelliti and colleagues, for example, only one person said that they were more biased than average [1]. While the blind spot bias does not affect everyone equally, it is unrelated to intelligence, decision-making ability, and several personality traits. As marketing professor Carey Morewedge said:

> People seem to have no idea how biased they are. Whether a good decision-maker or a bad one, everyone thinks that they are less biased than their peers. This susceptibility to the bias blind spot appears to be pervasive, and is unrelated to people's intelligence, self-esteem, and actual ability to make unbiased judgments and decisions [2].

Clinicians, of course, are not immune to the blind spot bias. As Erin McCormick, a student of behavioral decision, pointed out:

> When physicians receive gifts from pharmaceutical companies, they may claim that the gifts do not affect their decisions about what medicine to prescribe because they have no memory of the gifts biasing their prescriptions. However, if you ask them whether a gift might unconsciously bias the decisions of other physicians, most will agree that other physicians are unconsciously biased by the gifts, while continuing to believe that their own decisions are not. This disparity is the bias blind spot, and occurs for everyone, for many different types of judgments and decisions [2].

A consequence of this is that many clinicians are overly confident. According to one study, 94% of academic doctors believed themselves to be above average and many have difficulty recalling any error they made [3]. Importantly, people with a large blind spot bias are the least likely to engage in strategies to improve their thinking and performance. As Dr. Scopelliti and colleagues wrote:

> People who believe that they are relatively immune to bias are less likely to enact corrective strategies, even when correcting strategies are explained and explicitly suggested. In the work place, the results suggest that employees high in bias blind spot may be less receptive to training designed to improve their decision making, and may need more or different kinds of training [1].

While the attention given to cognitive biases in medicine and society at large is great, there is one important point to be learned from studying biases that many people miss. To the brain, biases feel like knowledge or even wisdom, and simply becoming aware of a particular bias doesn't help you to tell the difference. No one should expect that because they know about a particular bias, they will be able to recognize it when it influences their thoughts. To the brain, biased thinking feels just like normal thinking. You have learned that a blind spot exists in your vision. You could further study everything that is known about how your brain fills in the blind spot to create a coherent visual image. However, this knowledge won't change your visual perception one bit. Unless you specifically look for it, you will never notice your blind spot. Instructing people to be "fair and unbiased" in their thinking is like telling them to notice their visual blind spot; it's not possible.

Samuel McNerney, a science writer, even wrote that texts such as this contribute to the blind-spot bias, stating:

> Too often, readers finish popular books on decision making with the false conviction that they will decide better... We are plagued by systematic biases, and reflecting on those biases only exacerbates the problem. Like knifing Hydra, every time we think about thinking errors we commit even more errors. It's an epistemic Chinese finger trap.... The common sendoff, "now that you know about these biases, perhaps you'll decide better," instills a false confidence - it's the trick we're all failing to notice [4].

Being inclined to think that you can avoid a bias because you aware of it is a bias itself. Laurie Santos and Tamar Gendler called this notion the G. I. Joe Fallacy after a cartoon that claimed that "knowing is half the battle" [5]. To the extent that learning about biases is half the battle, this is because your knowledge will help you to recognize cognitive errors in *others*. This can give you the false impression that your thinking has improved while other people remain hopelessly misguided. This can contribute to something called naive realism, in which people believe only they see the world objectively, as it truly is, while others are ignorant, misinformed, or deluded. Instead of making us wise, knowledge of cognitive biases may make it easier to simply dismiss people with whom we disagree when we should actually be paying attention to their arguments.

There is evidence that clinicians can learn about cognitive biases and heuristics [6]. However, it is not clear how much can be done to teach rational thought and minimize the impact of biases on clinicians' decisions. Daniel Kahneman, whose study of cognitive biases earned him a Nobel Prize, shared this pessimism, writing:

> Except for some effects that I attribute mostly to age, my intuitive thinking is just as prone to overconfidence, extreme predictions, and the planning fallacy as it was before I made a study of these issues. I have improved only in my ability to recognize situations in which errors are likely...And I have made much more progress in recognizing the errors of others than my own [7].

Certainly, there are several suggestions to minimize cognitive biases that sound entirely reasonable. However, as we have seen, interventions that seem entirely plausible are often found to be useless or even harmful. Several studies by Silvia Mamede and colleagues found that such reflective practice improved diagnostic accuracy in complex cases in residents [8a, b]. Aside from these studies, however, there is precious little evidence that clinicians can overcome their biases with training or conscious effort any more than they can will themselves not to be tired or teach themselves to require less sleep. Several studies by Jonathan Sherbino and colleagues found that cognitive forcing strategies did nothing to reduce errors in students during a four-week rotation in emergency medicine [9, 10]. Geoffrey Norman and colleagues found no improvement in the performance of residents who were told to be thoughtful and reflective compared to those who were told to be rapid but accurate [11]. Their study concluded that "that simply encouraging slowing down and increasing attention to analytical thinking is insufficient to increase diagnostic accuracy."

As I hope this book has demonstrated, many cognitive biases are inverses of each other. For example, A yin-yang error occurs when patients have had multiple, unrevealing tests and procedures, causing clinicians to erroneously feel that nothing more can be done. This is the opposite of the failure-to-close error, which occurs when physicians are unable to put the brakes on an unrevealing diagnostic work-up, subjecting patients to unnecessary tests. Given this, a case can be made that there is a risk in trying to correct for certain cognitive biases. As Justin Morgenstern, an emergency doctor, wrote:

> Many of the described biases exist at opposite ends of a spectrum. Therefore, if you are consciously correcting for one form of bias you may be simultaneously increasing your chance of falling for another. For example, if you recognize that you are retreating from the diagnosis of a 'zebra' and actively attempt to correct your thinking, you may quickly shift into a scenario in which you are ignoring the base-rate of this rare condition. You can't save the patient with a rare disease unless you think about it, but it if you think about it too often you will harm the many patients with common diseases [12].

An ideal clinician is essentially like the baby bear in the story *Goldilocks and the Three Bears*. They will not do too much or too little, but rather they will do everything just right.

So now what? Are we hopelessly flawed, destined to make the same errors over and over again? Can we do anything to improve our flaws and biases? While there is disagreement amongst psychologists about the degree to which individuals can correct for their cognitive biases, all hope is not lost. We can all engage in metacognition, which is essentially thinking about how we think. We can strive to adjust our attitudes and work environments to either minimize some biases or at least increase the likelihood that others will point them out to us. A review by Mark Graber and colleagues found three categories of interventions to improve clinicians' decision-making [13]:

1. Interventions to improve knowledge and experience, such as simulation-based training, improved feedback and education focused on a single disease.
2. Interventions to improve clinical reasoning and decision-making skills, such as reflective practice and active metacognitive review.
3. Interventions that provide cognitive 'help' that included use of electronic records and integrated decision support, informaticians and facilitating access to information, second opinions and specialists.

Fig. 29.1 The PAT criteria facilitate thinking by helping clinicians focus on diagnoses that are probable, alarming, and treatable

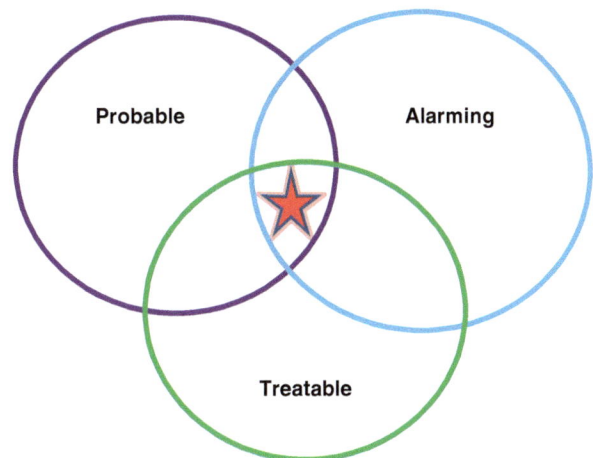

Although I fully recognize that there is little evidence that they are helpful, below are 15 suggestions that clinicians may use to minimize the impact of cognitive biases and improve their diagnostic accuracy and treatment algorithms.

1. Clinicians may want to use cognitive forcing strategies, which are conscious strategies that attempt to force clinicians to think about their decisions in a systematic way, hopefully improving the results.

   One such cognitive forcing strategy is to think about a potential diagnosis using the PAT criteria, whereby a clinician judges a potential diagnosis by a combination of how **P**robable is it, how **A**larming it is, and how **T**reatable it is. For example, a clinician who meets a patient with a severe headache might first consider that that they have a subarachnoid hemorrhage. This type of headache is certainly possible given this complaint, it is often fatal, and if recognized early is eminently treatable. Only after ruling out a dire condition would a clinician entertain a relatively benign entity such as a migraine. Dr. Morgenstern also suggested including an unusual diagnosis in this algorithm so that zebras are not forgotten (Fig. 29.1) [14].

Another cognitive forcing strategy is the VINDICATE mnemonic. It lists categories of diseases that may force clinicians to broaden their differential diagnosis.

V – Vascular
I – Infectious
N – Neoplastic
D – Degenerative
I – Iatrogenic/intoxication
C – Congenital
A – Autoimmune
T – Traumatic
E – Endocrine/metabolic

A clinician using this mnemonic on a patient with confusion might come up with the following potential diagnoses.

Vascular: Stroke (ischemic or hemorrhagic), subarachnoid hemorrhage, posterior reversible encephalopathy syndrome
Infectious: Meningitis, encephalitis, sepsis
Neoplastic: Primary brain tumor, metastasis, paraneoplastic disorder
Degenerative: Alzheimer's disease, frontotemporal dementia, Lewy body dementia
Iatrogenic/intoxication: Opioids, anticholinergics, alcohol intoxication/ withdrawal
Congenital: Epilepsy (post-ictal state)
Autoimmune: Multiple sclerosis, limbic encephalitis
Traumatic: Traumatic brain injury, epidural or subdural hematoma
Endocrine/metabolic: Adrenal or thyroid dysfunction, abnormalities of glucose, sodium, or calcium, renal or hepatic failure.

Although this list (which is incomplete) may seem intimidatingly long, almost all of these conditions, and certainly the most treatable ones, can be rapidly evaluated in an ER.

Another similar strategy is to employ a "time-out" procedure before rendering a diagnosis [15]. Time-outs are now routinely done before surgeries and procedures to help ensure the right intervention is being performed on the right person in the right location. Clinicians can employ a similar strategy, asking themselves "What else might this be?" before finalizing their diagnosis. Dr. Morgenstern suggests asking the following five questions with every patient.

- What traps might I be falling into?
- What else can it be?
- Is there anything that doesn't fit (disconfirmation)?
- Is there more than one thing going on?
- Is this a case where I need to slow down?

Clinicians should also be amenable to periodically asking these questions for patients they diagnosed long ago. All too often, incorrect diagnostic labels stick to patients like Velcro.

Sometimes, a cognitive forcing strategy can help mitigate against a specific bias. For example, a clinician who knows they mistrust prisoners, may force themselves to spend extra time and effort with inmates.

2. Clinicians should feel comfortable asking for help. Given that learning about cognitive biases allows you to see the cognitive biases of others, the natural corollary is that others are in the best position to reveal your biases to you. If someone says, "you are wrong," you should learn to resist the strong temptation to immediately defend yourself and instead try to listen to what your critic is saying.

Clinicians should strive to surround themselves with trusted colleagues who won't criticize them for asking them help. They should also recognize that someone asking them for help is a sign of strength. While generally continuity of care is beneficial for patients, it may be wise for a second opinion to be a standard part of treatment. At my multiple sclerosis center, patients occasionally alternate between providers, allowing for a fresh consideration of the diagnosis and treatment.

3. Clinicians should actively seek out feedback from respected peers. The world's best athletes and singers have coaches. Yet clinicians are generally expected to be entirely self-sufficient immediately after completing their training. Surgeon Atul Gawande has advocated that other professions should emulate these professions by using coaches [16]. After having a respected surgeon watch and comment on one of his operations, Dr. Gawande wrote "That one 20-minute discussion gave me more to consider and work on than I'd had in the past 5 years." To my knowledge, only some psychiatrists routinely employ this practice, using supervisors after their formal training has ended. While few clinicians will formally employ a coach, most clinicians can find a trusted mentor to help them continually improve.

4. When working in a team, the leader should assign someone to play "devil's advocate" and argue that the current diagnosis or treatment plan is wrong. This will free at least one team member from the burden of groupthink and allow dissenting opinions to be heard.

5. Clinicians should familiarize themselves with Bayesian reasoning and the important statistics relevant to their field. They should know which diseases are common, which diseases are rare, and which are in the middle. They should have a sense of the sensitivity and specificity of the tests they use, and based on the frequency of the disease, their positive/negative predictive values and likelihood ratios.

6. Clinicians should keep a list of the mistakes they made and a list of cases with suboptimal outcomes. This may prevent them from repeating their mistakes and may help them detect unexpected patterns of error. Institutions should similarly keep track of their metrics to see how they compare against national averages in potentially avoidable errors such as infections and fall prevention.

7. When presenting cases to others, clinicians should be aware that the information presented first and last is the most likely to be remembered. Information that could potentially bias the other people should not be presented before the essential details.

8. Institutions should establish formal feedback mechanisms and conferences to discuss errors and how they can be avoided in the future. The goal should to prevent future errors, not to embarrass or penalize clinicians. Cases with poor outcomes should be discussed in morbidity and mortality conferences. When possible, challenging cases should be discussed in regularly scheduled case-conferences to solicit a variety of opinions. It is also important to review cases where everything went right. Learning from these cases can increase the likelihood that the good outcome is repeated.

9. Clinicians should be aware of how patients make them feel. If a sympathetic patient leads them to pursuing futile or even harmful treatments in the mis-

guided spirit of doing "everything," they should be aware of this. Similarly, if they minimize the concerns of a patient they resent, they should do their best to be aware of this as well.

10. Clinicians should remember that all outcomes are viewed in hindsight. When viewing the potential errors of others, they should know that the poor outcome will influence their appraisal of the case. This is also true when clinicians reflect upon their own mistakes.

11. If a clinician is tired, hungry, ill, or distracted for personal reasons, they should take a break if possible, or even go for home for the day if necessary. No one performs well under physical or emotional duress. Clinicians who continue to work when they are feeling unwell are not likely doing their patients any favors. Although clinicians may have little control over this (especially in ER), they should try to work in a quiet environment with few interruptions.

12. Clinicians should decrease reliance on memory, which historically has been one of the most valued skills in medicine. Medical students are largely admitted based on their ability to memorize information, not their critical thinking skills. Yet, rote memory matters less than ever before. With modern technology, the entirety of medical knowledge is instantly available at our fingertips. Clinicians who are unfamiliar with a medication or diagnosis should not hesitate to look it up. The palest ink is better than the best memory.

    Additionally, the recognition of the fallibility of human memory has led to the development of checklists and "time-outs" prior to the start of operations. Similar procedures in the aviation industry have largely eliminated human error as a cause of crashes.

13. When there is a bad outcome, team members should write down their recollection of the event as soon as possible, prior to any group discussion. As we have seen, memories are malleable and can be easily distorted by the impressions of others.

14. Clinicians should practice when possible. Simulation centers offer clinicians the opportunity to practice emergency situations and procedures so that they are more familiar when the real situation occurs. Practice can shift clinicians from type II (slow and deliberative) to type I thinking (reflexive and automatic). In emergency situations especially, type I thinking is preferable to type II thinking.

15. Clinicians should avoid unnecessary interactions with pharmaceutical companies. This will make them less vulnerable to the mere-exposure effect. Clinicians who reject financial relationships with pharmaceutical companies will be immune to the norm of reciprocity.

Given the highly speculative nature of these suggestions, it is clear that more research is needed in how to best minimize cognitive biases in medicine and improve diagnostic accuracy. Only a few small studies have been done. A review in 2012 found only 42 studies that tested interventions to reduce the likelihood of cognitive errors [13]. Many of these were done in students and residents, not expert clinicians.

Moreover, many of these studies evaluate clinicians' performance in artificial environments, such as case vignettes, which often differ dramatically from real-world patient care. Many of them are likely too short to conclude that critical thinking skills cannot be learned. A program aimed at teaching someone a new language or a musical instrument would not be declared a failure, if at the end of four weeks, its students had not mastered the material. Critical thinking, the ability to make balanced decisions without jumping to false conclusions, is most likely analogous to these skills in that it takes years to learn and must be continually practiced and reinforced.

Even if debiasing strategies turn out to be of minimal use in adults, the same may not be true for children. In the same way children can learn multiple languages with no effort at all, an impossible task for done adults, children's thought processes are more malleable as well. Allen Nsangi and colleagues conducted a randomized trial of over 10,000 children in Uganda. They found that children aged 10–12 years-old could be taught to critically assess health effect claims [17]. One researcher involved with this study said:

> In a time of rapidly spreading fake news, it is more important than ever that people are able to distinguish the truth from "alternative facts." In addition, we need to be able to assess what is a sensible interpretation of facts, particularly when facts are used to argue for or against implementing measures. This applies to claims about what causes better or worse health [18].

Heather Butler and colleagues have shown that critical thinking skills are more important than overall intelligence in determining a variety of real-life outcomes [19]. Clearly, in this era of "fake news," internet miracle cures, and fearmongering over the greatest achievements science and medicine have to offer, critical thinking skills should be taught with the same urgency as reading, writing, and arithmetic (Fig. 29.2).

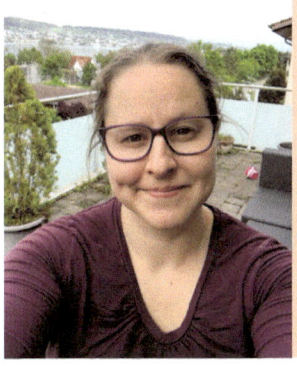

Why science? Because the world is unimaginably interesting and complex, much too complex for us to assume that we know what it is about, and how it works. We can choose that we do not wish to understand any of that, of course. The alternative is always there – to go ahead and continue fooling ourselves.
Iida Ruishalme

Fig. 29.2 Iida Ruishalme gets it right. (Ruishalme I. (n.d.) Personal photograph.)

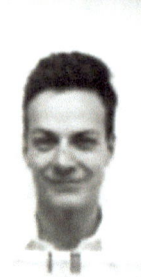

**The first principle is
that you must not fool
yourself —
and you are the easiest
person to fool.**

Richard Feynman

Fig. 29.3 Richard Feynman gets it right. (Fastfission. Los Alamos ID badge photograph: Richard Feynman [Image file]. In: Wikimedia commons. 2011. Retrieved from https://commons.wikimedia.org/wiki/Richard_Feynman#/media/File:Richard_Feynman_ID_badge.png.)

Conclusion

The brain is a self-affirming spin-doctor with a bottomless bag of tricks and millions of years of practice at its disposal. Our brains are pattern-seeking machines, filling in the gaps in our perception and knowledge consistent with our expectations, beliefs, and wishes. Essentially by definition, we are blind to our own biases. If we were aware of them, they would cease to exist. Cognitive biases can best be thought of as cognitive blind spots. Like the blind spot in your vision, it's impossible to notice without them being pointed out to you. Further, once you do notice them, there isn't really much you can do to avoid those biases. At best, you can understand the mistake the bias is likely to lead to, the information it is preventing you from having, or the perspective it obscures, and attempt to mitigate it. This is easier to do with some biases than others, but preventing bias all together is not an option.

So why care about biases if there is little to be done about them? First of all, learning about cognitive biases and the quirks of how our minds work is fascinating. The other reason is more practical—to keep yourself from embracing them. While it may be very difficult, if not impossible, to see past our biases, we can avert the urge to run with them and eagerly allow them to distort our view. We can stop ourselves from relying on them as a defense for our positions.

However, a warning is in order when learning about cognitive biases. Your brain will tend to use this knowledge to add yet another trick to its arsenal. We don't learn about biases as a means of helping us ensure that our thinking is right, but to understand the particular ways in which it could be wrong. Knowledge of bias should contribute to your humility, not your confidence (Fig. 29.3).

References

1. Scopelliti I, Morewedge CK, McCormick E, Min HL, Lebrecht S, Kassam KS. Bias blind spot: structure, measurement, and consequences. Manag Sci. 2015;61(10):2468–86. https://doi.org/10.1287/mnsc.2014.2096.

2. Rea S. (2015, June 8). Researchers find everyone has a bias blind spot. Carnegie Mellon University. Retrieved from https://www.cmu.edu/news/stories/archives/2015/june/bias-blind-spot.html.

3. Mele AR. Real self-deception. Behav Brain Sci. 1997;20(1):91–102.

4. McNerney S. (2013, May 15). The bias within the bias [Blog post]. Scientific American. Retrieved from https://blogs.scientificamerican.com/mind-guest-blog/the-bias-within-the-bias/.

5. Santos LR, Gendler T. (2014). 2014: what scientific idea is ready for retirement? Edge. Retrieved 15 Sept 2018 from https://www.edge.org/response-detail/25436.

6. Reilly JB, Ogdie AR, Von Feldt JM, Myers JS. Teaching about how doctors think: a longitudinal curriculum in cognitive bias and diagnostic error for residents. BMJ Qual Saf. 2013;22(12):1044–50. https://doi.org/10.1136/bmjqs-2013-001987.

7. Kahneman D. Thinking, fast and slow. New York: Farrar, Straus and Giroux; 2011.

8a. Mamede S, Schmidt HG, Penaforte JC. Effects of reflective practice on the accuracy of medical diagnoses. Med Educ. 2008;42(5):468–75. https://doi.org/10.1111/j.1365-2923.2008.03030.x.

8b. Mamede S, Schmidt HG, Rikers RMJP, Penaforte JC, Coelho-Filho JM. Influence of perceived difficulty of cases on physicians' diagnostic reasoning. Acad Med. 2008;83(12):1210–6. https://doi.org/10.1097/ACM.0b013e31818c71d7.

9. Sherbino J, Kulasegaram K, Howey E, Norman G. Ineffectiveness of cognitive forcing strategies to reduce biases in diagnostic reasoning: a controlled trial. CJEM. 2014;16(1):34–40. https://doi.org/10.2310/8000.2013.130860.

10. Sherbino J, Dore KL, Siu E, Norman GR. The effectiveness of cognitive forcing strategies to decrease diagnostic error: an exploratory study. Teach Learn Med. 2011;23(1):78–84. https://doi.org/10.1080/10401334.2011.536897.

11. Norman G, Sherbino J, Dore K, Wood T, Young M, Gaissmaier W, Kreuger S, Monteiro S. The etiology of diagnostic errors: a controlled trial of system 1 versus system 2 reasoning. Acad Med. 2014;89(2):277–84. https://doi.org/10.1097/ACM.0000000000000105.

12. Morgenstern J. (2015, Sept 22). Cognitive theory in medicine: some problems [Blog post]. In: First10EM. https://first10em.com/cognitive-problems/.

13. Graber ML, Kissam S, Payne VL, Meyer AND, Sorensen A, Lenfestey N, Tant E, Henriksen K, Labresh K, Singh H. Cognitive interventions to reduce diagnostic error: a narrative review. BMJ Qual Saf. 2012;21(7):535–57. https://doi.org/10.1136/bmjqs-2011-000149.

14. Morgenstern J. (2015, Sept 21). Cognitive errors in medicine: mitigation of cognitive errors [Blog post]. In: First10EM. https://first10em.com/mitigation-of-errors/.

15. Trowbridge RL. Twelve tips for teaching avoidance of diagnostic errors. Med Teach. 2008;30:496–500. https://doi.org/10.1080/01421590801965137.

16. Gawande A. (2011, Oct 3). Top athletes and singers have coaches. Should you? The New Yorker. Retrieved from https://www.newyorker.com/magazine/2011/10/03/personal-best.

17. Nsangi A, Semakula D, Oxman AD, Austvoll-Dahlgren A, Oxman M, Rosenbaum S, Morelli A, Glenton C, Lewin S, Kaseje M, Chalmers I, Fretheim A, Ding Y, Sewankambo NK. Effects of the informed health choices primary school intervention on the ability of children in Uganda to assess the reliability of claims about treatment effects: a cluster-randomised controlled trial. Lancet. 2017;390(10092):374–88. https://doi.org/10.1016/S0140-6736(17)31226-6.

18. Norwegian Institute of Public Health. (2017, May 23). Critical thinking can be taught. ScienceDaily. Retrieved from https://www.sciencedaily.com/releases/2017/05/170523084439.htm.

19. Butler HA, Pentoney C, Bong MP. Predicting real-world outcomes: critical thinking ability is a better predictor of life decisions than intelligence. Think Skills Creat. 2017;25:38–46. https://doi.org/10.1016/j.tsc.2017.06.005.

Research Errors

Introduction

A key theme of this book is that the scientific method is required for clinicians to minimize their biases and make optical decisions for their patients. While there is often not enough evidence to guide every decision a clinician must make, clinicians should use scientific evidence as much as possible in their treatment recommendations. Patients are poorly served when clinicians use their intuition, personal experience, and unquestioned traditions. The push to formally use evidence-based medicine (EBM) began in earnest in the 1990s. As David Sackett, who is considered the father of EBM, and colleagues wrote, EBM involves "the conscientious, explicit and judicious use of current best evidence in making decisions about the care of individual patients (Fig. 30.1)" [1].

While the scientific method may help minimize cognitive errors, researchers themselves and the institutions that support them are not immune from biases.

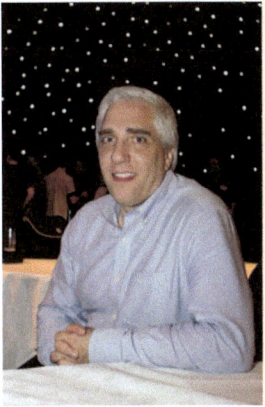

What do you think science is? There's nothing magical about science. It is simply a systematic way for carefully and thoroughly observing nature and using consistent logic to evaluate results. Which part of that exactly do you disagree with? Do you disagree with being thorough? Using careful observation? Being systematic? Or using consistent logic?

Steven Novella

Fig. 30.1 Steven Novella gets it right. (RIchardc39. Steve Novella [Image file]. In: Wikimedia commons. 2011. Retrieved from https://commons.wikimedia.org/wiki/File:Steve_Novella.jpg.)

© Springer International Publishing AG, part of Springer Nature 2019   537
J. Howard, *Cognitive Errors and Diagnostic Mistakes*,
https://doi.org/10.1007/978-3-319-93224-8_30

Critics of science, as it is practiced today, have raised doubts as to how much of the medical literature can be trusted. In 2005, John Ioannidis, an epidemiologist, published a paper titled *Why Most Published Research Findings Are False* [2]. In this provocative paper, Ioannidis posited that, due to flaws in research methodology, "it is more likely for a research claim to be false than true." He wrote that, because of conflicts of interest, flexibility of designs, definitions, outcomes, and analytical modes, "claimed research findings may often be simply accurate measures of the prevailing bias." In a later "report to David Sackett," Dr. Ioannidis claimed that EBM was a noble idea that had been "hijacked." He wrote:

> As EBM became more influential, it was also hijacked to serve agendas different from what it originally aimed for. Influential randomized trials are largely done by and for the benefit of the industry. Meta-analyses and guidelines have become a factory, mostly also serving vested interests. National and federal research funds are funneled almost exclusively to research with little relevance to health outcomes. We have supported the growth of principal investigators who excel primarily as managers absorbing more money. Diagnosis and prognosis research and efforts to individualize treatment have fueled recurrent spurious promises. Risk factor epidemiology has excelled in salami-sliced data-dredged articles with gift authorship and has become adept to dictating policy from spurious evidence. Under market pressure, clinical medicine has been transformed to finance-based medicine. In many places, medicine and health care are wasting societal resources and becoming a threat to human well-being [3].

In another article, Dr. Ioannidis and Davod Chavalarias wrote there were 235 (!) biases in biomedical research that lead to potential erroneous results [4]. Leonard Freedman and colleagues posit that, due to untrustworthy study designs, poor research techniques and data analysis that similar problems plague pre-clinical research as well. They wrote that "the cumulative (total) prevalence of irreproducible preclinical research exceeds 50%." The total cost of this research was of $28 billion a year [5].

This chapter will cover some of the biases and flaws in the current structure of the scientific research that can make it difficult for patients and clinicians to know the truth. Unfortunately, not all of these flaws are the result of unconscious and unintentional biases. Pharmaceutical companies and academic researchers have been known to hide unwanted results, spin them in a favorable light, and occasionally fabricate them altogether. Potential solutions will also be discussed.

Expectation Bias

All researchers must make decisions about how to design their studies and collect and analyze the data. Their choices can have a profound effect on the results. Researchers are vulnerable to a phenomenon known as the expectation bias. In the words of Pat Croskerry:

> The expectation bias occurs when researchers tend to believe, certify and publish data that are in accord with their own expectations for the outcome of an experiment, or downgrade or minimize data that appear to be in conflict with those expectations. It can lead to researchers unconsciously manipulating their data to obtain an expected or desired result [6].

The entire reason many medical studies are randomized and blinded is to minimize such bias. A double-blind study means that neither the study subject nor the investigator knows whether or not the subject received the investigational treatment or a placebo until after the study is over. Certain procedures and surgeries have even been studied in a double-blind fashion. In such studies, surgeons perform the actual surgery in some subjects. In others, they will simulate a surgery, even making an incision and then have an evaluator, who is blinded to which patient has had or has not had the surgery, judge whether the subject improved or not.

A well-known example of the expectation bias was provided by René Blondlot and his research team. Blondlot was a French physicist who believed that he had discovered a new type of radiation, which he called N-rays after his hometown. In 1903, Blondlot fired X-rays through a prism and saw that an electric spark in a detector had gotten got brighter. He photographed the finding and attributed it to N-rays. Over 100 scientists published over 300 papers claiming to detect N-rays emanating from every substance except green wood and some treated metals (Fig. 30.2).

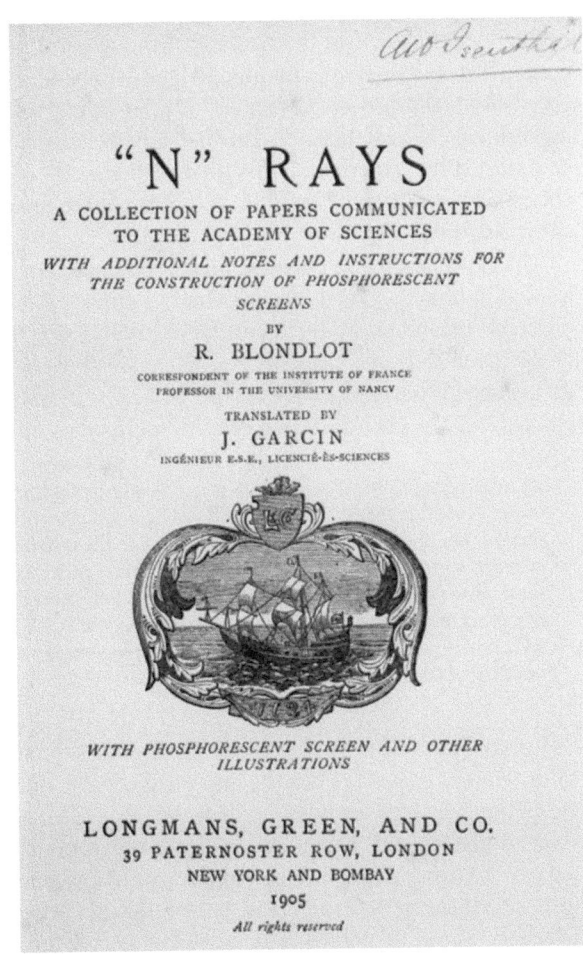

Fig. 30.2 René Blondlot's 156-page monograph on N-rays. (Blondlot R, Garcin JFW. "N" rays: a collection of papers communicated to the Academy of Sciences: with additional notes and instructions for the construction of phosphorescent screens. London, United Kingdom: Longmans, Green, and Co. 1905. (Scanned version retrieved from https://archive.org/stream/nrayscollectiono00blon#page/n9/mode/2up.)

When other eminent European physicists were unable to replicate his results, American physicist Robert Wood was summoned to investigate Blondlot's claim and definitively determine whether or not N-rays existed. In a dark room, unbeknownst to Blondlot and his team, Wood removed the prism from the experimental setup. He also exchanged a file that supposedly emitted N-rays with a piece of inert wood. Despite this, in each instance, the experimenters still insisted they observed N-rays. Having convinced themselves that N-rays existed, the experimenters saw what they expected to see. Wood published his findings disproving the existence of N-rays, which have since become a cautionary tale of how researchers may "observe" findings that meet their expectations.

More recently, Daniel Klein, a professor of economics, wrote about a time when he was victimized by the expectation bias. He created a series of questions to determine the economic literacy of people across the political spectrum. Subjects were asked whether they agreed with statements such as, "Restrictions on housing development make housing less affordable." Eight such statements were given, and he discovered that people who were economic conservatives like him outperformed liberals on basic economic questions. The results pleased him and received considerable media attention, particularly from gleeful right-wing organizations. He wrote, "I'm a libertarian, and I found it easy to believe that people on the left had an especially bad grasp of economics" [7]. However, his survey was flawed, as Klein unwittingly chose statements that challenged cherished liberal beliefs. To his credit, he repeated the experiment, this time with a series of statements that contradicted cherished conservative beliefs. With these statements, liberals outperformed conservatives.

The expectation bias may also affect clinicians, not in how they design their studies, but in how they analyze data that has already been collected. To examine how different researchers might get different results using the same raw data set, a group of 29 research teams consisting of 61 analysts were asked to determine whether dark-skinned soccer players were more likely to receive red cards than light-skinned players [8]. The core of the study was described as follows:

> All teams were given the same large data set collected by a sports-statistics firm across four major football leagues. It included referee calls, counts of how often referees encountered each player, and player demographics including team position, height and weight. It also included a rating of players' skin colour...The teams independently tested their hypotheses. Each made its own decisions about how to best analyse the data set. We then took an inventory of all the approaches. Each team provided details such as which statistical model they used — everything from Bayesian clustering to logistic regression and linear modelling — what variables they used and why.

It may seem a simple matter to see if dark-skinned players received more red cards. However, as there may be important confounders, this approach might not be the optimal way to analyze the data. For example, perhaps there were few dark-skinned goalies and, being isolated from rough play, goalies almost never receive red cards. Perhaps dark-skinned players were concentrated on teams whose games were officiated by strict referees, known for giving out red cards. I have no idea if any of this is true, but it shows that researchers must make choices when examining data sets and that these choices can lead to different results.

While most research teams had similar results (darker skin players were found to be slightly more likely to receive red cards) there were some outliers. Some research teams found a large difference between dark and light-skinned players. One group even found that dark-skinned players were less likely to receive red cards. Twenty research teams found a statistically significant correlation between skin color and red cards, while nine teams did not find a statistically significant difference.

As Raphael Silberzahn and Eric Uhlmann, who conducted the experiment noted, "Had any one of these 29 analyses come out as a single peer-reviewed publication, the conclusion could have ranged from no race bias in referee decisions to a huge bias" [8].

P-Hacking and HARKing

One of the most common ways that the expectation bias manifests is through misuse of a statistical measure knows as the p-value. In the words of neurologist Steven Novella, the p-value is defined:

> As the probability of the results of an experiment deviating from the null by as much as they did or greater if the null hypothesis is true...To put it more simply, what are the odds that you would have gotten the results you did (or greater) if your hypothesis is not true? [9].

As science journalist Brian Resnick wrote, "The p-value quantifies this rareness. It tells you how often you'd see the numerical results of an experiment — or even more extreme results — if the null hypothesis is true and there's no difference between the groups" [10]. (In statistics the "null hypothesis" posits that there is no relationship between two variables.) The lower the p-value, the less likely a finding is due to chance alone. By convention, a p-value less than 0.05 is considered "significant."

No single statistical measure has led to a greater number of erroneous and false positive results than the p-value. Many researchers misunderstand its meaning, thinking that a low p-value means a particularly finding is unlikely due to chance alone and is therefore true. However, the p-value must be interpreted with regards to the original study hypothesis and design. As Ronald Wasserstein and Nicole Lazar wrote:

> P-values do not measure the probability that the studied hypothesis is true, or the probability that the data were produced by random chance alone. Researchers often wish to turn a p-value into a statement about the truth of a null hypothesis, or about the probability that random chance produced the observed data. The p-value is neither. It is a statement about data in relation to a specified hypothetical explanation, and is not a statement about the explanation itself [11].

Additionally, a statistically significant result may not be clinically significant. For example, a medication may lower blood pressure by a trivial amount. If a large enough group of people are studied, this finding can reach statistical significance.

Vaccine	Broken bone N = 85,151		Open wound N = 73,290		OCD N = 3,222		Anorexia nervosa N = 551		Anxiety disorder N = 23,462		Tic disorder N = 2,547		ADHD N = 46,640		Major depression N = 13,295		Bipolar disorder N = 5,892	
	Hazard ratio (HR)	95% CI	HR	95% CI	HR	95% CI	HR	95% CI	HR	95% CI	HR	95% CI	HR	95% CI	HR	95% CI	HR	95% CI
Any vaccine																		
3 months	1.04	1.00 1.08	0.96	0.92 1.00	1.23	1.02 1.49	1.80	1.21 2.68	1.12	1.04 1.20	1.11	0.90 1.38	1.06	1.00 1.12	0.88	0.80 0.97	0.87	0.75 1.01
6 months	1.08	1.05 1.11	0.97	0.94 1.01	1.27	1.10 1.47	1.63	1.17 2.27	1.13	1.07 1.19	1.25	1.06 1.47	1.04	1.00 1.09	0.92	0.86 0.99	0.82	0.73 0.91
12 months	1.07	1.04 1.09	0.97	0.94 1.00	1.23	1.09 1.38	1.47	1.12 1.93	1.14	1.09 1.19	1.19	1.04 1.36	1.08	1.05 1.12	0.89	0.84 0.95	0.87	0.79 0.95
Influenza																		
3 months	1.03	0.96 1.11	0.93	0.86 1.01	1.36	1.02 1.82	2.20	1.10 4.38	1.23	1.10 1.38	1.24	0.91 1.67	0.98	0.91 1.07	0.81	0.68 0.96	0.71	0.55 0.92
6 months	1.07	1.02 1.13	0.96	0.91 1.02	1.48	1.21 1.83	1.83	1.07 3.15	1.24	1.14 1.35	1.27	1.02 1.58	0.97	0.91 1.02	0.89	0.79 1.00	0.84	0.70 1.00
12 months	1.06	1.02 1.09	0.97	0.93 1.01	1.35	1.16 1.59	1.52	0.99 2.34	1.27	1.19 1.35	1.28	1.08 1.50	1.04	0.99 1.09	0.93	0.84 1.02	0.87	0.76 1.00
TD																		
3 months	1.02	0.94 1.11	0.92	0.83 1.02	1.15	0.72 1.84	1.70	0.78 3.71	0.95	0.80 1.13	0.86	0.47 1.60	1.04	0.91 1.19	0.95	0.78 1.16	0.83	0.62 1.12
6 months	1.07	1.00 1.14	0.94	0.87 1.01	1.07	0.75 1.51	1.77	0.90 3.49	0.91	0.80 1.03	1.24	0.82 1.88	1.03	0.93 1.13	0.96	0.83 1.10	0.82	0.66 1.02
12 months	1.07	1.02 1.12	0.93	0.88 0.98	0.99	0.77 1.26	1.63	1.05 2.52	0.98	0.90 1.07	0.93	0.66 1.30	1.04	0.97 1.11	0.90	0.82 1.00	0.80	0.68 0.93
HepA																		
3 months	1.02	0.94 1.12	0.97	0.88 1.07	1.47	0.92 2.33	1.60	0.52 4.84	1.00	0.85 1.18	1.13	0.70 1.83	1.03	0.92 1.17	0.86	0.68 1.08	1.03	0.73 1.47
6 months	1.05	0.98 1.12	0.99	0.92 1.07	1.43	1.02 2.01	1.09	0.48 2.51	1.08	0.95 1.22	1.35	0.92 1.98	1.05	0.96 1.15	0.95	0.81 1.13	0.79	0.60 1.03
12 months	1.08	1.02 1.13	0.99	0.93 1.05	1.40	1.07 1.82	1.73	0.89 3.37	1.00	0.91 1.10	1.17	0.88 1.56	1.09	1.02 1.18	0.97	0.86 1.11	0.81	0.66 1.00
HepB																		
3 months	1.09	0.93 1.25	1.05	0.89 1.24	0.71	0.32 1.61	3.00	0.61 14.86	1.01	0.76 1.34	1.40	0.44 4.41	1.13	0.91 1.39	1.05	0.77 1.43	0.97	0.61 1.56
6 months	1.07	0.92 1.13	1.02	0.91 1.15	0.80	0.45 1.44	1.71	0.68 4.35	1.01	0.83 1.23	1.17	0.54 2.52	1.07	0.92 1.24	0.89	0.71 1.11	0.91	0.64 1.29
12 months	1.03	0.91 1.11	1.00	0.91 1.09	0.93	0.60 1.44	1.56	0.72 3.30	1.01	0.89 1.16	1.19	0.61 2.31	1.06	0.95 1.18	1.00	0.85 1.18	1.07	0.83 1.38
Meningitis																		
3 months	1.05	0.95 1.17	1.04	0.92 1.19	1.10	0.67 1.80	1.71	0.68 4.35	1.06	0.88 1.27	1.46	0.72 2.95	1.16	0.98 1.38	0.89	0.70 1.13	0.87	0.57 1.33
6 months	1.08	1.00 1.17	1.02	0.92 1.12	1.15	0.78 1.71	1.75	0.86 3.56	1.12	0.97 1.29	1.94	1.08 3.46	1.08	0.95 1.23	0.88	0.73 1.05	0.82	0.61 1.11
12 months	1.08	0.99 1.14	1.02	0.94 1.10	1.34	0.96 1.87	1.42	0.79 2.56	1.14	1.01 1.29	1.73	1.07 2.80	1.06	0.95 1.18	0.81	0.70 0.94	0.85	0.67 1.09
Varicella																		
3 months	0.88	0.79 0.99	0.90	0.79 1.03	1.33	0.79 2.26	1.00	0.20 4.96	1.06	0.85 1.31	0.73	0.42 1.27	1.06	0.90 1.24	0.85	0.58 1.24	1.08	0.63 1.87
6 months	0.97	0.86 1.06	0.96	0.87 1.07	1.38	0.89 2.15	2.66	0.71 10.04	1.17	0.99 1.38	0.91	0.59 1.40	1.09	0.97 1.23	0.85	0.64 1.14	0.79	0.52 1.21
12 months	1.00	0.93 1.08	0.93	0.85 1.01	1.36	0.92 1.99	1.23	0.48 3.45	1.11	0.97 1.28	0.97	0.67 1.40	1.06	0.95 1.17	0.84	0.66 1.06	0.74	0.53 1.05

Cases and controls matched on date (±15 days, see text) of the start of continuous enrollment, year of birth, gender, and three-digit zip code. N's represent cases only. Results in bold are statistically significant at p < 0.05.
OCD, obsessive-compulsive disorder, ADHD, attention deficit hyperactivity disorder, TD, tetanus and diphtheria, Hep, hepatitis

Fig. 30.3 When enough variables are studied, statistically significant findings are more likely than not. (Leslie DL, Kobre RA, Richmand BJ, Guloksuz SA, Leckman JF. Temporal association of certain neuropsychiatric disorders following vaccination of children and adolescents: a pilot case-control study [Table 2]. Front Psych 2017;8:3. https://doi.org/10.3389/fpsyt.2017.00003.)

However, as this medication is unlikely to have an impact on any particular person's health, this finding will be clinically insignificant.

Despite the confusion that surrounds it, the p-value reigns supreme in the medical literature. A p-value less than 0.05 is the magic number by which a researcher is felt to have found a meaningful result and can submit their finding for publication. Unfortunately, this means researchers often feel compelled to chase p-values less than 0.05. As one scientist said, "I feel torn between asking questions that I know will lead to statistical significance and asking questions that matter" [10].

Additionally, unethical, careless, or simply misguided researchers can explore their data and invariably find statistically significant results, a practice known as p-hacking or data dredging. P-hacking occurs when a researcher takes a large data set, goes on a fishing expedition, and publishes the statistically significant findings. When enough endpoints are studied, researchers can easily find something that reaches statistical significance. Importantly, when p-values less than 0.05 are considered significant, this implies that up to 5% of statistically significant findings may be due to chance alone.

Figure 30.3 is the data set from a study which purported to find an association between vaccines and several neuropsychiatric conditions [12].

As science journalist Tara Haelle pointed out, the study examined nine conditions (seven psychiatric conditions and two "controls"), six vaccines, and three administration dates [13]. This equates to 162 possibilities, meaning it is virtually guaranteed that a statistically significant finding will emerge. At least this study was upfront about the multiple possibilities it studied. Some researchers may only report the results that produced significant findings, neglecting to publish multiple negative results.

The problem of p-hacking is compounded by the fact that, by tinkering with their data, researchers can virtually guarantee a statistically significant finding, and even obtain results with very low p-values (less than 0.01). Joseph Simmons and colleagues termed this "researcher degree of freedom" [14]. They wrote:

> In the course of collecting and analyzing data, researchers have many decisions to make: Should more data be collected? Should some observations be excluded? Which conditions should be combined and which ones compared? Which control variables should be considered? Should specific measures be combined or transformed or both?

> It is rare, and sometimes impractical, for researchers to make all these decisions beforehand. Rather, it is common (and accepted practice) for researchers to explore various analytic alternatives, to search for a combination that yields "statistical significance," and to then report only what "worked." The problem, of course, is that the likelihood of at least one (of many) analyses producing a falsely positive finding at the 5% level is necessarily greater than 5%.

A variant of p-hacking is known as subgroup analysis. Let's say a study is done showing a drug has no effect on a disease. The researchers may find a statistically significant result if they only look at a subset of the study participants. Perhaps the drug was effective in men but not women. Perhaps it was effective in people between of 20 and 40 years of age. Perhaps it was effective in people born on a Tuesday. This technique is sometimes known as salami slicing as researchers attempt to look at thinner slices of their data. By the law of small numbers, researchers can be virtually guaranteed to find a significant value if they look hard enough. There is not necessarily anything wrong with performing a subgroup analysis if it is done as the first step to performing another investigation. After all, perhaps a medication does work in men but not women. However, a separate study should be done to determine this.

Yet another method of p-hacking is to examine results at multiple different times, publishing only the positive results. Let's say a company tests a medication to see if it can lower glucose levels in people with diabetes. The study lasts six months, and at the end of that time there is no difference between people who take the medication and those who take placebo. But perhaps at the three-month period, there was a statistically significant difference. Voila! This result can be published and the medication declared a success.

Due to widespread misunderstandings, the American Statistical Association wrote a position paper (its first in 177 years), with six principles underlying the proper use and interpretation of the p-value. The statement's six principles are:

1. P-values can indicate how incompatible the data is with a specified statistical model.
2. P-values do not measure the probability that the studied hypothesis is true, or the probability that the data was produced by random chance alone.
3. Scientific conclusions and business or policy decisions should not be based only on whether a p-value passes a specific threshold.
4. Proper inference requires full reporting and transparency.

5. A p-value, or statistical significance, does not measure the size of an effect or the importance of a result.
6. By itself, a p-value does not provide a good measure of evidence regarding a model or hypothesis [11].

A phenomenon related to p-hacking occurs when researchers either formulate or alter their hypothesis after a study is complete. This is colloquially known as Hypothesizing After the Results are Known (HARKing) [15]. Statisticians Andrew Gelman and Erik Loken have called this "the garden of forking paths," meaning if a researcher doesn't specify their study design, outcome of interest, and statistical methods, *until after* a study is complete, many results can seem meaningful and planned-out after the fact [16]. This does not imply maleficence on the part of the researchers. As Gelman and Loken wrote:

> *We are starting to feel that the term "fishing" was unfortunate, in that it invokes an image of a researcher trying out comparison after comparison, throwing the line into the lake repeatedly until a fish is snagged. We have no reason to think that researchers regularly do that. We think the real story is that researchers can perform a reasonable analysis given their assumptions and their data, but had the data turned out differently, they could have done other analyses that were just as reasonable in those circumstances.*

Science journalist John Bohannon performed a devious prank to show how p-hacking and HARKing can be exploited to create erroneous results [17]. He created a pseudonym, Johannes Bohannon Ph.D, who was said to be the research director of the Institute of Diet and Health. While this title and institute were fabricated, he and a general practitioner named Gunter Frank, actually did perform a small study on five men and 11 women, randomizing them to one of three diets: a low-carbohydrate diet, a low-carbohydrate diet plus a daily chocolate bar, and a control group who was told to eat their usual diet. After three weeks, both of the treatment groups lost about five pounds, and those who ate chocolate lost weight 10% faster. They submitted their paper for publication and it was accepted in multiple journals in less than one day, often without peer-review. The authors chose a journal (International Archives of Medicine), paid a fee of 600 Euros, and their study was published.

The authors then hoped to take advantage of what they considered "journalists' incredible laziness." They created an appealing press release and a promotional video to tout their findings. Soon thereafter, multiple media outlets were credulously reporting the happy news that chocolate caused weight loss. They were interviewed by several journalists eager to spread the news. No journalist questioned their findings.

So, what's the catch? After all, the researchers actually performed the experiment. There was no fraud, and their findings were statistically significant. The problem is that they p-hacked and HARKed. Their study measured 18 different outcomes. With this many outcomes, there was a 60% chance of obtaining a statistically significant result by chance alone. The researchers were then able to say they made a meaningful discovery, when in fact all they did was collect a large amount of data and take advantage of random chance. Dr. Bohannon did not start out to investigate whether or not a daily chocolate bar causes weight loss. Rather once his study "discovered" this, he was able to retroactively able to "explain" why.

While p-hacking and HARKing are common and pollute the scientific literature, most commonly they are not done in a purposefully fraudulent manner. As Dr. Bohannon wrote, "Most scientists are honest and do it unconsciously. They get negative results, convince themselves they goofed, and repeat the experiment until it 'works.' Or they drop 'outlier' data points" [17].

As a result of p-hacking and HARKing, highly implausible results, such as the existence of ESP (also known as psi), can be made to seem highly plausible. In 2011 Daryl Bem, a psychology professor, published a paper titled *Feeling the Future: Experimental Evidence for Anomalous Retroactive Influences on Cognition and Affect* [18]. It reported the results of nine experiments involving over 1,000 participants and claimed to prove people had conscious awareness of future events. Eight of the nine studies had statistically significant results and the average effect size in psi performance across all nine experiments was 0.22. The paper was published in a highly-respected journal, the *Journal of Personality and Social Psychology*. The decision to publish this paper created significant controversy. If his results were true, fundamental tenets of physics and neuroscience would be turned on their head.

Critics of Bem's work noticed that it likely involved a combination of p-hacking, salami slicing, and HARKing. As science writer Daniel Engber wrote:

> If you give yourself a dozen different ways to slice and dice your data, you're at much greater risk of finding patterns in a set of random blips. That's not so bad at the start of your research, when you're working out the best approach for your experiments, but later on it can be disastrous. If Bem hadn't decided well ahead of time exactly how he planned to crunch his numbers, all his findings would be suspect [19].

None of Bem's critics suggested he was dishonest or fraudulent. They also recognized that his methodology and statistical analysis did not significantly differ from more conventional psychological papers that are regularly published without controversy. Rather, like many researchers, he made decisions in how he collected and analyzed his data that were to confirm his biases. Not surprisingly, later researchers were utterly unable to replicate Bem's results with experiments of over 3,000 subjects [20]. Bem is not alone in using research to "prove" implausible findings. A randomized, controlled trial published in 1999 found "evidence" that "remote, intercessory prayer" improved outcomes in patients admitted to a coronary care unit [21].

P-hacking is not necessarily inappropriate as a starting point to launch future investigations. Such results are considered hypothesis-generating, rather than hypothesis-confirming. For example, if a researcher examines a large data set and finds that patients with a particular disease share a common exposure, it would be reasonable to do a separate study to specifically investigate the relationship between these two variables.

File Drawer Effect/Publication Bias

Another unfortunate aspect of the scientific culture is that negative findings, such as a study finding *no* link between an exposure and a disease, are unlikely to be published in prestigious journal providing it is published at all. Negative studies are often intentionally not published, most commonly when they are done by pharmaceutical companies. This phenomenon is known as the file drawer effect or publication bias, and it can lead to gross distortions in the medical literature.

To see how the file drawer effect may influence results, imagine a pharmaceutical company that ran ten trials showing a drug failed to treat a disease and one showing it worked. If only the one positive study is published while the ten negative studies are hidden away, this would create a very misleading picture of the drug's efficacy. Although by definition, the true incidence of hidden studies cannot be known, Erick Turner and colleagues found that "Among 74 FDA-registered studies, 31%, accounting for 3,449 study participants, were not published" [22]. They found that "Not only were positive results more likely to be published, but studies that were not positive, in our opinion, were often published in a way that conveyed a positive outcome." The problem appears particularly dire in pediatrics. Natalie Pica and Florence Bourgeois examined 559 clinical trials that were registered with the US federal government from 2008-2011 [23]. Of these, 19% were stopped prematurely, mostly because it was difficult to recruit children. Of the 455 completed trials, 30% were not published. Over 77,000 children participated in studies that vanished into the scientific ether.

Additionally, research teams may not report failed experiments, creating a misleading impression of their results. Social psychologist Michael Inzlicht wrote of a time he received two submissions for a journal he edits [24]. As he wrote:

> *The first paper contained 7 experiments, often with outliers removed and covariates included, and reported effect sizes in the medium to large range all supporting the main hypothesis. The second paper contained 18 experiments, didn't exclude anyone or add any covariates, and reported small effect sizes that sometimes were contrary to the hypothesis. The first paper found 7 out of 7 significant results; the second paper contained 2 significant effects out of 18.*

However, there was a catch. There really weren't two papers. Rather, there were two versions of the same paper, titled *The Propagation Of Self-Control: Self-Control In One Domain Simultaneously Improves Self-Control In Other Domains* [25]. The first paper took advantage of the file-drawer effect to make its results seem more impressive. As Dr. Inzlicht explained:

> *The first (paper) was emblematic of the old way of doing business, with 7 studies that were scrubbed clean to be near-perfect. The second is emblematic of the new ways we are trying to do business, with studies that were raw, unvarnished, and true... File drawering studies warps our sense of how real, robust, and large an effect is. Because researchers file drawer papers—be that because they choose to or because the review process leads them to—there is a growing sense that we cannot fully trust the published record.*

Poor Surrogate Outcomes

In a clinical trial, a surrogate endpoint is an outcome measure that is not important by itself, but is felt to strongly correlate with a meaningful clinical endpoint. The National Institutes of Health (NIH) defined a surrogate endpoint as "a biomarker intended to substitute for a clinical endpoint," while clinical endpoints are "a characteristic or variable that reflects how a patient feels, functions, or survives" [26]. With their health, people are generally only interested in two things, living longer and feeling well. Ideally, all medical studies would measure these outcomes in some way. However, many medical studies measure things that don't matter except to the extent they are accurate markers for a longer, healthier life.

The use of surrogate outcomes and biomarkers is extremely common in medicine. This is because they are relatively easy to measure [26]. For example, a short trial with a small number of people may be able to demonstrate that a medication lowers blood pressure. However, a longer and larger trial will be needed to demonstrate that this medication prevents more meaningful outcomes such as strokes, heart attacks, and death. Since such studies may take decades before they are complete, medications are often approved based on surrogate endpoints.

One study examined clinical trials of diabetes treatments. It found that patient-important outcomes, such as cardiovascular events, death, pain, function, and quality of life were reported as primary or secondary outcomes in just 201 of 436 studies [27]. Patient-important outcomes were the primary outcome measured in only 18% of the studies.

Of course, no one feels better when their cholesterol, glucose level, or blood pressure is lowered, though it is hoped that by lowering these parameters clinicians can prevent cardiovascular disease. Yet, surrogate endpoints do not always correlate with clinically meaningful outcomes. For example, some brain tumors can nearly vanish on MRIs when treated with steroids, and any clinical trial that used imaging data as a primary outcome would be declared a great success [28]. Yet the tumor eventually comes roaring back, and patients treated with steroids don't live any longer. Additionally, intensive blood pressure lowering in patients with type 2 diabetes did not prevent death or cardiovascular events compared to a somewhat higher blood pressure and the lowering was associated with more side effects [29]. Similarly, diabetics treated with intensive control of blood sugar had a 22% higher death rate, increased weight gain, and more episodes of low blood sugar compared to patients treated with standard therapy.

Medications have caused damage after being approved based on surrogate outcomes. Torcetrapib had beneficial effects on patient's lipid profile, but increased the risk of mortality and morbidity through an unknown mechanism [30]. Rosiglitazone lowered blood sugar in people with diabetes, but caused heart attacks and death [31]. The medication bevacizumab shrank malignant brain tumors, though patients did not live any longer, and there were significant side effects [32].

Several cancer-studies have received similar criticism. Many clinical trials of metastatic solid tumors use a metric known as progression-free survival (PFS) as a primary endpoint. While PFS is easily measurable, it may fail to capture more meaningful outcomes such overall survival and quality of life. Indeed, clinical trials that have shown an improvement in PFS without a corresponding improvement in overall survival, have led to approval of new medications and changes in practice [33]. As Robert Kemp and Vinay Prasad wrote, the use of surrogate outcomes in oncology, "means that numerous drugs are now approved based on small yet statistically significant increases in surrogates of questionable reliability. In turn, this means the benefits of many approved drugs are uncertain" [34].

This practice of using relatively easy-to-measure numbers of questionable significance while ignoring more important but harder to measure outcomes is known as the quantitative fallacy. It is also called the McNamara fallacy, which named after the US Secretary of Defense from 1961 to 1968. He measured the "success" of the Vietnam War mainly by the number of dead enemy combatants, while ignoring more important, but harder to quantify endpoints [35].

Non-Representative Study Populations:

One of the most important questions a clinician must ask about a study is how well the study population adequately represents the patient in front of them. All too often, study subjects are poorly representative of the general population. Depending on the disease being studied, it can be very difficult to recruit subjects into medical studies because many of them are suspicious and do not want to be "guinea pigs." As journalist David Freedman wrote:

> Patient recruitment is an enormous problem in many medical studies, and researchers often end up paying for the participation of students, poor people, drug abusers, the homeless, illegal immigrants, and others who may not adequately represent the population in terms of health or lifestyle [36].

For many conditions, a large percentage of potential research subjects are excluded from clinical trials because they have one of many exclusion criteria. The unhealthiest patients are often excluded from clinical trials because they may make the medication appear less effective or more dangerous than it actually is. As Rafat Abonour, an oncologist, said:

> There's a joke that you have to be able to run a marathon before you can participate in a clinical trial...We don't really know how tolerable or effective a drug in clinical trials will be in the patients we see day-to-day because they so often have disease complications and other health problems. I am usually disappointed to find that drugs are less effective and have more side effects than reported in the studies [37].

Additionally, certain groups, such as women and minorities are often underrepresented in research studies. For ethical reasons, some populations, such as pregnant women, are excluded from almost every trial. Even a flawless study is of little use if its subjects do not represent a clinician's patients.

Citation Plagiarism

Citation plagiarism, a termed coined by social anthropologist Ole Bjorn Rekdal, occurs when researchers continually site a flawed source or one that does not accurately support their claim [38]. As a result of citation plagiarism, academic "urban legends" can be spawned. One of his original examples showed how a decimal point error mislead researchers into believing that spinach is a good source of iron [39]. In an article titled *Bad Footnotes Can Be Deadly*, Daniel Engber showed where a single paragraph helped spawn the opioid epidemic [40]. In 1980, a one-paragraph letter was published in the *New England Journal of Medicine* titled *Addiction Rare in Patients Treated with Narcotics* [41]. In this letter, two doctors examined their files and concluded that "despite widespread use of narcotic drugs in hospitals, the development of addiction is rare in medical patients with no history of addiction." In the ensuing decades, this letter was sited hundreds of times as evidence that opioid medications were generally safe. It was later referred to as an "extensive" and "landmark" study, though it was nothing of the sort. It wasn't even a study. As Engber wrote:

> When you try to trace the provenance of any given, referenced fact—on addiction rates, for example—you may well find yourself tangled in a nest of secondary sources, with each paper claiming to have pulled the fact from another. These daisy-chained citations make it very hard—and at times impossible—to locate original source material. They also lead to a game of research telephone, in which the context of a fact gets stripped away, and its meaning morphed as it gets transmitted from one citation to the next.

Lack of Replication

Replication is a hallmark of the scientific process. A single study almost never provides a definitive answer to a scientific question. Although different underlying patient populations may confound the results, generally speaking, if researchers find that a treatment works in Denver, it should work in Boston as well. If researchers from Boston successfully replicate findings from a group in Denver, then the value of the original research is magnified. If they fail to do so, then more research is needed. Unfortunately, there is less incentive for researchers to replicate the results of their colleagues than to produce new findings. Exciting, new discoveries are likely to be published in prominent medical journals and receive splashy headlines in the media. In contrast, replication studies are much less likely to be published in prominent journals and almost never receive media attention. Replication studies that fail to confirm the initial study are much less likely to receive the attention of the initial study itself. Indeed, in a study by G. N. Martin and Richard Clarke, only 33 out of 1150 psychology journals specifically stated in their aims or instructions to authors that they accepted replications [42]. Some researchers have privately expressed dismay that others might try to replicate their work, fearing that the effort is more an attempt to debunk them rather than a good-faith effort to determine the truth [43].

However, there is a "crisis" in psychology as many research studies, some of them well-known and influential, were unable to be replicated. Psychologist Brian Nosek, along with almost 300 of his colleagues, endeavored to reproduce about 100 of the most important findings in psychology, an endeavor known as the Reproducibility Project [44]. The results were sobering. Only 40% of the studies could be replicated. I have little doubt that some of the studies referenced in this book would fail the reproducibility rest, though I am obviously not sure which ones.

Some core findings of psychology failed the reproducibility test. For example, the concept of ego depletion held that people have a finite supply of willpower. Researchers found that people who successfully resisted eating cookies in favor of radishes were less willing to work on difficult puzzles afterwards [45]. The paper had been cited thousands of times and many other papers found evidence of ego depletion in other spheres [46]. A best-selling book was written on how people could use the concept of ego depletion to improve their willpower. However, evidence emerged that questioned the existence of ego depletion. In 2014, a meta-analysis found that due to publication bias and small studies, ego depletion might not be a real thing [47]. Then in 2016, a replication effort involving over 20 labs in several countries and 2,141 participants found no evidence that ego depletion existed [48]. One dismayed social psychologist, Michael Islincht, wrote:

> As someone who has been doing research for nearly twenty years, I now can't help but wonder if the topics I chose to study are in fact real and robust. Have I been chasing puffs of smoke for all these years? I have spent nearly a decade working on the concept of ego depletion, including work that is critical of the model used to explain the phenomenon. I have been rewarded for this work and I am convinced that the main reason I get any invitations to speak at colloquia and brown-bags these days is because of this work. The problem is that ego depletion might not even be a thing [49].

Not surprisingly, there was significant debate in the scientific literature about these findings and the Reproducibility Project as a whole. Psychologist Daniel Gilbert and colleagues responded to the Reproducibility Project by arguing that it was affected by several statistical errors and that in reality, "the reproducibility of psychological science is quite high" [50]. While the debate will continue, it is nonetheless unarguable that replication is undervalued compared to original research.

Other fields have similarly suffered a reproducibility crisis. For example, C. Glenn Begley and scientists in the hematology and oncology department at Amgen, a biotechnology company, attempted to reproduce 53 "landmark," preclinical research studies [51]. The results were sobering. The findings were confirmed in just six (11%) of the studies. Some of the studies that could not be reproduced had been sited nearly 2,000 times by other researchers. Similarly, researchers from Bayer HealthCare were only able to validate 20–25% of published preclinical studies. Many projects ended because of an inability to reproduce the results, and the success rates of medications in Phase II clinical trials is as low as 18% [52].

Editorial Board Invitation- Neurology

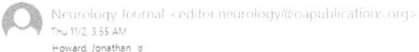

Dear Dr. **Jonathan Howard**,

Greetings from Neurology Journal.

OA Journal of Neurology is an open-access, peer-reviewed journal, that publishes original research, reviews, opinions and interviews.

We enthralled with your research and inviting you to be a part of our Editorial Board member.
To join in our Editorial Board list, kindly send your Biography, Research interest along with a recent photograph to display in our Editorial Board page.
Please feel free to contact me for further details.

Warm regards,
Sherlyn Sethia
OA Journal of Neurology

Fig. 30.4 An invitation I received to be on the editorial board of a predatory journal

Predatory Publishers

A recent, unfortunate trend in medicine and science is the proliferation of predatory journals. These are open-access journals that have the appearance and names (such as *International Archives of Medicine*) of legitimate scientific journals, but will publish almost anything as long as the authors have paid a hefty fee. These journals are the scientific version of fake news. I receive invitations daily to publish papers in these journals and am occasionally asked to sit on their editorial boards. One study found there are nearly 8,000 such journals, publishing about 400,000 articles annually (Fig. 30.4) [53].

According to the NIH, predatory journals have several characteristic attributes including [54]:

- Misleading pricing (e.g., lack of transparency about article processing charges).
- Failure to disclose information to authors.
- Aggressive tactics to solicit article submissions.
- Inaccurate statements about editorial board membership.
- Misleading or suspicious peer-review processes.

Others have identified several other red flags, such as [53]:

- Low article-processing fees (less than $150).
- Spelling and grammar errors on the website.
- An overly broad scope.
- Language that targets authors rather than readers.
- Promises of rapid publication.
- A lack of information about retraction policies, manuscript handling, or digital preservation.
- Manuscript submissions by e-mail and the inclusion of distorted images.

According to medical librarian Jeffrey Beall, who kept a list of predatory journals, up to 10% of open-access articles are published in such journals [55]. Pharmaceutical companies have published their work in these journals, possibly unaware they are not legitimate. The Federal Trade Commission (FTC) estimated that over a six-year span, researchers spent $26.6 million on publication and conference registration fees for predatory journals [56].

Devious authors have exposed predatory journals by managing to publish hoaxes and utter nonsense in these journals. These pranksters showed the peer-review process for predatory journals is worthless or non-existent. Philip Davis, a graduate student in communication sciences, used a computer program "that generates grammatically correct but nonsensical text." He hoped to discover whether a journal would be willing to "accept a completely nonsensical manuscript if the authors were willing to pay." He and his colleagues used pseudonyms to successfully published a paper in *The Open Information Science Journal*, leading its editor to resign when the hoax was revealed [57]. It gets worse. A blogger by the name of Neuroskeptic wrote a "Star Wars-themed spoof paper… an absurd mess of factual errors, plagiarism, and movie quotes" [58]. The methods section was largely plagiarized from Wikipedia. Though several journals rejected the paper, four accepted it, and three published it. It gets even worse. Christoph Bartneck managed to get a paper accepted at the *International Conference on Atomic and Nuclear Physics* [59]. He wrote the paper by starting a sentence with "Atomic" or "Nuclear" and then randomly hitting the auto-complete suggestions on his phone. The opening sentence of his paper was "Atomic Physics and I shall not have the same problem with a separate section for a very long long way." It gets even worse. In 2005, two scientists, David Mazières and Eddie Kohler, frustrated at receiving invitations to publish in predatory journals, wrote a paper consisting entirely of the sentence "Get me off your fucking mailing list" [60]. It included several diagrams with this sentence as well. In 2014, another frustrated researcher, Peter Vamplew, submitted the paper to the *International Journal of Advanced Computer Technology* [61]. Much to his surprise, the paper received an "excellent" rating and was accepted for publication (Fig. 30.5).

While it may seem that researchers are the victims of such journals, this is not necessarily the case. Given that researchers receive promotions and tenure based largely on their publication record, many are able to advance their careers by publishing their papers in predatory journals with legitimate-sounding names. As science journalist Gina Kolata wrote:

> Along the way they earned the "predatory" epithet, because they were thought to be taking advantage of innocent scientists. But, I learned, predation is only a small part of the story. Many — probably most — academics who publish in these journals know exactly what they are doing. They are padding their résumés, taking advantage of the fact that colleges may not know if a journal is legitimate or not. When the number of publications a person has can determine his or her chances for advancement, some decide to take the easy route [62].

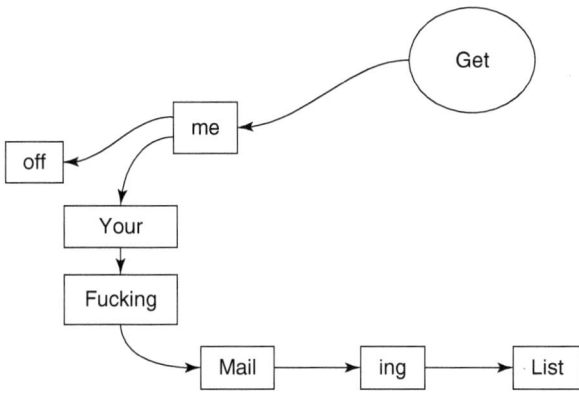

Fig. 30.5 Figure 1 from the paper "Get Me Off Your Fucking Mailing List." (Mazières D, Kohler E. Get me off your fucking mailing list [Figure 1, PDF file]. (n.d.). Retrieved from http://www.scs.stanford.edu/%7Edm/home/papers/remove.pdf.)

Conflicts of Interest

When researchers have a vested interest in a trial's result, they are more likely to get the result they want. Few players have more at stake in the outcome of many clinical trials than pharmaceutical and device companies. Billions of dollars can be at stake.

Not surprisingly, there is overwhelming evidence that clinical trials are more likely to be positive when they are sponsored by industry. A study by Florence Bourgeois and colleagues examined 546 drug trials and found that 85% of studies conducted by pharmaceutical companies or commercial interests had positive results. This fell to 72% when nonprofits or non-federal organizations funded trials, and to 50% for government-funded trials [63]. A reasonable interpretation of these findings is that pharmaceutical companies are more likely to carry out studies of drugs that have already shown promise in earlier studies. However, even when taking this into account, studies funded by pharmaceutical companies were still more likely to be positive. Dr. Bourgeois said about the findings:

> I wouldn't say these things are necessarily deliberate. Our findings simply raise concerns about whether there is an inherent conflict of interest if you have pharmaceutical companies designing and conducting trials to validate drugs they are also seeking to market, and standing to gain quite a bit from good results [64].

Paula Rochon and colleagues studied 56 trials of anti-inflammatory drugs for arthritis funded by pharmaceutical companies. In all of the studies, the company's drug was equal to or better than the comparison drug [65]. A review of 30 trials by Joel Lexchin and colleagues found that research funded by pharmaceutical companies was less likely to be published, but more likely to have positive results compared to studies funded by other sources [66]. A study by Nathaniel Smilowitz and colleagues found that randomized trials of devices used in interventional cardiology were more likely to be positive if at least one author was an industry employee [67].

Assuming that outright fraud is rare, then how do pharmaceutical companies do it? Richard Smith, an editor of the *British Medical Journal (BMJ)*, revealed several techniques they use to achieve their remarkable outcomes [68]:

1. Conduct a trial of your drug against a treatment known to be inferior.
2. Trial your drugs against too low a dose of a competitor drug.
3. Conduct a trial of your drug against too high a dose of a competitor drug (making your drug seem less toxic).
4. Conduct trials that are too small to show differences from competitor drugs.
5. Use multiple endpoints in the trial and select for publication those that give favorable results.
6. Do multicenter trials and select for publication results from centers that are favorable.
7. Conduct subgroup analyses and select for publication those that are favorable.
8. Present results that are most likely to impress — for example, reduction in relative rather than absolute risk.

Importantly, many of these pharmaceutical trials are published in the most prestigious scientific journals, such as *The Lancet* and *New England Journal of Medicine* [69]. Publishing positive results from trials sponsored by pharmaceutical companies can be lucrative for all parties. Pharmaceutical companies often order reprints of journal articles, which can result in substantial printing fees paid to the journals. Dr. Smith wrote:

> *Editors, too, know that publishing such studies is highly profitable, and editors are increasingly responsible for the budgets of their journals and for producing a profit for the owners. Many owners—including academic societies—depend on profits from their journals. An editor may thus face a frighteningly stark conflict of interest: publish a trial that will bring US$100,000 of profit or meet the end-of-year budget by firing an editor* [68].

Recognizing this conflict of interest, the editor of *The Lancet*, Richard Horton, wrote in 2004, "Journals have devolved into information laundering operations for the pharmaceutical industry" [70].

Legal Threats

While companies most often push for favorable research, at other times, companies and ideologically motivated organizations may try to entirely suppress unfavorable research. For example, with support of the National Rifle Association (NRA), the CDC has been prohibited from studying gun violence. According to journalist Todd Zwillich:

> *The NRA complained to Congress that the CDC was using the results of its research to essentially advocate for gun control. They called it propaganda. And back at that time, Congress slashed the CDC's funding by the exact amount that was used for gun-related public health research* [71].

In 2015, Pieter Cohen and colleagues published a study showing that a stimulant (BMPEA) commonly used in dietary supplements had no evidence for its efficacy or safety [72]. Several weeks later, The FDA alerted consumers to these results and asked supplement makers to remove it from their products. One supplement maker sued Dr. Cohen for $200 million in damages for libel, alleging that his paper and public comments afterwards were untrue [73]. The company likely never intended to win the trial but hoped to intimidate and silence Dr. Cohen and researchers like him. Such lawsuits are known as strategic lawsuit against public participation (SLAPP). SLAPP lawsuits can be incredibly expensive, lengthy, and emotionally-draining. As Dr. Cohen, said:

Preparation for the trial included a six-hour deposition, a mock trial and a review of more than 4,000 pages of studies, emails, correspondences, drafts and depositions. The trial itself lasted seven days, and put my family through the wringer [73].

Unfortunately, Dr. Cohen's experience is not unique, and other researchers who have published unfavorable results have found themselves targeted by industry [74].

Ghostwriting

Ghostwriting is another deceptive practice of pharmaceutical and device companies. It occurs when they hire writers to produce favorable articles for publication. Prominent researchers receive a fee for being listed as authors, even if they had nothing to do with the actual research or writing of the manuscript. As philosopher Sergio Sismondo wrote:

In extreme cases, drug companies pay for trials by contract research organizations (CROs), analyze the data in-house, have professionals write manuscripts, ask academics to serve as authors of those manuscripts, and pay communication companies to shepherd them through publication in the best journals. The resulting articles affect the conclusions found in the medical literature, and are used in promoting drugs to doctors [75].

Not surprisingly, ghostwritten articles are often extremely misleading. Perhaps the most infamous case of ghostwriting is known as Study 329, which was published in 2001. The study examined the use of the antidepressant paroxetine in adolescents. It concluded, "Paroxetine is generally well tolerated and effective for major depression in adolescents" [76]. The medication became a blockbuster for the pharmaceutical company with nearly $12 billion in sales. In 2015, a reanalysis of the original data was performed using previously confidential court documents. It found that paroxetine was both ineffective at treating depression and likely unsafe, as it led to more suicidal thoughts and behavior [77]. These findings were known to the manufacturers at the time of publication, though they were not included in the final publication. Psychiatrist Martin Keller and 21 other researchers were listed as authors on the original study. It reality, it was ghostwritten by Scientific Therapeutics Information, a company that specializes in communications for the pharmaceutical industry [78]. This also was not known until a lawsuit was filed against the company.

This was by no means an isolated incident. Adriane Fugh-Berman, a professor of pharmacology and physiology, explained that ghostwriting was also used to deceive clinicians and the public about hormone therapy (HT) for menopausal women [79]. As she wrote:

> The pharmaceutical company Wyeth used ghostwritten articles to mitigate the perceived risks of breast cancer associated with HT, to defend the unsupported cardiovascular "benefits" of HT, and to promote off-label, unproven uses of HT such as the prevention of dementia, Parkinson's disease, vision problems, and wrinkles.

A total of 26 papers were ghostwritten, appearing in 18 medical journals [80]. Wyeth's role in paying for the research and writing the papers was not disclosed, and the scandal came to light only when a lawsuit revealed the paper trail.

A similar scandal occurred with a paper about the painkiller Vioxx™. It was later revealed that this paper had omitted crucial information, including the deaths of several patients due to cardiac causes. Jeffrey Lisse, a rheumatologist who was credited as the first author on the paper, defended himself by saying, essentially, that he had nothing to do with the study. "Merck designed the trial, paid for the trial, ran the trial" he said. "Merck came to me after the study was completed and said, 'We want your help to work on the paper.' The initial paper was written at Merck, and then it was sent to me for editing" [81].

Fraud

The most egregious form of scientific misconduct is outright fabrication (making up data) and falsification (altering or selecting data). While such cases are relatively rare, they are not unheard of. According to science writer Christopher Wanjek:

> This past year (2017), hundreds of scientific papers were retracted from professional journals. In the majority of cases involving these retractions, the reason was an innocent, yet sloppy, error in the methodology of the experiment that the authors themselves caught. But for quite a few papers, the retractions reflected scientific misconduct and a not-so-innocent attempt to tweak the data — or make it up entirely [82].

According to the website Retraction Watch, 39 researchers were criminally charged for fraudulent work between 1979 and 2016 [83]. Many others were disgraced, though not criminally charged. In addition to this, since 2012, over 500 papers have been retracted due to fraudulent peer review, almost all of them from China [82].

Specific examples of fraudulent research include:

• In 2015, Dong-Pyou Han, a former biomedical scientist in Iowa, was found to have fabricated data in trials of an HIV vaccine [84]. He used human blood to spike the blood of rabbits he was studying to make it appear as if his vaccine was effective. James Bradac, who oversaw AIDS vaccine grants for the NIH, had awarded Dr. Han's lab nearly $19 million. Dr. Bradac said it was the worst case of fraud he had seen in twenty years at the agency [85]. Dr. Han was fined over seven million dollars for his crime and sentenced to nearly five years in prison.

- In 2014, a revolutionary method of generating stem cells, known as stimulus-triggered acquisition of pluripotency, was found to be based on fraudulent research by Japanese scientist Haruko Obokata. The findings were published in the prestigious journal *Nature*. Her mentor, who was not implicated in the fraud, committed suicide.

- In 2014, Michael LaCour, a political science graduate student, published a paper titled *When Contact Changes Minds: An Experiment on Transmission of Support for Gay Equality*. It reportedly found that in-person conversations could increase support for gay marriage in people formally against it. It was retracted after its research was found to be fraudulent [86].

- In 2016, Caroline Barwood, a researcher at the University of Queensland, obtained or tried to obtain hundreds of thousands of dollars to conduct a study on Parkinson's disease. The study never took place, and Dr. Barwood admitted to investigators that she had "not even met a single patient" [87]. Instead, she used the work of another academic and portrayed it as her own.

- Dutch social psychologist Diederik Stapel, a dean of the School of Social and Behavioral Sciences and head of the social psychology department of Tilburg University, was an academic star who published dozens of influential papers. In 2011, his work was revealed to be based on falsified data. The fraud lasted nearly ten years and affected nearly 60 publications. Though "red-flags" had surfaced about his too-good-to-be true results, concerns were either ignored or dismissed. A subsequent investigation revealed that:

> *Stapel was known as a charismatic leader with great dedication to his students and colleagues. There was often a phase of intensive preparation of the research with the student. After developing experimental materials, the data collection was completely in the hands of Stapel. The so-called data collection occurred at secondary schools where Stapel had connections, and occurred under his sole supervision. He enlisted the help of unknown (fictitious) paid research assistants for data collection. After a few weeks, a complete, coded data set would be made available to the collaborator for further analysis. The collaborator could then immediately focus on manuscript writing. Stapel justified doing the research at secondary schools because students there were more naïve and therefore "better research participants." He did not allow collaborators to approach the schools, as schools might be overwhelmed with research requests and this would jeopardize his access. Stapel was described as intimidating and not tolerating questions from students regarding his refusal to have them involved in data collection [88].*

- South Korean stem-cell scientist Hwang Woo Suk achieved international fame and was considered the "Pride of Korea" for his pioneering work in cloning and creating human embryonic stem cells. His work was published in some of the most prominent scientific journals. In 2005 much of his work was revealed to be an elaborate fraud [89]. In 2009, he was convicted of fraud, embezzlement, and illegally purchasing human eggs.

- Marc Hauser, a Harvard psychology professor and evolutionary biologist, was forced to resign in 2011. An internal review found:

> *Hauser's shortcomings in respect to research integrity have in the main consisted instead of repeated instances of cutting corners, of pushing analyses of data further in the direction of significance than the actual findings warranted, and of reporting results as he may have wished them to have been, rather than as they actually were [90].*

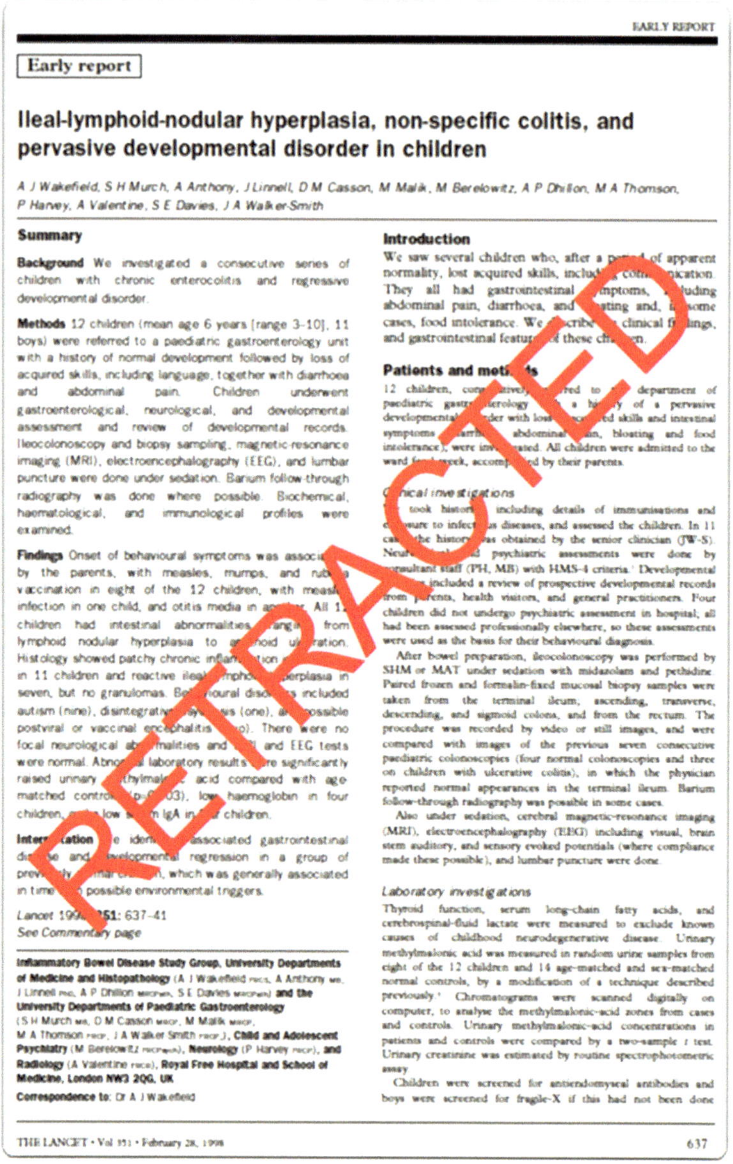

Fig. 30.6 The paper that started the modern-day anti-vaccine movement. (First page of the redacted study. Lancet 351(9103):637–641. https://doi.org/10.1016/S0140-6736(97)11096-0.)

- British gastroenterologist Andrew Wakefield started the modern-day anti-vaccine movement in 1998 with a paper published in *The Lancet* titled *Ileal-Lymphoid-Nodular Hyperplasia, Non-Specific Colitis, and Pervasive Developmental Disorder in Children* [91]. This study, based on 12 children, purportedly identified a new diagnosis called autistic enterocolitis and posited that the measles, mumps, and rubella (MMR) vaccine was responsible. Based on this paper and even more dramatic press conferences that followed, vaccine rates dropped in many parts of the world, leading to a predictable risk in vaccine-preventable diseases, with avoidable suffering and deaths. Large studies from around the world of hundreds of thousands of children have clearly demonstrated that vaccines do not cause autism, debunking Wakefield's claim (Fig. 30.6) [92].

A later investigation by the journalist Brian Deer described Wakefield's work as an "elaborate fraud." He found that Wakefield hoped to make tens of millions of dollars with "litigation driven testing" for autistic enterocolitis [93]. Lawyers had already paid him hundreds of thousands of pounds [94]. Another report in the *BMJ* revealed that the children in Wakefield's study did not even have inflammatory bowel disease [95]. In 2010, *The Lancet* and almost all of Wakefield's coauthors retracted the paper, writing:

We wish to make it clear that in this paper no causal link was established between (the) vaccine and autism, as the data were insufficient. However, the possibility of such a link was raised, and consequent events have had major implications for public health. In view of this, we consider now is the appropriate time that we should together formally retract the interpretation placed upon these findings in the paper, according to precedent [96].

In 2010, the British Medical Council found Dr. Wakefield guilty of multiple counts of dishonesty and the abuse of developmentally challenged children. They wrote to him, "you showed a callous disregard for the distress and pain that you knew or ought to have known the children involved might suffer." Dr. Wakefield was "struck off" the medical register. Unlike almost all researchers found guilty of such fraud, to this day Wakefield defends his work. He has instigated failed lawsuits against his critics [97]. He remains the unrepentant leader of the anti-vaccine movement: making documentaries, giving speeches, and writing books — all of which spread fears about vaccines. After he spoke to the Somali community in Minnesota, for example, vaccination rates plummeted. This lead to a measles outbreak in 2017 that sickened dozens of children [98]. Twenty-one children became sick enough to require hospitalization [99]. The consequences have been worse elsewhere. From 2016-2017, over 19,000 people in Europe contracted measles. Forty-six people died, the vast majority of them unvaccinated children in Romania [100].

Solutions

Before discussing potential solutions to the problems plaguing scientific research today, it is important to recognize that the vast majority of researchers are dedicated, honest people who work hard to learn more about the natural world in order to improve our lives. Doing science is not easy. As Albert Einstein said, "If we knew what we were doing, it wouldn't be called research, would it?" Research takes time, money, and effort. There is no guarantee of success. Though there are certainly some well-known superstars, most scientists are underpaid and underappreciated.

Importantly, many influential studies are of very high quality. Consider, for example, the studies for the newest drug for relapsing-remitting multiple sclerosis (MS), ocrelizumab, which were published in the prestigious *New England Journal of Medicine* [101]. They involved 1,656 subjects in two separate but identical trials lasting ninety six weeks. These studies were preceded by smaller studies that showed efficacy of the drug. Its mechanism of action is consistent with our understanding of the disease. The studies were registered on clinicaltrials.gov before they began. They were randomized, double-blind, double-dummy, parallel-group studies that involved 141 trial sites across 32 countries. They used clinically meaningful outcomes (lowering the relapse rate and preventing disability progression). The drug was tested against an older, but powerful medicine used to treat MS. The p-value for the primary outcome was highly statistically significant ($P < 0.001$). All authors filled out easily accessible disclosure forms where interested readers can explore potential conflicts of interest [102]. These two studies were not outliers in being done well, and they are representative of recent drug trials for MS. Now that the medication has been approved, its safety is continually monitored for adverse effects that may not have been detected in these trials. The manufacturer of the medication has already reached out to me to discuss post-approval safety concerns.

While this chapter opened with the provocative claim that half of all medical studies are wrong, other researchers have come to more optimistic conclusions. Leah Jager and Jeffrey Leek examined the p-values from 5,322 papers published in the most prestigious journals from 2000-2010. They estimated the false positive rate was only 14% [103]. While some may argue that this is still unacceptably high (especially given that only the top-tier journals were studied), Jager and Leek concluded that "the medical literature remains a reliable record of scientific progress."

It is clear, however, that there is much room for improvement, and an entire new field, meta-research, is devoted in identifying and fixing problems in scientific research [104]. Some relatively simple solutions can, and already have, had a large impact in minimizing the problems described in this chapter.

- An important guard against the file draw effect, p-hacking, and HARKing is the registration of planned clinical studies before they begin. In 2004, the International Committee of Medical Journal Editors, an organization that includes some of the most influential medical journals, released a statement that they will not accept any studies that are not publically registered ahead of time [105]. According to the statement:

  The registry must be accessible to the public at no charge. It must be open to all prospective registrants and managed by a not-for-profit organization. There must be a mechanism to ensure the validity of the registration data, and the registry should be electronically searchable. An acceptable registry must include at minimum the following information: a unique identifying number, a statement of the intervention (or interventions) and comparison (or comparisons) studied, a statement of the study hypothesis, definitions of the primary and secondary outcome measures, eligibility criteria, key trial dates (registration date, anticipated or actual start date, anticipated or actual date of last follow-up, planned or actual date of closure to data entry, and date trial data considered complete), target number of subjects, funding source, and contact information for the principal investigator.

- Primary Registry and Trial Identifying Number
- Date of Registration in Primary Registry
- Secondary Identifying Numbers
- Source(s) of Monetary or Material Support
- Primary Sponsor
- Secondary Sponsor(s)
- Contact for Public Queries
- Contact for Scientific Queries
- Public Title
- Scientific Title
- Countries of Recruitment
- Health Condition(s) or Problem(s) Studied
- Intervention(s)
- Key Inclusion and Exclusion Criteria
- Study Type
- Date of First Enrollment
- Target Sample Size
- Recruitment Status
- Primary Outcome(s)
- Key Secondary Outcomes

Fig. 30.7 WHO Trial Registration Data Set

The World Health Organization currently has a list of 20 items that must be completed before a trial is considered registered (Fig. 30.7) [106].

Since 2007, the US government has required that certain studies be registered and the results reported on the public website clinicaltrials.gov. If a company or researcher starts a trial and either fails to complete it, fails to publish it, or deviates from the original study design, the scientific community will be aware that something is amiss. Similarly, Ben Goldacre, a doctor and vocal critic of the pharmaceutical industry and junk science, founded an organization known as AllTrials. It has the support of many prominent journals and scientific bodies. Its ambitious mission includes the retrospective registration of all published trials. Its petition states that "All trials past and present should be registered, and the full methods and the results reported" [107].

AllTrials has also launched an initiative called Restoring Invisible and Abandoned Trials (RIAT). Its goal is to "publish, or update already published findings" from missing and abandoned trials [108]. Through court records, the *BMJ*, which is part of RIAT, has access to hundreds of thousands pages of previously unreleased trial data for several medications [109]. It was partly through the RIAT program that hidden data about paroxetine Study 329 came to light. The Center for Open Science's Open Science Framework is another site where researchers register both trial design and their plans for data analysis. According to its founders, about 7,000 studies have been preregistered [110].

There is evidence that the registration of trials has had its intended effect. Robert Kaplan and Veronica Irvin studied trials funded by the National Heart, Lung, and Blood Institute. Starting in 2000, it required that investigators publicly register their research analysis plan before beginning their clinical trials [111]. They found that "17 of 30 studies (57%) published prior to 2000 showed a significant benefit of intervention on the primary outcome in comparison to only 2 among the 25 (8%) trials published after 2000." However, other investigators have found that a minority of studies are in full compliance with the US government law and policies of clinicaltrials.gov, with a majority of studies failing to be registered or failing to report their outcomes in a timely manner [112–114]. Interestingly, studies sponsored by pharmaceutical companies were in better compliance than those sponsored by governmental agencies.

Joseph Simmons and colleagues made the following suggestions for both authors and reviewers looking to maintain the integrity of the scientific literature [14]:

Requirements for Authors
1. Authors must decide the rule for terminating data collection before data collection begins and report this rule in the article.
2. Authors must collect at least 20 observations per cell or else provide a compelling cost-of-data-collection justification.
3. Authors must list all variables collected in a study.
4. Authors must report all experimental conditions, including failed manipulations.
5. If observations are eliminated, authors must also report what the statistical results are if those observations are included.
6. If an analysis includes a covariate, authors must report the statistical results of the analysis without the covariate.

Guidelines for Reviewers
1. Reviewers should ensure that authors follow the requirements.
2. Reviewers should be more tolerant of imperfections in results.
3. Reviewers should require authors to demonstrate that their results do not hinge on arbitrary analytic decisions.
4. If justifications of data collection or analysis are not compelling, reviewers should require the authors to conduct an exact replication.

Some researchers have gone a step further than this, suggesting that studies should be accepted for publication before they even start. As long as the study question is interesting and the design is sound, the trial will be published before the results are known if it is carried out in a competent manner. This policy would help eliminate the publication bias, where positive findings are more likely to be published and receive more attention than negative ones.

- As another tool to combat p-hacking and false positive results, several prominent researchers have suggested lowering the threshold of statistical significance to 0.005 [115]. Of course, lowering the p-value for significance will result in fewer false positive results, but at the cost of more false negatives. One psychology journal banned the use of p-value altogether [116]. The journal editors explained, "We believe that the $p < .05$ bar is too easy to pass and sometimes serves as an excuse for lower quality research." Statistical tools exist to minimize false positive rates. A Bonferroni correction, for example, is an adjustment intended to account for the fact that, in large enough data sets, statistically significant results are mathematically more likely than not.

- Medical schools need to improve the statistical literacy of their students so they both spot p-hacking and not do it themselves. Before entering medical school, students are required to pass intense courses in calculus, organic chemistry, and physics. While I am not disparaging these subjects, their relevance to the practice of medicine is minimal. Once in medical school, many hours are spent learning gross anatomy, physiology, pharmacology, and histology. While these subjects have much more clinical relevance, in reality only a few clinicians need to know the anatomy of the thoracic inlet or the Frank-Starling law on a daily basis. Most students spend hours memorizing such information only to forget most of it, as it has little relevance to their clinical practice. In contrast, courses in medical statistics and epidemiology are much shorter and are often perceived by students as afterthoughts. However, unlike the anatomy of the brachial plexus, knowing how to read a scientific paper is a skill that every clinician will need at every stage of their careers. As shown in several chapters in this book, confusion over how to properly interpret statistics means that many clinicians have a very poor grasp of the efficacy of their tests and treatments. Medical educators should teach and reinforce these concepts throughout medical training. An entire lecture could be devoted the p–value alone. Ideally, statistic will become a core part of the math curriculum throughout a child's education.

- One novel suggestion to minimize the expectation bias is known as blind analysis. Medical researchers routinely blind themselves and study subjects in data collection. It is routine for subjects to receive a placebo (or active comparator) in drug trials, and multiple procedures and surgeries have been compared to "sham" treatments. As neither the researchers nor the study subjects know which treatment the subject receives, bias can be minimized during this phase of the study. However, once the data is revealed during the analysis of the study, p-hacking and the removal of "inconvenient" results can occur. To combat this problem, particle physicists and cosmologists routinely use blind analysis, which "avoids the possibility of experimenters biasing their result toward their own preconceptions by preventing them from knowing the answer until the analysis is complete" [117]. Robert MacCoun, a psychologist, and Saul Perlmutter, a physicist, suggested that other scientific fields could adopt this approach [118]. They wrote:

Blind analysis ensures that all analytical decisions have been completed, and all programmes and procedures debugged, before relevant results are revealed to the experimenter. One investigator — or, more typically, a suitable computer program — methodically perturbs data values, data labels or both, often with several alternative versions of perturbation. The rest of the team then conducts as much analysis as possible 'in the dark'. Before unblinding, investigators should agree that they are sufficiently confident of their analysis to publish whatever the result turns out to be, without further rounds of debugging or rethinking.

- It is clear that researchers who seek to replicate the work of others should be afforded more respect and attention. Most prestigious medical journals want to publish new, revolutionary findings. Replication studies, in contrast, might not bet published at all. However, replication studies, whether they support or contradict the original research, are as often as important as the original research itself.

- Surrogate outcomes are not inappropriate in medical trials. However, as Robert Kemp and Vinay Prasad wrote, "the use of surrogate outcomes should be limited to situations where a surrogate has demonstrated robust ability to predict meaningful benefits, or where cases are dire, rare or with few treatment options" [34].

- All authors on medical publications should disclose potential conflicts of interest. Although it relies on the honor system, all journals require that authors report when they or an immediate family member have a financial interest in any entity remotely related to the publication. These disclosure statements are then prominently displayed on the publication. Speakers are required to make disclosure statements prior to speaking at continuing medical education conferences.

- Many top medical schools prohibit their faculty members from being listed as authors on ghostwritten papers [119]. Similarly, the International Committee of Medical Journal Editors has taken steps to prevent ghostwriting. It requires that anyone who makes a "substantial contribution" to the design of a study, data acquisition, or writing the manuscript should be included as an author, with their potential conflicts of interest available for all to see [120]. Non-author contributors, who may have played a smaller role, should be acknowledged as well. The federal government has taken notice as well. In 2010, Senator Charles E. Grassley issued a 31-page report titled *Ghostwriting in Medical Literature* [119]. Researchers should refuse all offers to have their name attached to ghostwritten papers.

- Many journals have taken steps to facilitate commenting on scientific papers. Until recently, anyone hoping to dispute a paper's conclusions or correct an error had to write a letter to the journal. Such letters often required the same review process as the original paper, and they might not be seen by those who had read the original. In 2014, the US National Library of Medicine began allowing anyone who has published a paper listed on the PubMed database to comment on the papers listed there. Other forums, such as pubpeer.com, allow researchers to discuss and debate papers in a public forum. As a demonstration of the power of this process, an anti-vaccine paper by Christopher Shaw and Lucija Tomljenovic was retracted in less than a month after careful readers noticed certain important results had been omitted and even improperly manipulated [121].

- A small number of computer scientists are specializing in detecting videos and images that have been improperly manipulated [122]. Their work has been and will continue to be instrumental in detecting the small number of researchers who commit such fraud.

- Governmental agencies are taking action against predatory journals. In 2013, the US Health and Human Services department demanded that the publisher of hundreds of purported online academic journals, known as Omics, stop misusing the names of the NIH and the agency's employees in its promotional material [123]. In 2016, the FTC charged Omics with deceiving researchers with its publications and hiding publication fees of thousands of dollars [56]. The same year, the Federal Trade Commission (FTC) warned researchers about such journals an invited them to contact the FTC with their concerns [124]. In 2017, the NIH made a statement on articles resulting from research they funded. They encouraged authors to [54]:
  - Adhere to the principles of research integrity and publication ethics.

- Identify journals that follow best practices promoted by professional scholarly publishing organizations.
- Avoid publishing in journals that do not have a clearly stated and rigorous peer review process.

Of course, clinicians should not knowingly submit their research to predatory journals.

Conclusion

Much of medical science is filled with contradictions, conflicts of interests, reversals, and retractions. Clinicians and the general public find the current situation frustrating and confusing. It often seems as though something that cures cancer one day causes it the next. Medical reversals are common enough that Vinay Prasad and Adam Cifu were able to write an entire book on the subject, listing over 150 such reversals [125]. This has led some pessimists to declare that science, as is it practiced today is not "self-correcting," as many would like to believe, but rather fundamentally broken [126]. Even worse, the rare cases of outright scientific fraud can have an outsized impact, leading some people to believe that large swaths of academic medicine are fraudulent and dishonest. Others believe that even well-intentioned researchers are mere dupes of greedy corporations and evil governments. Some conspiracy theorists believe that pharmaceutical companies are purposefully hiding cures or even making people ill, hoping to profit from their suffering. As science journalist Tom Siegfried wrote, "If people stop trusting medical science, they turn to those even worse sources of knowledge that lead to serious consequences (such as children not getting proper vaccinations)" (Fig. 30.8) [127].

Certainly, complementary and alternative medicine (CAM) advocates revel in the confusion. Their livelihood depends on spreading fear, uncertainty, and doubt about the motivations of mainstream clinicians. Sayer Ji, founder of the CAM site greenmedinfo.com, for example, wrote an essay based on the work of Dr. Ioannidis titled *Evidence-Based' Medicine: A Coin's Flip Worth of Certainty*. In it, he wrote:

> The very life's blood of 'evidence-based' medicine – peer-reviewed and published clinical research results – which legitimizes the entire infrastructure and superstructure upon which conventional medical knowledge and practice is erected, has been revealed as **mostly and patently false**.

Mr. Ji advocated a return to pre-scientific time, when medical decisions were made based on feelings and tradition. He wrote, "Perhaps we would do equally well for ourselves if we went back to our intuition, drawing from ancient dietary and natural medical practices to take back control of our health." However, science-denialists like Mr. Ji are missing the point. Dr. Ioannidis and like-minded critics do not suggest that the scientific method should be replaced with anecdotes, tradition, and faith. Rather, Dr. Ioannidis feels that "evidence-based medicine still remains an unmet goal, worthy to be attained." He warned that "science denialism and quacks are also flourishing and leading more people astray in their life choices, including health" [3]. Legitimate critics of science want researchers to recognize the biases and flaws in their work in order to improve it. They want

Fig. 30.8 A conspiracy
theory meme.
(GreenMedInfo.com. The
plant that could save millions
[Image file, Facebook status
update]. 2017. Retrieved
from https://www.facebook.
com/greenmedinfo/photos/a.1
72939738489/101557445933
63490/?type=3.)

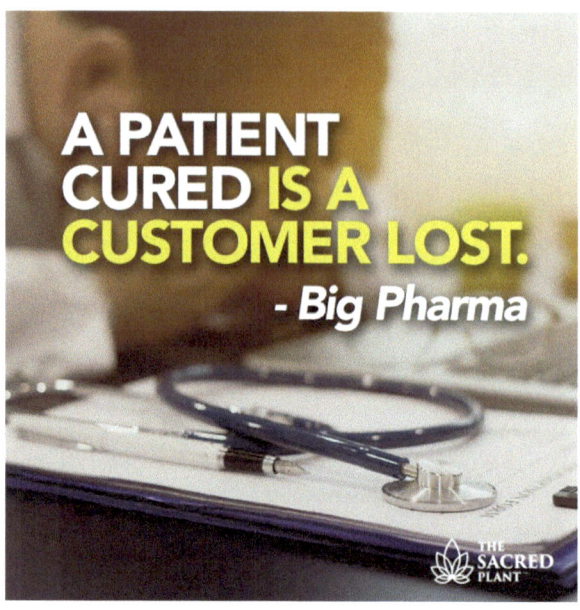

to improve statistical literacy. They want to improve the structure of science to encourage collaboration, as well as the publication of negative findings and replication studies (Fig. 30.9).

Moreover, the most strident critics and reformers of both medical research and clinical practice are themselves medical insiders. It is to the credit of mainstream medicine that it is willing to investigate its practices, acknowledge its failures, and take steps to correct them. The Meta-Research Innovation Center at Stanford (METRICS) is devoted to "reimagining science for the twenty-first century with the goal of strengthening the research enterprise to improve the quality of scientific studies in biomedicine and beyond" [104].

The drive to register trials came from within the medical community. The AllTrials project was founded by medical insiders. The blog Retraction Watch, which documents retracted research papers and fraud, was founded by Ivan Oransky, a doctor and journalist at New York University. Dr. Fugh-Berman directs PharmedOut at Georgetown University Medical Center. It is a "project that advances evidence-based prescribing and educates healthcare professionals about pharmaceutical marketing practices" [128]. Mainstream clinicians have written multiple books exposing the deceptions and chicanery of the pharmaceutical industry. The drive to make sure screening tests are effective is lead by medical insiders at the US Preventative Task Force. The Choosing Wisely campaign, which seeks to limit overtesting and overtreatment, was launched by medical insiders. Medical insiders investigate cherished practices, such as coronary artery stenting and surgery for osteoarthritis of the knee. When these practices are found to be ineffective, medical insiders publish the results in prominent medical journals (Fig. 30.10).

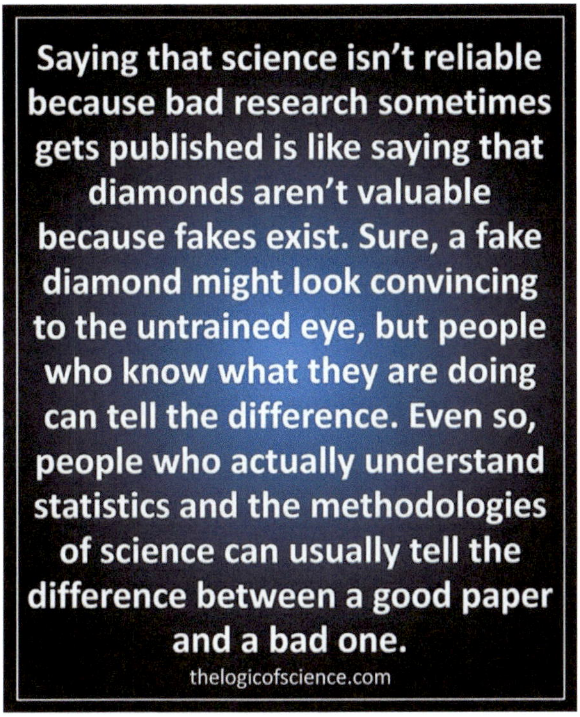

Fig. 30.9 I agree. (The Logic of Science. Note: the word "valuable" here is very clearly being used to refer to monetary value [Image file, Facebook status update]. 2017. Retrieved from https://www.facebook.com/thelogicofscience/posts/2048369678727758:0.)

In contrast, CAM practitioners almost never encourage scientific investigations into their practices, instead suggesting their treatments should be exempt from scientific scrutiny. The idea of a CAM practitioner abandoning a treatment that has been proven ineffective is almost laughable on its face. While mainstream critics of medicine are often embraced, Britt Hermes, a former naturopath who has exposed pseudoscientific practices in the field (Fig. 30.11), had her criticisms met with insults and legal threats [129].

When medical paradigms get reversed and scientific studies get retracted, it does not mean that the entire scientific process should be abandoned. Rather this is a sign that science is working. As one science-blogger wrote:

> From a public relations standpoint, it would be better if there were no retractions in science at all. It would look better if all scientists agreed with one another about everything, and never criticized published work (at least not in public). But that wouldn't really be science. It would be a cult. We shouldn't be concerned about retractions – quite the reverse. We should be concerned about people and groups that never admit their mistakes [130].

I could not agree more (Fig. 30.12).

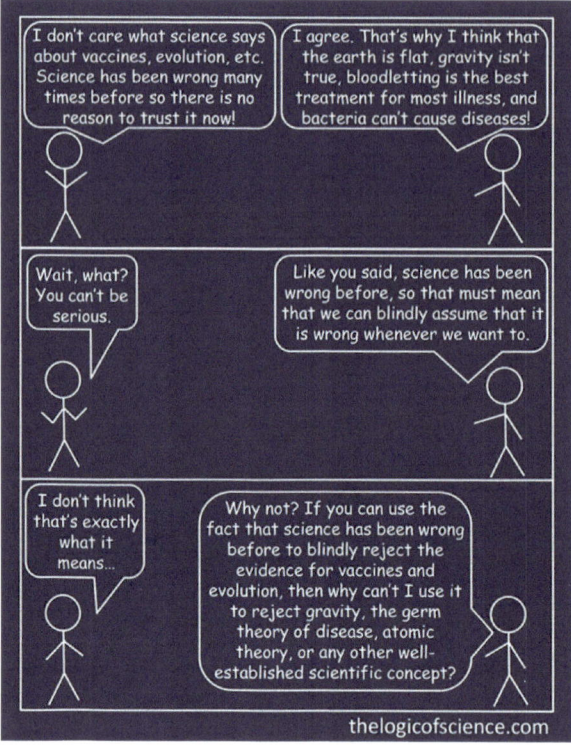

Fig. 30.10 Just because science has been wrong before, doesn't mean it is wrong now. (The Logic of Science. Reductio ad absurdum logic [Image file, Facebook status update]. 2016. Retrieved from https://www.facebook.com/thelogicofscience/posts/1869501483281246:0.)

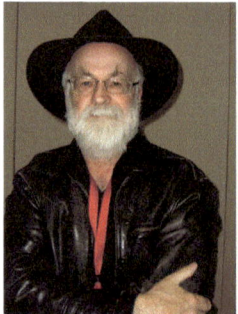

Sometimes scientists change their minds. New developments cause a rethink. If this bothers you, consider how much damage is being done to the world by people for whom new developments do not cause a rethink.

Terry Pratchett

Fig. 30.11 Terry Pratchett gets it right. (Novi L. (Luigi). Novelist Terry Pratchett on day 2 of the 2012 New York Comic Con [Image file]. In: Wikimedia commons. 2012. Retrieved from https://commons.wikimedia.org/wiki/Category:Terry_Pratchett#/media/File:10.12.12TerryPratchettByLuigiNovi1.jpg.)

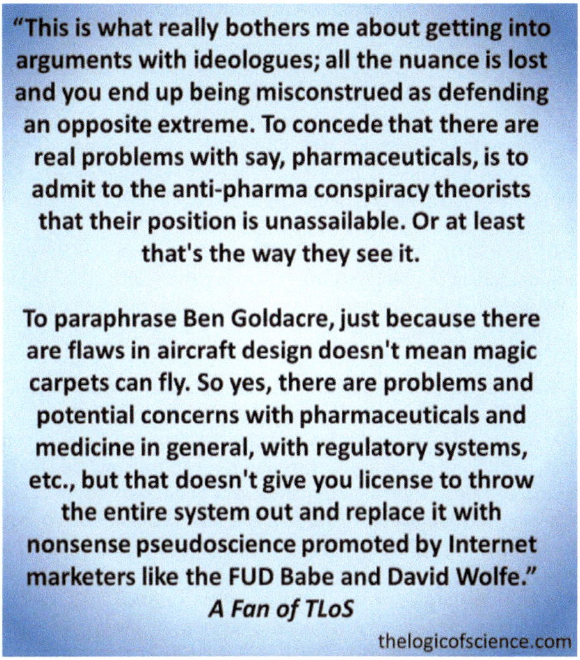

> "This is what really bothers me about getting into arguments with ideologues; all the nuance is lost and you end up being misconstrued as defending an opposite extreme. To concede that there are real problems with say, pharmaceuticals, is to admit to the anti-pharma conspiracy theorists that their position is unassailable. Or at least that's the way they see it.
>
> To paraphrase Ben Goldacre, just because there are flaws in aircraft design doesn't mean magic carpets can fly. So yes, there are problems and potential concerns with pharmaceuticals and medicine in general, with regulatory systems, etc., but that doesn't give you license to throw the entire system out and replace it with nonsense pseudoscience promoted by Internet marketers like the FUD Babe and David Wolfe."
> *A Fan of TLoS*
>
> thelogicofscience.com

Fig. 30.12 I agree. (The Logic of Science. [Image file, Facebook status update]. 2015. Retrieved from https://www.facebook.com/thelogicofscience/posts/1779978982233497:0.)

References

1. Sackett DL, Rosenberg WM, Gray JA, Haynes RB, Richardson WS. Evidence based medicine: what it is and what it isn't. BMJ. 1996;312(7023):71–2.
2. Ioannidis JPA. Why most published research findings are false. PLoS Med. 2005;2(8):e124. https://doi.org/10.1371/journal.pmed.0020124.
3. Ioannidis JPA. Evidence-based medicine has been hijacked: a report to David Sackett. J Clin Epidemiol. 2016;73:82–6. https://doi.org/10.1016/j.jclinepi.2016.02.012.
4. Chavalarias D, Ioannidis JPA. Science mapping analysis characterizes 235 biases in biomedical research. J Clin Epidemiol. 2010;63(11):1205–15. https://doi.org/10.1016/j.jclinepi.2009.12.011.
5. Freedman LP, Cockburn IM, Simcoe TS. The economics of reproducibility in preclinical research. PLoS Biol. 2015;13(6):e1002165. https://doi.org/10.1371/journal.pbio.1002165.
6. Croskerry P. (2013). 50 cognitive and affective biases in medicine [PDF file]. Retrieved from http://sjrhem.ca/wp-content/uploads/2015/11/CriticaThinking-Listof50-biases.pdf.
7. Klein DB. I was wrong, and so are you. The Atlantic. 2011;2011(12). Retrieved from https://www.theatlantic.com/magazine/archive/2011/12/i-was-wrong-and-so-are-you/308713/.
8. Silberzahn R, Uhlmann EL. Crowdsourced research: many hands make tight work. Nature. 2015;526:189–91. https://doi.org/10.1038/526189a.
9. Novella S. (2017, Aug 2). 0.05 or 0.005? P-value wars continue. Science-Based Medicine. Retrieved from https://sciencebasedmedicine.org/0-05-or-0-005-p-value-wars-continue/.

10. Resnick B. (2017, July 31). What a nerdy debate about p-values shows about science – and how to fix it. Vox. Retrieved from https://www.vox.com/science-and-health/2017/7/31/16021654/p-values-statistical-significance-redefine-0005.

11. Wasserstein RL, Lazar NA. The ASA's statement on *p*-values: context, process, and purpose. Am Stat. 2016;70(2):129–33. https://doi.org/10.1080/00031305.2016.1154108.

12. Leslie DL, Kobre RA, Richmand BJ, Guloksuz SA, Leckman JF. Temporal association of certain neuropsychiatric disorders following vaccination of children and adolescents: a pilot case-control study [Table 2]. Front Psych. 2017;8:3. https://doi.org/10.3389/fpsyt.2017.00003.

13. Haelle T. (2017, Mar 13). Assessing the red flags in a study…annotated [Blogpost]. Retrieved from https://healthjournalism.org/blog/2017/03/assessing-the-red-flags-in-a-study-annotated/.

14. Simmons JP, Nelson LD, Simonsohn U. False-positive psychology: undisclosed flexibility in data collection and analysis allows presenting anything as significant. Psychol Sci. 2011;22(11):1359–66. https://doi.org/10.1177/0956797611417632.

15. Kerr NL. HARKing: Hypothesizing after the results are known. Personal Soc Psychol Rev. 1998;2(3):196–217. https://doi.org/10.1207/s15327957pspr0203_4.

16. Gelman A, Loken E. (2013). The garden of forking paths: why multiple comparisons can be a problem, even when there is no "fishing expedition" or "p-hacking" and the research hypothesis was posited ahead of time [PDF file]. Department of Statistics, Columbia University. Retrieved from http://www.stat.columbia.edu/%7Egelman/research/unpublished/p_hacking.pdf.

17. Bohannon J. (2015, May 27). I fooled millions into thinking chocolate helps weight loss. Here's how. Retrieved from https://io9.gizmodo.com/i-fooled-millions-into-thinking-chocolate-helps-weight-1707251800.

18. Bem DJ. Feeling the future: experimental evidence of anomalous retroactive influences on cognition and affect. J Pers Soc Psychol. 2011;100(3):407–25. https://doi.org/10.1037/a0021524.

19. Engber D. (2017, May 17). Daryl Bem proved ESP is real. Which means science is broken. Slate. Retrieved from https://slate.com/health-and-science/2017/06/daryl-bem-proved-esp-is-real-showed-science-is-broken.html.

20. Galak J, LeBoeuf RA, Nelson LD, Simmons JP. Correcting the past: failures to replicate psi. J Pers Soc Psychol. 2012;103(6):933.

21. Harris WS, Gowda M, Kolb JW, Strychacz CP, Vacek JL, Jones PG, Forker A, O'Keefe JH, McCallister BD. A randomized, controlled trial of the effects of remote, intercessory prayer on outcomes in patient admitted to the coronary care unit. Arch Intern Med. 1999;159(19):2273–8. https://doi.org/10.1001/archinte.159.19.2273.

22. Turner EH, Matthews AM, Linardatos E, Tell RA, Rosenthal R. Selective publication of antidepressant trials and its influence on apparent efficacy. N Engl J Med. 2008;358(3):252–60. https://doi.org/10.1056/NEJMsa065779.

23. Pica N, Bourgeois F. Discontinuation and nonpublication of randomized clinical trials conducted in children. Pediatrics. 2016;138(3):e20160223.

24. Inzlicht M. (2015, Nov). A tale of two papers [Blog post]. Sometimes I'm wrong. Retrieved 15 Sept 2018 from http://sometimesimwrong.typepad.com/wrong/2015/11/guest-post-a-tale-of-two-papers.html.

25. Tuk MA, Zhang K, Sweldens S. The propagation of self-control: self-control in one domain simultaneously improves self-control in other domains. J Exp Psychol Gen. 2015;144(3):639–54. https://doi.org/10.1037/xge0000065. (Erratum published 2015, J Exp Psychol Gen, 144(3).).

26. Aronson JK. Biomarkers and surrogate endpoints. Br J Clin Pharmacol. 2005;59(5):491–4. https://doi.org/10.1111/j.1365-2125.2005.02435.x.

27. Gandhi GY, Murad MH, Fujiyoshi A, Mullan RJ, Flynn DN, Elamin MB, Swiglo BA, Isley WL, Guyatt GH, Montori VM. Patient-important outcomes in registered diabetes trials. JAMA. 2008;299(21):2543–9. https://doi.org/10.1001/jama.299.21.2543.

28. Weller M. Glucocorticoid treatment of primary CNS lymphoma. J Neuro-Oncol. 1999;43(3):237–9.

29. The ACCORD Study Group. Effects of intensive blood-pressure control in type 2 diabetes mellitus. N Engl J Med. 2010;362(17):1575–85. https://doi.org/10.1056/NEJMoa1001286.

30. Barter PJ, Caulfield M, Eriksson M, Grundy SM, Kastelein JJ, Komajda M, Lopez-Sendon J, Mosca L, Tardif JC, Waters DD, Shear CL, Revkin JH, Buhr KA, Fisher MR, Tall AR, Brewer B. Effects of torcetrapib in patients at high risk for coronary events. N Engl J Med. 2007;357(21):2109–22. https://doi.org/10.1056/NEJMoa0706628.

31. Nissen SE, Wolski K. Effect of rosiglitazone on risk of myocardial infarction and death from cardiovascular causes. N Engl J Med. 2007;356(24):2457–71. https://doi.org/10.1056/NEJMoa072761.

32. Khasraw M, Ameratunga MS, Grant R, Wheeler H, Pavlakis N. Antiangiogenic therapy for high-grade glioma. Cochrane Database Syst Rev. 2014;2014(9). https://doi.org/10.1002/14651858.CD008218.pub3

33. Booth CM, Eisenhauer EA. Progression-free survival: meaningful or simply measurable. J Clin Oncol. 2012;30(10):1030–3. https://doi.org/10.1200/JCO.2011.38.7571.

34. Kemp R, Prasad V. Surrogate endpoints in oncology: when are they acceptable for regulatory and clinical decisions, and are they currently overused? BMC Med. 2017;15:134. https://doi.org/10.1186/s12916-017-0902-9.

35. Salem Baskin J. (2014, July 25). According to U.S. big data, we won the Vietnam War. Forbes. Retrieved from https://www.forbes.com/sites/jonathansalembaskin/2014/07/25/according-to-big-data-we-won-the-vietnam-war.

36. Freedman DH. (2010, Dec 10). Why scientific studies are so often wrong: the streetlight effect. Discover Magazine. Retrieved from http://discovermagazine.com/2010/jul-aug/29-why-scientific-studies-often-wrong-streetlight-effect.

37. Swartz A. (2017). Cancer clinical trials exclude many desperate patients – should that change? Chicago Tribune. Retrieved from http://www.chicagotribune.com/lifestyles/health/ct-cancer-clinical-trials-exclude-desperate-patients-20171218-story.html.

38. Rekdal OB. Academic citation practice: a sinking sheep? Portal: Libr Acad. 2014;14(4):567–85.

39. Rekdal OB. Academic urban legends. Soc Stud Sci. 2014;44(4):638–54. https://doi.org/10.1177/0306312714535679.

40. Engber D. (2017, June 11). Bad footnotes can be deadly. Slate. Retrieved from http://www.slate.com/articles/health_and_science/science/2017/06/how_bad_footnotes_helped_cause_the_opioid_crisis.html.

41. Porter J, Jick H. Addiction rare in patients treated with narcotics. N Engl J Med. 1980;302(2):123. https://doi.org/10.1056/NEJM198001103020221.

42. Martin GN, Clarke RM. Are psychology journals anti-replication? A snapshot of editorial practices. Front Psychol. 2017;8:523. https://doi.org/10.3389/fpsyg.2017.00523.

43. But I don't want people to try to replicate my research. (2013, Mar 5). In: My perspectives [Blog post]. Retrieved 15 Sept 2018 from https://morepops.wordpress.com/2013/03/05/but-i-dont-want-people-to-try-to-replicate-my-research/.

44. Open Science Collaboration. (n.d.). Estimating the reproducibility of psychological science. In: OSFHome: reproducibility project: psychology: Wiki. Retrieved 15 Sept 2018 from https://osf.io/ezcuj/wiki/home/.

45. Baumeister RF, Bratslavsky E, Muraven M, Tice DM. Ego depletion: is the active self a limited resource. J Pers Soc Psychol. 1998;74(5):1252–65.

46. Hagger MS, Wood C, Stiff C, Chatzisarantis NLD. Ego depletion and the strength model of self-control: a meta-analysis. Psychol Bull. 2010;136(4):495–525. https://doi.org/10.1037/a0019486.

47. Carter EC, McCullough ME. Publication bias and the limited strength model of self-control: has the evidence for ego depletion been overestimated? Front Psychol. 2014;5:823. https://doi.org/10.3389/fpsyg.2014.00823.

48. Hagger MS, Chatzisarantis NLD, Alberts H, Anggono CO, Batailler C, Birt AR, Brand R, Brandt MJ, Brewer G, Bruyneel S, Calvillo DP, Campbell WK, Cannon PR, Carlucci M, Carruth NP, Cheung T, Crowell A, De Ridder DTD, Dewitte S, Elson M, Evans JR, Fay BA, Fennis BM, Finley A, Francis Z, Heise E, Hoemann H, Inzlicht M, Koole SL, Koppel L, Kroese F, Lange F, Lau K, Lynch BP, Martijn C, Merckelbach H, Mills NV, Michirev A, Miyake A, Mosser AE, Muise M, Muller D, Muzi M, Nalis D, Nurwanti R, Otgaar H, Philipp MC, Primoceri P, Rentzsch K, Ringos L, Schlinkert C, Schmeichel BJ,

Schoch SF, Schrama M, Schütz A, Stamos A, Tinghög G, Ullrich J, van Dellen M, Wimbarti S, Wolff W, Yusainy C, Zerhouni O, Zwienenberg M. A multilab preregistration replication of the ego-depletion effect. Perspect Psychol Sci. 2016;11(4):546–73. https://doi.org/10.1177/1745691616652873.

49. Inzlicht M. (2016, Feb 29). Reckoning with the past [Blog post]. Retrieved from http://michaelinzlicht.com/getting-better/2016/2/29/reckoning-with-the-past.

50. Gilbert DT, King G, Pettigrew S, Wilson TD. Comment on "Estimating the reproducibility of psychological science". Science. 2016;351(6227):1037. https://doi.org/10.1126/science.add7243.

51. Begley CG, Ellis LM. Raise standards for preclinical cancer research. Nature. 2012;483:531–3. https://doi.org/10.1038/483531a.

52. Arrowsmith J. Phase II failures: 2008-2010. Nat Rev Drug Discov. 2011;10:328–9. https://doi.org/10.1038/nrd3439.

53. Moher D, Shamseer L, Cobey KD, Lalu MM, Galipeau J, Avey MT, Ahmadzai N, Alabousi M, Barbeau P, Beck A, Daniel R, Frank R, Ghannad M, Hamel C, Hersi M, Hutton B, Isupov I, McGrath TA, McInnes MDF, Page MJ, Pratt M, Pussegoda K, Shea B, Srivastava A, Stevens A, Thavorn K, van Katwyk S, Ward R, Wolfe D, Yazdi F, Yu AM, Ziai H. Stop this waste of people, animals and money. Nature. 2017;549:23–5. https://doi.org/10.1038/549023a.

54. U.S. Department of Health and Human Services, National Institutes of Health, Office of Extramural Research. (2017). Statement on article publication resulting from NIH funded research. (NIH Notice No. NOT-OD-18-011). Retrieved from https://grants.nih.gov/grants/guide/notice-files/NOT-OD-18-011.html?platform=hootsuite.

55. Butler D. Investigating journals: the dark side of publishing. Nature. 2013;495:433–5. https://doi.org/10.1038/495433a.

56. Deprez EE, Chen C. (2017, Aug 29). Medical journals have a fake news problem. Bloomberg Businessweek. Retrieved from https://www.bloomberg.com/news/features/2017-08-29/medical-journals-have-a-fake-news-problem.

57. Gilbert N. Editor will quit over hoax paper. Nature. 2009; https://doi.org/10.1038/news.2009.571.

58. Neuroskeptic. (2017, July 22). Predatory journals hit by 'Star Wars' sting [Blog post]. Retrieved from http://blogs.discovermagazine.com/neuroskeptic/2017/07/22/predatory-journals-star-wars-sting/#.W5qD2PZRfs2.

59. Bartneck C. (2016, Oct 20). iOS just got a paper on nuclear physics accepted at a scientific conference [Blog post]. Retrieved from http://www.bartneck.de/2016/10/20/ios-just-got-a-paper-on-nuclear-physics-accepted-at-a-scientific-conference/.

60. Mazières D, Kohler E. (n.d.). Get me off your fucking mailing list [PDF file]. Retrieved from http://www.scs.stanford.edu/%7Edm/home/papers/remove.pdf.

61. Safi M. (2014, Nov 25). Journal accepts bogus paper requesting removal from mailing list. The Guardian. Retrieved from https://www.theguardian.com/australia-news/2014/nov/25/journal-accepts-paper-requesting-removal-from-mailing-list.

62. Kolata G. (2017, Oct 30). How to report when the science is sketchy. The New York Times. Retrieved from https://www.nytimes.com/2017/10/30/insider/reporting-open-access-journals-sketchy-science.html.

63. Bourgeois FT, Murthy S, Mandl KD. Outcome reporting among drug trials registered in ClinicalTrials.gov. Annu Intern Med. 2010;153(3):158–66.

64. Pfeiffer S. (2010, Aug 3). Study: Industry-funded drug trials produce more favorable results. WBUR News. Retrieved from http://www.wbur.org/news/2010/08/03/drug-studies.

65. Rochon PA, Gurwitz JH, Simms RW, Fortin PR, Felson DT, Minaker KL, Chalmers TC. A study of manufacturer-supported trials of nonsteroidal anti-inflammatory drugs in the treatment of arthritis. Arch Intern Med. 1994;154(2):157–63. https://doi.org/10.1001/archinte.1994.00420020059007.

66. Lexchin J, Bero LA, Djulbegovic B, Clark O. Pharmaceutical industry sponsorship and research outcome and quality: systematic review. BMJ. 2003;326(7400):1167. https://doi.org/10.1136/bmj.326.7400.1167.

67. Smilowitz NR, Pirmohamed A, Weisz G. Published articles reporting studies by industry employees on interventional cardiology devices: scope and association with study outcomes. JAMA Intern Med. 2016;176(5):706–8. https://doi.org/10.1001/jamainternmed.2016.0367.
68. Smith R. Medical journals are an extension of the marketing arm of pharmaceutical companies. PLoS Med. 2005;2(5):e138. https://doi.org/10.1371/journal.pmed.0020138.
69. Egger M, Bartlett C, Jüni P. Are randomised controlled trials in the *BMJ* different? BMJ. 2001;323(7323):1253. https://doi.org/10.1136/bmj.323.7323.1253a.
70. Horton R. The dawn of McScience. New York Rev Books. 2004;51(4):7–9.
71. Zwillich T. (Producer). (2015, Oct 5). Quietly, congress extends a ban on CDC research on gun violence. The Takeaway. Retrieved from https://www.pri.org/stories/2015-07-02/quietly-congress-extends-ban-cdc-research-gun-violence.
72. Cohen PA, Bloszies C, Yee C, Gerona R. An amphetamine isomer whose efficacy and safety in humans has never been studied, β-methylphenylethylamine (BMPEA), is found in multiple dietary supplements. Drug Test Anal. 2016;8(3-4):328–33. https://doi.org/10.1002/dta.1793.
73. Carroll AE. (2017, Dec 4). Why a lot of important research is not being done. The New York Times. Retrieved from https://www.nytimes.com/2017/12/04/upshot/health-research-lawsuits-chilling-effect.html.
74. Bagley N, Carroll AE, Cohen PA. Scientific trials – in the laboratories, not the courts. JAMA Intern Med. 2018;178(1):7–8. https://doi.org/10.1001/jamainternmed.2017.5730.
75. Sismondo S. Ghost management: how much of the medical literature is shaped behind the scenes by the pharmaceutical industry? PLoS Med. 2007;4(9):e286. https://doi.org/10.1371/journal.pmed.0040286.
76. Keller MB, Ryan ND, Strober M, Klein RG, Kutcher SP, Birmaher B, Hagino OR, Koplewicz H, Carlson GA, Clarke GN, Emslie GJ, Feinberg D, Geller B, Kusumakar V, Papatheodorou G, Sack WH, Sweeney M, Wagner KD, Weller EB, Winters NC, Oakes R, McCafferty JP. Efficacy of paroxetine in the treatment of adolescent major depression: a randomized, controlled trial. J Am Acad Child Adolesc Psychiatry. 2001;40(7):762–72.
77. Le Noury J, Nardo JM, Healy D, Jureidini J, Raven M, Tufanaru C, Abi-Jaoude E. Restoring study 329: efficacy and harms of paroxetine and imipramine in treatment of major depression in adolescence. BMJ. 2015;351:h4320. https://doi.org/10.1136/bmj.h4320.
78. Laden SK, Romankiewicz JA. (1998). Adolescent depression study 329: proposal for a journal article [PDF file]. Retrieved from https://www.industrydocumentslibrary.ucsf.edu/drug/docs/#id=npfw0217.
79. Fugh-Berman AJ. The haunting of medical journals: how ghostwriting sold "HRT". PLoS Med. 2010;7(9):e1000335. https://doi.org/10.1371/journal.pmed.1000335.
80. Singer N. (2009, Aug 5). Medical papers by ghostwriters pushed therapy. The New York Times. Retrieved from https://www.nytimes.com/2009/08/05/health/research/05ghost.html.
81. Berenson A. (2005, Apr 24). Evidence in Vioxx suits shows intervention by Merck officials. The New York Times. Retrieved from https://www.nytimes.com/2005/04/24/business/evidence-in-vioxx-suits-shows-intervention-by-merck-officials.html.
82. Wanjek C. (2017, Dec 27). Lies, mistakes & more: these scientific papers got nixed in 2017. Live Science. Retrieved from https://amp.livescience.com/61275-scientific-retractions-2017.html.
83. Oransky I, Abritis A. (n.d.). Who faces criminal sanctions for scientific misconduct? [PDF file]. Retrieved from https://wcrif.org/images/2017/documents/1.%20Monday%20May%2029,%202017/1.%20Aula/I.%20Oransky%20-%20Who%20faces%20criminal%20sanctions%20for%20scientific%20misconduct.pdf.
84. Reardon S. US vaccine researcher sentenced to prison for fraud. Nature. 2015;523:138–9. https://doi.org/10.1038/nature.2015.17660.
85. Lestch C. (2013, Dec 27). Iowa professor cops to faking results of big-bucks AIDS vaccine research. New York Daily News. Retrieved from http://www.nydailynews.com/news/national/professor-cops-faking-aids-vaccine-research-data-article-1.1559245.
86. LaCour MJ, Green DP. When contact changes minds: an experiment on transmission of support for gay equality. Science. 2014;346(6215):1366–9. https://doi.org/10.1126/science.1256151. (Retraction published 2015, Science, 348(6239), 1100. https://doi.org/10.1126/science.aac6638).

87. Ex-UQ academic found guilty of fraud. (2016, Oct 24). On 9News. Retrieved from https://www.9news.com.au/national/2016/10/24/17/05/ex-uq-academic-found-guilty-of-fraud.
88. Verfaellie M, McGwin J. The case of Diederik Stapel. Psychol Sci Agenda. 2011;25(12). Retrieved from http://www.apa.org/science/about/psa/2011/12/diederik-stapel.aspx.
89. The cloning scandal of Hwang Woo-Suk (n.d.). Retrieved 15 Sept 2018 from http://stemcell-bioethics.wikischolars.columbia.edu/The+Cloning+Scandal+of+Hwang+Woo-Suk.
90. Johnson CY. (2014, May 29) Harvard report shines light on ex-researcher's misconduct. The Boston Globe. Retrieved from https://www.bostonglobe.com/metro/2014/05/29/internal-harvard-report-shines-light-misconduct-star-psychology-researcher-marc-hauser/maSUow-PqL4clXrOgj44aKP/story.html.
91. Wakefield AJ, Murch SH, Anthony A, Linnell J, Casson DM, Malik M, Berelowitz M, Dhillon AP, Thomson MA, Harvey P, Valentine A, Davies SE, Walker-Smith JA. Ileal-lymphoid-nodular hyperplasia, non-specific colitis, and pervasive developmental disorder in children. Lancet. 1998;351(9103):637–41. https://doi.org/10.1016/S0140-6736(97)11096-0. (Retraction published 2010, Lancet, 375(9713), 445. https://doi.org/10.1016/S0140-6736(10)60175-4).
92. Taylor LE, Swerdfeger AL, Eslick GD. Vaccines are not associated with autism: an evidence-based meta-analysis of case-control and cohort studies. Vaccine. 2014;32(29):3623–9. https://doi.org/10.1016/j.vaccine.2014.04.085.
93. Deer B. How the vaccine crisis was meant to make money. BMJ. 2011;342:c5258. https://doi.org/10.1136/bmj.c5258.
94. Deer B. (2006, Dec 31). MMR doctor given legal aid thousands [Reprint]. Retrieved from https://briandeer.com/mmr/st-dec-2006.htm.
95. Deer B. Pathology reports solve "new bowel disease" riddle. BMJ. 2011;343:d6823. https://doi.org/10.1136/bmj.d6823.
96. Ross E. (2004, Mar 3). Media investigation forces retractions of bogus vaccine research [Reprint]. Retrieved from https://briandeer.com/mmr/lancet-retraction.htm.
97. Carey M. (2014, Sept 19). Andrew Wakefield loses frivolous defamation lawsuit. To pay court costs. [Blog post]. Retrieved from https://leftbrainrightbrain.co.uk/2014/09/19/andrew-wakefield-loses-frivolous-defamation-lawsuit-to-pay-court-costs/.
98. Sun LH. (2017, May 4). Anti-vaccine activists spark a state's worse measles outbreak in decades. The Washington Post. Retrieved from https://www.washingtonpost.com/national/health-science/anti-vaccine-activists-spark-a-states-worst-measles-outbreak-in-decades/2017/05/04/a1fac952-2f39-11e7-9dec-764dc781686f_story.html.
99. Pearson C. (2017, June 29). Minnesota hoping for all-clear after measles outbreak in Somali-American community. Voice of America. Retrieved from https://www.voanews.com/a/minnesota-measles-outbreak-somali-community/3921139.html.
100. European Centre for Disease Prevention and Control. (2017, Nov 10). Measles in the EU/EEA: Current outbreaks, latest data and trends – November 2017. Retrieved from https://ecdc.europa.eu/en/news-events/measles-eueea-current-outbreaks-latest-data-and-trends-november-2017.
101. Hauser SL, Bar-Or A, Comi G, Giovannoni G, Hartung H-P, Hemmer B, Lublin F, Montalban X, Rammohan KW, Selmaj K, Traboulsee A, Wolinsky JS, Arnold DL, Klingelschmitt G, Masterman D, Fontoura P, Belachew S, Chin P, Mairon N, Garren H, Kappos L. Ocrelizumab versus interferon beta-1a in relapsing multiple sclerosis. N Engl J Med. 2017;376(3):221–34. https://doi.org/10.1056/NEJMoa1601277.
102. Hauser SL, Bar-Or A, Comi G, Giovannoni G, Hartung H-P, Hemmer B, et al. ICMJE Form for disclosure of potential conflicts of interest [PDF file]. N Engl J Med. 2017;376(3):221–34. Retrieved from https://www.nejm.org/doi/suppl/10.1056/NEJMoa1601277/suppl_file/nejmoa1601277_disclosures.pdf.
103. Jager LR, Leek JT. An estimate of the science-wise false discovery rate and application to the top medical literature. Biostatistics. 2014;15(1):1–12. https://doi.org/10.1093/biostatistics/kxt007.
104. Meta-Research Innovation Center at Stanford. (n.d.). Why meta-research matters. Retrieved 15 Sept 2018 from https://metrics.stanford.edu/.
105. De Angelis C, Drazen JM, Frizelle FA, Haug C, Hoey J, Horton R, Kotzin S, Laine C, Marusic A, Overbeke AJ, Schroeder TV, Sox HC, Van Der Weyden MB. Clinical trial regis-

tration: a statement from the International Committee of Medical Journal Editors. N Engl J Med. 2004;351(12):1250–1. https://doi.org/10.1056/NEJMe048225.

106. World Health Organization. (2018). International clinical trials registry platform: WHO data set (Version 1.3.1). Retrieved 15 Sept 2018 from http://www.who.int/ictrp/network/trds/en/.

107. AllTrials. (n.d.) Petition. Retrieved 15 Sept 2018 from http://www.alltrials.net/petition/.

108. AllTrials. (2013). RIAT initiative for publication of historical clinical trial findings [Purpose statement]. Retrieved 15 Sept 2018 from http://www.alltrials.net/news/riat-initiative-for-publication-of-historical-clinical-trial-findings/.

109. Doshi P, Dickersin K, Healy D, Vedula SS, Jefferson T. Restoring invisible and abandoned trials: a call for people to publish the findings. BMJ. 2013;346:f2865. https://doi.org/10.1136/bmj.f2865.

110. Zamzow R. (2017, Dec 5). Spotting shady statistics. The OPEN Notebook. Retrieved from https://www.theopennotebook.com/2017/12/05/spotting-shady-statistics/.

111. Kaplan RM, Irvin VL. Likelihood of null effects of large NHLBI clinical trials has increased over time. PLoS One. 2015;10(8):e0132382. https://doi.org/10.1371/journal.pone.0132382.

112. Law MR, Kawasumi Y, Morgan SG. Despite law, fewer than one in eight completed studies of drugs and biologics are reported on time on ClinicalTrials.gov. Health Aff. 2011;30(12) https://doi.org/10.1377/hlthaff.2011.0172.

113. Prayle AP, Hurley MN, Smyth AR. Compliance with mandatory reporting of clinical trial results on ClinicalTrials.gov: cross sectional study. BMJ. 2012;344:d7373. https://doi.org/10.1136/bmj.d7373.

114. Anderson ML, Chiswell K, Peterson ED, Tasneem A, Topping J, Califf RM. Compliance with results reporting at ClinicalTrials.gov. N Engl J Med. 2015;372(11):1031–9. https://doi.org/10.1056/NEJMsa1409364.

115. Benjamin DJ, Berger J, Johannesson M, Nosek BA, Wagenmakers E, Berk R, et al. Redefine statistical significance. Nat Hum Behav. 2017; https://doi.org/10.31234/osf.io/mky9j.

116. Woolston C. Psychology journal bans P values. Nature. 2015;519 https://doi.org/10.1038/519009f.

117. Klein JR, Roodman A. Blind analysis in nuclear and particle physics. Annu Rev Nucl Part Sci. 2005;55:141–63. https://doi.org/10.1146/annurev.nucl.55.090704.151521.

118. MacCoun R, Perlmutter S. Blind analysis: hide the results to seek the truth. Nature. 2015;526:187–9. https://doi.org/10.1038/526187a.

119. United States Senate Committee on Finance. (2010). Ghostwriting in medical literature [PDF file]. Retrieved from https://www.grassley.senate.gov/sites/default/files/about/upload/Senator-Grassley-Report.pdf.

120. International Committee of Medical Journal Editors. (n.d.). Defining the roles of authors and contributors. Retrieved 15 Sept 2018 from http://www.icmje.org/recommendations/browse/roles-and-responsibilities/defining-the-role-of-authors-and-contributors.html.

121. Han AP. (2017, Oct 9). Journal to retract paper called "anti-vaccine pseudoscience" [Blog post]. Retraction Watch. Retrieved from https://retractionwatch.com/2017/10/09/journal-retract-paper-called-anti-vaccine-pseudoscience/.

122. Gibney E. The scientist who spots fake videos. Nature. 2017; https://doi.org/10.1038/nature.2017.22784.

123. Kaiser J. (2013, May 9). U.S. government accuses open access publisher of trademark infringement. Science. Retrieved from http://www.sciencemag.org/news/2013/05/us-government-accuses-open-access-publisher-trademark-infringement.

124. Lake L. (2016, Aug 26). Academics and scientists: beware of predatory journal publishers [Blog post]. Retrieved from https://www.consumer.ftc.gov/blog/2016/08/academics-and-scientists-beware-predatory-journal-publishers.

125. Prasad VK, Cifu AS. Ending medical reversal: improving outcomes, saving lives. Baltimore: Johns Hopkins University Press; 2015.

126. Engber D. (2017, Aug 21). Is science broken? Or is it self-correcting? Slate. Retrieved from http://www.slate.com/articles/health_and_science/science/2017/08/science_is_not_self_correcting_science_is_broken.html.

127. Siegfried T. (2014, Feb 7). To make science better, watch out for statistical flaws [Blog post]. Science News. Retrieved from https://www.sciencenews.org/blog/context/ make-science-better-watch-out-statistical-flaws.
128. PharmedOut. (2006). About us. Retrieved 15 Sept 2018 from http://www.pharmedout.org/ aboutus.html.
129. Mehta H. (2017, July 30). Naturopathic school accuses blogger, a former student, of defamation. Retrieved from http://friendlyatheist.patheos.com/2017/07/30/ naturopathic-school-accuses-blogger-a-former-student-of-defamation/.
130. Neuroskeptic. (2017, June 19). Is science broken, or is it self-correcting? [Blog post]. Retrieved from http://blogs.discovermagazine.com/neuroskeptic/2017/06/19/science-broken-self-correcting/#.

Index

© Springer International Publishing AG, part of Springer Nature 2019   577
J. Howard, *Cognitive Errors and Diagnostic Mistakes*,
https://doi.org/10.1007/978-3-319-93224-8